Your roadmap to...

MATERNAL-NEWBORN

DAVIS ESSENTIAL NURSING CONTENT
+ **PRACTICE QUESTIONS**

STEP 1 | Not enough time to read your textbook?

- Succinct summaries focus on must-know information.
- "Alerts" highlight important information at a glance.
- "Key Terms" at the beginning of each chapter make reference quick and easy.

I. Maternal Nutrition Description

Maternal nutrition includes co[...]
foods in appropriate amounts t[...]
weight gain, including vitamin[...]
tion during pregnancy. By usin[...]
fered through the United States[...]
pregnant women can learn mor[...]
to plan healthy meals during p[...]
fessionals can also utilize this[...]

ALERT Maternal obesity increases the risk for gestational diabetes, maternal hypertension, preeclampsia, and delivery complications, including increased rate of cesarean delivery. Babies born to obese mothers are more likely to suffer from macrosomia, or large for gestational age, which can place them at greater risk for birth injuries and other neonatal complications, including stillbirth.

KEY TERMS

Anorexia nervosa—An eating disorder involving starvation of the body based on the fear of gaining weight
Body mass index (BMI)—An estimate of body fat that is calculated based upon the patient's height and weight values
Bulimia nervosa—An eating disorder characterized by compulsive consumption and purging of food
[...]ed to convert food into
[...]so known as *folate*). Ade-
[...]n pregnancy can help to

CASE STUDY: Putting It All Together

Amanda is a 24-year-old G1 P0000 who presents to your prenatal clinical for her first prenatal visit. She has a good relationship with her significant other, and this pregnancy was not planned. She took a pregnancy test at home and believes she is 10 weeks pregnant. Amanda offers a history of anxiety and worries that she will "gain a lot of weight during the pregnancy." As you collect her health history, you document a history of mild depression as a teenager treated with therapy and medication. She currently denies being on any medication except for prenatal vitamins. She offers a history of iron deficiency anemia as a child and recalls taking iron tablets daily. Socially, she works full-time as an administrative assistant and runs about 4 miles daily as her form of exercise. She denies smoking, drinking, or using drugs. Her family history is unremarkable. She has tried a [...]

- She occasionally feels out of breath and tired during running but pushes herself to continue her goal.

Vital Signs
Temp: 98.7°F
Pulse: 50
Respiration: 16
Blood pressure: 90/60
Height: 5'4"
Weight: 107 lb
BMI: 18.4
Pain scale: 0/10
General appearance: appropriate affect and responsive to questions
Integumentary: skin is cool to touch, no apparent lesions or aberrations, decreased skin turgor, lips and mucous membranes pink, nail beds pallor
HEENT: hair thinning and short [...]

STEP 2 | Worried about clinical?

- "Putting It All Together," a case study at the end of most chapters, connects your knowledge to a common clinical scenario.
- Questions on the relevant objective and subjective data in the study ask you to identify a nursing diagnosis, interventions, and client evaluation.

STEP 3 | Struggling with your exams?

- 650 NCLEX®-style questions in the book and online at Davis*Plus*—including alternate-format questions—feature answers and rationales for both correct and incorrect responses to identify areas for additional study.
- 100-question final examination at the end of the text assesses your progress and prepares you for classroom tests.

REVIEW QUESTIONS

Be sure to read the Introduction for valuable test-taking tips.

1. A nurse is assessing the weight gain of a client who is 16 weeks pregnant. The nurse understands that inadequate weight gain is associated with a high risk for which complication?
   1. Delivering an infant with macrosomia
   2[...]
   3[...]
   4[...]

REVIEW QUESTION ANSWERS

1. **ANSWER: 2**
   Rationale
   1. Macrosomia is associated with an increase in weight gain and gestational diabetes.
   2. Inadequate weight gain is associated with an increased risk for giving birth to a low-birth-weight infant.
   3. Congenital anomalies are associated with high maternal weight gain early in pregnancy.
   4. Giving birth to a low-birth-weight infant does not automatically cause the infant to be admitted to the intensive care unit.

Unlock your Davis*Plus* Resources Online

Follow the instructions on the inside front cover to use the access code to unlock the questions online at Davis*Plus*.com.

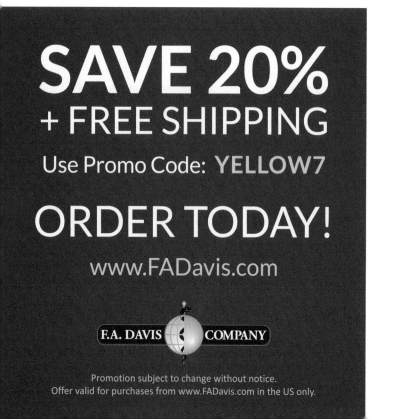
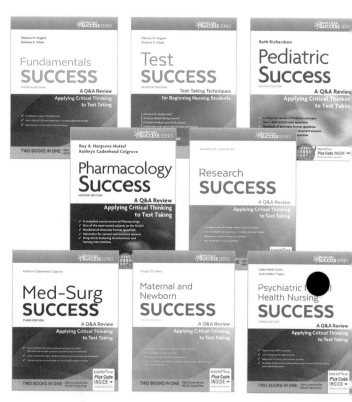

DAVIS ESSENTIAL NURSING CONTENT
+ PRACTICE QUESTIONS

Maternal-Newborn

Sheila C. Whitworth, DNP, RN
Assistant Professor
University of South Alabama College of Nursing
Mobile, Alabama

Taralyn McMullan, DNP, RN, CNS-BC
Assistant Professor
University of South Alabama College of Nursing
Mobile, Alabama

F.A. Davis Company • Philadelphia

F. A. Davis Company
1915 Arch Street
Philadelphia, PA 19103
www.fadavis.com

Copyright © 2017 by F. A. Davis Company

Printed in the United States of America

Last digit indicates print number: 10 9 8 7 6 5 4 3 2 1

Publisher, Nursing: Terri Wood Allen
Content Project Manager II: Amy M. Romano
Illustration and Design Manager: Carolyn O'Brien

As new scientific information becomes available through basic and clinical research, recommended treatments and drug therapies undergo changes. The author(s) and publisher have done everything possible to make this book accurate, up to date, and in accord with accepted standards at the time of publication. The author(s), editors, and publisher are not responsible for errors or omissions or for consequences from application of the book, and make no warranty, expressed or implied, in regard to the contents of the book. Any practice described in this book should be applied by the reader in accordance with professional standards of care used in regard to the unique circumstances that may apply in each situation. The reader is advised always to check product information (package inserts) for changes and new information regarding dose and contraindications before administering any drug. Caution is especially urged when using new or infrequently ordered drugs.

Library of Congress Cataloging-in-Publication Data

Names: Whitworth, Sheila C., author. | McMullan, Taralyn, author.
Title: Davis essential nursing content + practice questions. Maternal-newborn
  / Sheila C. Whitworth, Taralyn McMullan.
Other titles: Essential nursing content + practice questions.
  Maternal-newborn | Davis essential nursing content and practice questions.
  Maternal-newborn | Maternal-newborn
Description: Philadelphia : F. A. Davis Company, [2017] | Includes
  bibliographical references.
Identifiers: LCCN 2016033605 | ISBN 9780803644250 (pbk.)
Subjects: | MESH: Maternal-Child Nursing | Obstetric Nursing | Pregnancy
  Complications—nursing
Classification: LCC RG951 | NLM WY 157.3 | DDC 618.2/0231—dc23 LC record available at https://lccn.loc.gov/2016033605

Dedicated to my husband, Terry, for his love and support as I progressed through my nursing career and his enduring patience while writing this book.
—Sheila Whitworth

To my husband, Paul, for his support and constant motivation while dedicating long hours to work on this book. His love and encouragement were truly appreciated. Additionally, I would like to thank my parents, Lynne and Rich Wood, with a special thank you to my father for his endless mentoring and exemplifying his passion for education and writing.
—Taralyn McMullan

Why This Book Is Necessary

Most beginning nursing students have information over-load. They must possess knowledge about a variety of subjects, including anatomy and physiology, psychology, sociology, medical terminology, diagnostic and laboratory tests, and growth and development, to mention a few. In addition, with the expanding roles and responsibilities of the nursing profession, the nursing information that beginning nursing students must learn is growing exponentially in depth and breadth. Maternal-newborn nursing concepts are either taught in abbreviated sessions as a specialty course or integrated into the entire nursing curriculum. Therefore, additional educational support is critical to promote the understanding of maternal-newborn health nursing concepts. These concepts can be applied in all fields of nursing. *Davis Essential Nursing Content + Practice Questions Maternal-Newborn* provides that additional educational support.

Who Should Use This Book

Davis Essential Nursing Content + Practice Questions Maternal-Newborn provides beginning nursing students with need-to-know information as well as questions to practice their ability to apply the information in a simulated clinical situation. This textbook is designed to be:

- The sole textbook for a maternal-newborn health nursing course and used in conjunction with reliable primary Internet sources for nursing information.
- Required or recommended by a nursing program and used in conjunction with a traditional maternal-newborn health nursing textbook.
- Used by beginning nursing students who want to focus on essential information contained in a maternal-newborn health nursing course.
- Used by nursing students to learn how to be more successful when answering National Council Licensure Examination (NCLEX)–type multiple-choice and alternate-format nursing questions early in their nursing education.
- Used by nursing students preparing for the NCLEX-RN or NCLEX-PN examination to review basic nursing theory and practice.

What Information Is Presented in This Textbook

This textbook begins with an introduction, which includes information to help students maximize their ability to study effectively and achieve success when studying maternal-newborn content and when taking nursing examinations. General study strategies, specific study strategies, test-taking tips for answering multiple-choice questions and alternate-format questions, and the test plan categories for the NCLEX examinations are discussed. The content is divided into 22 chapters.

The first 18 chapters outline the critical need-to-know information related to maternal health nursing, while Chapters 19 through 22 focus on newborn nursing. All chapters are in outline format, eliminating extraneous information. Only essential information is included, limiting the challenge of wading through excessive material. This approach assists students to focus on what is most important:

- Each chapter includes definitions of key words to assist the student in understanding the context of the information presented.
- All chapters include at least 15 high-level questions related to the content covered in the chapter. Each question contains rationales for correct and incorrect answers. Studying rationales for the right and wrong answers to practice questions helps students learn new or solidify previously learned information.
- Multiple-choice questions and alternate-format questions included on NCLEX examinations are incorporated.
- Each question is coded according to the NCLEX-RN test plan categories: Integrated Processes, including the Nursing Process, Client Need, and Cognitive Level.
- For added flexibility, every question in the book appears online at www.DavisPlus.com. Students can create targeted quizzes by sorting the questions by Content Area, Concept, and/or Question Type. The online questions are formatted to use on a tablet, mobile device, or laptop.
- To provide even more opportunities to practice NCLEX-type questions, the book includes two 75-question comprehensive tests posted online at www.DavisPlus.com. Like the practice questions in

the book, each question includes rationales for correct and incorrect answers and coding for the NCLEX test plan categories.

- Each chapter ends with a Putting It All Together case study, encouraging students to put the content into practice. Students are quizzed on the relevant objective and subjective information presented in the scenario and are asked to identify a nursing diagnosis, interventions, and client evaluation.

- Chapter 23 is a 100-item maternal-newborn health comprehensive nursing examination that integrates questions spanning content throughout the textbook.

Students should use every resource available to facilitate the learning process. The authors believe that this textbook will assist nursing students to master maternal-newborn health concepts and use this understanding to succeed on the NCLEX.

DIANE ANDRONACO, DNP, RNC-OB, CNE
Instructor of Nursing
Ramapo College of New Jersey
Mahwah, New Jersey

LOUISE AURILLO, PhD, RN-BC, CNE
Professor Emeritus
Youngstown State University
Youngstown, Ohio

CHRISTY DALLENBACH, MN, RNC-OB
Nursing Instructor
Swedish Medical Center
Seattle, Washington

AMY E. DAVIS, RNC-MNN, MSN
Instructor
University of South Alabama
Mobile, Alabama

JULIA FITZGERALD, PhD, RN, CNE
Assistant Professor
Ramapo College of New Jersey
Mahwah, New Jersey

PENNI COATES HUFFMAN, DNP, APRN, NNP-BC
Assistant Professor
University of South Alabama
Mobile, Alabama

ANGELA M. KELLY, DNP, RNC-OB, APN, WHNP-BC
Clinical Assistant Professor
Rutgers, The State University of New Jersey
Camden, New Jersey

VICTORIA KYARSGAARD, DNP, RNC, PHN, CNE
Associate Professor
Crown College
St. Bonifacius, Minnesota

ASHLEY MARASS, DNP, CPNP
Assistant Professor
University of South Alabama
Fairhope, Alabama

SHARON McELWAIN, DNP, RN, FNP-BC
Instructor
University of Mississippi Medical Center School
 of Nursing
Jackson, Mississippi

LEIGH A. MINCHEW, DNP, RN, WHNP-BC, CRNP
Assistant Professor
University of South Alabama
Mobile, Alabama

TERESA GAYLE NEWBY, DNP, RNC
Associate Professor
Crown College
Saint Bonifacius, Minnesota

TERRI PLATT, DNP, RN, WHNP-BC
Assistant Professor
University of South Alabama
Mobile, Alabama

JEANANN SOUSOU, DNP, RN, CNM, CNE
Assistant Professor
Rutgers, The State University of New Jersey
Camden, New Jersey

CHRISTINA THOMPSON, RNC, DNP
Assistant Professor
University of South Alabama
Mobile, Alabama

MARTA ANDERSON, MSN, RN
Clinical Instructor
University of Texas Austin
Austin, Texas

LAURIE D. BARCUS, RN, MSN
Assistant Professor
Kent State University
New Philadelphia, Ohio

SCHVON BUSSEY, RN, MSN, FNP
Director
Albany Technical College
Albany, Georgia

PAULA BYLASKA-DAVIES, PhD, RN
Associate Professor
MCPHS University
Worcester, Massachusetts

SUSAN M. CANTRELL, MSN, RNC-HROB
Assistant Professor of Nursing
Samuel Merritt University
Oakland, California

CARLA CRIDER, MSN, RNC OB & EFM
Associate Professor
Weatherford College
Weatherford, Texas

GAYLE CUDÉ, PhD, MS, BSN, CNE
Assistant Professor
Tulsa Community College
Tulsa, Oklahoma

COLETTE DIEUJUSTE, RN, MS
Associate Professor
Simmons College
Boston, Massachusetts

SUSAN ELLISON, MS, RNC, CNE
Course Coordinator
Middlesex County College
Edison, New Jersey

ANGELA ERICKSON, MSN, RN
Assistant Professor
Mineral Area College
Park Hills, Missouri

CATHERINE FOLKER-MAGLAYA, MSN, APN-CNM, IBCLC
Assistant Professor
Truman College City of Colleges of Chicago
Chicago, Illinois

MARCIA L. GASPER, EdD, MSN, RN
Associate Professor
East Stroudsburg University
East Stroudsburg, Pennsylvania

SHARLENE GEORGESEN, PhD, MSN, RN
Associate Professor
Morningside College
Sioux City, Iowa

MARY E. HANCOCK, PhD, RNC-OB
Assistant Professor
Shepard University
Shepherdstown, West Virginia

SUELANE Y. HANNAH, RN, MS
Assistant Professor
Bob Jones University
Greenville, South Carolina

THERESA H. JACKSON, PhDc, RN
Associate Professor
Shawnee State University
Portsmouth, Ohio

BRENDA LENNON, MS, RN, BC
Course Chair
Memorial School of Nursing
Albany, New York

BARBARA McCLASKEY, PhD, APRN, CNS-BC, RNC
University Professor
Pittsburg State University
Pittsburg, Kansas

ANNE NEZ, MSN, CNE, RN
Professor of Nursing
Central Wyoming College
Riverton, Wyoming

MICHELLE NORRIS, RN, MSN, CMSRN
Nursing Faculty
Bladen Community College
Dublin, North Carolina

ALISSA PARRISH, MSN, RN
Assistant Professor
University of Tennessee at Martin
Martin, Tennessee

JESSICA M. PARROTT, DNP, RN, CPNP-PC, CNE
Associate Professor
Norfolk State University
Norfolk, Virginia

REBECCA PRESSWOOD, RN, MSN
Professor of Nursing
Blinn College
Bryan, Texas

JENNIFER RODRIGUEZ, RN, MSN
Nursing Faculty
Kellogg Community College
Battle Creek, Michigan

LAURA R. RODRIGUEZ, DNP, RN, MCH-CNS
Clinical Assistant Professor
University of Texas at El Paso
El Paso, Texas

MARTHA C. RUDER, RN, MSN
Coordinator of Nursing
Gulf Coast State College
Panama City, Florida

PAULA SCHERER, MSN, RNC
Director, Lower Division Nursing
Arizona College-Mesa Campus
Mesa, Arizona

REBECCA SHABO, PhD
Associate Professor
Kennesaw State University
Kennesaw, Georgia

CHRISTINA SIMON, MSN, CRNP, RNC
Associate Professor
Luzerne County Community College
Nanticoke, Pennsylvania

GLADDI TOMLINSON, RN, MSN
Professor of Nursing
Harrisburg Area Community College
Harrisburg, Pennsylvania

VICKI J. VAWTER, ARNP, MS
Assistant Professor
Hillsborough Community College
Plant City, Florida

ANNE VOGTLE, MS, RNC
Assistant Professor
Monroe Community College
Rochester, New York

LAURA J. WALLACE, RN, CNM, PhD
Associate Professor
Brenau University
Gainesville, Georgia

CONNIE WATSON, RN, BSN, MSN
Associate Professor of Nursing
Anne Arundel Community College
Arnold, Maryland

NANCY WILK, DNS, WHNP-C
Associate Professor of Nursing
St. John Fisher College
Rochester, New York

POLLY GERBER ZIMMERMAN, RN, MS, MBA, CEN, FAEN
Associate Professor
Harry S. Truman College
Chicago, Illinois

We would like to acknowledge the following individuals who helped us to develop and write this book:

Penni Huffman, who contributed her time and expertise. Her friendship has been inspirational, and her knowledge of the material will encourage students to seek specialties in the field of neonatal nursing.

All the maternal-nurse educators who contributed to this book and shared their expertise.

Our colleagues at the University of South Alabama College of Nursing for their suggestions and support.

SHEILA C. WHITWORTH
TARALYN MCMULLAN

Contents

Planning for a child is equally as important as the pregnancy period itself. While caring for a mother during pregnancy until delivery of her newborn is a specialty focus, general knowledge of care is essential to maintaining a healthy transition to life outside the womb. Teaching students how to successfully prepare for a healthy pregnancy and delivery, while caring for a newborn and mother during the postpartum days characterizes the essential focus of having a course concentrate on maternal-newborn health. The ability to care for both mother and child during this acute phase of life is built upon the growing knowledge that a student gains during foundational courses such as adult, pediatric, psychiatric, and community health. Regardless of future career aspirations, at some point in a nurse's life, he or she will encounter a pregnant mother, a mother who has just delivered a baby, or a newborn in practice. Establishing a framework of care, therefore, has to be learned during the educational process prior to graduating from nursing school.

Maternal-newborn content is tested on the NCLEX and therefore reflects the essential components of why this content is integral to a nursing student's curriculum. Students must possess the knowledge to answer general questions that provide a holistic view on caring for a mother and/or newborn while not compromising basic care standards. These standards are essential to learn in a course that provides information that is required for the nursing student to understand. Comprehension of course content will be integrated with personal experiences, readiness to learn, and willingness to seek further understanding.

This text presents various teaching strategies that can help maximize learning. The content of each chapter is concisely presented in outline form, including all the "need to know" information, while eliminating extraneous "nice to know" content. The questions presented are meant to generate critical thinking as you review both the questions and answer options. It is important to review the rationales for all the answer choices in order to fully understand the often-complex maternal-newborn content. Don't ignore the rationales for the incorrect answers. Learning has truly occurred when you can explain *why* an answer is incorrect.

In addition, this book presents test-taking tips that will help you understand what a test question is asking, identify key words that affect the meaning of both the question and the answer, practice how to examine options in a multiple-choice question, and determine how to eliminate incorrect options (distractors). At the beginning of each chapter, key terms are presented that help you focus on understanding concepts and terminology needed to choose correct answers.

For additional information on the studying and test-taking strategies presented in this introduction, refer to *Test Success: Test-Taking Techniques for Beginning Nursing Students* published by the F.A. Davis Company.

Use General Study Strategies to Maximize Learning

1. Set short- and long-term learning goals because doing so promotes planned learning with a purpose.
2. Control internal and external distractors.
   a. Select a study environment that allows you to focus on your learning and is free from external interruptions.
   b. Limit internally generated distractions by challenging negative thoughts. For example, rather than saying to yourself, "This is going to be a hard test," say, "I can pass this test if I study hard."
   c. Establish a positive internal locus of control. For example, say, "I can get an A on my next test if I study hard and I am prepared," rather than blaming the instructor for designing "hard" tests.
   d. Use controlled-breathing techniques, progressive muscle relaxation, and guided imagery to control anxious feelings.
3. Review content before each class because doing so supports mental organization and purposeful learning.
4. Take class notes.
   a. Review class notes within 48 hours after class because doing so ensures that the information is still fresh in your mind.
   b. Use one side of your notebook for class notes and use the opposite page to jot down additional, clarifying information from the textbook or other sources.
   c. After reviewing your notes, identify questions that you still have and ask the instructor for clarification.
5. Balance personal sacrifice and time for relaxation. A rigorous course of study requires sacrifices in terms of postponing vacations, having less time to spend with family members and friends, and having less time to engage in personal leisure activities. However, you

should find a balance that supports your need to meet course requirements and yet allows you time to rest and reenergize.

6. Treat yourself to a reward when you meet a goal because doing so supports motivation. Your long-term reward is to graduate and become a nurse. However, that reward is in the distance, so to stimulate motivation now, build in rewards when short-term goals are achieved.
   a. An external reward might be watching a television program that you enjoy, having a 10-minute break with a snack, or calling a friend on the phone.
   b. An internal reward might be saying to yourself, "I feel great because I now understand the principles presented in this chapter."

7. Manage time effectively.
   a. Examine your daily and weekly routines to identify and eliminate barriers to your productivity, such as attempting to do too much, lacking organization, or being obsessive compulsive.
   b. Learn to delegate household tasks.
   c. Learn to say no to avoid overcommitting yourself to activities that take you away from what you need to do to meet your learning needs.
   d. Get organized. Identify realistic daily, weekly, and monthly "to do" calendars. Work to achieve deadlines with self-determination and self-discipline.
   e. Maintain a consistent study routine because doing so eliminates procrastination and establishes an internal readiness to learn.

8. Recognize that you do not have to be perfect. If every waking moment is focused on achieving an A, your relationship with family members and friends will suffer. The key is to find a balance and accept the fact that you do not have to have an A in every course to become a nurse.

9. Capitalize on small moments of time to study by carrying flash cards, a vocabulary list, or a small study guide, such as one of the products in the *Notes* series by F.A. Davis.

10. Study in small groups. Sharing and listening increases understanding and allows for correction of misinformation.

Use Specific Study Strategies to Maximize Learning

1. Use acronyms, alphabet cues, acrostics, and mnemonics to help learn information that must be memorized for future recall.
2. When studying, continually ask yourself how and why, because the nurse must comprehend how a

process occurs and why a particular intervention is or is not appropriate. Many questions on nursing examinations require the nurse to comprehend the how and why in order to decide what he or she should do first or next or what not to do.

3. Relate new information to something you already know to enhance learning. When trying to remember the meaning of the positive and negative symptoms of gestational diabetes, relate "positive" to "added" (beyond the normal) and relate "negative" to "missing" (less than the normal).

4. Identify and study principles that are common among different nursing interventions because doing so maximizes the application of information in client situations. For example, trust is the common denominator in all interpersonal relationships. No progress in client care can occur without a mutual feeling of trust.

5. Identify and study differences. For example, three patients may have an increase in blood pressure for three different reasons, such as anxiety, acute pain stimulating the sympathetic nervous system, and side effects of medications.

Use Test-Taking Tips to Maximize Success on Nursing Examinations

1. There is no substitute for being prepared for a test. However, when you are uncertain of a correct answer, test-taking tips are strategies you can use to be test wise.

2. By being test wise you may be better able to identify what a question is asking and to eliminate one or more distractors. Your chances of selecting the correct answer increase when you are able to eliminate distractors from consideration. For example, when answering a traditional multiple-choice question that has four answer options, if you can eliminate one distractor from further consideration, you increase your chances of selecting the correct answer to 33%. If you are able to eliminate two distractors from further consideration, you increase your chances of selecting the correct answer to 50%.

Test-Taking Tips for Multiple-Choice (One-Answer) Items

1. A traditional multiple-choice item typically presents a statement (stem) that asks a question. Usually, four statements that are potential answers follow the stem (options), one of which is the correct answer and three of which are incorrect answers (distractors). The test taker must select the option that is the correct answer to receive credit.

2. Test-taking tips describe strategies that can be used to analyze a traditional multiple-choice item and improve a test taker's chances of selecting the correct answer.

Test-Taking Tip #1: Identify Positive Polarity of a Stem

1. A stem with positive polarity is asking, "What should the nurse do when . . . ?"
2. The correct answer may be based on understanding what is accurate or comprehending the principle underlying the correct answer. For example, a stem with positive polarity might say, "Which nursing action should a nurse implement when a pregnant client presents to labor and delivery with bright red vaginal bleeding?"
3. **Study tip:** Change the stem so that it reflects a negative focus and then answer the question based on a stem with negative polarity. For example, "Which action should a nurse *not implement* when a pregnant client presents to labor and delivery with bright red bleeding?"

Test-Taking Tip #2: Identify Key Words in the Stem That Indicate Negative Polarity

1. A stem with negative polarity asks such questions as, "What should the nurse *not* do?" "What is contraindicated, unacceptable, or false?" "What is the exception?"
2. Words in a stem that indicate negative polarity include *not, except, never, contraindicated, unacceptable, avoid, unrelated, violate,* and *least.*
3. **Study tip:** As with test-taking tip #1, change the word that indicates negative polarity to a positive word and then answer the question based on a stem with positive polarity.

Test-Taking Tip #3: Identify Words in the Stem That Set a Priority

1. The correct answer is something that the nurse should do first.
2. Words in the stem that set a priority include *first, best, main, greatest, most, initial, primary,* and *priority.* For example, a stem that sets a priority might ask, "What should a nurse do first when administering an anticonvulsant medication to a pre-eclamptic pregnant client?"
3. **Study tip:** After identifying the first step in a procedure, place the remaining steps in order of importance.

Test-Taking Tip #4: Identify Options That Are Opposites

1. Options that are opposites generally reflect extremes on a continuum.
2. More often than not, an option that is an opposite is the correct answer.
3. If you are unable to identify the correct answer, select one of the opposite options.
4. Some opposites are easy to identify, such as positive and negative symptoms of schizophrenia, whereas others are more obscure, such as psychosis and neurosis.
5. **Study tip:** Make flash cards that reflect the clinical indicator on one side and identify all situations that can cause that sign or symptom on the other side.

Test-Taking Tip #5: Identify Client-Centered Options

1. Client-centered options focus on feelings, opportunities for clients to make choices, and actions that empower clients or support client preferences.
2. More often than not, a client-centered option is the correct answer. For example, a client-centered option might ask, "What genetic question would you like to discuss with your health care provider?" This example option gives a client an opportunity to make a choice, which supports independence. A nursing action that supports a client's independence is an example of a client-centered option.
3. **Study tip:** Compose your own client-centered options that would be a correct answer for the scenario presented in your test question.

Test-Taking Tip #6: Identify Options That Deny Clients' Feelings, Needs, or Concerns

1. Options that avoid clients' feelings, change the subject, offer false reassurance, or encourage optimism cut off communication.
2. Options that deny clients' feelings, needs, or concerns are always distractors unless the stem has negative polarity. For example, an option that says, "You will feel better tomorrow," fails to recognize the client's concerns about the pain that he or she is feeling today.
3. If a stem with negative polarity asks, "What should the nurse *avoid* saying when clients express concerns about the pain they are experiencing?" the option that says, "You will feel better tomorrow" is the correct answer. *It is important to ensure that you identify the polarity of the stem.*

4. **Study tip:** Construct additional options that deny clients' feelings, needs, or concerns that relate to the scenario in the stem, such as, "Cheer up because things could be worse," "Why are you crying? Having a new baby should be a happy time," or "Having a miscarriage is sad, but you can always get pregnant again."

Test-Taking Tip #7: Identify Equally Plausible Options

1. Equally plausible options are those that are so similar that one option is no better than the other.
2. Equally plausible options can both be deleted from further consideration.
3. **Study tip:** Construct equally plausible options for the correct answer and identify equally plausible options for those that are distractors.

Test-Taking Tip #8: Identify Options with Specific Determiners (Absolutes)

1. A specific determiner is a word or phrase that indicates no exceptions.
2. Words that are specific determiners place a limit on a statement that generally is considered correct.
3. Words in options that are specific determiners include *all, none, only, always,* and *never.* For example, options with a specific determiner might say, "Always use Methergine to stop postpartum bleeding."
4. Most of the time, options with specific determiners are distractors.
5. **Study tip:** Construct examples of options with specific determiners so that you are able to recognize when an option has a specific determiner. Next, identify whether the option should be deleted or whether it is an exception to the rule.

Test-Taking Tip #9: Identify the Unique Option

1. When one option is different from the other three options that are similar, examine the unique option carefully.
2. More often than not, an option that is unique is the correct answer. For example, if a question is asking you to identify an expected client response to a problem and three of the options identify an increase in something and one option identifies a decrease in something, examine the option that identifies the decrease in something because it is unique.

3. **Study tip:** Construct options that are similar to the distractors and construct options that are similar to the unique option. Doing so can help you to distinguish among commonalities and differences.

Test-Taking Tip #10: Identify the Global Option

1. Global options are more broad and wide ranging than specific options.
2. One or more of the other options might be included under the umbrella of a global option.
3. Examine global options carefully because they are often the correct answer. For example, a global option might say, "Maintain client confidentiality" versus a specific option, which might say, "Do not release client information over the telephone."
4. **Study tip:** Construct as many specific options as possible that could be included under the umbrella of a global option. Construct as many global options as possible in relation to the content presented in the stem. Doing so will increase your ability to identify a global option.

Test-Taking Tip #11: Use Client Safety and Maslow's Hierarchy of Needs to Identify the Option That Is the Priority

1. This technique is best used when answering a question that asks what the nurse should do first or which action is most important.
2. Examine each option and identify which level need it meets according to Maslow's hierarchy. Identify whether any of the options is associated with maintaining a client's safety. For example, in a question associated with hemorrhage, an option that addresses client safety and prevents harm is the priority.
3. **Study tip:** Start by identifying the action that is least important and work backward toward the option with the action that is most important. Then identify the reasoning behind the assigned order. This technique focuses on the how and why and helps you to clarify the reasoning underlying your critical thinking. This technique is often done best when working in a small study group.

Test-Taking Tip #12: Identify Duplicate Facts in Options

1. Some options contain two or more facts. The more facts that are contained in an option, the greater your chances of selecting the correct answer.

2. If you identify an incorrect term, definition, or dosage, eliminate all options that contain the incorrect item.
3. After you eliminate options that you know are incorrect, move on and identify any fact(s) of which you are sure.
4. Focus on the options that contain at least one fact of which you are sure.
5. By eliminating options, you increase your chances of selecting the correct answer.
6. By the process of elimination, you may arrive at the correct answer even when unsure of all the facts in the correct answer.
7. **Study tip:** Identify all the facts you can that are associated with what the question is asking.

Test-Taking Tip #13: Practice Test-Taking Tips

Practicing test taking is an effective way to achieve five outcomes:
1. You can desensitize yourself to the discomfort or fear that you might feel in a testing situation.
2. You can increase your stamina if you gradually increase the time that you spend practicing test taking to 2 to 3 hours. This practice will enable you to concentrate more effectively for a longer period of time.
3. You will learn how to better manage your time during a test so that you have adequate time to answer all the questions.
4. You will increase your learning when studying the rationales for the right and wrong answers. Also, by practicing the application of test-taking techniques and employing the study tips presented, you will learn how to maximize your learning associated with each test-taking tip.
5. You will become more astute in determining what a question is asking and better able to identify when a test-taking tip might help you eliminate a distractor and focus on an option that might be the correct answer.

Test-Taking Tip #14: Use Multiple Test-Taking Techniques When Examining Test Questions and Options

1. If using one test-taking technique to analyze a question is beneficial, think how much more beneficial it would be to use two or more test-taking techniques to analyze a question.
2. Examine the stem first. For example, ask yourself, "Does the stem have negative polarity?" or "Is the

stem setting a priority?" Read closely to see if the language of the stem suggests a test-taking tip to use.
3. Next, examine the answer options. For example, ask yourself, "Do any of the options contain a specific determiner?" or "Is there a global option?" or "Is there a client-centered option?"
4. By using more than one test-taking tip, you can usually increase your success in selecting the correct answer.

Test-Taking Tips for Alternate-Format Items

Alternate-format items are purported by the National Council of State Boards of Nursing to evaluate some nursing knowledge more readily and authentically than is possible with traditional multiple-choice items. To accomplish this, an alternate-format item does not construct a question with the same organization as a multiple-choice item. Each type of alternate-format item presents information along with a question using a distinctive format and requires you to answer the item in a unique manner. Some alternate-format items use multimedia approaches, such as charts, tables, graphics, sound, and video. Understanding the composition of alternate-format items and having strategies to analyze these items can increase your chances of selecting the correct answer.

Multiple-Response or Select All That Apply (SATA) Item

1. A multiple-response or SATA item presents a stem that asks a question.
2. It presents five or six options as potential answers.
3. You must identify all (two or more) correct answers to the question posed in the stem.
4. On a computer, each answer option is preceded by a circle. You must place the cursor in the circle and click the mouse to select the desired answers.
5. **Test-taking tip:** Before looking at the options, quickly review information you know about the topic. Then compare what you know against the options presented. Another approach is to eliminate one or two options that you know are wrong, identify one option you know is correct, and then eliminate another one or two options that you know are wrong. Finally, you should identify all the options you believe are correct. To do this, you can use some of the test-taking tips that apply to traditional multiple-choice questions, such as identifying options that are opposites; identifying client-centered options; identifying options that deny clients' feelings, needs, or concerns; and identifying options with specific determiners (absolutes) to either eliminate options or focus on potential correct answers.

Drag-and-Drop (Ordered Response) Item

1. A drag-and-drop item makes a statement or presents a situation and then asks you to prioritize five or six options.
2. The item may ask you to indicate the order in which nursing interventions should be performed, the order of importance of concerns, or actual steps in a procedure.
3. To produce a correct answer, you must place all of the options in the correct order.
4. When answering a drag-and-drop item on a computer, you may highlight and click on the option or actually drag the option from the left side of the screen to a box on the right side of the screen. When practicing a drag-and-drop item in a textbook, you can indicate the priority order only by listing the options in order by number.
5. **Test-taking tip:** Use client safety, Maslow's hierarchy of needs, and the nursing process to help focus your ordering of options. Identify the option that you consider to be the priority, and identify the option that you consider to be the least important. Then, from the remaining options, select the next priority option and the next least priority option. Keep progressing along this same line of thinking until all the options have received a placement on the priority list.

Fill-in-the-Blank Calculation Item

1. A fill-in-the-blank calculation item presents information and then asks you a question that requires the manipulation or interpretation of numbers.
2. Computing a medication dosage, intake and output, or the amount of IV fluid to be administered are examples of fill-in-the-blank calculation items.
3. You must answer the item with either a whole number or within a specified number of decimal points as requested by the item.
4. **Test-taking tip:** Before answering the question, recall the memorized equivalents or formulas that are required to answer the item; then perform a calculation to answer the item.

Hot-Spot Item

1. A hot-spot item presents an illustration or photograph and asks a question about it.
2. You must identify a location on the visual image presented to answer the question.
3. The answer must exactly mirror the correct answer to be considered correct.

4. When answering a hot-spot item on a computer, you place the cursor on the desired location and left-click the mouse. These actions place an *X* on the desired location to answer the question. When answering a hot-spot item in a textbook, you are asked to either place an *X* on the desired location or to identify an option indicated by an *a, b, c,* or *d* label presented in the illustration or photograph.
5. **Test-taking tip:** Read and reread the item to ensure that you understand what the item is asking. When attempting to answer a question that involves anatomy and physiology, close your eyes and picture in your mind the significant structures and recall their functions before answering the item.

Exhibit Item

1. An exhibit item presents a scenario, usually a client situation.
2. You are then presented with a question.
3. You must access information from a variety of sources. The information must be analyzed to determine its significance in relation to the question being asked to arrive at an answer.
4. These items require the highest level of critical thinking (analysis and synthesis).
5. On a computer, each option is preceded by a circle. You must place the cursor in the circle and click the mouse to select the desired answers.
6. **Test-taking tip:** Identify exactly what the item is asking. Access the collected data and dissect, analyze, and compare and contrast the data collected in relation to what you know and understand in relation to what the item is asking.

Graphic Item

1. A graphic item presents a question with several answer options that are illustrations, pictures, photographs, charts, or graphs rather than text.
2. You must select the option with the illustration that answers the question.
3. On a computer, each option is preceded by a circle. You must place the cursor in the circle and click the mouse to select the desired answer. When answering a graphic item in a textbook, you are presented with an illustration and must select one answer from among several options, or you are asked a question and must select one answer from among several options, each having an illustration.
4. **Test-taking tip:** When reading your textbook or other resource material, visual images are

presented to support written content. Examine these images in relation to the content presented to reinforce your learning. Oftentimes, similar illustrations may be used in either hot-spot or graphic alternate test items.

Audio Item

1. An audio item presents an audio clip that must be accessed through a headset. After listening to the audio clip, you must select the answer from among the options presented.
2. On a computer, each option is preceded by a circle. You must place the cursor in the circle and click the mouse to select the desired answer.
3. **Test-taking tip:** Listen to educational resources that provide audio clips of sounds that you must be able to identify such as breath, heart, and bowel sounds. Engage in learning experiences using simulation mannequins available in the on-campus nursing laboratory. When in the clinical area, use every opportunity to assess these sounds when completing a physical assessment of assigned clients.

NCLEX-RN Test Plan and Classification of Questions

The National Council Licensure Examinations for Registered Nurses (NCLEX-RN) and for Licensed Practical/Vocational Nurses (NCLEX-PN) test plans were primarily designed to facilitate the classification of examination items and guide candidates preparing for these examinations. These test plans were developed to ensure the formation of tests that measure the competencies required to perform safe, effective nursing care as newly licensed, entry-level registered nurses or licensed practical/vocational nurses. These test plans are revised every 3 years after an analysis of the activities of practicing nurses and after input from experts on the NCLEX Examination Committees and National Council of State Board of Nursing's content staff and member boards of nursing to ensure that the test plans are relevant and consistent with state nurse practice acts. The detailed test plans for the NCLEX-RN and NCLEX-PN differ due to differences in the scope of practice for these professions. Each of these test plans can be found on the National Council of State Board of Nursing's website at www.ncsbn.org/nclex.htm.

Integrated Processes Categories

Integrated processes are the basic factors essential to the practice of nursing, which are the nursing process, caring, communication and documentation, and teaching and learning. Because the nursing process provides a format for critical thinking, it is included for each question.

Nursing Process

Assessment: Nursing care that collects objective and subjective data from primary and secondary sources.
Nursing Diagnosis (Analysis): Nursing care that groups significant data, interprets data, and comes to conclusions.
Planning: Nursing care that sets goals, objectives, and outcomes; prioritizes interventions; and performs calculations.
Implementation: Nursing care that follows a regimen of care prescribed by a primary health care provider, such as administration of medications; this also covers providing nursing care for procedures and providing care within the legal scope of the nursing profession.
Evaluation: Nursing care that identifies a client's responses to medical and nursing interventions.

Client Need Categories

Client needs reflect activities most commonly performed by entry-level nurses.

Safe and Effective Care Environment

Management of Care: Nursing care that provides or directs the delivery of nursing activities to clients, significant others, and other health care personnel. Management of care items account for 17% to 23% of the items on the NCLEX-RN examination.

Safety and Infection Control: Nursing care that protects clients, significant others, and health care personnel from health and environmental hazards. Safety and infection control items account for 9% to 15% of the items on the NCLEX-RN examination.

Health Promotion and Maintenance: Nursing care that assists clients and significant others to prevent or detect health problems and achieve optimum health, particularly in relation to their developmental level. Health promotion and maintenance items account for 6% to 12% of the items on the NCLEX-RN examination.

Psychosocial Integrity: Nursing care that supports and promotes the emotional, mental, and social well-being of clients and significant others as well as those with acute or chronic mental health problems. Psychosocial integrity items account for 6% to 12% of the items on the NCLEX-RN examination.

Physiological Integrity

Basic Care and Comfort: Nursing care that provides support during the performance of the activities of daily living, such as hygiene, rest, sleep, mobility, elimination, hydration, and nutrition. Basic care and comfort items account for 6% to 12% of the items on the NCLEX-RN examination.

Pharmacological and Parenteral Therapies: Nursing care that relates to the administration of medication, intravenous fluids, and blood and blood products. Pharmacological and parenteral therapies items account for 12% to 18% of the items on the NCLEX-RN examination.

Reduction of Risk Potential: Nursing care that limits the development of complications associated with health problems, treatments, or procedures. Reduction of risk potential items account for 9% to 15% of the items on the NCLEX-RN examination.

Physiological Adaptation: Nursing care that meets the needs of clients with acute, chronic, or life-threatening physical health problems. Physiological adaptation items account for 11% to 17% of the items on the NCLEX-RN examination.

Cognitive Level Categories

This category reflects the thinking processes necessary to answer a question.

Knowledge: Information must be recalled from memory, such as facts, terminology, principles, and generalizations.

Comprehension: Information and the implications and potential consequences of information identified must be understood, interpreted, and paraphrased or summarized.

Application: Information must be identified, manipulated, or used in a situation, including mathematical calculations.

Analysis: A variety of information must be interpreted, requiring the identification of commonalities, differences, and the interrelationship among the data.

Human Reproduction

Chapter 1

Anatomy and Physiology of Female and Male Reproduction Systems

KEY TERMS

Androgens—Male sex hormones (primarily testosterone); produced in cells in the testes and responsible for the development of primary and secondary male sex characteristics

Cervix—The lowest section of the uterus (sometimes referred to as the *neck*) that opens into the posterior vagina

Corpus Luteum—A small, yellow body that develops within a ruptured ovarian follicle and is an endocrine structure secreting progesterone

Embryo—Stage of development between the second and eighth weeks

Endometrial cycle—Responding to the hormonal changes of the ovarian cycle, the lining (endometrium) of the uterus undergoes three phases resulting in either the reception and nourishing of the developing embryo or menstruation if pregnancy does not occur

Endometrium—The mucous membrane lining the inner surface of the uterus

Estrogen—The primary female sex hormone; is released by the ovaries and the placenta during pregnancy and is responsible for the development of the secondary sex characteristics in females and the monthly changes in the endometrium in the uterus

Fallopian tube—The hollow structure extending from the right and left lateral angles of the uterine fundus; these narrow tubes end near each ovary

Fimbriae—The fine, fringelike ends of the fallopian tubes

Follicle—Structure in an ovary that contains the egg prior to ovulation (primary, secondary, and graafian phases)

Follicle-stimulating hormone (FSH)—A gonadotrophic hormone that is released by the anterior pituitary; is essential to the pubertal development and the growth of the ovarian follicle before the release of the egg from the follicle at ovulation

Gamete—The mature female ovum or male sperm, capable of uniting in fertilization

Labia majora/minora—The inner and outer fleshy structures that cover the vagina and urethra in women

Luteinizing hormone (LH)—A gonadotrophic hormone released by the anterior pituitary; the increase in levels of LH precedes the release of an egg from an ovarian follicle

Menstrual cycle—Averaging 28 days in length, the cycle of changes in the uterus and ovaries, controlled by regulatory sex hormones

Oocyte—The early or primitive ovum before it has developed completely

Ovarian cycle—Cycle of specific changes in the ovary that occur during the menstrual cycle whereas follicle swells with a maturing ovum (egg) ruptures, releasing the egg, and shrinks into an increasingly smaller **corpus luteum** by the beginning of menses

Ovulation—The periodic ripening and rupture of the mature graafian follicle and discharge of the ovum from the ovary

Continued

Ovum—The female reproductive or germ cell that is capable of developing into a new organism of the same species

Oxytocin—A hormone secreted by the hypothalamus and stored in the pituitary gland; stimulates the uterus to contract during labor, postpartum, and during breastfeeding to stimulate milk letdown

Pituitary gland—Produces the stimulating hormones that regulate the hormones produced by the ovaries and the adrenal glands

Progesterone—A hormone obtained from the corpus luteum and placenta

Prolactin—Produced by the pituitary gland and stimulates breast development and the formation of milk during pregnancy

Prostaglandins—Hormones responsible for the contraction and relaxation of smooth muscle; in the female reproductive system, regulate contraction of the uterus

Prostate gland—Surrounds the neck of the bladder and urethra in males; restricts bladder function and contributes to seminal fluid during sexual arousal and ejaculation

Puberty—Physiological life stage when the release of gonadotropic hormone begins the process of sexual maturation and the development of secondary sex characteristics; ends when female or male is capable of reproducing

Seminal vesicles—Produce the final additions to the seminal fluid that empties into the ejaculatory ducts, mixing with sperm prior to ejaculation

Sperm—The ejaculate from the male containing spermatozoa

Spermatogenesis—The development of spermatids into fully functional sperm

Testis (testes, pl.)—Spurred to maturity by testosterone, the sperm-producing glands, exterior to the male body at the base of the penis

Testosterone—An anabolic (steroidal) hormone that is the main male sex hormone; responsible for the maturation of male reproductive organs and the maturation of sperm

Uterus—A muscular organ lying behind the bladder in the female pelvis, approximately 5 cm long and 2.5 cm in diameter, consisting of a "body," the top of which is the fundus; layers include the inner lining called the **endometrium**, a thicker middle layer of smooth muscle called the *myometrium,* and an outer serosal layer known as the *perimetrium*

Vagina—The fibromuscular tube that surrounds the cervix at the distal portion and opens into the vestibule protected by the labia; sometimes called the *birth canal*

Vas deferens—A long section of the epididymis that transports the sperm to the ejaculatory duct

I. Female Reproductive System

The female reproductive system is formed in the fetus, differentiated from the male system by the lack of a Y chromosome. This system is responsible for the production and maintenance of the egg cells, or **oocytes.** Each oocyte has the capacity to become a mature **ovum,** which, if surrounded by viable **sperm,** will become fertilized. If functioning as expected, the female reproductive organs then protect and allow the embryo to grow into a human being. The maturation and cycles of the female reproductive system are controlled by a series of hormonal activities. The success of human reproduction relies on a complex series of events in order to continue the species.

A. External structures

1. Unlike the male reproductive system, the female system has few external structures; the majority of the system is internal.

2. The external structures, or genitals (referred to as the *external accessory organs*), consist of the labia (major and minora), the clitoris, and the vestibular glands. Above the symphysis pubis and anterior to

the labia is the mons pubis, a pad of fatty tissue covered by pubic hair. These structures, known as the **vulva,** surround the openings of the urethra and the vagina. Lastly, on the anterior chest wall, the mammary glands (breasts) are located midthorax on each side of the midline.

a) The **labia majora** are fleshy folds of epithelium and adipose cells that close over the labia minora. Hair grows on the outer surface.

b) The **labia minora** are thinner, hairless folds of epithelial tissue located just under the labia majora.

c) These folds of tissue also form a hood around the clitoris, the female erectile organ. The clitoris is similar to the male penis in function but does not contain the urethra. Its only function is sensory, engorging during sexual activity.

d) Together the labia cover the vestibule, including the openings of the urethra and the vagina. Vestibular glands, also known as Bartholin's glands, are located on either side of the vaginal opening and secrete fluids that lubricate the vestibule. They provide lubrication for the vagina and vulva.

e) Mammary glands provide the unique means by which female mammals feed their young. The mammary glands are the least consistent in size of all the external female reproductive organs. They are located on both sides of the anterior center thoracic region and are stimulated to growth during **puberty**. They consist of alveolar glands that produce nourishing milk specifically formulated for human infants. Lactiferous ducts transport the milk to the nipple for extraction either manually or by a suckling infant. Breasts also contain varying amounts of fatty tissue and differ in size from woman to woman, but regardless of size, they are capable of producing enough milk to adequately feed an infant (or two or three). The milk-producing cells and glands begin to prepare for milk production at the time of conception. Production is stimulated by the pituitary hormones **prolactin** and **oxytocin**.

B. Internal structures

1. Female internal reproductive organs are responsible for maturing the human egg, or ovum, facilitating the fertilization process and nurturing the developing **embryo** through the fetal stage until the fetus is capable of living on its own outside the **uterus**. The female internal accessory reproductive organs include the uterus, the **fallopian tubes,** and the **ovaries**. All of these structures lie within the female pelvic cavity and are supported in the pelvis by the broad, round, ovarian, and suspensory ligaments. Female internal reproductive organs are stimulated by the pituitary hormones **estrogen, progesterone, luteinizing hormone,** and **follicle-stimulating hormone (FSH)** (Table 1.1).

a) The uterus is a single hollow, muscular organ located midline, superior to the urinary bladder in the female pelvis. Isolated, it looks like an upside-down pear. It consists of three layers:
   • The perimetrium, or outer peritoneal tissue
   • The myometrium in the middle
   • The endometrium is the inner layer

The upper two-thirds of the uterus have the thickest myometrium, or muscle layer. Three layers of involuntary smooth muscle are uniquely designed to expand to accommodate a growing fetus and work together to contract, causing the descent and expulsion of the fetus during labor. This muscular layer extends through the entire uterus into the fallopian tubes and the vagina. Though these structures have distinct functions, the continuity of the muscle serves to ensure that

Table 1.1 Female Reproductive Hormones

Hormone	Source	Actions
Gonadotropin-releasing hormone (GnRH)	Hypothalamus	Stimulates the anterior pituitary gland to secrete follicle-stimulating hormone (FSH) and luteinizing hormone (LH)
Estrogen	Ovarian follicle Placenta during pregnancy	Promotes maturation of the ovarian follicle Stimulates the growth of endometrial blood vessels Stimulates secondary sex characteristics development
FSH	Anterior pituitary	Initiates ovarian follicle development Stimulates estrogen secretion by follicular cells
LH	Anterior pituitary	Causes the release of the mature ovum (ovulation) Stimulates progesterone secretion by the corpus luteum
Oxytocin	Secreted by hypothalamus; stored in the pituitary	Stimulates the uterus to contract Stimulates breast milk letdown
Prolactin	Anterior pituitary	Stimulates breast development Stimulates formation of milk following pregnancy
Progesterone	Corpus luteum of ovary Placenta during pregnancy	Stimulates changes in the endometrium during the second half of the menstrual cycle Facilitates implantation by decreasing uterine motility Inhibits myometrial contraction during pregnancy Stimulates development of the mammary glands
Prostaglandin (E & F)	Cells of the endometrium	PGE relaxes smooth muscle; vasodilator PGF increases muscle contractility; vasoconstrictor
Relaxin	Corpus luteum of ovary Placenta during pregnancy	Inhibits myometrial contraction, promoting embryo implantation Promotes relaxation of the uterine ligaments during pregnancy

the system responds and functions as a whole. The top of the uterus is known as the *fundus.* At the narrow lower (inferior) end of the uterus, the **cervix** opens into the distal portion of the vagina (birth canal). With pregnancy, the uterus grows in size and weight, stretching to hold 9 to 10 lb of fetus, placenta, and fluid. Following pregnancy, it never again achieves its prepregnancy size. Prostaglandins, progesterone, and oxytocin exert hormonal influences on the myometrium, either causing it to relax or contract throughout the reproductive cycle and pregnancy. The inner lining of the uterus is called the *endometrium,* which consists of a base layer and a functional layer. Endometrial tissue is very vascular and builds up a spongy layer of blood-rich glandular tissue each month. This endometrial buildup is shed during menstruation if pregnancy does not occur.

b) Attached to the peritoneal and myometrium of the uterus are ligaments that support the other reproductive structures. A portion of the broad ligaments support the thin tubes that open up from the uterus in the upper medial angle and extend outward on both sides of the uterus. The fallopian tubes extend about 10 cm, opening with **fimbriae** covering the lateral aspect of the ovaries. An ovum released from the ovary is gently scooped into the tube. Smooth muscle waves move the ovum to the uterus. Fertilization of the ovum by motile sperm occurs as it moves along the fallopian tubes.

c) The ovaries are the walnut-shaped female gonads that hold, mature, and release the female **gamete** or ovum following maturation during the **ovarian cycle.** They are supported laterally to the uterus by the broad and ovarian ligaments. Thousands of **follicles,** each containing an oocyte, are present in the ovaries at the birth of a female infant. These follicles are responsible for the secretion of estrogen into the female bloodstream. As the female matures, the increased release of estrogen spurs the development of the secondary female reproductive organs. Normally, during the **menstrual cycle,** a mature graafian follicle releases one ovum per month **(ovulation).** The corpus luteum that remains after ovulation produces the steroidal hormone progesterone.

d) The **vagina** surrounds the cervix at the inferior end of the uterus and leads to the external vulva in the peritoneum. It is approximately 4 in. (9 cm) long and consists of specialized smooth muscle with a lining of stratified squamous epithelial cells that resist colonization by harmful bacteria. The normal microbial flora of the vagina create an acidic environment that also helps to resist infectious microbes. Moist lubricants, secreted by the cells, aid in the insertion of the penis during intercourse, provide a favorable environment for sperm, and help cleanse potentially harmful microbes from the vaginal wall. The epithelial mucosa lining is "folded" into rugae attached to specialized connective tissue. The purpose of the folds and the uniquely stretchy tissues is that the vagina must stretch without tearing in order to allow the birth of a baby.

C. Female reproductive cycle

1. The menstrual cycle is the monthly process that regulates female fertility. It is actually a combination of several hormonal cycles acting on the ovaries and the uterine lining (endometrium). There are three interactive cycles occurring in relation to the 28-day menstrual cycle: the hypothalamic–pituitary cycle, the ovarian cycle, and the **endometrial cycle.** The cycles begin on the first day of the start of the menstrual flow, on or about the 28th day of the cycles. They end just before the next menses if fertilization has not occurred.

a) The hypothalamic–pituitary axis forms the master control for the associated ovarian and uterine changes. It begins in the hypothalamus

---

MAKING THE CONNECTION

Patient Education and Reproductive Health

The structure of the female reproductive system is critical to the process of reproduction, the function for which the system exists. Abnormal development of the organs or damage to any part of the system may result in the inability to conceive or carry a fetus. Because most of the system is internal, signs of abnormality may not be evident until puberty or an attempt to conceive. It is important for nurses to understand the normal structure and function of the female system in order to educate women about how to care for their reproductive organs.

In addition, nurses play an important role in teaching and encouraging young women to seek regular care for their reproductive health. Regardless of whether the young woman is sexually active, it is important for her to understand her body and its normal functioning. The woman's health nurse is in a position to teach women about reproductive health and the importance of routine examinations with age-appropriate screening. Standardized reproductive health questions should be part of annual examinations as soon as the development of secondary sex characteristics becomes evident.

with the release of gonadotropin-releasing hormone (GnRH). GnRH acts on the anterior **pituitary gland,** which releases luteinizing hormone (LH) and follicle-stimulating hormone (FSH). These hormones are peptide compounds that cannot cross cell membranes; instead they attach to specific cell receptors on the outside of a follicle within the ovary. Granulosa material within the follicle is converted to estrogen, stimulating the rapid maturation of the oocyte. Typically, only one of the two ovaries matures one ova per cycle.

b) The ovarian cycle, controlled by increasing stimulation from the LH and FSH, undergoes the follicular phase of the ovarian cycle. As estrogen levels rise, a spike in the pituitary's production of both LH and FSH around the 14th day of the new menstrual cycle induces the release of a mature ovum from the now-matured graafian follicle. Following ovulation, the former follicle becomes the **corpus luteum,** often called the *luteal phase* of the cycle. As LH and estrogen decrease, the newly formed corpus luteum begins to produce progesterone, which emerges as the primary hormone influencing the cycle at this point. The level and influence of progesterone increase until about the 22nd to 23rd day of the cycle. If fertilization has not occurred, the corpus luteum shrinks, producing less and less progesterone and estrogen. If ovulation does not lead to fertilization and implantation, the corpus luteum disintegrates into connective tissue. However, if implantation does occur, the corpus luteum continues to produce progesterone and estrogen. The higher levels of these hormones provide negative feedback to the pituitary gland, suppressing the release of LH and FSH. As long as these stimulating hormones are suppressed, further ovulation will not occur.

c) In the uterus, the endometrial cycle is defined by changes to the **endometrium** on the uterine walls, which occur in response to the changes and hormone production in the ovaries. There are four distinct phases of the endometrial cycle: the menstrual phase, the proliferative phase, the secretory phase, and the ischemic phase.

   (1) Following menstruation, the endometrium, influenced by the increase in estrogen production by the maturing graafian follicle, begins to thicken and continues to do so over the first 14 days of the cycle. This is the proliferative phase.

   (2) Around the 14th day of the menstrual cycle, following the release of the ovum,

MAKING THE CONNECTION

Identifying Ovulation

Knowledge about the neurohormonal control of the female reproductive cycle is critical to an understanding of normal versus abnormal complex actions of releasing hormones from the hypothalamus and anterior pituitary hormones that act directly on the ovarian development of mature ova. The nurse should understand that interruption in any of these hormone and stimulation pathways may affect the female's ability to reproduce. The presence of adequate amounts of the primary female hormone estrogen does not necessarily indicate or ensure healthy reproductive function.

Understanding and identifying ovulation occurrence can be useful in determining if ovulation has occurred. A common, noninvasive method to identify ovulation is the measurement of a woman's basal body temperature (BBT). This method involves training a woman how and when to measure her temperature and record the results over the course of her monthly cycle. When ovulation has occurred, the BBT typically rises 0.4° to 1°F. This rise in temperature is caused by the increase in progesterone production during the ovarian luteal phase. However, since the rise in temperature occurs following ovulation, and coitus to achieve pregnancy appears to be most effective in the 24 to 48 hours prior to or the day of ovulation, the rise in basal temperature may not be helpful when attempting to become pregnant. Some women also experience pain in the right or left pelvic region during ovulation. Referred to as *mittelschmerz,* it is thought to be a localized response to the release of the mature ovum.

the resulting corpus luteum produces increasing amounts of the hormone progesterone. Progesterone causes an increase in both the vascularity and the glandular characteristics of the endometrium. This is called the *secretory phase* because the glands in the endometrium begin to secrete more sugars and fats, engorging the endometrial tissues with fluids that can nourish a developing embryo.

   (3) By the 24th day of the cycle, if fertilization and implantation have not occurred, the shrinking corpus luteum produces fewer and fewer hormones; the blood- and nutrient-rich endometrium begins to break down and slough, in a process known as *menstruation.* As levels of estrogen and progesterone begin to fall rapidly, the levels of LH and FSH begin to rise, and the entire cycle begins again (Fig. 1.1).

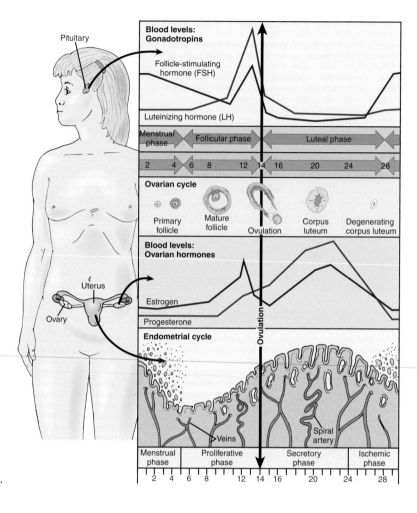

Fig 1.1 The female reproductive cycle.

d) The glandular cells of the uterus also produce small amounts of **prostaglandin.** Prostaglandins (PGs) are produced in several areas in the body, often related to the process of tissue damage when vasodilation is required to get necessary repair materials to the injured site. There are two types of prostaglandin: E and F (PGE and PGF). The effects of PGE are smooth muscle relaxation and vasodilation. However, PGF increases the contractility of muscles and arteries. Prostaglandins are found in increased amounts around the follicle at the time of ovulation. Uterine-produced prostaglandins serve two purposes. During menstruation, they cause the body of the uterus to contract and simultaneously cause vascular dilation and softening of the cervix. This aids in the effective expulsion of the unneeded endometrial lining. Unfortunately, because of the effects of prostaglandin, nerve endings in the area of activity may transmit increased pain sensation, resulting in very painful uterine cramping. Prostaglandin is also thought to be the cause of headaches, nausea,

---

MAKING THE CONNECTION

Menarche

Menarche, or the beginning of menstrual cycle, may be seen in girls as young as 9 or 10 years of age or it may be delayed into the teens. A menstrual cycle is normally 28 to 32 days long. However, differences among women and monthly cycles may be noted. Menstrual cycle length may be affected by fatigue, illness, stress, nutrition, or excessive illness. A nurse needs to be prepared to perform thorough examinations that include a reproductive history for all women. If a girl is showing outward signs of sexual maturation, menarche is often not far behind. The teen who has not experienced menarche by her 16th birthday, or within 4 years of breast development, may require a thorough assessment to try to identify any factors for the delay. In addition, all young women need to understand that regular menstruation means that they are releasing ova (eggs) that may be fertilized. An active reproductive system means that pregnancy is possible, regardless of age.

and diarrhea that can occur during menstruation. This is referred to as *dysmenorrhea* and is a monthly experience for up to half of all menstruating women.

II. The Male Reproductive System

Unlike the female reproductive system, the majority of the male organs are located externally. The male reproductive system is controlled by hormones called **androgens,** though not in the cyclical manner that regulates female reproduction. The **testes** are the primary sex organs or gonads. They produce the sperm cells and the male sex hormone **testosterone.** The other organs, some internal and others external, in the male reproductive system are considered to be secondary or accessory sex organs. The pathway of the male gametes—called *sperm*—begins in the testes, travels through the accessory organs internally, and ends in the urethra of the penis, the other external organ.

A. Testes
1. The gamete-producing testes lie side by side in the soft saclike scrotum, each suspended by a spermatic cord. They are approximately 2.5 to 3 cm in diameter in the adult male. Although formed internally during fetal development, they normally descend into the scrotal sac through the inguinal canal just prior to birth. A testicle that remains inside the male body cannot produce viable sperm because the body's normal temperature is too warm for **spermatogenesis.** Each testicle is encapsulated by a tough membrane called the *tunica albuginea.* Inside each testicle are numerous lobes, each containing up to four seminiferous tubules. It is within these tubules that spermatids begin to become mature sperm. Unlike females who are born with a plentiful but finite number of potential ova, healthy males are capable of producing millions of sperm continuously from puberty well into old age. Testosterone, the primary male sex hormone, is produced by interstitial cells that lie within the loops of the seminiferous tubules.

   The seminiferous tubules lead toward the posterior surfaces of the testes to a network of vessels, the rete testis, where sperm continue toward maturity. From there, efferent tubules transport the yet immature sperm to the epididymis.
2. The coiled epididymis, located on the outside of the testicle (still within the scrotal sack), heads downward to the testicular base where thousands of mature sperm are stored in the "tail" of the epididymis for 40 to 60 days. Any sperm remaining after that time break down and are absorbed back into the system. Active sperm leave the epididymis

when sexual stimulation propels them toward the vas deferens, which continue upward through the spermatic cord into the internal structures of the male reproductive system. The vas deferens continue to the posterior, loop downward over each ureter, and finally join with the seminal vesicle. From there, the two structures form the ejaculatory ducts, travel through the prostate gland, and empty into the urethra.

B. Internal structures (facilitating sperm ejaculation)
1. At the base of the bladder are the **seminal vesicles.** They release a thick fluid that nourishes the sperm, giving them the energy to navigate the female system during coitus. This fluid comprises the bulk of semen's volume.
2. The **prostate gland** lies just beyond the ejaculatory ducts and surrounds both the ejaculatory ducts and the urethra, just past the bladder. This walnut-shaped gland performs two functions: It secretes additional fluid into the semen and contracts to shut off the urethra at the bladder and it assists in propelling the semen externally through the urethra. The fluid aids in sperm motility and counteracts the more acidic environment of the vagina. Cowper's or bulbourethral glands, located at the base of the prostate gland, secrete a clear lubricant that serves to neutralize any urine acid remaining in the urethra. In order for sperm to remain healthy and mobile, they require a more alkaline environment.

C. The penis
1. The male urethra travels from the bladder through the external male sex organ, the penis. In adult males, an entire urethra is approximately 17 cm long from the bladder through the external opening. (The female urethra is

---

MAKING THE CONNECTION

Testosterone

The male hormone testosterone is responsible for most of the masculine physical attributes. In addition to affecting the development of the male genital tract, it stimulates the growth and strength of the long bones of the male. Testosterone promotes muscle development and mass. It affects the vocal cords, enlarging them and deepening the voice. The distribution and appearance of body hair in the male is also influenced by testosterone. Unlike female hormonal fluctuations, testosterone's action is steady, continuing throughout a man's life. Men are capable of fathering children long beyond the age at which women cease their normal childbearing capacity.

about one-third the length of the male's.) The penis lies in front of the scrotum, is cylindrical in shape, and varies in size in its flaccid and erect states. From its base, the shaft extends to the distal head of the penis, also known as the glans penis. Three cylinders of tissue are contained within the penis: two corpus cavernosa situated anterolaterally and the corpus spongiosum surrounding the urethra. During sexual excitement, the cavernous or erectile tissues fill with blood, causing the penis to elongate and stiffen. This is to ensure that the semen containing sperm has the best chance of being deposited inside the vagina near the cervix during coitus, or intercourse.

MAKING THE CONNECTION

Conception and Fertilization

Ejaculated semen contains between 40 million and 1 billion sperm per episode. However, only one sperm will be allowed to enter the female ovum. For conception to occur, the male sperm need to connect with the female ovum. If there is any barrier or inability for the two to meet, there will be no conception. In the same manner, purposely preventing conception involves breaking the cycle of gamete production or blocking the connection. The nurse's understanding of the anatomy and physiology of reproduction will enable the nurse to effectively assist patients in controlling their fertility.

CASE STUDY: Putting It All Together

Subjective Data

Julia Crenshaw is 18 years old. She began menstruating shortly after turning 13 and has had fairly regular 28- to 30-day cycles since her 14th birthday. Although she has had sports physicals for school, she has declined to have regular pelvic examinations or screening, explaining that she has not been sexually active and intends to wait until marriage.

However, today during a precollege physical, she complains that her periods have become heavier in the past year and that she has increasing discomfort prior to the start of her periods. This discomfort includes slight weight gain, headaches, fatigue, and mood swings. For the first 2 days of her period, she has painful cramps and takes ibuprofen, which offers some relief.

Objective Data

Julia is 5'5" tall and weighs 54.5 kilogram (kg) (BMI 19.9). Her pulse is 62, blood pressure (BP) is 117/64, respirations (RR) is 16, Hgb = 11.6, and Hct = 34. She is up to date on all recommended vaccines except the papillomavirus vaccine, Gardasil, which she has declined.

Case Study Questions

1. What should be reviewed in Julia's past history?

2. Which current findings should be addressed by the nurse?

3. What health information should the nurse offer in regard to Julia's complaints? (Are her periods and symptoms "normal," or what is important for Julia to understand?)

REVIEW QUESTIONS

Be sure to read the Introduction for valuable test-taking tips.

1. What is the primary function of the endometrial layer of the uterus?
   1. Increase in density and content during each menstrual cycle
   2. Prepare to receive and nourish a fertilized ovum (blastocyst)
   3. Produce the hormones that regulate ovulation
   4. Maintain pregnancy

2. For both males and females, which is the first hormone secreted to initiate puberty?
   1. Follicle-stimulating hormone (FSH)
   2. Estrogen
   3. Testosterone
   4. Gonadotropin-releasing hormone (GnRH)

3. Ova and sperm are also known as which of the following?
   1. Gonads
   2. Gametes
   3. Stem cells
   4. Hormones

4. What is the primary function of the corpus luteum?
   1. Produce a mature ovum
   2. Produce progesterone and estrogen
   3. Stimulate initial growth of the endometrium
   4. Promote maturation of the next follicle

5. The vulva consists of which structure?
   1. Labia majora, minora, clitoris, mons pubis, and vestibular glands
   2. Penis, scrotum, and prostate gland
   3. Internal female structures, including the uterus and ovaries
   4. Openings of the urethra and vagina

6. During which phase of the ovarian cycle is progesterone circulating in high amounts?
   1. Proliferative phase
   2. Menstrual phase
   3. Ovulatory phase
   4. Luteal phase

7. Which is true regarding the endometrium? *Select all that apply.*
   1. It consists of a single layer of epithelial glandular cells.
   2. Estrogen stimulates the functional layer to thicken.
   3. Progesterone stimulates the functional layer to thicken.
   4. There are no changes once implantation occurs.
   5. If fertilization and implantation do not occur, the functional layer is shed.

8. The myometrium of the uterus responds to which hormone?
   1. Prostaglandins and oxytocin
   2. Progesterone and estrogen
   3. Oxytocin, relaxin, and prostaglandin E
   4. Progesterone and testosterone

9. A patient who is experiencing trouble becoming pregnant reported that she has only two to three menstrual periods per year. What is an initial explanation for this problem?
   1. Ovulation is difficult to predict.
   2. There is a definite lack of gonadotropin-releasing hormone.
   3. Something is blocking one or both fallopian tubes.
   4. Only one ovary is functioning.

10. After Sam fathers five children, he and his wife decide that he should have a vasectomy, which is a cutting and removal of a small section of each vas deferens. Why will this cause Sam to be infertile?
    1. It will become impossible for him to ejaculate during coitus.
    2. The sperm will not be able to get from the epididymis to the urethra.
    3. He will no longer produce sperm.
    4. The seminal fluid will be too acidic for the sperm to survive.

11. A young woman experienced signs of secondary sexual development (puberty) beginning at age 12. She is now approaching her 17th birthday but has not yet begun menstruating. What is the clinic nurse's *best* response?
    1. "Don't worry, your periods should start soon."
    2. "This is a cause for great concern. You could have difficulty conceiving in the future."
    3. "Given that other signs of sexual development have occurred, we should schedule an appointment for further assessment."
    4. "This is fairly normal. Some young women are just 'late bloomers,' and there is no real cause for concern."

12. Arrange the steps of the female menstrual cycle in the correct order of occurrence.
    1. Menstrual phase
    2. Premenstrual phase
    3. Secretory phase
    4. Proliferative phase

13. What does FSH primarily act to stimulate?
    1. Development of the uterine endometrium
    2. Release of the mature ovum
    3. Maturation of the ovarian follicle
    4. Development of the ovary

14. Testosterone is responsible for the development of which of the following? *Select all that apply.*
    1. The male reproductive organs
    2. Male secondary sex characteristics
    3. Male muscle mass
    4. Male height
    5. Male weight

15. Which phases are included in the ovarian cycle?
    1. Proliferative and secretory phases
    2. Estrogen and progesterone phases
    3. Endometrial and luteal phases
    4. Follicular and luteal phases

16. The stimulation of initial milk production and release in the breast is accomplished by which hormones? *Select all that apply.*
    1. Oxytocin
    2. Progesterone
    3. Prolactin
    4. Luteinizing hormone
    5. Estrogen

17. A woman who is charting her basal temperature during her cycle notes a sudden increase of 0.6°F in her waking temperature on the 15th day of her menstrual cycle. Which hormone is the cause of this finding?
    1. FSH
    2. Progesterone
    3. Estrogen
    4. Prostaglandin

18.

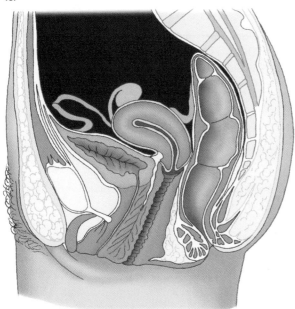

Mark an *X* on the cervix in the diagram.

19. A young woman is giving her menstrual history to the nurse. She is concerned about a short-lived pain that sometimes occurs on either the right or left side of her lower abdomen about 2 weeks before her period is due to begin. What is the nurse's *best* response?
    1. "This pain is probably related to ovulation and is not uncommon."
    2. "The pain may be caused by abnormal hormone levels, so the levels should be checked."
    3. "Don't worry, this is to be expected in young women."
    4. "There might be some structural abnormality that should be assessed further."

20. What is the primary structural difference between the male and female urethra?
    1. The male urethra has two functions, whereas the female urethra has one.
    2. The male urethra is up to three times as long as the female urethra.
    3. The female urethra is less protected than the male urethra.
    4. The female urethra is connected directly to the bladder.

REVIEW QUESTION ANSWERS

1. ANSWER: 2
Rationale
1. While it is true that the endometrium increases in density and content during the menstrual cycle, this is not its primary physiological function.
2. The endometrium exists to receive a fertilized ovum at the blastocyst stage. If implantation occurs, the functional layer thickens and begins to produce glycogen; if implantation does not occur, the functional layer of the endometrium is shed during menses.
3. The hormones that initiate ovulation originate in the pituitary gland.
4. Progesterone, which helps to maintain pregnancy, is initially produced by the corpus luteum if implantation occurs. Once developed, the placenta takes over this function.
TEST-TAKING TIP: There is a difference between what occurs to or within a physical structure and its function. (Why does the structure exist?) In this case, the functional layer of the uterine lining changes in a cyclical manner, depending on whether its purpose is served or not. It is important to recall the sequence and influences on the ovulatory cycle versus the endometrial cycle.
Content Area: Structure and Function of the Female Reproductive Organs—Endometrium
Integrated Process: Nursing Process—Assessment
Client Need: Physiological Integrity
Cognitive Level: Knowledge
Concept: Female Reproduction
Reference: Durham, R. F., & Chapman, L. (2014). Maternal-newborn nursing: The critical components of nursing care. 2nd ed. Philadelphia, PA: F.A. Davis Company.

2. ANSWER: 4
Rationale
1. The release of FSH from the anterior pituitary in both genders stimulates the hormones (estrogen in females, testosterone in males) that stimulate the development of the secondary sex characteristics. However, the release of GnRH begins the processes that define puberty.
2. Following the release of FSH and LH, estrogen produced in the ovarian follicle is the primary female hormone inducing secondary sex characteristics and menarche.
3. Following the release of FSH and LH, which stimulate enlarging of the testes, testosterone is the primary male hormone produced in the testes. Testosterone influences the development of secondary sex characteristics in the male.
4. Initially, the release of GnRH from the hypothalamus stimulates the release of FSH and LH from the anterior pituitary. This begins the cascade of hormonal influence over the development and maturing of the reproductive systems.
TEST-TAKING TIP: Recall that "tropins" are hormones that stimulate other hormones—initiators of many hormonal processes in the endocrine system.
Content Area: Physiology of Male and Female Reproductive Systems—Hormones
Integrated Process: Nursing Process—Assessment
Client Need: Physiological Integrity
Cognitive Level: Knowledge
Concept: Female/Male Reproduction

Reference: Thompson, G. S. (2015). Understanding anatomy & physiology: A visual, auditory, interactive approach. 2nd ed. Philadelphia, PA: F.A. Davis Company.

3. ANSWER: 2
Rationale
1. Gonads are the physical structures in males and females that produce and store the gametes, or ova and sperm.
2. Gametes are cells with one-half of the chromosomes (23) contained in the human cell (46), including the unique chromosomes (X or Y) that determine gender in the fertilized ovum. Gametes, or ova and sperm, are capable of uniting to form a new human.
3. Stem cells are the undifferentiated cells that, through mitosis, form germ cells that undergo meiosis to form a mature ovum or sperm.
4. Hormones are the chemicals that act on the gonads to stimulate gamete production and release.
TEST-TAKING TIP: A basic knowledge of anatomical and physiology terms is necessary to understand physiological processes. These terms are used frequently when discussing the concerns that reproductive health care professionals have when treating reproductive disorders and making recommendations for safe reproduction and embryonic development.
Content Area: Anatomical/Biological Terminology
Integrated Process: Nursing Process—Assessment
Client Need: Physiological Integrity
Cognitive Level: Knowledge
Concept: Female/Male Reproduction
Reference: Thompson, G. S. (2015). Understanding anatomy & physiology: A visual, auditory, interactive approach. 2nd ed. Philadelphia, PA: F.A. Davis Company.

4. ANSWER: 3
Rationale
1. The corpus luteum is formed from the graafian follicle, following the release of the mature ovum in the middle of the ovulatory cycle. It does not "mature" the ovum.
2. The corpus luteum takes on an endocrine role, producing significant amounts of progesterone and some estrogen until implantation of the fertilized ovum does (or does not) occur. If fertilization occurs, the production of progesterone continues until the placenta matures and begins producing progesterone. If fertilization does not occur, the corpus luteum degenerates, forming connective tissue.
3. The initial increase in the depth and amount of the functional layer of the endometrium in the first half of the menstrual cycle occurs prior to the formation of the corpus luteum. It is true that following ovulation, the progesterone produced by the corpus luteum induces continued thickening of the endometrial layer unless implantation of a fertilized ovum does not occur.
4. The maturation of the next follicle (prepared to release another mature ovum) is stimulated by estrogen forming within the maturing follicle, having been acted upon by FSH from the pituitary gland.
TEST-TAKING TIP: The monthly physiological process of producing and releasing a mature female gamete or ovum is an orderly hormonal process. Nurses should have a basic knowledge of the order of the process and the functions

of the involved structures. Understanding when the corpus luteum forms and its specific function determines the response to this question.
Content Area: Physiology of the Female Reproductive System—Hormones
Integrated Process: Nursing Process—Assessment
Client Need: Physiological Integrity
Cognitive Level: Knowledge
Concept: Female Reproduction
Reference: *Durham, R. F., & Chapman, L. (2014). Maternal-newborn nursing: The critical components of nursing care. 2nd ed. Philadelphia, PA: F.A. Davis Company.*

5. ANSWER: 1
Rationale
1. These structures form the external female genitalia, or the vulva. The vulvar structures protect the opening of the urethra and the vagina, provide lubrication, and respond to sexual stimulation.
2. The penis, scrotum, and prostate gland are parts of the male reproductive system.
3. The vulva includes external female structures, not the internal organs, which include the uterus and ovaries.
4. The vulva surrounds the openings of the urethra and vagina, but these structures do not form the vulva.
TEST-TAKING TIP: The nurse needs to know the terms and be able to identify the internal and external structures of the reproductive system. Injuries and disorders affecting reproductive health will require assessment of all parts of the reproductive anatomy. Assessment of the female reproductive system will require descriptions of these structures.
Content Area: Male and Female Reproductive Anatomy—Structure
Integrated Process: Nursing Process—Assessment
Client Need: Physiological Integrity
Cognitive Level: Knowledge
Concept: Female Reproduction
Reference: *Thompson, G. S. (2015). Understanding anatomy & physiology: A visual, auditory, interactive approach. 2nd ed. Philadelphia, PA: F.A. Davis Company.*

6. ANSWER: 4
Rationale
1. The proliferative phase is part of the endometrial/menstrual cycle, occurring during the follicular phase of the ovarian cycle; estrogen is the primary hormone driving these actions.
2. The menstrual phase is marked by significant decreases in both progesterone and estrogen; the corpus luteum in the ovary shrinks and becomes inactive.
3. The ovulatory phase of the ovarian cycle follows a sudden surge in the secretion of LH, causing the follicle to rupture and release the mature ovum into the fimbriae of the fallopian tube.
4. The luteal phase of the ovarian cycle occurs following ovulation, when the corpus luteum begins to produce and secrete high levels of progesterone and lesser amounts of estrogen.
TEST-TAKING TIP: Although the phases of the menstrual cycle and ovarian cycle occur in tandem and are physiologically coordinated, the nurse needs to understand that they

are separate cycles, influenced by unique hormonal processes. During these cycles, progesterone is produced during a specific phase and either continues to be produced if implantation occurs or plummets in the absence of implantation, causing ischemia in the endometrial lining that leads to shedding the tissue and blood during menstruation.
Content Area: Female Reproductive Physiology—Ovarian Cycle
Integrated Process: Nursing Process—Assessment
Client Need: Physiological Integrity
Cognitive Level: Knowledge
Concept: Female Reproduction
Reference: *Thompson, G. S. (2015). Understanding anatomy & physiology: A visual, auditory, interactive approach. 2nd ed. Philadelphia, PA: F.A. Davis Company.*

7. ANSWER: 2, 3, 5
Rationale
1. There are two layers of cells: One attaches the endometrium to the myometrium and assists in the monthly increase in the thickness or regeneration of the second layer of cells, and the second layer is the functional layer.
2. In the proliferative phase of the menstrual cycle, estrogen produced by the graafian follicle in the ovary stimulates the initial thickening of the endometrium.
3. Following ovulation, during the secretory phase of the menstrual cycle, progesterone produced by the corpus luteum induces further thickening of the endometrium.
4. On the contrary, following implantation, the endometrium continues to thicken to provide protection for the implanted embryo.
5. This is the response of the functional layer of the endometrium to the reduction in progesterone production by the shrinking corpus luteum.
TEST-TAKING TIP: Look for limiters in question responses; they are often associated with incorrect responses. However, if there is an understanding of the structure and function of the endometrium, the correct responses should be related.
Content Area: Female Reproductive Structure and Function—Endometrium
Integrated Process: Nursing Process—Assessment
Client Need: Physiological Integrity
Cognitive Level: Comprehension
Concept: Female Reproduction
Reference: *Thompson, G. S. (2015). Understanding anatomy & physiology: A visual, auditory, interactive approach. 2nd ed. Philadelphia, PA: F.A. Davis Company.*

8. ANSWER: 3
Rationale
1. Prostaglandin E inhibits smooth muscle contraction, while PGF increases muscle contractility. Oxytocin causes myometrial contraction, but these are only two of the hormones that act on the uterine myometrium.
2. Progesterone, produced by the placenta, inhibits myometrial contraction during pregnancy; estrogen, whose production is reduced during pregnancy when the ovulatory cycle is halted, has no effect on the myometrium.

3. Each of these hormones acts on the myometrium, though in different ways. Oxytocin, produced in increasing amounts toward the end of pregnancy, initiates uterine myometrial contractions and drives the uterine forces of labor. It also ensures the contraction of the empty uterus following delivery to prevent bleeding from the placental insertion site. Relaxin also inhibits myometrium contraction, promoting implantation of the blastocyst in the endometrium; it also promotes relaxation of the uterine ligaments. Prostaglandin E relaxes smooth muscle, including the myometrium.
4. Progesterone is a correct response, but testosterone, the primary male hormone, has no part in myometrial function.

TEST-TAKING TIP: When test item responses include more than one correct answer, look for known incorrect responses within the choices. Realize that the answers may not all have similar relationships to the object of the question—in this case the question refers only to a general "response," not the type of response.

Content Area: Female Hormonal Function—Myometrium
Integrated Process: Nursing Process—Assessment
Client Need: Physiological Integrity
Cognitive Level: Knowledge
Concept: Female Reproduction
Reference: *Scanlon, V. C., & Saunders, T. (2011). Essentials of anatomy and physiology. 6th ed. Philadelphia, PA: F.A. Davis Company.*

9. **ANSWER: 1**
Rationale
1. Normally, ovulation occurs in conjunction with a woman's menstrual cycle. Since it is only possible to become pregnant if ovulation takes place, the fact that she seems to be ovulating only two or three times per year will make timing conception within the 24 hours on either side of ovulation difficult.
2. There may be any number of explanations for the limited menstrual cycles for this patient. However, barring a number of tests and other assessments, it cannot be stated that gonadotropin-releasing hormone deficiency is the problem.
3. Again, there could be a physiological problem, but regular menses may occur in spite of a blocked fallopian tube. A key symptom is limited menstrual cycles.
4. This, too, could be an issue, but further assessment is needed to see if this is an underlying cause of the problem.

TEST-TAKING TIP: While there may be one or more underlying issues in any failure of normal physiological processes, the initial observation may also be the most relevant explanation. Related underlying causes require further investigation. The nurse understands the basic relationship between regular ovulatory and menstrual cycles and the ability to become pregnant.

Content Area: Female Reproductive System/Anatomy and Physiology of Female and Male Reproduction
Integrated Process: Nursing Process—Assessment
Client Need: Safe and Effective Care/Management of Care
Cognitive Level: Application
Concept: Female Reproduction
Reference: *Thompson, G. S. (2015). Understanding anatomy & physiology: A visual, auditory, interactive approach. 2nd ed. Philadelphia, PA: F.A. Davis Company.*

10. **ANSWER: 2**
Rationale
1. The vas deferens are the tubes that connect the epididymis to the ejaculatory duct in the prostate gland. Cutting them does not affect the male sexual response.
2. Cutting the vas deferens will prevent mature sperm from traveling from the epididymis in the scrotum to the ejaculatory duct and the urethra during ejaculation. No sperm means no pregnancy.
3. The production of sperm is not regulated or affected by the cutting of the vas deferens. Sperm production will continue, but the sperm will not be able to travel past the "disconnect."
4. The cutting of the vas deferens will not affect the prostate or its production of the alkaline fluid that normally comprises male ejaculate; the sperm will not reach the ejaculatory duct in the prostate.

TEST-TAKING TIP: The nurse needs to understand the anatomical structure and function of a system in order to understand what will happen if that structure or function changes. Think about the path of the sperm from the scrotum to the end of the male urethra, or the path of any substance through the anatomy. Interruption of that pathway will block the passage of the substance.

Content Area: Male Reproductive Structure and Function—Sperm Ejaculation
Integrated Process: Nursing Process—Assessment
Client Need: Physiological Integrity
Cognitive Level: Comprehension
Concept: Male Reproduction
Reference: *Thompson, G. S. (2015). Understanding anatomy & physiology: A visual, auditory, interactive approach. 2nd ed. Philadelphia, PA: F.A. Davis Company.*

11. **ANSWER: 3**
Rationale
1. Although intended to reassure the patient, this is not the best or most accurate response.
2. This statement is not factual. There is no indication that later menarche causes or is related to difficulty conceiving in the future.
3. This is the most correct statement, relaying the facts without creating alarm. Though menarche may occur in the later teens, it may warrant further assessment in order to detect an abnormality versus normal development for that young woman. Menarche is expected to begin within 4 years of the start of breast development.
4. This statement is not entirely factual. The fact that this young woman began breast development over 4 years ago places menarche for her outside the expected parameters. Though there may be no underlying issues, it cannot be stated that there is no cause for concern.

TEST-TAKING TIP: When responding to patients, the nurse should avoid false reassurances, unsubstantiated suppositions, or personal opinions. Responses that state facts and share a correct understanding of the plan of care are the most appropriate.

Content Area: Female Reproductive Development—Menarche
Integrated Process: Nursing Process—Implementation
Client Need: Health Promotion and Maintenance

Cognitive Level: Application
Concept: Female Reproduction
Reference: Thompson, G. S. (2015). Understanding anatomy & physiology: A visual, auditory, interactive approach. 2nd ed. Philadelphia, PA: F.A. Davis Company.

12. ANSWER: 1, 4, 3, 2

Rationale

The menstrual cycle begins on days 1 through 5 with the shedding of the functional layer of the endometrium that has not received a fertilized blastocyst. Following this, the endometrium begins to build up during the proliferative phase over days 6 through 14. The endometrium continues to thicken during the secretory phase, days 15 through 25. If implantation of a blastocyst does not occur, the endometrium goes into a premenstrual phase, where the functional layer breaks down quickly over days 26 through 28. The cycle begins again.

TEST-TAKING TIP: When faced with ordinal questions, begin by determining which step comes first. Do not assume that terms will help to identify the first step; in this case, the prefix *pre-* does not indicate that it is the first step in the process. Understanding a process may help to recall an ordinal process rather than memorizing the steps or phases.

Content Area: Female Reproductive Development— Menstrual Cycle
Integrated Process: Nursing Process—Assessment
Client Need: Physiological Integrity
Cognitive Level: Knowledge
Concept: Female Reproduction
Reference: Thompson, G. S. (2015). Understanding anatomy & physiology: A visual, auditory, interactive approach. 2nd ed. Philadelphia, PA: F.A. Davis Company.

13. ANSWER: 3

Rationale

1. The development of the uterine endometrium is stimulated by estrogen produced by ovarian follicular cells, not FSH.
2. The mature ovum is released from the graafian follicle following a spike in LH.
3. FSH is responsible for stimulating the maturation of the ovarian follicle.
4. The development of the ovaries occurs during fetal development, influenced by estrogen.

TEST-TAKING TIP: Hormones are often named based on the tissues or organs on which they act. Look for terms in questions that may help to identify the correct response. In this case, *follicle* is a key term.

Content Area: Female Hormonal Function—Ovarian Cycle
Integrated Process: Nursing Process—Assessment
Client Need: Physiological Integrity
Cognitive Level: Knowledge
Concept: Female Reproduction
Reference: Scanlon, V. C., & Saunders, T. (2011). Essentials of anatomy and physiology. 6th ed. Philadelphia, PA: F.A. Davis Company.

14. ANSWER: 1, 2, 3

Rationale

1. Increases in testosterone stimulate the development of the male reproductive organs.

2. Testosterone is also responsible for development of male secondary sex characteristics.
3. As an anabolic steroid, testosterone increases protein synthesis, specifically building skeletal muscle.
4. & 5. Testosterone is not a growth hormone and does not affect male height or weight.

TEST-TAKING TIP: Testosterone stimulates the growth and strength of the long bones of the male, promotes muscle development and mass, thickens vocal cords, and is responsible for the distribution and appearance of body hair.

Content Area: Male Hormones—Testosterone
Integrated Process: Nursing Process—Assessment
Client Need: Physiological Integrity
Cognitive Level: Knowledge
Concept: Male Reproduction
Reference: Scanlon, V. C., & Saunders, T. (2011). Essentials of anatomy and physiology. 6th ed. Philadelphia, PA: F.A. Davis Company.

15. ANSWER: 4

Rationale

1. The proliferative and secretory phases are part of the menstrual cycle, not the ovarian cycle.
2. Estrogen and progesterone are hormones that stimulate the female reproductive cycles but are not phases in the ovarian cycle.
3. The endometrium experiences its own phases, though the luteal phase is part of the ovarian cycle.
4. "Follicular" and "luteal" are both phases of the ovarian cycle. The follicular phase involves the maturation of a follicle within the ovary. The luteal phase follows ovulation at the end of the follicular phase.

TEST-TAKING TIP: When test item responses include more than one correct answer, look for known incorrect responses within the choices. The pairs in this question need to be associated with ovarian processes and differentiate between the phases and the hormones that stimulate the changes in question.

Content Area: Physiology of the Female Reproductive System—Ovarian Cycle
Integrated Process: Nursing Process—Assessment
Client Need: Physiological Integrity
Cognitive Level: Knowledge
Concept: Female Reproduction
Reference: Durham, R. F., & Chapman, L. (2014). Maternal-newborn nursing: The critical components of nursing care. 2nd ed. Philadelphia, PA: F.A. Davis Company.

16. ANSWER: 1, 3

Rationale

1. In addition to inducing uterine myometrial contraction, oxytocin promotes the release of milk from the milk-producing glands in the breast.
2. Progesterone stimulates the endometrium and inhibits myometrial contraction during pregnancy. It promotes the growth of secretory cells within the breast, but the question asks about milk production and release.
3. Prolactin is released in the female body following several stimulating activities; however, after delivery, it is secreted by the pituitary gland and acts on the glands in the breast that produce human milk.
4. Luteinizing hormone stimulates the graafian follicle to release the mature ovum.

5. Estrogen promotes growth of the duct system in the breast; it is thought to cause the "swelling" of the breasts in early pregnancy but has no effect on milk production.

TEST-TAKING TIP: Multiple answer or "select all that apply" questions may require the test taker to first eliminate the responses they know to be incorrect. It is rarely helpful to guess or change your responses. In this case, "prolactin" contains a clue that it is related to "lactation," and oxytocin is a primary hormone released during and following delivery. Progesterone and estrogen are present during pregnancy.

Content Area: Female Hormonal Function—Breast (Lactation)
Integrated Process: Nursing Process—Assessment
Client Need: Physiological Integrity
Cognitive Level: Knowledge
Concept: Female Reproduction
Reference: Scanlon, V. C., & Saunders, T. (2011). Essentials of anatomy and physiology. 6th ed. Philadelphia, PA: F.A. Davis Company.

17. **ANSWER: 2**
Rationale
1. FSH and LH surge and drop immediately prior to ovulation. The basal body temperature rises after ovulation. So, on the 15th day, ovulation has presumably occurred.
2. Progesterone begins to rise immediately following ovulation, stimulating the thickening of the endometrium. It is thought to be the reason why basal body temperature rises and remains elevated up to the premenstrual phase of the menstrual cycle.
3. Estrogen rises and falls through the menstrual cycle. It is not related to basal body temperature.
4. Prostaglandins are not involved in these reproductive cycles.

TEST-TAKING TIP: The question relates to hormone levels during the ovulatory and menstrual cycles. Aside from recalling the specific information about these hormones, studying diagrams may be helpful when learning the relationships of physiological stimulators or causes of physical changes or processes. Pictures in memory may help the test taker to recall important information.

Content Area: Female Hormonal Function—Ovarian Cycle
Integrated Process: Nursing Process—Assessment
Client Need: Physiological Integrity
Cognitive Level: Application
Concept: Female Reproduction
Reference: London, M. L., Ladewig, P. A., Davidson, M. R., Ball, J. W., Bindler, R. C., & Cowen, K. J. (2014). Maternal & child nursing care. 4th ed. Upper Saddle River, NJ: Pearson.

18. **ANSWER: X over the inferior aspect of the diagram of the uterus**
Rationale
The cervix is located past the lower uterine segment at the inferior end of the uterus.

TEST-TAKING TIP: Locating anatomical landmarks is one of the questioning formats in nursing examinations. Understanding and recalling anatomical structures is necessary for nursing assessment. Look carefully at any test diagram and recall the location of key structures. When studying, it may help to label the structures on a blank diagram.

Content Area: Female Reproduction—Uterine Anatomy
Integrated Process: Nursing Process—Assessment
Client Need: Physiological Integrity
Cognitive Level: Knowledge
Concept: Female Reproduction
Reference: Thompson, G. S. (2015). Understanding anatomy & physiology: A visual, auditory, interactive approach. 2nd ed. Philadelphia, PA: F.A. Davis Company.

19. **ANSWER: 1**
Rationale
1. Statement of fact. "Mittelschmerz," or middle pain, is believed to be a localized response to the release of the mature ovum. It is characterized by brief lower abdominal discomfort halfway through the menstrual cycle. It occurs in some women but is not universal.
2. This is not a factual statement.
3. Though there is probably nothing concerning in this woman's history, this is not "expected."
4. This is not in evidence or factually related to the patient's symptoms. Only further assessment could support this statement.

TEST-TAKING TIP: When addressing patients, use responses that state facts and share a correct understanding of known physiological symptoms. Assuming concerns not in evidence is to be avoided. Sometimes there may appear to be two responses that are not incorrect, but the response that is most true or accurate should be chosen as the most correct answer.

Content Area: Female Reproduction—Ovarian Cycle
Integrated Process: Nursing Process—Implementation
Client Need: Health Promotion and Maintenance
Cognitive Level: Application
Concept: Female Reproduction
Reference: London, M. L., Ladewig, P. A., Davidson, M. R., Ball, J. W., Bindler, R. C., & Cowen, K. J. (2014). Maternal & child nursing care. 4th ed. Upper Saddle River, NJ: Pearson.

20. **ANSWER: 2**
Rationale
1. Although this is a true statement, it refers to the function of the urethra, not the structure.
2. This answer does pertain to the structure of the urethra and is correct. The length of the male urethra is related to its dual function and is one reason that males experience fewer urinary infections than females. The female urethra is much shorter and is completely located internally, with the external opening covered within the vulva, just in front to the vaginal opening. The anatomical location and length of the female urethra seems to place females at higher risk for urinary tract infections.
3. This statement is not correct. Though the female urethra is shorter, it is protected by virtue of its internal location. However, it is prone to injury during childbirth or sexual violence.
4. The male and female urethras are connected to the bladder. In the male, the prostate gland controls the flow of urine exiting the bladder and contributes to the composition and release of semen during coitus.

TEST-TAKING TIP: Read questions such as this to determine precisely what the question is asking. It is important to differentiate between structure and function. In addition, two of the possible responses refer only to one of the options involved—the female. The other options include both characteristics for comparison, so the difference comes down to structure versus function.

Content Area: Male and Female Anatomy—Urethra
Integrated Process: Nursing Process—Assessment
Client Need: Physiological Integrity
Cognitive Level: Knowledge
Concept: Female/Male Reproduction
Reference: *Scanlon, V. C., & Saunders, T. (2011).* Essentials of anatomy and physiology. *6th ed. Philadelphia, PA: F.A. Davis Company.*

Chapter 2

Infertility

KEY TERMS

Asherman's syndrome—Secondary amenorrhea related to endometrial scarring. Causes include endometritis and aggressive curettage for purposes of removing the products of conception, such as in abortion or removal of retained placental fragments.

Azoospermia—Absence of spermatozoa in the semen

Cryopreservation—The preservation at very low temperatures of biological materials such as blood or plasma, embryos or sperm, or other tissues. After thawing, the preserved material can be used for its original biological purpose.

Cryptorchidism—Failure of the testicles to descend into the scrotum

Ectopic pregnancy—Implantation of the fertilized ovum outside the uterine cavity, most frequently in the fallopian tube

Endometriosis—Presence of functioning ectopic endometrial glands and stroma outside the uterine cavity

Gonadotropin—A gonad-stimulating hormone, including follicle-stimulating hormone (FSH), luteinizing hormone (LH), and human chorionic gonadotropin (hCG)

Hyperprolactinemia—An excess secretion of prolactin thought to be due to hypothalamic–pituitary dysfunction. This is usually associated with amenorrhea with or without galactorrhea

Hypogonadotropic hypogonadism—Occurs when there is a disturbance in the hypothalamic–pituitary axis resulting in low levels of gonadotropins with inadequate production of sex hormones

Hysterosalpingography—Radiography of the uterus and oviducts after injection of a contrast medium

Infertility—Inability to achieve pregnancy during a year or more of unprotected intercourse. The condition may be present in either or both partners and may be reversible.

Myoma—A tumor that contains muscle tissue

Oligospermia—A temporary or permanent deficiency of spermatozoa in seminal fluid

Ovarian hyperstimulation syndrome—Medical complication that may result from ovulation induction characterized by enlargement of the ovaries, extravascular fluid accumulation, and intravascular volume depletion. Symptoms include intermittent abdominal pain, abdominal bloating, nausea, vomiting, diarrhea, and pelvic tenderness. Signs of increasing severity include severe abdominal pain, persistent nausea and vomiting, decreased urination, shortness of breath, and dizziness.

Ovarian reserve—The capacity of the ovary to provide oocytes capable of fertilization, resulting in a healthy and successful pregnancy

Ovulation—The periodic ripening and rupture of the mature graafian follicle and the discharge of the ovum from the cortex of the ovary

Ovulation induction—Stimulating ovulation by the use of drugs

Pelvic inflammatory disease (PID)—Infection of the uterus, fallopian tubes, and adjacent pelvic structures that is not associated with surgery or pregnancy. Chlamydia trachomatis and Neisseria gonorrhea are the most frequent causes of PID.

Varicoceles—Enlargement of the veins of the spermatic cord, commonly occurring above the left testicle

I. Infertility

Infertility is defined as the inability to achieve pregnancy during a year or more of unprotected intercourse. The cause for the infertility can be related to factors in the female partner, the male partner, or both. A progressive decline in fertility occurs in women after the age of 30 to 32. Lifestyle also affects fertility in both the female and male partner. Promotion of normal reproduction includes maintaining a normal body mass index (BMI), avoiding sexually transmitted infections, adequately treating sexually transmitted infections, and avoiding the use of tobacco and other substances. This section focuses on the main causes of female and male factor infertility.

A. Female factor infertility
 1. Ovulatory factors
  a) **Ovarian reserve** refers to the capacity of the ovary to provide oocytes capable of fertilization, resulting in a healthy and successful pregnancy (Box 2.1). Ovarian reserve steadily declines with increasing age.

DID YOU KNOW?
A woman's fertility begins to decline in her early 30s, and the decline accelerates during her late 30s and early 40s.

  b) Polycystic ovary syndrome (PCOS) is the most common endocrine disorder among women of reproductive age and the leading cause of female factor infertility. Young women affected by PCOS may present with menstrual dysfunction, infertility, hirsutism (male pattern hair growth), alopecia, and acne. Obesity is a common feature and appears to play a central role in the etiology of PCOS by leading to the development of insulin resistance. Disturbance of the hypothalamic-pituitary-gonadal hormonal axes leads to anovulation. Luteinizing hormone (LH) levels are high when the menstrual cycle starts and remain higher than follicle-stimulating hormone (FSH) levels. This imbalance of LH and FSH may cause the ovaries to fill with multiple tiny cysts. Because the LH levels are already quite high, there is no LH surge. Without the surge in LH, **ovulation** does not occur and periods are often irregular. High levels of LH signal the ovary to produce more androgens or male hormones.

  c) **Hyperprolactinemia** or an excess secretion of prolactin leads to low levels of **gonadotropin** secretion. The result is anovulation and amenorrhea.

  d) **Hypogonadotropic hypogonadism** describes low levels of gonadotropins with inadequate production of sex hormones and is the result of a disturbance in the hypothalamic–pituitary axis. The cause may be acquired or congenital. Potential causes are stress, extreme weight loss, excessive exercise, and hyperprolactinemia.

 2. Tubal/pelvic factors
  a) **Endometriosis** is a condition characterized by the presence of functioning ectopic endometrial glands and stroma outside the uterine cavity. The response of the ectopic endometrial cells to hormonal stimuli leads to cyclic bleeding and local inflammation. This response results in fibrosis, adhesions, and fallopian tube occlusion.

  b) Tubal disease involves anatomic abnormalities that prevent the union of sperm and ovum. **Pelvic inflammatory disease (PID)** is considered the leading cause of tubal factor infertility. Other potential causes are developmental anomalies, **ectopic pregnancy**, surgical trauma, and endometriosis.

 3. Uterine factors
  a) Congenital uterine anomalies are associated with pregnancy loss and complications during pregnancy. The anomalies may result in obstructions that present in adolescence with amenorrhea and cyclic pain.

  b) Endometrial polyps are hyperplastic growths on the lining of the uterus and are thought to interfere with implantation. Risk factors for the development of polyps include obesity and PCOS.

  c) **Asherman's syndrome** is most commonly the result of surgical trauma to the uterus followed by the formation of uterine adhesions. Most women with Asherman's syndrome

---

Box 2.1 **Female Factor Infertility**

Ovulatory Factors

Ovarian reserve
Polycystic ovary syndrome (PCOS)
Hyperprolactinemia
Hypogonadotropic hypogonadism

Tubal/Pelvic Factors

Endometriosis
Tubal disease
  Pelvic inflammatory disease
  Ectopic pregnancy

Uterine Factors

Congenital uterine anomalies
Endometrial polyps
Asherman's syndrome
Myomas (fibroids)

present with decreased or absent menstrual flow, dysmenorrhea, recurrent pregnancy loss, or infertility.

d) **Myomas** (or fibroids) are benign uterine tumors that can contribute to infertility by obstructing or distorting the uterine cavity. The location of myomas determines the effect on fertility and pregnancy outcomes. Intramural (within the wall) and submucosal (in the connective tissue below the mucosa) myomas are linked to lower implantation and live birth rates. Subserosal (beneath the serosa) myomas have minimal impact on conception rates and pregnancy outcomes.

4. Unexplained

B. Male factor infertility
  1. Genetic
     a) Klinefelter syndrome (47 XXY) is the most common sex chromosome disorder among males. Low testosterone levels result in small testes and **azoospermia** (Box 2.2).
     b) Noonan syndrome is an autosomal-dominant genetic disorder resulting in undescended testicles and diminished spermatogenesis.
  2. Congenital
     a) **Cryptorchidism** is the failure of the testes to descend into the scrotum. It is the most common birth defect of male genitalia and results in **oligospermia** if left untreated.

Box 2.2 Male Factor Infertility

Genetic Factors

Klinefelter syndrome
Noonan syndrome

Congenital Factors

Cryptorchidism
Varicocele

Acquired Factors

Testicular torsion
Infections
  STIs
  Mumps
Trauma
Medications and drugs of abuse
Sperm transport
Ejaculatory disorders
  Spinal cord injuries
  Neurological diseases
  Medications
Erectile dysfunction
  Cardiovascular disease
  Diabetes
  Depression, anxiety, stress
  Medications

---

b) **Varicocele** is an abnormal dilation of the veins within the spermatic cord and is the most common correctable cause of male infertility. The varicocele is usually on the left side and has a progressive adverse effect on spermatogenesis.

3. Acquired
   a) Testicular torsion is rotation of the testis, resulting in twisting of the blood vessels in the spermatic cord. Correction within 6 hours of the onset of symptoms will preserve testicular function and prevent impaired sperm production.
   b) Infections such as orchitis, epididymitis, and prostatitis can lead to tissue damage and ductal obstruction. Bacterial epididymitis is often caused by chlamydia and gonorrhea in males younger than age 35. A possible complication of the mumps in males is orchitis. Infections can result in ductal obstruction.
   c) Trauma resulting in testicular injury may decrease sperm production and affect sperm transport.
   d) Medications and drug abuse can impact male fertility.
      (1) Chemotherapy
      (2) Ionizing radiation
      (3) Ketoconazole
      (4) Exogenous testosterone supplementation
      (5) Marijuana, opiates, heroin
      (6) Alcohol and tobacco
4. Sperm transport
   a) Ejaculatory disorders may be caused by surgery, spinal cord injuries, neurological diseases, or medications. Retrograde ejaculation—discharge of seminal fluid into the bladder—can occur as a consequence of radical prostatectomy. Antihypertensives, antidepressants, antihistamines, sedatives, and narcotics can all decrease ejaculatory ability. The effect of spinal cord injuries is determined by the location of the injury.
   b) Erectile dysfunction is the inability to achieve or maintain an erection suitable for sexual intercourse and can be caused by the following:
      (1) Cardiovascular disease
      (2) Diabetes
      (3) Neurological disease
      (4) Hypogonadism
      (5) Depression, anxiety, stress
      (6) Medications

DID YOU KNOW?

Pregnancy rates decrease when the male partner is older than age 40 to 45. Increasing paternal age is associated with structural chromosome abnormalities in the sperm, higher rates of autosomal-dominant diseases in offspring, and recurrent pregnancy loss.

II. Assessment

Assessment of the infertile couple includes a complete medical history, an interview, and a thorough physical examination. With the multiplicity of factors that may affect a couple's ability to conceive, assessment should be conducted simultaneously for both partners. Initial assessment of male partners will include a sperm analysis. A thorough assessment will require commitment to the process by both partners and considerable financial resources. This section focuses on diagnostic testing available for the assessment of the infertile couple.

A. Female factors
1. Evaluation of ovulatory factors
   a) Basal body temperature (BBT) is a cost-effective method for determining if ovulation has occurred and the approximate time it occurred. The woman should be instructed to take an oral temperature every morning before getting out of bed and prior to eating or drinking. This temperature should be recorded on a BBT chart. Temperature rises approximately 0.5°F in the luteal phase; this temperature rise occurs 1 to 5 days after the midcycle LH surge and up to 4 days after ovulation.
   b) Estrogenic cervical and vaginal discharge is clear, stretchy, and slippery and is the result of an increase in estrogen levels 5 to 6 days prior to ovulation. The optimal time for intercourse to achieve conception is 1 to 2 days prior to ovulation. Recognition of estrogenic cervical and vaginal mucus provides women with a cost-efficient method for tracking ovulation. Spinnbarkeit is the elasticity of cervical mucus discharge at ovulation. Spinnbarkeit is measured by placing cervical mucus on a slide and pulling upward on the mucus with a forceps. Elasticity will measure at least 12 to 24 cm during the fertile period leading up to ovulation.
   c) The progesterone level obtained during the midluteal phase is the most widely used laboratory assessment for evidence that ovulation has occurred. The serum level of progesterone drawn 1 week prior to anticipated start of menstruation (day 21 of a 28-day cycle) should be greater than 3 ng/mL if ovulation has occurred.
   d) FSH level is useful in the evaluation of ovarian reserve. The FSH level is obtained on day 3 of the menstrual cycle, and a level of 10 mIU/mL or lower indicates normal ovarian reserve.
   e) The estrogen level obtained on the third day of the menstrual cycle is also useful in evaluating ovarian reserve. An estradiol level of 80 pg/mL or higher is considered normal.
   f) The LH level typically surges 18 to 36 hours prior to ovulation. A woman's interval of greatest fertility is the day of the surge and the following 2 days. Ovulation predictor kits test urine for the LH surge and are available over the counter.
   g) Serum prolactin levels are useful in detecting hyperprolactinemia as a cause of ovulatory dysfunction.
   h) Androgen levels, including DHEA-S and testosterone, can be useful in the evaluation of women with signs of hyperandrogenism, including hirsutism, acne, and male pattern hair loss.
   i) Vaginal ultrasound is useful in the assessment of ovarian reserve and in the identification of uterine pathology, including myomas, endometrial polyps, and congenital uterine anomalies.
2. Evaluation of tubal/pelvic factors
   a) **Hysterosalpingography** is an x-ray test that is useful in evaluating the uterine cavity and the fallopian tubes. Radioactive dye is placed in the uterus to aid visualization. The test is performed after menses but prior to ovulation. Cramping may occur during this procedure.
   b) Laparoscopy is performed as an outpatient surgical procedure to evaluate the fallopian tubes and ovaries. The procedure allows the surgeon to treat endometriosis, pelvic adhesions or scarring, and some tubal diseases. The laparoscope is inserted through the navel, allowing visualization of the pelvis.
3. Evaluation of uterine factors
   a) Hysteroscopy utilizes a special endoscope for inspection of the uterine cavity and surgical correction of uterine pathology. The uterus is accessed through the vagina. The procedure may be performed in either the office or operating room setting.

B. Male factors
1. Semen
   a) Semen analysis is the basic test in the evaluation of male fertility. Collection should occur after 2 to 3 days of abstinence and be collected by masturbation directly into a clean container. Exposure of the semen sample to extremes of temperature should be avoided and delivery to the laboratory should occur within 1 hour (Table 2.1).
2. Endocrine
   a) Serum FSH and total testosterone levels are included in the basic endocrine evaluation of the infertile male. Endocrine evaluation is considered following an abnormal semen analysis, with sexual dysfunction, or to evaluate clinical symptoms.

Table 2.1	**Normal Reference Values for Semen Analysis**
Parameter	**Normal Values**
Volume	1.5–5 mL
pH	>7.2
Sperm concentration	>20 million/mL
Total sperm number	>40 million/ejaculate
Percent motility	>50%
Normal morphology	>50% normal

3. Ultrasound
   a) Transrectal ultrasound is useful in the diagnosis of ejaculatory duct obstruction.
   b) Transscrotal ultrasound is useful in the evaluation of scrotal masses.

III. Methods of Management

The determination of treatment choices will follow a thorough physical, psychosocial, and cultural assessment of both partners. Treatment of medical conditions that may impact fertility is a priority. Patients must be fully informed of available treatments and the risks and benefits of each. A couple's religious and cultural beliefs may dictate acceptable infertility treatment choices. This section focuses on the available management choices for the couple experiencing infertility.

A. Nonmedical treatments
   1. Lifestyle changes
      a) Extremes of body weight have been found to impact both female and male fertility. Being overweight or obese is associated with reduced fertility in the male and with ovulatory dysfunction in the female. Anorexic women and female athletes have an increased incidence of menstrual cycle disturbances and amenorrhea.

DID YOU KNOW?

A loss of 5% to 10% of body weight in obese women with PCOS is often sufficient to restore ovulation.

      b) Dietary supplementation for the female should include 0.4 mg/day of folic acid.
      c) Excessive consumption of alcohol negatively impacts both male and female fertility. Alcohol consumption during pregnancy has the potential to harm a developing fetus. Heavy alcohol use, defined as two drinks or more a day, should be discouraged. The couple should be encouraged to abstain from alcohol and recreational drug use while attempting to conceive.
      d) Smoking is considered a reproductive system toxin in both the female and male. Fertility is lowered in male and female smokers. A smoking cessation strategy is crucial for any couple attempting to conceive.
      e) Stress management techniques should be discussed with couples experiencing infertility. The emotional impact of infertility evaluation and treatment may evoke feelings of depression, loss, and isolation. Treatment choices may conflict with religious and cultural beliefs and create a financial burden for the couple.
      f) Many of the commonly used lubricants have been shown to have spermicidal properties. If lubricant is desired during intercourse, couples should be advised to choose a water-soluble one.
   2. Environmental
      a) Heat exposure with increases in scrotal temperature can adversely affect spermatogenesis. Males should be advised to avoid hot baths, saunas, tight underwear, and resting a laptop computer directly on the lap for extended periods of time.
      b) Exposure to occupational or environmental toxins, including herbicides and fungicides, has been shown to impact both female and male fertility. A thorough assessment should be completed to identify a couple's potential risk for exposure.

B. Pharmacological treatments
   1. Ovulation induction agents
      a) Clomiphene citrate is an estrogen agonist/antagonist. The method of administration is oral. The body perceives estrogen levels to be low and signals the hypothalamus and pituitary gland to increase FSH and LH secretion. This stimulates the ovaries, which results in follicular development. Women taking clomiphene

---

MAKING THE CONNECTION

Low BMI and Infertility

Decreased fertility is linked to women with low BMIs, eating disorders, or extreme exercise regimens. A BMI less than 17 is associated with infertility. It may prove more challenging to convince an underweight woman than an obese woman that her lifestyle is contributing to her infertility. Slender women often view diet and exercise as a healthy lifestyle. Underweight women should be encouraged to increase their weight to 100% of predicted ideal body weight for their height. The recommended rate of weight gain is one-half pound per week.

citrate should be informed that the drug may cause abdominal bloating, nausea, visual disturbances, insomnia, and **ovarian hyperstimulation syndrome.** There is an increased risk of multiple births associated with the use of clomiphene citrate. May also be used to stimulate spermatogenesis in males with hypogonadism.

b) Letrozole is an aromatase inhibitor and leads to a decrease in estrogen production. Method of administration is oral. The resultant increase in FSH secretion stimulates the ovaries and follicular development. Side effects of letrozole include hot flashes, headache, and depression.

c) Menotropins, also referred to as *human menopausal gonadotropins,* are derived from the urine of menopausal women. The drugs are a combination of FSH and LH and are used to promote ovarian follicle development. Method of administration is intramuscular. The risks associated with menotropins are multiple births and thromboembolism. The adverse effects include dizziness, nausea, vomiting, and ovarian hyperstimulation syndrome. May also be used to stimulate spermatogenesis in males with hypogonadism.

d) Follitropins are synthetically manufactured FSHs, which have a stimulatory effect on ovarian follicles. Method of administration is subcutaneous or intramuscular. Risks include an increased incidence of multiple births and of premature delivery. Adverse effects include breast tenderness, mood swings, depression, and ovarian hyperstimulation syndrome. May also be used to stimulate spermatogenesis in males with hypogonadism.

e) Human chorionic gonadotropin (hCG) is given the first day following the last dose of menotropin to induce ovulation. Method of administration is intramuscular. Direct action on the ovarian follicle stimulates meiosis and rupture of the follicle. Adverse effects include headaches, irritability, edema, depression, and fatigue.

🛑 **ALERT Ovulation induction** carries the risk of ovarian hyperstimulation syndrome, which can be life-threatening. In moderate cases, the women experience abdominal distention and gastrointestinal upset, which can be managed on an outpatient basis. Patients are instructed to weigh daily, maintain fluid intake of at least 1 liter a day of mostly electrolyte-balanced fluid, and monitor output. Excessive weight gain, ascites, electrolyte disturbances, hemoconcentration, coagulation abnormalities, respiratory failure, and renal dysfunction are characteristic of more severe cases. Management will require hospitalization. Patients should be made aware of the symptoms. Mild to moderate ovarian hyperstimulation syndrome is characterized by intermittent abdominal pain, abdominal bloating, nausea, vomiting, diarrhea, and pelvic tenderness. Signs of increasing severity include severe abdominal pain, persistent nausea and vomiting, decreased urination, dark urine, shortness of breath, and dizziness.

2. Suppression of premature ovulation
   a) GnRH antagonists suppress the secretion of LH during ovulation induction cycles, preventing ovulation prior to harvesting eggs or oocytes for in-vitro fertilization. Method of administration is subcutaneous. Adverse effects include temporary symptoms of menopause, including hot flashes, mood swings, and vaginal dryness.

3. Luteal phase support
   a) Progesterone prepares and maintains the endometrium for implantation to occur. Pharmacological preparations of progesterone administered vaginally are useful for luteal phase support through the first 10 to 12 weeks of pregnancy. Adverse effects include headaches and breast tenderness.

4. Insulin sensitizing agent
   a) Metformin decreases glucose production in the liver and increases glucose utilization in peripheral tissues. Method of administration is oral. Metformin has been found to help restore cyclic ovulation in women with PCOS and insulin resistance. Normal liver and renal function should be confirmed prior to administration of metformin. Adverse effects include diarrhea, nausea, metallic taste, and anorexia.

5. Reduction of prolactin levels in hyperprolactinemia
   a) Cabergoline is a dopamine agonist and is effective in reducing prolactin levels. Patients are instructed to take one or two tablets orally twice a week. Treatment with a dopamine agonist should be stopped during pregnancy. Possible adverse effects include nasal congestion, fatigue, drowsiness, headaches, nausea, vomiting, syncope, vertigo, and hypotension. Long-term use of cabergoline increases the risk of hypertrophic valvular heart disease.
   b) Bromocriptine is also a dopamine agonist and is an alternative to cabergoline. Method of administration is oral. Dosing is once a day at bedtime with food. Possible adverse effects are nasal congestion, fatigue, drowsiness,

headaches, nausea, vomiting, syncope, vertigo, and hypotension. Treatment of hyperprolactinemia with bromocriptine avoids the risk of hypertrophic valvular heart disease.

C. Assisted reproductive therapies
  1. Intrauterine insemination (IUI)
    a) Indications for the use of IUI include:
      (1) Scarring of the cervix following surgical procedures
      (2) Male partner with a low sperm count
      (3) Improved chances of conceiving with ovulation induction cycles
      (4) Male partner with ejaculatory disorder or erectile dysfunction
      (5) To facilitate use of donor sperm
      (6) Use of previously collected and frozen (cryopreserved) sperm
    b) IUI requires collection of the sperm sample and preparation of the sample in the laboratory. The IUI is timed to coincide with spontaneous or induced ovulation. A catheter is inserted through the cervix into the uterus and the prepared semen sample is injected into the uterus. Placement of sperm in the uterus makes the journey to the fallopian tubes much shorter.

ALERT Vasovagal syncope is common following manipulation of the cervix and is a risk associated with intrauterine insemination. The woman should be instructed to remain in a supine position for a minimum of 10 minutes following the procedure.

  2. Assisted reproductive technology
    a) In-vitro fertilization and embryo transfer (IVF-ET) is a method of assisted reproduction in which the oocyte and sperm are combined in the laboratory. The process includes the following steps: ovarian stimulation, oocyte retrieval, fertilization, embryo culture, and transfer of embryo(s) to the woman's uterus. Timing is critical during IVF-ET cycles. Transvaginal ultrasound examinations and estrogen levels are utilized to monitor the female's response to ovulation induction medications. The goal is to retrieve mature oocytes prior to ovulation. Retrieval is performed as an outpatient procedure and is accomplished by transvaginal ultrasound–guided aspiration. Fertilization and maturation of the embryos occur in the laboratory prior to embryo transfer. Embryo(s) are transferred through a catheter directly into the uterus. The characteristics of the embryos and the individual patient are considered prior to determining how many embryos to transfer. The goal is to decrease the number of IVF-ET cycles that result in high-order multiple pregnancies (triplets and higher). Extra embryos may be cryopreserved (frozen) for future use. The risks associated with IVF-ET include ovarian hyperstimulation syndrome, bleeding, infection, and damage to the bowel, bladder, or a blood vessel during retrieval.

    b) Variations of IVF
      (1) Intracytoplasmic sperm injection (ICSI) is performed when there is poor semen quality or history of failed fertilization in a previous cycle. A single sperm cell is selected and injected directly into a mature oocyte.
      (2) Gamete intrafallopian transfer (GIFT) is an option if the woman has normal fallopian tubes. The gametes (oocyte and sperm) are transferred to the fallopian tube, where fertilization takes place. GIFT provides an alternative for the couples whose religious doctrine prohibits fertilization outside the body. A laparoscopic procedure is required for the transfer.
      (3) Zygote intrafallopian transfer (ZIFT) is similar to IVF-ET, but the zygote (fertilized egg) is placed in the fallopian tube instead of the uterus. As with GIFT, this procedure requires a laparoscopy.
      (4) Donor oocytes are an option in cases of decreased ovarian reserve, absent ovaries, or autosomal or sex-linked disorders. The oocytes are fertilized and the embryo(s) are transferred into the uterus of the recipient following hormonal preparation with estrogen and progesterone.
      (5) Donor embryo(s) may be unused frozen embryos donated by other infertile couples and may be required if both the male and female are infertile. The embryo(s) are transferred to the recipient's uterus at the appropriate time during a normal or induced menstrual cycle.
      (6) Gestational carrier is an option for the woman without a uterus, with a uterine abnormality, or a medical condition that would make pregnancy dangerous to her health and well-being. The infertile couple goes through an IVF cycle and the embryo(s) are placed in the uterus of the gestational carrier.
      (7) Donor sperm is available through sperm banks for both IUI and assisted reproductive cycles. Donated sperm is frozen and quarantined for a minimum of 6 months. Donors are screened and rescreened for

sexually transmitted infections. A thorough personal and family health history is obtained and a thorough physical examination is performed prior to donation. The donor is also screened for genetic diseases such as cystic fibrosis and other carrier states.

c) **Cryopreservation** of embryos, oocytes, or sperm requires freezing at very low temperatures to maintain viability. The option of freezing embryos can make future assisted reproductive therapies simpler, less invasive, and less expensive than initial IVF cycles. Cryopreservation of extra embryos should be discussed with couples prior to the start of IVF cycles. The couple should also consider the possible dilemma of how to dispose of frozen embryos they choose not to use. Cryopreservation of oocytes or sperm is an option for young women or men preparing to undergo medical treatments or procedures, such as chemotherapy, that may affect future fertility.

DID YOU KNOW?

A couple's religion may place restrictions on the acceptable methods of management. For Roman Catholics, human existence begins with the embryo, and fertilization outside the body is prohibited, limiting use of IVF, donor sperm, and cryopreservation of embryos. Christian Scientists are opposed to surgical procedures, excluding the use of IVF.

CASE STUDY: Putting It All Together

Subjective Data

A 24-year-old female presents to a women's health center with complaint of irregular menses. On her intake paperwork, she reports a 15-pound weight gain over the past year. Additional concerns listed are acne and hair loss. During her intake interview, she expresses concern about the dark hair on her upper lip requiring waxing every 2 weeks. She has been married for 2 years, and 1 year ago she discontinued her combined oral contraceptive pills. She and her husband are ready to start a family and have not used birth control for the past year. She has no known drug allergies and current medications and supplements include a prenatal vitamin once daily.

Objective Data

Nursing Assessment

Vital Signs	
Current weight:	172 lb
Height:	65 in.
BMI:	28.6
Temperature:	98.6
Blood pressure:	130/84
Heart rate:	172
Respiratory rate:	14

1. Skin tags and dark velvety areas visible on neck and in axillary area
2. Cystic acne on face and chest
3. Dark hair on chin and upper lip

Health Care Provider Orders

1. Laboratories Urine pregnancy test, prolactin level, DHEA-S, total and free testosterone, fasting insulin, fasting glucose, estrogen and FSH on third day of cycle
2. Transvaginal ultrasound
3. Semen analysis, male partner

CASE STUDY: Putting It All Together (Continued)

_____ **Case Study Questions** _____

A. What assessment findings indicate that the client is experiencing an alteration in reproductive health?

1. _____

2. _____

3. _____

4. _____

5. _____

B. What interventions should the nurse plan and/or implement to meet the needs of this client and her partner?

1. _____

2. _____

3. _____

4. _____

5. _____

C. What client outcomes should the nurse use to evaluate the effectiveness of the nursing interventions?

1. _____

2. _____

3. _____

4. _____

5. _____

REVIEW QUESTIONS

Be sure to read the Introduction for valuable test-taking tips.

1. A man has been instructed to make an appointment with the laboratory for sperm analysis. Which instruction should the nurse provide?
   1. Keep the sample in a cooler for transport.
   2. Deliver the sample to the laboratory within 1 hour of collection.
   3. Collect the sample during a period of frequent sexual activity.
   4. An acceptable collection method is withdrawal prior to ejaculation.

2. A provider has ordered several diagnostic procedures for a couple with suspected infertility. Which diagnostic procedure is useful for determining if ovulation has occurred?
   1. FSH level
   2. Progesterone level
   3. Estrogen level
   4. Vaginal ultrasound

3. A nurse is instructing a woman on the use of ovulation predictor kits. What should the nurse tell the client?
   1. "A prescription is required."
   2. "The kit will determine a serum LH level."
   3. "The LH surge usually occurs 12 hours prior to ovulation."
   4. "Your interval of greatest fertility is on the day of the LH surge and the following 2 days."

4. Lisa, a 35-year-old practicing attorney and marathon runner, presents to the clinic with a complaint of irregular menses. She tells the nurse, "My husband and I want to start a family but it hasn't happened yet. We stopped using birth control 6 months ago. Should we be concerned?" What is the nurse's *best* response?
   1. "Relax and it will happen."
   2. "No, infertility is the failure to conceive after 1 year of unprotected intercourse."
   3. "Aging and extreme exercise regimens may impact fertility. You should address your concerns with your provider during today's visit."
   4. "Decreasing your exercise frequency and intensity will increase your chances of conceiving."

5. Karen, a 28-year-old female patient, has a hysterosalpingogram ordered but not scheduled. What should the nurse tell the patient? *Select all that apply.*
   1. "When your next menses starts, call the office to schedule your procedure."
   2. "You may experience uterine cramping during the procedure."
   3. "Radiation exposure will be avoided through the use of ultrasound imaging."
   4. "The purpose of the test is to evaluate the inside of your uterus and your fallopian tubes."
   5. "The test will be scheduled during the interval following menses and prior to midcycle."

6. Lori, who is 32 years old, is taking clomiphene citrate to induce ovulation and presents to the office for a vaginal ultrasound. As the nurse is walking Lori to ultrasound, Lori mentions that over the past 12 hours she has experienced abdominal bloating, nausea, and weight gain of 5 pounds. The nurse recognizes these signs and symptoms to be associated with what condition?
   1. Ovulation
   2. Premenstrual syndrome
   3. Ovarian hyperstimulation syndrome
   4. Failed ovulation induction

7. A nurse is evaluating the effectiveness of preconception education. Which statement by the client indicates that additional education is needed?
   1. "I know smoking is harmful in pregnancy, so I plan to quit soon. My husband has agreed to avoid smoking in my presence."
   2. "I have started taking a daily prenatal vitamin with folic acid."
   3. "My husband bought a small desk for his laptop computer."
   4. "We plan to avoid the use of chemicals in our garden this year."

8. Cindy, a 36-year-old, has been prescribed Follistim AQ, a follitropin. What information should the nurse include in Cindy's education? *Select all that apply.*
   1. Eggs or oocytes develop within ovarian follicles. The purpose of the medication is to stimulate development of ovarian follicles.
   2. Follistim is a manufactured form of FSH, a hormone released from the pituitary gland during the menstrual cycle.
   3. Rapid weight gain is typical during ovulation induction.
   4. Typical side effects include breast tenderness, changes in mood, and depression.
   5. Take one pill orally 30 minutes prior to breakfast.

9. The nurse responsible for completing the medical history during a couple's initial visit to the reproductive medicine clinic recognizes which of the following as the leading cause of tubal factor infertility in the female?
   1. History of endometriosis
   2. History of pelvic inflammatory disease
   3. History of ectopic pregnancy
   4. History of Asherman's syndrome

10. A nurse is offering preconception counseling in a primary care clinic. Which statement by a patient indicates a need for correction?
   1. "Pregnancy rates are not related to the age of the male partner."
   2. "Sexually active males should be routinely tested for STIs and treated appropriately."
   3. "Maintaining a healthy weight is important for the reproductive health of both female and male partners."
   4. "Certain medications, such as testosterone supplementation and chemotherapy, can impact male fertility."

11. A 36-year-old female patient presents to the reproductive medicine clinic for a follow-up appointment. Initial laboratory results are available and indicate diminished ovarian reserve, and her partner's semen analysis is within normal parameters. Which infertility options may be appropriate for this client? *Select all that apply.*
   1. Donor oocytes
   2. Ovulation induction with clomiphene citrate
   3. Follitropin injections to stimulate ovarian follicles
   4. In-vitro fertilization and embryo transfer
   5. IUI—intrauterine insemination

12. A 25-year-old female tells the nurse, "I have always planned on having children, but now I have been diagnosed with leukemia. I will start chemotherapy treatments soon." The nurse should discuss which fertility preservation options with this patient? *Select all that apply.*
   1. Donor oocytes
   2. Gestational carrier
   3. Ovulation induction with oocyte retrieval
   4. Cryopreservation
   5. Sperm banking

13. The nurse is counseling a couple about infertility. Which piece of assessment data may affect the woman's ability to become pregnant?
   1. The woman exercises three times a week for 1 hour.
   2. The couple each consumes a glass of wine each night.
   3. The couple has a sauna in their backyard.
   4. The male partner works on heavy machinery.

14. The nurse is instructing a client on taking her basal body temperature. The nurse understands that this test is used to determine which of the following?
   1. If the client's cervical mucus contains enough estrogen to support sperm motility
   2. If the client's temperature rises 1 to 5 days after the midcycle
   3. If surgical correction of uterine pathology is needed
   4. If the client is experiencing blockage of the uterine cavity and the fallopian tubes

15. The nurse is educating a client about hysterosalpingograms. Which information should the nurse include in her discussion prior to this procedure?
   1. This procedure is always performed under general anesthesia.
   2. This procedure should be performed after ovulation has occurred.
   3. This procedure involves instillation of a radiopaque dye into the uterine cavity.
   4. After the procedure, the client should take Tylenol to decrease cramping.

REVIEW QUESTION ANSWERS

1. ANSWER: 1
Rationale
1. Extremes of temperature are avoided during transport of sperm to the laboratory. Ideally the sample will be collected near the laboratory, minimizing transport time.
2. The sample should be delivered to the laboratory within 1 hour.
3. Collection should follow 2 to 3 days of abstinence.
4. Acceptable methods of collection are masturbation with collection in a clean container or in a spermicidal-free plastic sheath worn during intercourse.
TEST-TAKING TIP: Review the assessment of male factors if you had difficulty with this question. The accuracy of the sperm analysis is dependent on a complete sample and timely analysis following collection. Recollection is often necessary to confirm an analysis in the subfertile range.
Content Area: Reproductive Health—Male Factor Infertility
Integrated Process: Teaching/Learning
Client Need: Health Promotion and Maintenance
Cognitive Level: Knowledge
Concept: Male Reproduction
Reference: Durham, R. F., & Chapman, L. (2014). Maternal-newborn nursing: The critical components of nursing care. *Philadelphia: F.A. Davis.*

2. ANSWER: 2
Rationale
1. The FSH level is useful for determining ovarian reserve.
2. A progesterone level drawn in the midluteal phase is useful for determining if ovulation has occurred.
3. An estrogen level drawn on the third day of the menstrual cycle is useful in the evaluation of ovarian reserve.
4. A vaginal ultrasound may be used to perform an antral follicle count as a measure of ovarian reserve. Vaginal ultrasound is also useful in identifying uterine pathology.
TEST-TAKING TIP: Review evaluation of ovulatory factors if you had difficulty with this question. A serum progesterone level drawn at the appropriate time will help determine if ovulation has occurred.
Content Area: Reproductive Health—Female Factor Infertility
Integrated Process: Nursing Process—Assessment
Client Need: Physiological Integrity
Cognitive Level: Application
Concept: Female Reproduction
Reference: Perry, S. E., Hockenberry, M. F., Lowdermilk, D. L., & Wilson, D. (2014). Maternal child nursing care. *St. Louis, MO: Elsevier.*

3. ANSWER: 4
Rationale
1. Ovulation predictor kits are sold over the counter.
2. The kit determines the level of LH in the urine.
3. The LH surge occurs 18 to 36 hours prior to ovulation.
4. The day of the surge and the following 2 days are the interval of greatest fertility for the female.
TEST-TAKING TIP: Review evaluation of ovulatory factors if you had difficulty with this question. The surge of LH during the menstrual cycle signals ovulation or the release of the oocyte from the follicle. Prediction of the interval of greatest fertility in the female is possible with detection of the LH surge.

Content Area: Reproductive Health—Female Menstrual Cycle
Integrated Process: Teaching/Learning
Client Need: Health Promotion and Maintenance
Cognitive Level: Application
Concept: Female Reproduction
Reference: Perry, S. E., Hockenberry, M. F., Lowdermilk, D. L., & Wilson, D. (2014). Maternal child nursing care. *St. Louis, MO: Elsevier.*

4. ANSWER: 3
Rationale
1. Stress level may impact fertility but several identified factors, including advanced maternal age, may impact this couple's ability to conceive.
2. The definition of infertility is the failure to conceive following a year or more of unprotected intercourse when the woman is less than 35 years of age and 6 months if the woman is older than 35 years of age.
3. Aging and extreme exercise regimens may negatively impact fertility, and this couple has failed to conceive following 6 months of unprotected intercourse.
4. This approach fails to acknowledge other factors that may impact this couple's ability to conceive.
TEST-TAKING TIP: Review infertility and methods of management if you had difficulty with this question. A multiplicity of factors may affect a couple's ability to conceive.
Content Area: Reproductive Health—Female Factor Infertility
Integrated Process: Nursing Process—Assessment
Client Need: Health Promotion and Maintenance
Cognitive Level: Application
Concept: Female Reproduction
Reference: Durham, R. F., & Chapman, L. (2014). Maternal-newborn nursing: The critical components of nursing care. *Philadelphia: F.A. Davis.*

5. ANSWER: 1, 2, 4, 5
Rationale
1. Hysterosalpingogram is performed early in the menstrual cycle and prior to ovulation.
2. Uterine cramping often occurs during this procedure.
3. Radioactive dye is placed in the uterus and x-rays are taken of the uterus and fallopian tubes.
4. Hysterosalpingography is useful in evaluation of the uterine cavity and the fallopian tubes.
5. Performing this test following menses avoids the interference of intrauterine blood and clots; performing it prior to midcycle avoids the possibility of interfering with conception.
TEST-TAKING TIP: Review evaluation of tubal/pelvic factors if you had difficulty with this question. Hysterosalpingography should be scheduled following the start of menses but prior to ovulation. Injection of radioactive dye requires manipulation of the cervix, which often causes uterine cramping and discomfort for the client.
Content Area: Reproductive Health—Female Factor Infertility
Integrated Process: Nursing Process—Implementation
Client Need: Reduction of Risk Potential
Cognitive Level: Comprehension
Concept: Female Reproduction
Reference: Ward, S. L., & Hisley, S. M. (2011). Maternal-child nursing care: Optimizing outcomes for mothers, children, and families. *Philadelphia: F.A. Davis.*

6. ANSWER: 3

Rationale

1. Symptoms associated with ovulation are mild, localized abdominal pain and spotting. Women are often unaware that ovulation has occurred.

2. Abdominal bloating and weight gain are symptoms associated with premenstrual syndrome but nausea is not.

3. Induction of ovulation carries the risk of ovarian hyperstimulation syndrome. Abdominal bloating, gastrointestinal upset, and weight gain are all signs of this potentially life-threatening complication.

4. Determination of the success of ovulation induction is dependent on laboratories and pelvic ultrasound results.

TEST-TAKING TIP: Review pharmacological treatments if you had difficulty with this question.

Content Area: Reproductive Health—Ovulation Induction
Integrated Process: Nursing Process—Assessment
Client Need: Pharmacological and Parenteral Therapies
Cognitive Level: Application
Concept: Female Reproduction
Reference: Perry, S. E., Hockenberry, M. F., Lowdermilk, D. L., & Wilson, D. (2014). Maternal child nursing care. St. Louis, MO: Elsevier.

7. ANSWER: 1

Rationale

1. Tobacco has a negative effect on the reproductive health of females and males.

2. Folic acid supplementation in early pregnancy has been found to reduce the incidence of neural tube defects.

3. Males should avoid excessive heat to the scrotal area. Increases in scrotal temperature can adversely affect spermatogenesis.

4. Exposure to environmental toxins has been shown to impact female and male fertility.

TEST-TAKING TIP: Review nonmedical management of infertility if you had difficulty with this question. The multiplicity of the factors affecting a couple's ability to conceive requires consideration of female and male factors.

Content Area: Reproductive Health—Nonmedical Management
Integrated Process: Teaching/Learning
Client Need: Health Promotion and Maintenance
Cognitive Level: Knowledge
Concept: Female Reproduction
Reference: Durham, R. F., & Chapman, L. (2014). Maternal-newborn nursing: The critical components of nursing care. Philadelphia: F.A. Davis.

8. ANSWER: 1, 2, 4

Rationale

1. Follitropins are ovulation-induction agents that stimulate ovarian follicles.

2. FSH, a gonadotropin released by the pituitary gland during the menstrual cycle, stimulates the development of a dominant ovarian follicle.

3. Rapid weight gain is a sign of ovarian hyperstimulation syndrome, a life-threatening risk of ovulation induction.

4. Typical side effects of ovulation induction agents are breast tenderness, changes in mood, and depression.

5. Follitropins are administered intramuscularly or subcutaneously.

TEST-TAKING TIP: Review ovulation induction agents if you had difficulty with this question. Ovulation induction therapies often precede intrauterine insemination or assisted reproductive technologies such as in-vitro fertilization and embryo transfer.

Content Area: Reproductive Health—Ovulation Induction
Integrated Process: Teaching/Learning
Client Need: Pharmacological and Parenteral Therapies
Cognitive Level: Knowledge
Concept: Female Reproduction
Reference: Perry, S. E., Hockenberry, M. F., Lowdermilk, D. L., & Wilson, D. (2014). Maternal child nursing care. St. Louis, MO: Elsevier.

9. ANSWER: 2

Rationale

1. A potential cause of pelvic factor infertility is endometriosis. The body's reaction to endometrial glands and stroma outside the uterine cavity may result in fibrosis, adhesions, and fallopian tube occlusion.

2. Pelvic inflammatory disease is considered the leading cause of tubal factor infertility. Bacterial STIs are the most common cause of pelvic inflammatory disease. Identification of STIs and effective treatment reduces the risk of pelvic inflammatory disease and the potentially devastating effects on reproductive health.

3. Ectopic pregnancy is a potential cause of tubal factor infertility.

4. Asherman's syndrome is a potential cause of uterine factor infertility. Trauma to the uterus leads to the formation of uterine adhesions.

TEST-TAKING TIP: Review tubal/pelvic factors associated with female factor infertility if you had difficulty with this question. Carefully read the stem for key words such as "leading cause." Ectopic pregnancy is a potential cause of tubal factor infertility but not the leading cause.

Content Area: Reproductive Health—Female Factor Infertility
Integrated Process: Nursing Process—Assessment
Client Need: Health Promotion and Maintenance
Cognitive Level: Knowledge
Content: Female Reproduction
Reference: Durham, R. F., & Chapman, L. (2014). Maternal-newborn nursing: The critical components of nursing care. Philadelphia: F.A. Davis.

10. ANSWER: 1

Rationale

1. Pregnancy rates are related to the age of the male partner. Rates decrease when the male partner is older than 40 to 45 years of age.

2. Infections can lead to tissue damage and ductal obstruction and acquired male factor infertility.

3. Extremes of body weight impact both male and female infertility.

4. Testosterone supplementation has a negative effect on male fertility. Chemotherapy and other medication may also impact male fertility.

TEST-TAKING TIP: Review male factor infertility and nonmedical treatments of infertility if you had difficulty with this question.

Content Area: Reproductive Health—Preconception Counseling

Integrated Process: Teaching/Learning
Client Need: Health Promotion and Maintenance
Cognitive Level: Application
Concept: Male Reproduction
Reference: Durham, R. F., & Chapman, L. (2014). Maternal-newborn nursing: The critical components of nursing care. Philadelphia: F.A. Davis.

11. **ANSWER: 1, 4**
Rationale
1. Donor oocytes are an option for women with diminished ovarian reserve or absent ovaries.
2. The presence of diminished ovarian reserve predicts a poor response to clomiphene citrate.
3. The presence of diminished ovarian reserve predicts a poor response to follitropins.
4. Donor oocytes are fertilized and the embryo(s) are transferred into the uterus of the recipient following hormonal preparation with estrogen and progesterone.
5. In the presence of diminished ovarian reserve, intrauterine insemination is not indicated.
TEST-TAKING TIP: Review assisted reproductive technology if you had difficulty with this question.
Content Area: Reproductive Health—Female Factor Infertility
Integrated Process: Nursing Process—Implementation
Client Need: Health Promotion and Maintenance
Cognitive Level: Synthesis
Concept: Female Reproduction
Reference: Perry, S. E., Hockenberry, M. F., Lowdermilk, D. L., & Wilson, D. (2014). Maternal-child nursing care. St. Louis, MO: Elsevier.

12. **ANSWER: 3, 4**
Rationale
1. With the availability of cryopreservation, donor oocytes may not be necessary.
2. In the absence of a uterine abnormality, a gestational carrier may not be required.
3. In consultation with the client's oncologist, ovulation induction and oocyte retrieval may be an option to preserve future fertility.
4. Cryopreservation has made it possible to preserve oocytes and sperm for future use in in-vitro fertilization and embryo transfer cycles.
5. Cryopreservation of sperm will not be immediately necessary with a presumably healthy male partner or in the absence of a male partner.
TEST TAKING TIP: Review assisted reproductive technology if you had difficulty with this question.
Content Area: Reproductive Health—Female Factor Infertility
Integrated Process: Nursing Process—Implementation
Client Need: Health Promotion and Maintenance
Cognitive Level: Application
Concept: Female Reproduction
Reference: American Society for Reproductive Medicine. (2011). Assisted reproductive technologies: A guide for patients. Retrieved from www.reproductivefacts.org/uploadedFiles/ASRM_Content/Resources/Patient_Resources/Fact_Sheets_and_Info_Booklets/ART.pdf.

13. **ANSWER: 3**
Rationale
1. Regular moderate exercise does not have an effect on female reproduction.

2. Moderate intake of alcohol is not a cause of infertility.
3. The hot water of a sauna can cause testicular warming, resulting in a decrease in the life span of the sperm.
4. Working with heavy equipment does not have an effect on a male's fertility.
TEST-TAKING TIP: Factors that may be a cause of male infertility are active contact sports, smoking, tight constrictive underwear, and testicular warming.
Content Area: Reproductive Health—Male Factor Infertility
Integrated Process: Nursing Process—Teaching/Learning
Client Need: Health Promotion and Maintenance
Cognitive Level: Application
Concept: Male Reproduction
Reference: Ward, S. L., & Hisley, S. M. (2016). Maternal-child nursing care. 2nd ed. Philadelphia: F.A. Davis.

14. **ANSWER: 2**
Rationale
1. Spinnbarkeit is the elasticity of cervical mucus discharge at ovulation.
2. Basal body temperature (BBT) is a cost-effective method for determining if ovulation has occurred and the approximate time it occurred.
3. Laparoscopy is performed as an outpatient surgical procedure to evaluate the fallopian tubes and ovaries.
4. Hysterosalpingography is performed to evaluate the uterine cavity and the fallopian tubes.
TEST-TAKING TIP: Review testing for female factors in infertility if you missed this question.
Content Area: Reproductive Health—Female Factor Infertility
Integrated Process: Nursing Process—Teaching/Learning
Client Need: Health Promotion and Maintenance
Cognitive Level: Application
Concept: Female Reproduction
Reference: Ward, S. L., & Hisley, S. M. (2016). Maternal-child nursing care. 2nd ed. Philadelphia: F.A. Davis.

15. **ANSWER: 3**
Rationale
1. A hysterosalpingogram can be performed on an outpatient with anesthesia.
2. This procedure should be performed in the follicular phase of the cycle (prior to ovulation) to avoid interrupting a pregnancy.
3. This procedure involves instillation of a radiopaque dye into the uterine cavity.
4. This procedure may cause cramping and discomfort. The nurse should instruct the client to take an over-the-counter (OTC) prostaglandin synthesis inhibitor, such as ibuprofen, 30 minutes prior to the procedure.
TEST-TAKING TIP: Review this diagnostic tool if you missed this question.
Content Area: Reproductive Health—Female Factor Infertility
Integrated Process: Nursing Process—Implementation
Client Need: Physiological Integrity
Cognitive Level: Application
Concept: Female Reproduction
Reference: Lowdermilk, D. L., Perry, S. E., Cashion, K., & Alden, K. R. (2016). Maternity & women's health care. 11th ed. St. Louis, MO: Elsevier.

Chapter 3

Genetics

Alleles—Any of two or more different genes containing specific inheritable characteristics that occupy corresponding loci on paired chromosomes

Autosomes—Any chromosome other than the sex (X and Y) chromosomes

Chromosomes—A linear strand made of DNA (and associated proteins in eukaryotic cells) that carries genetic information

Deoxyribonucleic acid (DNA)—Molecule that encodes the genetic instructions used in the development and functioning of all known living organisms and many viruses

Diploid—In somatic cells, possessing two sets of chromosomes (46 chromosomes in humans)

Gene—The basic unit of heredity, made of DNA, the code for a specific protein. Each gene occupies a certain location on a chromosome.

Genotype—The total of the hereditary information present in an organism

Germ cells—The cells from which the gametes (the ova and sperm) originate

Haploid—In germ cells, possessing half the diploid or normal number of chromosomes found in somatic or body cells

Heterozygous—Alleles that are different

Homologous—Having the same genes or alleles, with loci usually in the same order

Homozygous—Alleles that are identical; both are either dominant or recessive

Karyogram—A photomicrograph of the chromosomes of a single cell, taken during metaphase, when each chromosome is still a pair of chromatids

Karyotype—The number and pattern of chromosomes in a cell

Meiosis—A process of two successive cell divisions, producing cells, egg or sperm, that contain half the number of chromosomes (haploid) in somatic cells. When fertilization occurs, the nuclei of the sperm and ovum fuse and produce a zygote with the full chromosome complement (diploid).

Mendelian inheritance—The laws governing the genetic transmission of dominant and recessive traits

Mitosis—A type of cell division of somatic cells in which each daughter cell contains the same number of chromosomes as the parent cell

Monosomy—Condition of having only one of a pair of chromosomes, as in Turner's syndrome, in which there is one X chromosome rather than the normal pair

Mosaicism—Presence of cells of two different genetic materials in the same individual

Mutation—Change; transformation. A permanent variation in genetic structure with offspring differing from parents in a certain characteristic. A change in a gene potentially capable of being transmitted to offspring

Pedigree—A chart, diagram, or table of an individual's ancestors used in genetics to analyze or reveal inherited traits and illnesses

Phenotype—The expression of the genes present in an individual. This may be directly observable or apparent only with specific tests. Some phenotypes are completely determined by heredity; others are readily altered by environmental agents.

Ribonucleic acid—A nucleic acid that controls protein synthesis in all living cells and takes the place of DNA in certain viruses

Somatic—Nonreproductive cells or tissues

Teratogen—Anything that adversely affects normal cellular development in the embryo or fetus. Certain chemicals, some therapeutic and illicit drugs, radiation, and intrauterine viral infections are known to adversely alter cellular development in the embryo or fetus.

Trisomy—Having three homologous chromosomes per cell instead of two

Zygote—Cell produced by the union of two gametes; the fertilized ovum

I. Genetic Principles

All individuals inherit a specific pattern of growth from their parents. The pattern of growth from one parent combines with that of the other and determines how their child will look and develop. The information that governs the pattern of growth is found in the genetic material that exists in each cell. In most cells, the genetic material is located inside the cell's nucleus. Within the nucleus of each cell, the genetic material is arranged into small units called **chromosomes.** Each chromosome contains several types of proteins and **deoxyribonucleic acid (DNA).** DNA consists of two strands, each composed of a long chain of subunits called *nucleotides.* These nucleotides form a double helix (the shape of two stretched, intertwined springs).

Inheritable traits are determined by **genes,** which are DNA segments that contain specific sequences of nucleotides. The gene is the functional unit of heredity. Gene replication, mutation, and expression are important to a person's individual characteristics. A person's gene constitution is known as the **genotype,** whereas the outward physical appearance, or expression of a person's genes, is known as the **phenotype.** The entire sequence of nucleotides in DNA is the genetic code. This code supplies the instructions on how cells make proteins, the chemical compounds that are necessary for all biological functions. To make proteins from the genetic code's instructions, the code must be transferred from DNA to another type of nucleic acid called **ribonucleic acid (RNA).** RNA transports the genetic message from the DNA to the protein-making parts of the cell. Sometimes a gene is missing or has an error in the coded instructions. When there are abnormalities of the genetic material, genetic diseases and/or birth defects occur.

II. Genetics and Reproduction

The **somatic** cells of all humans have a number of paired, **homologous** chromosomes. Each human somatic cell contains 46 chromosomes or 23 pairs; there are 22 pairs of **autosomes** plus one pair of sex chromosomes. The number of chromosomes in each somatic cell is called a **diploid.** In a process called **mitosis,** somatic cells separate and each chromosome duplicates, with exact copies going to each new cell.

At the moment of fertilization, a person's characteristics are determined by the alleles present. According to the law of **Mendelian inheritance,** two genes are provided—one from each parent. One gene is dominant and expressed, and one gene is recessive and not expressed. A person's characteristics are **homozygous** when the alleles are identical (both dominant [XX] or both recessive [xx]). A person is **heterozygous** when the alleles are different ([Xx]).

Genetics and Genomics

The terms *genetic* and *genomic* are often used interchangeably. However, genetics is the examination of DNA material in specific genes and their role in the biological influence of a trait or disease. Genetics research has identified genes that have led to the ability to diagnose and screen for numerous genetic disorders. Genomics is the study of the entire genetic makeup of an organism and its interaction with the environment. The study of genomics has the capability to improve the awareness of complex diseases and improve medical treatment.

A. Sex chromosomes

The sex chromosomes are referred to as *X* and *Y,* and their combination determines a person's sex. The sperm and egg cells are called *gametes.* All of the gametes that are the mother's eggs possess X chromosomes. The father's sperm contain about half X and half Y chromosomes. The sperm is the variable factor in determining the sex of the baby. If the sperm carries an X chromosome, it will combine with the egg's X chromosome to form a female **zygote.** If the sperm carries a Y chromosome, it will result in a male. A gamete contains only half the number of chromosomes as a somatic cell.

This reduced number of chromosomes occurs through the process of **meiosis.** Meiosis involves two successive cell divisions—the first and second meiotic divisions. During fertilization, a gamete that is a sperm combines with a gamete that is an egg to form a zygote. The zygote contains two sets of 23 chromosomes for the required 46. The zygote, therefore, has the same diploid number as a somatic cell. The zygote develops into a new organism, producing somatic cells by mitotic cell division. As the organism matures, certain cells are set aside for reproduction. These cells are diploid but divide through meiosis, producing haploid cells (gametes).

B. Karyotype

A **karyotype** is the number and pattern of chromosomes in a cell. Humans have 46 chromosomes (23 from each parent), which you can see in the **karyogram.** In karyograms, homologous chromosomes (or pairs of chromosomes that are the same size and shape) are grouped together. Humans have 22 of these pairs, called *autosomes.* Autosomes are chromosomes that have nothing to do with determining sex. A karyogram provides a photograph of an individual's chromosomes, sorted and arranged by size.

C. Pedigree

A **pedigree** is a diagram that shows the phenotype of a particular gene and its ancestors from one generation to the next. The diagram consists of family history information using standardized symbols and terminology. A phenotype is an individual's observable traits, such as height, eye and hair color, and blood type. The genetic influence to the phenotype is called the *genotype*. Some traits are determined by the genotype, while others may be determined by environmental factors.

D. Punnett square

A Punnett square is used to understand how genetic traits and disorders are predicted and the likelihood of inheritance (Fig 3.1) as well as predict the potential combinations and the odds of genotypes that can occur in children by using the genotypes of their parents.

III. Inheritance of Disease

A. Multifactorial inheritance

Multifactorial inheritance means that many factors, both genetic and environmental, may contribute to the cause of a genetic disease. One gender is usually affected more frequently. The possibility for a trait or disorder to happen more than once depends on how closely the family member with the trait or disorder is related. Other multifactorial inheritance disorders are cleft lip, cleft palate, neural tube defects, pyloric stenosis, and congenital heart disease. These disorders may range from mild to severe depending on the number of genes for the particular defect and the amount of the environmental influence.

🛑 **ALERT** The developing human is most vulnerable to the effects of **teratogens** during the first 8 weeks of

gestation. Preconception education is very important because most women do not confirm their pregnancy until 8 weeks or later.

B. Unifactorial inheritance

1. This results when a specific trait or disorder is caused by a single gene. Single-gene traits or disorders include autosomal-dominant, autosomal-recessive, X-linked dominant, and X-linked recessive modes of inheritance.

2. Autosomal-dominant inheritance **mutations** in genes are located on one of the 22 pairs of autosomes. Autosomal conditions occur in both men and women. A parent with an autosomal-dominant disorder will pass on either a changed mutation of the gene or a normal replica of the gene to each of his or her children. If a child inherits the changed replica of the gene, he or she is "affected" and therefore has the disorder. A child who inherits a normal (unchanged) replica of the gene will not inherit the disorder. A person needs to inherit only one changed replica of the gene pair in order to be affected with an autosomal-dominant disorder. The mutated gene "dominates" the pair of genes. In an autosomal-dominant disorder, one mutated gene from one parent causes the child to have the disorder. Examples of autosomal-dominant inheritance disorders include neurofibromatosis (Fig. 3.2), Marfan's syndrome, factor V Leiden mutation, Huntington disease, achondroplasia, and facioscapulohumeral muscular dystrophy.

3. Autosomal-recessive inheritance disorders exist when two mutated genes, one from each parent, are passed on to the parents' offspring. The affected child usually has unaffected parents who each carry a single copy of the mutated gene. The parents are referred to as *carriers* of the trait or disorder. When both parents carry the same

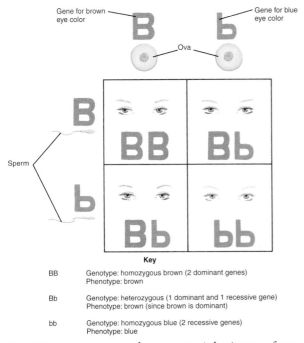

Key

BB	Genotype: homozygous brown (2 dominant genes) Phenotype: brown
Bb	Genotype: heterozygous (1 dominant and 1 recessive gene) Phenotype: brown (since brown is dominant)
bb	Genotype: homozygous blue (2 recessive genes) Phenotype: blue

Fig 3.1 Punnett square to demonstrate inheritance of eye color.

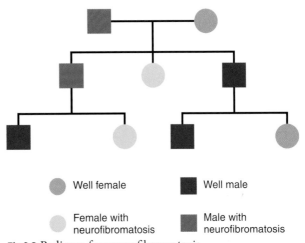

Well female   Well male

Female with neurofibromatosis   Male with neurofibromatosis

Fig 3.2 Pedigree for neurofibromatosis.

recessive mutated gene and have a child, they may pass on the mutated gene to that child. Autosomal-recessive inheritance is typically not seen in every generation of an affected family. Examples include sickle cell anemia (Fig. 3.3), galactosemia, phenylketonuria, maple syrup urine disease, Tay-Sachs disease, and cystic fibrosis (CF).

4. X-linked dominant inheritance is a disorder caused by a mutated gene on the X chromosome. As in autosomal-dominant inheritance, only one copy of a mutated gene on the X chromosome of a parent is required for a child to be susceptible to an X-linked dominant disorder. Both males and females can be affected, although males may be more severely affected because they carry only one copy of genes found on the X chromosome. Some X-linked dominant disorders are lethal in males. When a female is affected, each pregnancy will have a one in two, or 50%, chance for the off-spring to inherit the disorder. When a male is affected, all of his daughters but none of his sons will be affected. Examples of X-linked dominant inheritance disorders include hypophosphatemic rickets, oral-facial-digital syndrome type I, and fragile X syndrome (Fig. 3.4).

5. X-linked recessive inheritance traits or disorders appear when the gene responsible for the trait or the disorder is located on the X chromosome. As stated earlier, females have two X chromosomes, while males have one X and one Y. So genes on the X chromosome can be recessive or dominant, and the expression in females and males is not the same because the genes on the Y chromosome do

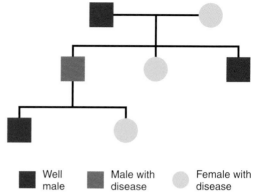

Key:
- ■ Well male
- ■ Male with disease
- ● Female with disease

Fig 3.4 Family pedigree for X-linked dominant inheritance.

not pair up with the genes on the X chromosome. X-linked recessive genes are expressed in females only if there are two copies of the gene (one on each X chromosome). However, for males, only one copy of an X-linked recessive gene is neces-sary for the trait or disorder to be expressed. Examples of X-linked recessive inheritance include hemophilia A and Duchenne muscular dystrophy.

IV. Abnormalities of Chromosomal Structure

Structural chromosome abnormalities occur when there is a change in the structure of a chromosome: the chro-mosome either has a part missing, an extra part, or a part that has switched places with another chromosome part. The total number of chromosomes per cell is 46. Abnor-malities of chromosome structure lead to the chromosome having too much or too little genetic material, resulting in birth defects. There are several types of abnormalities of chromosomal structure:

A. Translocation

Involves a chromosomal segment that has moved from one position to another, either within the same chro-mosome (intrachromosomal) or to another chromo-some (interchromosomal). In an intrachromosomal translocation, a segment breaks off the chromosome and rejoins it at a different location. A balanced translocation occurs when pieces from two different chromosomes switch places without loss or gain of any chromosome material. An unbalanced translocation involves the unequal loss or gain of genetic informa-tion between two chromosomes.

B. Duplication

Involves a chromosome that has duplicated. This re-sults in having extra genetic material, even though the total number of chromosomes is usually normal. A very small piece of a chromosome can contain many

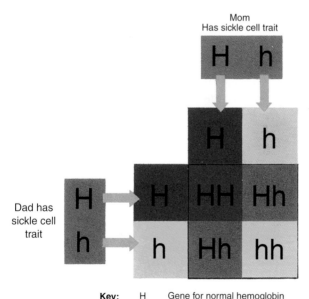

Mom
Has sickle cell trait

Dad has sickle cell trait

	H	h
H	HH	Hh
h	Hh	hh

Key: H   Gene for normal hemoglobin
h   Gene for sickle cell hemoglobin

Fig 3.3 Punnett square for sickle cell disease.

different genes; therefore, the extra genes present in a duplication and may cause those genes to not function properly.

C. Deletion

Involves a part of a chromosome that is missing a small piece. When genes are missing, there may be faults in the developing embryo.

D. Inversion

Involves a chromosome that has broken into two pieces. This breakage results in the DNA being reversed and reinserted into the chromosome. The genetic material may or may not be lost as a result of the chromosome breakage.

V. Abnormalities of Chromosome Number

An abnormal number of chromosomes is called *aneuploidy*. This occurs when an individual either is missing a chromosome from a pair (**monosomy**) or has more than two chromosomes of a pair (**trisomy**).

A. Monosomy

This occurs when a pair of chromosomes is missing a piece. Therefore, there are 45 chromosomes in each cell instead of the usual 46. Turner syndrome is an example of a monosomy and occurs when an infant is born with only one X sex chromosome, rather than the usual pair (either XX or XY).

B. Trisomy

This is the presence of an extra chromosome—meaning three chromosomes, instead of the usual pair. An example is trisomy 21, or Down syndrome, which occurs when a newborn has three copies of chromosome 21. In trisomy 18, there are three copies of chromosome 18 in every cell of the body rather than the usual pair.

C. Mosaicism

This is the occurrence of cells that differ in their genetic component and is caused when a mutation arises early in development. The resulting embryo will have a mixture of cells, some with and some without the mutation.

VI. Role of the Nurse

The nurse's role in genetics is very important. Nurses are responsible for obtaining a careful, detailed history, which provides the basis for future genetic counseling. This information establishes a foundation for risk assessment and future diagnosis confirmation. All patients benefit from a family history assessment for birth defects and gene mutations. Information may lead to detection of risk for chromosome disorders such as Down syndrome or for cancers related to gene mutations.

Couples identified as being at risk for a genetic disorder should be provided additional information about the genetic disorder, directed to support groups, and given Internet sites that contain accurate information. The nurse may serve as a liaison between the patient and a genetic counselor to ensure continuity of care. The couple should be encouraged to talk openly to each other about their feelings and concerns. The nurse should explain to the couple that they may experience grief and loss of their "perfect child." If the couple decides to terminate the pregnancy based on the outcomes of genetic testing, the nurse should be supportive by answering questions and clarifying information and options. Couples may also consider not pursuing pregnancy based on an assessment of a family pedigree and should also be given information on pregnancy prevention methods that meet their needs.

CASE STUDY: Putting It All Together

Richard and Katherine have been married for 3 years. They are now planning to start a family. Richard's younger sister had CF and died before she started high school. They have decided to have genetic tests before trying to conceive in order to determine whether they could have a child affected by the disease. Neither Richard nor Katherine show any signs of CF.

Case Study Questions

1. Is it possible for Richard to carry the gene for CF? Why?

2. If Richard is a carrier and Katherine is not, what are the chances that they could have a child with CF? Why?

Continued

CASE STUDY: Putting It All Together (Continued)

Richard and Katherine were both found to be carriers for the CF gene.

_____ **Case Study Questions** _____

3. Discuss the interpretation of risk as it applies to Richard and Katherine for giving birth to an infant who is normal, is a carrier, or is affected with CF.

4. Develop a pedigree chart indicating Richard's and Katherine's family histories for CF.

5. Draw a Punnett square for Richard and Katherine to illustrate the risk.

Two years later, Richard and Katherine become pregnant. After genetic testing for CF, the couple received news that their test results were positive and that they are both carriers.

_____ **Case Study Questions** _____

6. Discuss your role as the nurse in the education of and emotional support for Richard and Katherine.

REVIEW QUESTIONS

Be sure to read the Introduction for valuable test-taking tips.

1. The parents have just received news that their infant has sickle cell disease. They ask the nurse if this could happen to future children. Because this is an example of an autosomal-recessive inheritance, what should the nurse tell Tim and Katie? *Select all that apply.*
   1. "Because this child has sickle cell, there is a decreased chance none of your other children will have sickle cell disease."
   2. "Each time you get pregnant, there will be a 50/50 chance that your child will have sickle cell disease."
   3. "Each time you get pregnant, there will be a 25% chance that your child will inherit the gene from each parent and will have sickle cell disease."
   4. "Your next child will have a 50% chance of being a carrier for sickle cell disease."
   5. "Only your male children will have sickle cell disease."

2. A 4-month-old infant has been diagnosed with a rare genetic disease called *neonatal onset multisystem inflammatory disease* (NOMID). This disease occurs through an autosomal-dominant inheritance pattern. The parents ask the nurse, "Which of us passed this disease on to our child?" Which of the following is the nurse's *best* response?
   1. "Only the female carries the gene."
   2. "Only the father carries the gene."
   3. "Either the mother or the father can carry the gene."
   4. "Both the mother and the father have to be carriers."

3. The nurse is providing education to a pregnant woman whose genetic testing confirms her fetus has Down syndrome. The nurse understands that Down syndrome is an example of which abnormality?
   1. Chromosomal translocation
   2. Abnormality of chromosomal number
   3. Multifactorial monosomy inheritance
   4. Autosomal-recessive inheritance

4. The nurse educator is conducting a class for student nurses on X-linked recessive disorders. Which responses from a student nurse indicate that further education is needed? *Select all that apply.*
   1. "The male can't be a carrier if he doesn't have an X-linked disorder."
   2. "If the male doesn't have an X-linked disorder, then his children won't either."
   3. "If the female is a carrier, her daughter could be one too."
   4. "If the female is a carrier, her sons may have an X-linked recessive disorder."

5. The nurse is providing genetic counseling for an expectant couple who just found out that their child has Down syndrome. Which is the *best* way for the nurse to handle this?
   1. Be supportive by answering questions and clarifying information and options.
   2. Inform the parents that they should not tell anyone until they have made a decision concerning termination of the pregnancy.
   3. Refer the couple to another specialist for a second opinion.
   4. Tell the couple that there are a lot of parents who have children with Down syndrome and they all do fine.

6. A young couple is contemplating starting a family. Which is the *best* time for genetic counseling?
   1. Now, before they become pregnant
   2. As soon as they have a positive pregnancy test
   3. In the second trimester
   4. In the third trimester

7. The nurse in a genetic clinic interviews a couple and develops a pedigree chart. Which inheritance patterns does the pedigree chart portray?
   1. Autosomal recessive
   2. X-linked recessive
   3. Autosomal dominant
   4. X-linked dominant

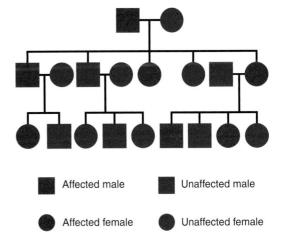

■ Affected male	■ Unaffected male
● Affected female	● Unaffected female

8. A couple has just seen a genetic specialist regarding genetic anomalies of their infant. The specialist has ordered a karyotype to be performed. What should the nurse inform the couple about karyotyping?
   1. "Karyotyping will reveal if your infant's head is growing appropriately."
   2. "Karyotyping will reveal if your baby will develop normally."
   3. "Karyotyping will provide information about the number and structure of the chromosomes."
   4. "Karyotyping will detect any present or future physical deformities your infant has or may have."

9. A patient is being interviewed by the nurse. During the family history assessment, the patient reports having had relatives with cancer. Which is the nurse's *best* response?
   1. Complete a pedigree, noting the types of cancer and which relatives were affected.
   2. Ask whether the cancer was in male or female relatives.
   3. Determine whether the cancer reported in the family history is pertinent to the patient's personal medical history.
   4. Schedule a consult with a genetic counselor to further assess the patient's risk.

10. A 44-year-old woman presents with an unexpected pregnancy. She asks the nurse, "Is my baby going to have a birth defect? My third cousin has Down syndrome." What is the nurse's *best* response?
    1. Tell the patient she is at risk for gene mutation because a birth defect in a distant relative places the woman at increased risk.
    2. Discuss the potential risk for intrauterine growth retardation due to the mother's advanced age.
    3. Discuss the patient's situation with the physician to ask for a referral to high-risk obstetrics.
    4. Discuss the potential risk for a chromosomal abnormality based on the patient's advanced age.

11. A patient and her husband request to view the results of their infant's karyotype. An aneuploidy was noted. The nurse understands the results to indicate what?
    1. An abnormal number of chromosomes were present on the karyogram.
    2. Translocations were noted on some of the chromosomes.
    3. The infant's chromosomes had broken areas, causing an abnormality in the picture of the chromosomes.
    4. Some of the infant's chromosomes were duplicated to total 46 chromosomes.

12. Of the following karyotype results, which indicates a finding of Turner syndrome?
    1. 46 XY
    2. 46 YY
    3. 46 XX
    4. 46 X

13. A nurse provides teaching for a patient scheduled for genetic testing. What should the nurse do to help the patient understand what is being taught? *Select all that apply.*
    1. Use simple vocabulary.
    2. Avoid the use of jargon.
    3. Speak slowly and clearly.
    4. Ask the patient to verbalize what was learned.
    5. Schedule a follow-up visit for the patient to ask questions related to the genetic testing procedure.

14. A patient asks for advice regarding whether to have children in the future after hearing she is a carrier for an autosomal-recessive disorder. What is the nurse's *best* response?
    1. Encourage the patient to avoid having children as the risk of having a child with a disorder is 50%.
    2. Explain that if the patient proceeds with a pregnancy, her risk of having a child with a disorder is 25% because she is only a carrier.
    3. Encourage the patient to pursue pregnancy, informing her that she can always terminate a pregnancy if the fetus is found to be affected.
    4. Ask the patient to describe her feelings about potentially having an affected infant.

15. A patient and her husband have just been told their unborn child has Down syndrome. The patient's husband becomes upset, stating, "There is no way this can be possible as we have no one in the family with this problem! You must run the test again because the results cannot be correct." What does the husband's behavior represent?
    1. Denial
    2. Sorrow
    3. Anger
    4. Bargaining

REVIEW QUESTION ANSWERS

1. ANSWER: 3, 4
Rationale
1. Sickle cell disease is an autosomal-recessive disease. Both parents must carry the mutated gene for their child to have sickle cell disease. If both parents carry the gene mutation, there is a 25% chance in each pregnancy that their child will inherit the mutated gene from each parent and have the disease, a 50% chance in each pregnancy that their child will receive one mutated gene and be a carrier, and a 25% chance in each pregnancy that their child will not receive the mutated gene and be neither a carrier nor have the disease.
2. Since the parents are both carriers for sickle cell disease, each time they get pregnant there will be a 25% chance that their child will have sickle cell disease.
3. This is a correct statement.
4. This is a correct statement.
5. Both male and female can be affected in an autosomal recessive disease.
TEST-TAKING TIP: When answering a question involving percentage of inheritance, it is helpful to do a Punnett square. Example for sickle disease:

Carrier parent

		A	a
Carrier parent	**A**	AA Normal child	Aa Carrier child
	a	Aa Carrier child	aa Affected child

Content Area: Autosomal-Recessive Disease/Genetics
Integrated Process: Nursing Process—Teaching/Learning
Client Need: Health Promotion and Maintenance—Health Screening
Cognitive Level: Application
Concept: Family
Reference: London, M. L., Ladewig, P. A., Davidson, M. R., Ball, J. W., Bindler, R. C., & Cowen, K. J. (2014). Maternal & child nursing care. 4th ed. Upper Saddle River, New Jersey: Pearson.

2. ANSWER: 3
Rationale
1. Translocations occur when DNA from one chromosome is swapped with the DNA of another chromosome.
2. Autosomal-dominant inheritance mutations in genes are located on one of the 22 pairs of autosomes. Autosomal conditions occur in both men and women.
3. Correct answer.
4. Autosomal-recessive inheritance disorders exist when two mutated genes, one from each parent, are passed on to their offspring.
TEST-TAKING TIP: Remember, with an autosomal-dominant disorder, a change or mutation in one copy of the gene is sufficient to impair cell function, leading to disease. The change is located on an autosome (a chromosome other than the sex [X and Y] chromosomes). A dominant genetic disorder is a characteristic or disorder a child will have if one of the parents has the changed or mutated gene.
Content Area: Autosomal-Dominant Disease/Genetics
Integrated Process: Nursing Process—Teaching/Learning
Client Need: Health Promotion and Maintenance—Health Screening
Cognitive Level: Application
Concept: Family
Reference: Perry, S. E., Hockenberry, M. F., Lowdermilk, D. L., & Wilson, D. (2014). Maternal child nursing care. 5th ed. St. Louis, MO: Elsevier.

3. ANSWER: 2
Rationale
1. Chromosome translocation occurs when there is a rearrangement of parts between chromosomes. A gene fusion may be created when the translocation joins two otherwise-separated genes.
2. Correct answer.
3. Multifactorial inheritance indicates that many factors (genetic and environmental) may be involved in causing a birth defect. A combination of genes from both parents along with unknown environmental factors produce the birth defect. Monosomy involves the absence of one member of a pair of chromosomes.
4. Autosomal-recessive inheritance disorders exist when two changed or mutated genes, one from each parent, is passed on to their offspring.
TEST-TAKING TIP: Remember, with an autosomal-dominant disorder, a change or mutation in one copy of the gene is sufficient to impair cell function, leading to disease. The change is located on an autosome (a chromosome other than the sex [X and Y] chromosomes). A dominant genetic disorder is a characteristic or disorder a child will have if one of the parents has the changed or mutated gene.
Content Area: Autosomal-Dominant Disease/Genetics
Integrated Process: Nursing Process—Teaching/Learning
Client Need: Health Promotion and Maintenance—Health Screening
Cognitive Level: Application
Concept: Family
Reference: Perry, S. E., Hockenberry, M. F., Lowdermilk, D. L., & Wilson, D. (2014). Maternal child nursing care. 5th ed. St. Louis, MO: Elsevier.

4. ANSWER: 1, 3, 4
Rationale
1. This is a correct statement. Females have two X chromosomes and males have an X and a Y. Males have only one X chromosome; therefore they will be affected with the X-linked disorder if they have the X-linked mutated gene. Likewise, if the male has a normal X chromosome, he cannot pass an X-linked disorder to his son.
2. This is an incorrect statement. A female who has a "recessive" gene variation in one of her X-linked chromosomes and whose other X-linked chromosome is normal is a carrier for the recessive mutated gene. The male passes a Y chromosome on to his son. If the son received the mutated gene, then he will be affected by the condition because of the X-linked recessive mutated gene he received from his mother.
3. This is a correct statement. The daughter has a one in four chance that she will inherit the normal X-linked gene

from her father and the mutated X-linked gene from her mother. She will be a genetic carrier of the disorder like her mother and will usually be unaffected.

4. This is a correct statement. The son has a one in four chance that he will inherit the mutated gene from his mother. In this case, he will not have a normal X chromosome and will be affected by the disorder.

TEST-TAKING TIP: Read carefully the wording in the question. Be aware of questions that have three right answers and you must choose the incorrect answer.

Content Area: X-Linked Recessive/Genetics
Integrated Process: Nursing Process—Teaching/Learning
Client Need: Health Promotion and Maintenance—Health Screening
Cognitive Level: Application
Concept: Family

Reference: Perry, S. E., Hockenberry, M. F., Lowdermilk, D. L., & Wilson, D. (2014). Maternal child nursing care. 5th ed. St. Louis, MO: Elsevier.

5. **ANSWER: 1**
Rationale
1. After the couple has seen the specialist, the nurse should review what the specialist has discussed with the family and clarify any doubts the couple might have.
2. The nurse should never make the decision for the client but rather should present all the relevant information and aid the couple in making an informed decision.
3. There is no need for the nurse to refer the client to another specialist or for further diagnostic and screening tests unless instructed to do so by the genetic specialist.
4. The couple should be encouraged to talk openly to each other about their feelings and concerns. The nurse should explain that the couple will experience grief and loss of their "perfect child."

TEST-TAKING TIP: The test taker should be sensitive to the needs of their clients and use good listening and communication techniques.

Content Area: Role of the Nurse/Genetics
Integrated Process: Nursing Process—Teaching/Learning
Client Need: Physiological Integrity—Basic Care and Comfort
Cognitive Level: Analysis
Concept: Family

Reference: Durham, R. F., & Chapman, L. (2014). Maternal-newborn nursing: The critical components of nursing care. 2nd ed. Philadelphia, PA: F.A. Davis.

6. **ANSWER: 1**
Rationale
1. The best time for genetic counseling is before the couple becomes pregnant. Preconception counseling allows the couple to discover possible pregnancy risks, plan for identified risks, and establish early prenatal care.
2. Genetic counseling should be presented prior to pregnancy.
3. Genetic counseling should be presented prior to pregnancy.
4. Genetic counseling should be presented prior to pregnancy.

TEST-TAKING TIP: The developing human is most vulnerable to the effects of teratogens during the first 8 weeks of

gestation. Preconception education is very important because most women do not confirm their pregnancy until 8 weeks gestation or later.

Content Area: Basics/Genetics
Integrated Process: Nursing Process—Planning
Client Need: Physiological Integrity—Reduction of Risk Potential
Cognitive Level: Application
Concept: Family

Reference: Durham, R. F., & Chapman, L. (2014). Maternal-newborn nursing: The critical components of nursing care. 2nd ed. Philadelphia, PA: F.A. Davis.

7. **ANSWER: 3**
Rationale
1. Autosomal-recessive disorders involve two unaffected parents, but each parent carries one copy of a gene mutation for an autosomal-recessive disorder. They have one affected child and three unaffected children, two of which carry one copy of the gene mutation.
2. X-linked recessive traits manifest in males because they have only one copy of the X chromosome. They do not have a normal copy of the gene to offset the mutated gene. Females are rarely affected by X-linked recessive diseases. Since the gene is on the X chromosome, there is no father-to-son transmission. There is a father-to-daughter and mother-to-daughter and -son transmission. If a man is affected with an X-linked recessive condition, all of his daughters will inherit one copy of the mutated gene from him.
3. Autosomal-dominant disorders are manifested in individuals who have just one copy of the mutated gene. Affected males and females have an equal chance of passing the trait to their offspring. Affected individuals have one normal copy of the gene and one mutated copy of the gene. Each offspring has a 50% chance of inheriting the mutated gene. As shown in the pedigree, approximately half of the children of affected parents inherit the condition and half do not.
4. X-linked dominant disorders have no transmission from father to son because the mutated gene is located on the X chromosome. Daughters of an affected male will have the disorder because the father has only one X chromosome to transmit to his daughter. Children of an affected woman have a 50% chance of inheriting the X chromosome with the mutated gene. X-linked dominant disorders are apparent when only one copy of the mutated gene is present.

TEST-TAKING TIP: Dominant genes produce dominant phenotypes in individuals who have one copy of the gene, which can come from just one parent. For a recessive allele to produce a recessive phenotype, the individual must have two copies, one from each parent.

Content Area: Basics/Genetics
Integrated Process: Nursing Process—Planning
Client Need: Physiological Integrity—Reduction of Risk Potential
Cognitive Level: Application
Concept: Family

Reference: Durham, R. F., & Chapman, L. (2014). Maternal-newborn nursing: The critical components of nursing care. 2nd ed. Philadelphia, PA: F.A. Davis.

8. ANSWER: 3
Rationale
1. Measuring head circumference will reveal if their infant's head is growing appropriately.
2. A karyotype is a photomicrograph of the chromosomes of a single cell and shows the number and appearance of chromosomes in the nucleus of a eukaryotic cell. Attention is paid to their length, the position of the centromeres, banding pattern, any differences between the sex chromosomes, and any other physical characteristics. The karyotype is no indication of how an infant will develop.
3. This is a correct statement.
4. Karyotyping will detect the number and structure of chromosomes in a single cell but will not provide any information on physical deformities present or deformities that may present in the future.
TEST-TAKING TIP: Karyotypes contain 22 pairs of autosomal chromosomes and one pair of sex chromosomes. Karyotypes for females contain two X chromosomes and are denoted 46 XX. Karyotypes for males have both an X and a Y chromosome, denoted 46 XY. Any variation from the standard karyotype may or may not lead to developmental problems.
Content Area: Basics/Genetics
Integrated Process: Nursing Process—Teaching/Learning
Client Need: Health Promotion and Maintenance
Cognitive Level: Application
Concept: Family
Reference: Perry, S. E., Hockenberry, M. F., Lowdermilk, D. L., & Wilson, D. (2014). Maternal child nursing care. 5th ed. St. Louis, MO: Elsevier.

9. ANSWER: 1
Rationale
1. Correct answer.
2. Gender, while important to some gene mutations, is not the priority. Establishing whether the relative is first (parent/sibling) or second (aunt/uncle/cousin) degree would provide more beneficial information.
3. All cancers reported during a family history assessment would be important. Some, however, would have greater chance of being hereditary.
4. Scheduling a consult with a genetic counselor would occur after a potential risk is identified. The nurse's priority role is to assess for risk.
TEST-TAKING TIP: Consider the answers in priority and applicability. Understanding which relatives are affected by cancers is important to the risk assessment. However, to fully evaluate potential for inherited disorders, a family tree, or pedigree, provides a picture of a family over time. Referral to a genetic counselor would be a later step than initial assessment within the care of the patient.
Content Area: Basics/Genetics
Integrated Process: Nursing Process—Reduction of Risk Potential
Client Need: Safe and Effective Care Environment—Management of Care
Cognitive Level: Analysis
Concept: Family
Reference: Littleton-Gibbs, L. Y., & Engebretson, J. C. (2013). Maternity nursing care. 2nd ed. Clifton Park, NY: Delmar Cengage Learning.

10. ANSWER: 4
Rationale
1. When a pedigree is created, autosomal-recessive disorders may alert the nurse to concern in distant relatives. However, chromosome alterations in distant relatives would not place the woman at greater risk.
2. Intrauterine growth restriction is not associated with a chromosomal abnormality's occurrence.
3. The nurse's role includes the ability to identify a patient at risk. Referral is not indicated at this point in the patient's care.
4. Correct answer.
TEST-TAKING TIP: Remember that chromosome disorders are the result of mutation, translocation, or increase or decrease in numbers of chromosomes. Alleles are responsible for traits (or disease) based on dominant and recessive expression.
Content Area: Basics/Genetics
Integrated Process: Nursing Process—Teaching/Learning
Client Need: Physiological Integrity—Reduction of Risk Potential
Cognitive Level: Application
Concept: Family
Reference: Littleton-Gibbs, L. Y., & Engebretson, J. C. (2013). Maternity nursing care. 2nd ed. Clifton Park, NY: Delmar Cengage Learning.

11. ANSWER: 1
Rationale
1. Correct answer.
2. Translocations do not affect the total number of chromosomes seen on the karyogram.
3. Broken areas do not affect the total number of chromosomes seen on the karyogram.
4. Chromosome duplications may be noted, but the total of 46 chromosomes does not define aneuploidy. A deletion or addition of a chromosome would be required to use this label.
TEST-TAKING TIP: The term *aneuploidy* means more or less than 46 chromosomes. A basic understanding of the vocabulary is required to answer this question. Look for common areas in the other answers. "Translocation" and "broken areas" have similarity but do not change the total number.
Content Area: Basics/Genetics
Integrated Process: Nursing Process—Teaching/Learning
Client Need: Physiological Integrity: Reduction of Risk Potential
Cognitive Level: Application
Concept: Family
Reference: Littleton-Gibbs, L. Y., & Engebretson, J. C. (2013). Maternity nursing care. 2nd ed. Clifton Park, NY: Delmar Cengage Learning.

12. ANSWER: 4
Rationale
1. 46 XY represents a normal male karyotype
2. 46 YY
3. 46 XX represents a normal female karyotype
4. Correct answer
TEST-TAKING TIP: Memorize normal karyotypes and consider whether an answer is providing more or less information than necessary to answer the question. A lack

of an X or Y chromosome on a karyotype renders the result monosomy in nature.

Content Area: Basics/Genetics
Integrated Process: Nursing Process—Teaching/Learning
Client Need: Safe and Effective Care Environment—Management of Care
Cognitive Level: Application
Concept: Family
Reference: Littleton-Gibbs, L. Y., & Engebretson, J. C. (2013). Maternity nursing care. *2nd ed. Clifton Park, NY: Delmar Cengage Learning.*

13. **ANSWER: 1, 2, 3, 4**
Rationale
1. This is a correct statement.
2. This is a correct statement.
3. This is a correct statement.
4. This is a correct statement.
5. Allow the patient to ask questions for clarification at the time of the discussion. Delaying an opportunity for the patient's questions to be answered may result in miscommunication or lack of understanding.

TEST-TAKING TIP: Remember that principles of communication allow the patient to have an opportunity to clarify any points that are unclear. Consider how allowing a patient to wait to have her questions answered will have a negative impact on her understanding and/or comfort with a testing procedure.

Content Area: Role of the Nurse/Genetics
Integrated Process: Nursing Process—Teaching/Learning
Client Need: Physiological Integrity—Basic Care and Comfort
Cognitive Level: Application
Concept: Family
Reference: Perry, S. E., Hockenberry, M. F., Lowdermilk, D. L., & Wilson, D. (2014). Maternal child nursing care. *5th ed. St. Louis, MO: Elsevier.*

14. **ANSWER: 4**
Rationale
1. Expressing an opinion places the focus on the nurse and negates the patient's concerns.
2. The risk for an affected future pregnancy depends on both partners' carrier status. If the partner is affected, the risk goes up to 50%. If the partner is unaffected, the risk remains 25%; however, the nurse is expressing an opinion that may not relieve the patient's concerns.
3. This answer may not align with the patient values.
4. This is the correct answer.

TEST-TAKING TIP: Ask the patient to describe her feelings about having an affected infant. This allows an opportunity for the patient to explore concerns and alternative solutions without others influencing her decision making. The nurse should avoid offering opinions that may involve judgment or inconsistency in values between the nurse and the patient.

Content Area: Basics/Genetics
Integrated Process: Nursing Process—Teaching/Learning
Client Need: Safe and Effective Care Environment—Management of Care
Cognitive Level: Application
Concept: Family
Reference: Littleton-Gibbs, L. Y., & Engebretson, J. C. (2013). Maternity nursing care. *2nd ed. Clifton Park, NY: Delmar Cengage Learning.*

15. **ANSWER: 1**
Rationale
1. Correct answer.
2. This is an assumption. There is insufficient information to reach this conclusion.
3. The husband is obviously upset, but he does not exhibit signs of anger.
4. While the husband is requesting that another test be performed, he is not offering anything in return.

TEST-TAKING TIP: Remember the stages of grief. Denial is an unconscious defense mechanism. The husband's request for repeat testing indicates that he does not agree or believe the results.

Content Area: Role of the Nurse/Genetics
Integrated Process: Nursing Process—Teaching/Learning
Client Need: Psychosocial Integrity
Cognitive Level: Application
Concept: Family
Reference: Perry, S. E., Hockenberry, M. F., Lowdermilk, D. L., & Wilson, D. (2014). Maternal child nursing care. *5th ed. St. Louis, MO: Elsevier.*

Conception and Fetal Development

Amnion—The innermost fetal membrane. It is a thin, transparent sac that holds the fetus suspended in amniotic fluid.

Blastocyst—In mammalian embryo development, the stage that follows the morula. It consists of an outer layer, or trophoblast, and an inner cell mass from which the embryo will develop.

Decidua basalis—The endometrium of the lining of the uterus and tissue around the ectopically located fertilized ovum that unites with the chorion to form the placenta

Decidua capsularis—The endometrium of the lining of the uterus and tissue around the ectopically located fertilized ovum that surrounds the chorionic sac

Ductus arteriosus—In the fetus, a blood vessel connecting the main pulmonary artery and the aortic arch.

In fetal circulation, it permits most of the blood to bypass the fetal lungs.

Ductus venosus—The smaller, shorter, and posterior of two branches into which the umbilical vein divides after entering the abdomen of the fetus

Ectoderm—The outer layer of cells of an embryo

Endoderm—The innermost of the three primary germ layers of a developing embryo

Foramen ovale—The opening in the septum between the two atria of the fetal heart that permits blood to bypass the lungs by flowing directly from the right to the left atrium

Morula—Solid mass of cells resulting from cleavage of ovum

Ovum—The female reproductive or germ cell

I. The Process of Fertilization

The process of fertilization is the joining of an egg and a sperm. This union also results in a fertilized egg or **zygote.** The process of fertilization consists of many sequential steps that are necessary in the development of the pre-embryo, embryo, and fetus. This chapter will describe the process of fertilization and embryonic and fetal development.

A. Mitosis

Mitosis is the division of somatic (body) cells into two cells containing two identical sets of chromosomes. These cells are termed *diploid cells* and contain 46 chromosomes. (See Chapter 3 for further discussion.)

B. Meiosis

Meiosis is the division of germ cells, which produces 23 chromosomes. These cells are termed *haploid cells,*

as they contain half the genetic material of a somatic cell. (See Chapter 3 for further discussion.)

C. Germ cells

Germ cells give rise to egg or sperm (gametes).

1. Gametogenesis

a) **Oogenesis: Ovum** (egg) formation begins during fetal life in a female. All a female's ova are present at the time of her birth (Fig. 4.1).

b) Ovulation: Throughout a woman's reproductive years, one oocyte is released, usually once every month. An oocyte contains 23 chromosomes (haploid): 22 autosomes and 1 sex chromosome, which in the female is an X chromosome.

c) Spermatogenesis: formation of sperm in the male testicles.

d) Mature sperm contain 23 chromosomes (haploid): 22 autosomes and 1 sex chromosome—either X

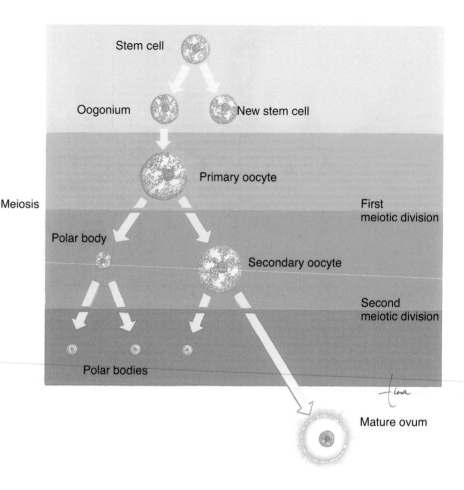

Fig 4.1 Oogenesis.

or Y; therefore, the male determines the sex (Fig. 4.2).
(1) XX = female
(2) XY = male

DID YOU KNOW?

The determination of sex is at the time of fertilization.

D. Fertilization
1. The union of an ovum and one sperm. This union creates a zygote, which contains 46 chromosomes (diploid).
2. Fertilization usually occurs in the ampulla (outer third) of the fallopian tube. At this point the ovum is impenetrable to other sperm, known as the *zona reaction.*

II. Pre-embryonic Stage

This stage is from conception to the end of the second week.
A. Cellular multiplication
1. After fertilization, a diploid number is restored in the resultant cell. Mitotic cell division (cleavage) of the zygote begins as the cell travels to the uterus. On day 3, a 16-cell

morula is produced, consisting of the following:
a) Inner solid mass of cells called the **blasto-cyst,** which contains an inner mass of cells called the *embryoblast.* The embryoblast

MAKING THE CONNECTION

Fertilization Process

After male ejaculation, the sperm cells go through several changes in the female genital before being able to penetrate the oocyte membrane. The first change is capacitation. The sperm cells accomplish this during the ascension through the female genital tract and uterine secretions. Capacitation changes take place with the removal of a glycoprotein layer in the acrosomal cap of the sperm. This process makes the acrosome reaction possible, which provides the sperm with enzymes that are able to penetrate the zona pellucida or outer layer of the oocyte. The constant force from the movement of the sperm's tail, along with acrosomal enzymes, allows the sperm to penetrate the zona pellucida and fuses with the plasma membrane of the oocyte. After fusion of the sperm with the oocyte, the sperm head is incorporated into the cytoplasm, resulting in a zygote.

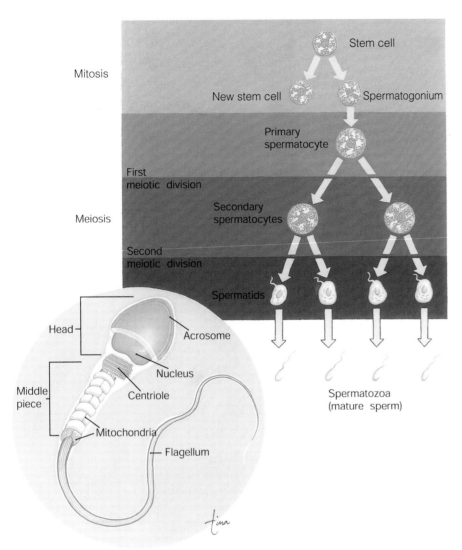

Mitosis

Stem cell

New stem cell

Spermatogonium

Primary spermatocyte

First meiotic division

Meiosis

Secondary spermatocytes

Second meiotic division

Spermatids

Spermatozoa (mature sperm)

Head

Acrosome

Nucleus

Centriole

Middle piece

Mitochondria

Flagellum

Fig 4.2 Spermatogenesis.

develops into an embryo that enters the uterus at 4 to 5 days.

b) The outer cell mass of the blastocyst is called the *trophoblast.* This outer cell mass becomes the placenta and chorionic villi.

c) Chorionic villi invade and destroy the uterine decidua while at the same time absorbing nutritive materials from it to support the growth of the embryo. Villi sprout from the chorion in order to give a maximum area of contact with the maternal blood.

B. Implantation (Nidation)

1. The blastocyst embeds into the endometrial wall at 6 to 10 days.

2. The woman may have implantation bleeding or spotting at this time. Implantation bleeding is one of the first pregnancy signs, but women often take this type of light spotting for their regular period (Fig. 4.3).

DID YOU KNOW?

The normal area of implantation is the upper posterior wall of the uterine mucosa.

C. Cellular differentiation

1. Two embryonic membranes form

a) Chorion—outer layer, covers fetal side of the placenta and contains chorionic villi.

b) **Amnion**—inner layer, which becomes a fluid-filled sac containing amniotic fluid (AF) that surrounds the embryo or fetus in the uterus.

2. Amniotic fluid

a) The volume is 600 mL to 800 mL at term.

b) The fetus swallows the fluid and urinates it, which increases fluid.

c) The fluid flows in and out of the fetal lungs, which helps in their development.

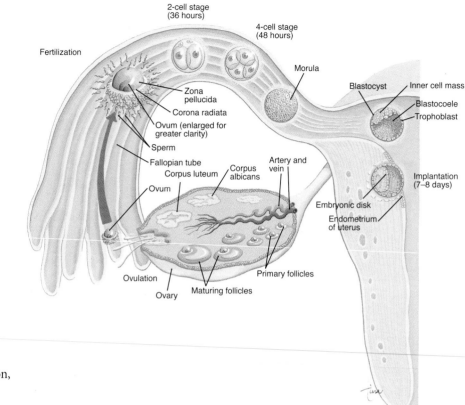

Fig 4.3 Ovulation, fertilization, and early embryonic development.

d) The functions of AF include temperature regulation, cushioning, musculoskeletal development, and as a repository for waste.
   (1) *Oligohydramnios* refers to a fluid volume of less than 300 mL due to a decrease in placental function. It is associated with renal abnormalities.
   (2) *Hydramnios* (polyhydramnios) refers to a fluid volume of more than 1,500 mL to 2,000 mL. It is associated with fetal gastrointestinal abnormalities and diabetes mellitus and causes overdistention of the uterus and can lead to postpartum hemorrhage.

MAKING THE CONNECTION

Amniotic Sac

The amniotic sac is filled with clear, pale, straw-colored fluid that provides an environment for the developing embryo/fetus. This environment allows for movement, temperature control, barrier from infection, detangling of the umbilical cord, and cushioning from trauma from outside forces, and it provides fluids to swallow. The amniotic sac starts to form and fill with fluid within days after fertilization. At about week 10, the fetus starts to pass small amounts of urine into the amniotic fluid. The amount of amniotic fluid increases gradually during pregnancy until about week 38. At this time the fluid reduces slightly until birth.

3. Umbilical cord
   a) The cord is 30 to 90 cm long (average 55 cm; 12–36 in./average 21 in.).
   b) It normally arises from the center of the placenta.
   c) It contains three vessels:
      (1) Two arteries that carry deoxygenated blood from embryo/fetus to placenta
      (2) One vein that carries oxygenated blood from placenta to embryo/fetus
      (3) Umbilical cord that contains Wharton's jelly, which protects the vessels
   d) A loop of umbilical cord around the fetal neck (nuchal cord) is a common finding at delivery.

🔔 **ALERT** An important nursing assessment after delivery is determining the number of vessels in the umbilical cord. A two-vessel cord may be associated with congenital abnormalities.

4. Twinning
   a) Dizygotic or fraternal twinning results from the fertilization of two ova with two different sperm.
      (1) The twins may be same sex or different sex.
      (2) They will be as alike as any two siblings.
      (3) They have two amnions, two chorions, and one placenta, which may be fused.
      (4) There is an increased incidence of twins due to use of fertility drugs.

b) Monozygotic ("identical") twinning results from one fertilized ovum, which later divides.
  (1) The twins are from the same genetic material, so must be the same sex.
  (2) The later the division occurs after fertilization, the more precarious the pregnancy becomes. Conjoined twins are monozygotic twins that divide later (13 to 15 days postconception).
  (3) The twins may have one or two amnions and one or two chorions, where possibilities include the following:
    (a) Diamnionic, dichorionic (di-di placenta), two placentae—may fuse
    (b) Diamnionic, monchorionic (di-mono placenta), one placenta
    (c) Monoamnionic, monchorionic (mono-mono placenta), one placenta. Least common and most dangerous, as umbilical cords may become entangled
c) Twin-to-twin transfusion syndrome (TTTS)
  (1) This is a rare condition that occurs in monchorionic, diamnionic twins.
  (2) Blood vessel connections are through a single placenta where blood flow becomes unbalanced.
    (a) One twin becomes the donor and gets decreased blood supply and is growth restricted and anemic, with resultant oligohydramnios from decreased urine output.
    (b) The other twin becomes the recipient and is larger, becomes fluid overloaded, and develops heart failure and hydramnios from increased urine output.
  (3) It is associated with high morbidity and mortality. All treatments are invasive.

III. Development and Function of the Placenta

A. Placenta
  1. The placenta starts to form at implantation and invades the decidua of the endometrium.
  2. Chorionic villi, projections of the chorion, become vascularized, which supports maternal–fetal circulation.
  3. The **decidua basalis** is the portion of the endometrium directly below the blastocyst and forms the maternal portion of the placenta.
  4. The **decidua capsularis** is the portion of the decidua covering the blastocyst.
  5. The decidua vera is the rest of the uterine lining.
  6. The functional unit of the placenta is made up of 15 to 20 lobes called *cotyledons.*
B. Fetal circulation (Fig. 4.4)
  1. The heart begins to beat around the 4th gestational week.

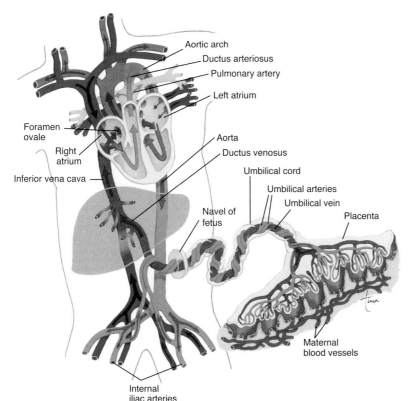

Fig 4.4 Fetal circulation.

2. Three shunts exist, which normally close after birth when lungs become functional:
   a) Ductus venosus—connects umbilical vein to inferior vena cava; delivers oxygenated blood to fetus while bypassing the fetal liver.
   b) Foramen ovale—blood flow delivers oxygenated blood from right atrium to left atrium while bypassing fetal lungs.
   c) **Ductus arteriosus**—blood flow delivers oxygenated blood from pulmonary artery to aorta.
C. Placental functions
   1. Metabolic and gas exchange
      a) Exchange of oxygen and carbon dioxide, delivery of glucose and amino acids
      b) Secretes hormones (endocrine function)
      c) Produces progesterone, which maintains the endometrium, decreases uterine contractility, stimulates maternal metabolism, prepares breasts for lactation (development of breast alveoli)
   2. Estrogen
      a) Stimulates uterine growth, prepares breasts for lactation (proliferation of glandular tissue)
      b) Stimulates myometrial contractility
         (1) Increase in estrogen and decrease of progesterone occur at beginning of labor
   3. Human chorionic gonadotropin (hCG)
      a) hCG can be detected 8 to 10 days after conception.
      b) hCG controls hormonal secretion of estrogen and progesterone by the corpus luteum until the placenta takes over.
      c) hCG is the basis for a positive pregnancy test.
      d) Human chorionic somatomammotropin (hCS) or human placental lactogen (hPL) regulates glucose available to the fetus, increases insulin resistance, and prepares breasts for lactation.

(!) **ALERT Teratogens** are agents capable of causing developmental abnormalities during the prenatal period. These agents may be environmental or chemical, such as medications, recreational drugs, and infections. The severity of damage is directly related to the timing and duration of the exposure during prenatal development. Most of the major organs are formed within the first 8 weeks of gestation when a woman may not even know she is pregnant. Exposure to teratogens during this time period can result in severe damage to the developing fetus.

IV. Embryonic and Fetal Stages

A. Embryonic and fetal development
   1. The embryonic stage is from 15 days until 8 weeks after conception.
      a) It is a critical time of development due to organogenesis (organ formation).
      b) Teratogens are substances such as drugs or environmental exposures such as x-rays that can cause congenital abnormalities.
      c) Primary germ layers form at around 14 days.
         (1) Ectoderm—nervous system, epidermis, enamel of the teeth
         (2) Mesoderm—dermis, bone and cartilage, muscles, heart and kidney, gonads
         (3) Endoderm (entoderm)—lining of gastrointestinal and respiratory tracts, liver, thyroid, pancreas, urinary bladder
      d) The yolk sac is a membranous sac attached to the embryo. It provides nutrients and produces blood cells in early pregnancy.
   2. The fetal stage is from completion of 8 weeks until birth (Table 4.1).
      a) By the beginning of the 9th week, the embryo has developed into a recognizable fetus.
      b) Crown-rump length is the measurement from the top of the head (crown) to the bottom of the buttocks (rump) of the embryo/fetus. It is determined by ultrasound imagery and used to estimate gestational age.

Table 4.1 Fetal Stage of Development	
Weeks Gestation	**Development**
12 weeks	Length is 7–9 cm.
	Weight is 20 g.
	Red blood cells are produced in the liver.
	Eyelids are closed.
	Fingers and toes are distinct.
	Placenta is complete.
	Fetal circulation is complete.
	Organ systems are complete.
	Fusion of the palate and nasal septum is complete.
	Fetal heart tone can be heard by Doppler device.

Table 4.1 **Fetal Stage of Development (Continued)**

Weeks Gestation	Development
16 weeks	Length is 10–17 cm. Weight is 55–120 g. Sex is differentiated. Rudimentary kidneys secrete urine. Meconium is formed in the intestines. Teeth begin to form. Sucking motions are made with the mouth.
20 weeks	Length is 25 cm. Weight is 223 g. Lanugo covers the entire body. Nails are formed. Brown fat begins to develop. Fetal movements are felt by mother (quickening).
24 weeks	Length is 28–36 cm. Weight is 680 g. Eyes are developed. Vernix caseosa appears. Alveoli begin to form in the lungs and surfactant production begins. Respiratory movement can be detected.
28 weeks	Length is 35–38 cm. Weight is 1,200 g. Eyes open and close. Adipose tissue develops rapidly. The respiratory system has developed to a point where the fetus has a good chance of survival if delivered at this time.
32 weeks	Length is 38–43 cm. Weight is 1,500 to 2,500 g. Bones are fully developed. Increased amounts of adipose tissue are present.
36 weeks	Length is 42–49 cm. Weight is 1,900 to 2,700 g. The face and body have a loose wrinkled appearance because of subcutaneous fat deposits. Lanugo disappears. Amniotic fluid decreases. Labia majora and minora are equally prominent. Testes are in upper portion of scrotum.
40 weeks	Length is 48 to 52 cm. Weight is 3,000 g. Skin is smooth. Eyes are uniformly slate colored. The bones of the skull are ossified and nearly together at the sutures. The fetus is considered full term at 38 weeks.

CASE STUDY: Putting It All Together

A 35-year-old gravida 3 para 1 female presents to the pre-natal clinic for an amniocentesis. Her first child was born 4 years ago and is healthy. The baby's father is a carrier for cystic fibrosis. She has a history of a spontaneous abortion (miscarriage) at 18 weeks in her second preg-nancy and is extremely nervous about the procedure. The patient also wants to know if her baby will have cystic fibrosis. She has no known allergies and her cur-rent medications are prenatal vitamins, one tablet daily.

Vital Signs

Height: 5'8" (172.7 cm)
Current weight: 185 lb (83.9 kg)
Prepregnancy weight: 145 lb (65.8 kg)
Temperature: 97.8°F (36.5°C)
Blood pressure: 110/68
Heart rate: 88 bpm, regular
Respiratory rate: 16 breaths per minute

Laboratory Data

Blood type and Rh: A negative
Antibody screen: Negative
Rubella: Immune
Hepatitis (HbsAg): Negative
HIV (3rd trimester): Negative
WBC: 8,000 wbc per mm^3

Objective Data

Nursing Assessment

Health Care Provider's Orders

1. Assess fetal heart rate prior and after the amniocentesis
2. Blood type and Rh on chart: Give RhoD immune globulin for Rh-negative client
3. Vital signs (V/S) prior and after the procedure

Case Study Questions

1. What *subjective* assessment findings indicate that the client is experiencing a change in clinical status?

2. What *objective* assessment findings indicate that the client is experiencing a change in clinical status?

3. After analyzing the data that has been collected, what *primary* nursing diagnosis should the nurse assign to this client?

4. What interventions should the nurse plan and/or implement to meet this client's needs?

5. What client outcomes should the nurse use to evaluate the effectiveness of the nursing interventions?

REVIEW QUESTIONS

Be sure to read the Introduction for valuable test-taking tips.

1. What are the number and type of chromosomes in a normal mature gamete?
   1. 22 autosomes
   2. 22 autosomes and one sex chromosome
   3. 46 chromosomes
   4. 23 autosomes

2. A 35-year-old woman is 34 weeks pregnant and is diagnosed with oligohydramnios. She asks the nurse to explain how this could affect the pregnancy. Which should the nurse explain to the client? *Select all that apply.*
   1. The baby's lungs may be underdeveloped.
   2. The umbilical cord may become compressed.
   3. The mother has developed diabetes mellitus.
   4. It is associated with fetal gastrointestinal abnormalities.
   5. The baby's limbs may be underdeveloped.
   6. The baby should be screened for renal abnormalities.

3. What is the point after which an ovum is fertilized and becomes impenetrable to any other sperm?
   1. The zona reaction
   2. Gametogenesis
   3. The zona pellucida
   4. Cleavage

4. Approximately 3 days after fertilization, what is the term for the developing zygote, which is a 16-cell mass?
   1. Trophoblast
   2. Morula
   3. Blastocyst
   4. Embryoblast

5. A 36-year-old G2P0 patient has been told that she has hydramnios. She asks what might have caused this and if it will cause complications. What is the nurse's correct response?
   1. "It is a decrease in the amount of amniotic fluid that occurs as a result of a neural tube defect."
   2. "It is an increase in the amount of amniotic fluid, which can compress the baby's cord."
   3. "It is an increase in amniotic fluid that can occur as a result of having diabetes mellitus."
   4. "It is a decrease in the amount of amniotic fluid that can cause preterm labor."

6. Expectant parents of twins tell the nurse they are having fraternal twins and are asking the nurse what that means. Which reply of the nurse is correct?
   1. "Your twins will both be boys."
   2. "Your twins are called *monozygotic*."
   3. "You have one placenta and one of each of the fetal membranes called the chorion and amnion."
   4. "Your twins will be as alike as any two siblings."

7. Conjoined twins are formed at which point of gestation?
   1. Immediately after fertilization
   2. At the time of implantation
   3. At about 13 to 15 days after conception
   4. In the blastocyst stage

8. Upon receiving report on a 36-week G1P0 patient, the nurse has been informed that the pregnancy is at high risk because the umbilical cords may become entangled. Which does the nurse understand about this pregnancy?
   1. It is a diamnionic, monochorionic twin gestation.
   2. It is a monoamnionic, monochorionic twin gestation.
   3. It is a monoamnionic, dichorionic twin gestation.
   4. It is a diamnionic, dichorionic twin gestation.

9. What is the portion of the endometrium beneath the blastocyst known as?
   1. Decidua basalis
   2. Chorionic villi
   3. Decidua vera
   4. Decidua capsularis

10. An expectant mother asks the nurse when her baby's heart will begin to beat. The nurse explains that this will occur at which time?
    1. The 8th gestational week
    2. The 4th gestational week
    3. The 12th gestational week
    4. The 16th gestational week

11. The time period immediately following fertilization results in which circumstance?
    1. Formation of a zygote that contains the haploid number of chromosomes
    2. Formation of an embryo that contains the haploid number of chromosomes
    3. Formation of a zygote that contains the diploid number of chromosomes
    4. Formation of a 16-cell morula

12. What is the hormone responsible for the mainte-
    nance of the endometrium during pregnancy and the
    maturation of mammary gland tissue?
    1. Estrogen
    2. Human chorionic gonadotropin (hCG)
    3. Prolactin
    4. Progesterone

13. The nurse is explaining fetal circulation to a student.
    Which statement by the nurse is correct?
    1. There is an opening between the atria that allows
       blood to flow directly to the lungs for oxygenation.
    2. There is a shunt between the aorta and the
       pulmonary vein that bypasses the lungs.
    3. The ductus arteriosus allows blood to flow from
       the pulmonary artery to the aorta.
    4. The foramen ovale closes just before birth.

14. During pregnancy, which structure secretes hormones
    until the placenta takes over?
    1. Decidua basalis
    2. Chorionic villi
    3. Corpus luteum
    4. Syncytiotrophoblast

15. Which immunoglobulin is the only one that crosses
    the placenta during pregnancy?
    1. IgG
    2. IgA
    3. IgM
    4. IgD

16. What is the function of the yolk sac in early
    pregnancy?
    1. Provides antibodies to the developing fetus
    2. Produces blood cells for the fetus
    3. Secretes hormones needed to support the pregnancy
    4. Becomes the placenta

17. The most critical time of development during preg-
    nancy is during organogenesis, where teratogens can
    cause congenital abnormalities. When is this time
    period?
    1. At the time of fertilization
    2. During the zygote period
    3. During the embryonic period
    4. At 20 weeks gestation

18. During formation of the germ layer in the embryo,
    which layer gives rise to the nervous system?
    1. Ectoderm
    2. Mesoderm
    3. Endoderm
    4. Entoderm

19. At which point in the pregnancy can a woman first
    feel fetal movement (quickening)?
    1. 12 weeks
    2. 16 weeks
    3. 20 weeks
    4. 24 weeks

20. At which point in the pregnancy are alveoli formed
    and fetal breathing movements noted?
    1. 12 weeks
    2. 6 weeks
    3. 20 weeks
    4. 24 weeks

REVIEW QUESTION ANSWERS

1. ANSWER: 2

Rationale

1. A cell with only 22 autosomes and no sex chromosome would not be normal.

2. A gamete is either an ovum or a sperm. These cells contain the haploid number (23) of chromosomes, which is half the normal number found in a somatic cell (46). There are 22 autosomes and 1 sex chromosome in each normal gamete.

3. There are 46 chromosomes in a normal somatic or body cell.

4. Twenty-three autosomes would not be normal in any cell.

TEST-TAKING TIP: Review the definition of germ cells (ova and sperm) if you answered this question incorrectly.

Content Area: Maternal Newborn

Integrated Process: Nursing Process—Assessment

Client Need: Health Promotion and Maintenance

Cognitive Level: Knowledge

Concept: Pregnancy

Reference: Lowdermilk, D. L., Perry, S. E., Cashion, K., & Alden, K. R. (2016). Maternity & women's health care. 11th ed. St. Louis, MO: Elsevier.

2. ANSWER: 1, 2, 5, 6

Rationale

1. Amniotic fluid is a necessary component of fetal lung development, and its absence may lead to pulmonary hypoplasia.

2. *Oligohydramnios* is defined as an amniotic fluid volume of less than 300 mL (normal is 600 mL to 800 mL at term). This can lead to compression of the umbilical cord due to the lack of cushioning from the fluid.

3. Diabetes mellitus is likely to lead to polyhydramnios or an increase in amniotic fluid.

4. Fetal gastrointestinal abnormalities are likely to lead to polyhydramnios or an increase in amniotic fluid.

5. Oligohydramnios can lead to decreased movement of the fetus, which can cause problems with musculoskeletal development.

6. A decrease in fluid may be due to a decline in urine output that stems from renal disease such as renal agenesis or malformed kidneys or urinary tract. The fetus/infant should be screened for renal abnormalities.

TEST-TAKING TIP: Review oligohydramnios and hydramnios with causes and effects. Rule out incorrect answers (3) and (4), which have the opposite results and produce hydramnios.

Content Area: Maternal Newborn

Integrated Process: Teaching/Learning

Client Need: Physiological Integrity—Reduction of Risk Potential

Cognitive Level: Analysis

Concept: Pregnancy

Reference: Lowdermilk, D. L., Perry, S. E., Cashion, K., & Alden, K. R. (2016). Maternity & women's health care. 11th ed. St. Louis, MO: Elsevier.

3. ANSWER: 1

Rationale

1. The zona reaction occurs after fertilization when the ovum is impenetrable to other sperm.

2. Gametogenesis is the process where cells divide and differentiate to form gametes.

3. The zona pellucida is one of the layers surrounding the ovum, which is essential for fertilization.

4. Cleavage is the division of cells that occurs in 3 to 4 days after fertilization.

TEST-TAKING TIP: Knowledge of the process of fertilization is needed to answer this question.

Content Area: Maternal Newborn

Integrated Process: Nursing Process—Assessment

Client Need: Health Promotion and Maintenance

Cognitive Level: Knowledge

Concept: Pregnancy

Reference: Lowdermilk, D. L., Perry, S. E., Cashion, K., & Alden, K. R. (2016). Maternity & women's health care. 11th ed. St. Louis, MO: Elsevier.

4. ANSWER: 2

Rationale

1. A trophoblast is the outer cell mass of the blastocyst, which is developed at 4 to 5 days after conception.

2. The morula is formed at day 3 and is a 16-cell mass.

3. A blastocyst is a developing embryo that enters the uterus at 4 to 5 days of gestation.

4. The embryoblast is the inner cell mass of the blastocyst, which is developed at 4 to 5 days after conception.

TEST-TAKING TIP: Review the process of fertilization and early fetal development if you were unable to answer the question correctly.

Content Area: Maternal Newborn

Integrated Process: Nursing Process—Assessment

Client Need: Health Promotion and Maintenance

Cognitive Level: Knowledge

Concept: Pregnancy

Reference: Lowdermilk, D. L., Perry, S. E., Cashion, K., & Alden, K. R. (2016). Maternity & women's health care. 11th ed. St. Louis, MO: Elsevier.

5. ANSWER: 3

Rationale

1. Neural tube defects are associated with an increase in amniotic fluid.

2. The baby's cord becoming compressed is more likely with oligohydramnios or a decrease in amniotic fluid.

3. Hydramnios or polyhydramnios is an increase in amniotic fluid volume. One cause of hydramnios could be diabetes mellitus.

4. Hydramnios or polyhydramnios is an increase in amniotic fluid volume, not a decrease.

TEST-TAKING TIP: Review the concepts regarding oligohydramnios and hydramnios if you were unable to answer the question correctly.

Content Area: Maternal Newborn

Integrated Process: Nursing Process—Analysis

Client Need: Physiological Integrity—Physiological Adaptation

Cognitive Level: Analysis

Concept: Pregnancy

Reference: Lowdermilk, D. L., Perry, S. E., Cashion, K., & Alden, K. R. (2016). Maternity & women's health care. 11th ed. St. Louis, MO: Elsevier.

6. ANSWER: 4

Rationale

1. A fraternal or dizygotic twin may be of the same sex or the opposite sex.

2. Monozygotic twins are derived from one zygote (one ova fertilized by one sperm) that later divides. They are genetically

identical and must be the same sex. Fraternal twins are dizygotic, as they are formed from two ova and two sperm.
3. Fraternal twins have two amnions, two chorions, and two placentae, which may be fused.
4. Fraternal twins will be as alike as any two siblings.
TEST-TAKING TIP: Review the cellular division in fraternal twinning if you missed this question.
Content Area: Maternal Newborn
Integrated Process: Nursing Process—Assessment
Client Need: Health Promotion and Maintenance
Cognitive Level: Application
Concept: Pregnancy
Reference: London, M. L., Ladewig, P. A., Davidson, M. R., Ball, J. W., Bindler, R. C., & Cowen, K. J. (2014). Maternal & child nursing care. 4th ed. New Jersey: Pearson.

7. ANSWER: 3
Rationale
1. A zygote is formed immediately after fertilization when it is too early for conjoined twins to be formed.
2. Implantation occurs at 6 to 10 days after fertilization when it is too early for conjoined twins to be formed.
3. Conjoined twins are monozygotic twins that divide later than normal (13 to 15 days postconception).
4. The blastocyst stage is at 4 to 5 days and is too soon for conjoined twins to form.
TEST-TAKING TIP: Review the process of twinning, including dizygotic and monozygotic zygotes, if you were unable to answer the question correctly.
Content Area: Maternal Newborn
Integrated Process: Nursing Process—Assessment
Client Need: Physiologic Integrity—Physiological Adaptation
Cognitive Level: Knowledge
Concept: Pregnancy
Reference: Durham, R. F., & Chapman, L. (2014). Maternal-newborn nursing: The critical components of nursing care. 2nd ed. Philadelphia: F.A. Davis.

8. ANSWER: 2
Rationale
1. The fetal membranes have two layers, the inner amnion and the outer chorion. In a diamnionic, monochorionic twin pregnancy, there is no chance of the cords becoming entangled since the fetuses have separate amniotic cavities.
2. In a monoamnionic, monochorionic twin gestation, there is a great chance of the cords becoming entangled since the fetuses share the same separate amniotic cavities.
3. A monoamnionic, dichorionic twin gestation cannot occur.
4. In a diamnionic, dichorionic twin pregnancy, there is no chance of the cords becoming entangled since the fetuses have separate amniotic cavities.
TEST-TAKING TIP: Review the anatomy and physiology of the amnion and chorion in a twin pregnancy if you were unable to answer the question correctly.
Content Area: Maternal Newborn
Integrated Process: Nursing Process—Analysis
Client Need: Physiologic Integrity—Physiological Adaptation
Cognitive Level: Analysis
Concept: Pregnancy
Reference: Lowdermilk, D. L., Perry, S. E., Cashion, K., & Alden, K. R. (2016). Maternity & women's health care. 11th ed. St. Louis, MO: Elsevier.

9. ANSWER: 1
Rationale
1. The portion of the endometrium directly beneath the blastocyst is known as the *decidua basalis.*
2. Chorionic villi develop from the trophoblast and become vascularized and provide nutrition to the fetus.
3. The decidua capsularis is the portion of the decidua covering the blastocyst.
4. The decidua vera is the rest of the uterine lining.
TEST-TAKING TIP: Review the process of fertilization and implantation if you were unable to answer the question correctly.
Content Area: Maternal Newborn
Integrated Process: Nursing Process—Assessment
Client Need: Health Promotion and Maintenance
Cognitive Level: Knowledge
Concept: Knowledge
Reference: Lowdermilk, D. L., Perry, S. E., Cashion, K., & Alden, K. R. (2016). Maternity & women's health care. 11th ed. St. Louis, MO: Elsevier.

10. ANSWER: 2
Rationale
1. The fetal heart has already begun to beat.
2. The fetal heart begins to beat in the 4th gestational week.
3. The fetal heart has already begun to beat, and at this time the heartbeat can be heard with a Doppler device.
4. The fetal heart should have already been heard by the 16th week.
TEST-TAKING TIP: Recall the fetal heart begins to beat in the 4th gestational week. Review fetal circulation if you were unable to answer the question correctly.
Content Area: Maternal Newborn
Integrated Process: Teaching/Learning
Client Need: Health Promotion and Maintenance
Cognitive Level: Comprehension
Concept: Pregnancy
Reference: Lowdermilk, D. L., Perry, S. E., Cashion, K., & Alden, K. R. (2016). Maternity & women's health care. 11th ed. St. Louis, MO: Elsevier.

11. ANSWER: 3
Rationale
1. Formation of a zygote creates a cell that contains the diploid number of chromosomes (46). Only gametes (ova or sperm) contain the haploid (23) number of chromosomes.
2. An embryo contains a diploid number of chromosomes (46) but the embryo stage does not begin until day 15.
3. A zygote is formed immediately after fertilization and contains 46 or diploid number of chromosomes, 23 from each parent.
4. The 16-cell morula is not formed until day 3.
TEST-TAKING TIP: Review the process of fertilization and the terms *haploid* and *diploid* if you were unable to answer the question correctly.
Content Area: Maternal Newborn
Integrated Process: Nursing Process—Assessment
Client Need: Health Promotion and Maintenance
Cognitive Level: Application
Concept: Pregnancy
Reference: Lowdermilk, D. L., Perry, S. E., Cashion, K., & Alden, K. R. (2016). Maternity & women's health care. 11th ed. St. Louis, MO: Elsevier.

12. ANSWER: 4

Rationale

1. Estrogen stimulates uterine growth and myometrial contractility. Its increase along with progesterone's decrease stimulates the onset of labor.
2. Human chorionic gonadotropin (hCG) is the hormone that increases after conception and regulates estrogen and progesterone until the developing placenta takes over.
3. Prolactin is a hormone secreted by the anterior pituitary that stimulates breast development and milk production.
4. Progesterone maintains the endometrium, decreases uterine contractility, and prepares the breasts for lactation.

TEST-TAKING TIP: Review the function of the four major hormones of pregnancy: progesterone, estrogen, hCG, and hCS/hPL if you were unable to answer the question correctly.

Content Area: Maternal Newborn
Integrated Process: Nursing Process—Assessment
Client Need: Health Promotion and Maintenance
Cognitive Level: Knowledge
Concept: Pregnancy
Reference: Lowdermilk, D. L., Perry, S.E., Cashion, K., Alden, K. R. (2016). Maternity & Women's Health Care. 11th ed. St. Louis, MO: Elsevier.

13. ANSWER: 3

Rationale

1. Fetal circulation allows for oxygenated blood to be supplied to the fetal body from the placenta. The vast majority of blood from the placenta bypasses the fetal lungs, as they are unable to oxygenate it before birth. The foramen ovale is the shunt that allows blood to flow from the right atrium to the left atrium to deliver oxygenated blood to the fetus.
2. The ductus arteriosus is the shunt from the aorta to the pulmonary artery, not the pulmonary vein.
3. The ductus arteriosus allows blood to flow from the pulmonary artery to the aorta.
4. The foramen ovale closes after birth, not before.

TEST-TAKING TIP: Review fetal circulation and the three shunts: ductus arteriosus, foramen ovale, and ductus venosus. Recall that the function of these shunts is to bypass the fetal lungs while the fetus is being oxygenated with placental blood.

Content Area: Maternal Newborn
Integrated Process: Teaching/Learning
Client Need: Health Promotion and Maintenance
Cognitive Level: Analysis
Concept: Pregnancy
Reference: Lowdermilk, D. L., Perry, S. E., Cashion, K., & Alden, K. R. (2016). Maternity & women's health care. 11th ed. St. Louis, MO: Elsevier.

14. ANSWER: 3

Rationale

1. The decidua basalis is the area of the endometrium directly below the developing blastocyst.
2. The chorionic villi develop from the trophoblast and become vascularized to provide nutrition to the fetus.
3. The corpus luteum develops from an ovarian follicle after it releases an oocyte in the luteal phase of the menstrual cycle.
4. The syncytiotrophoblast is the epithelial covering of the chorionic villi, both of which are part of the developing placenta.

TEST-TAKING TIP: Review the function of the four main hormones of pregnancy if you were unable to answer the question correctly.

Content Area: Maternal Newborn
Integrated Process: Nursing Process—Assessment
Client Need: Health Promotion and Maintenance
Cognitive Level: Knowledge
Concept: Pregnancy
Reference: Lowdermilk, D. L., Perry, S. E., Cashion, K., & Alden, K. R. (2016). Maternity & women's health care. 11th ed. St. Louis, MO: Elsevier.

15. ANSWER: 1

Rationale

1. IgG is the only immunoglobulin that crosses the placenta.
2. IgA does not cross the placenta to the fetus.
3. IgM does not cross the placenta to the fetus.
4. IgD does not cross the placenta to the fetus.

TEST-TAKING TIP: Review immunoglobulins in reference to pregnancy if you were unable to answer the question correctly.

Content Area: Maternal Newborn
Integrated Process: Nursing Process—Assessment
Client Need: Health Promotion and Maintenance
Cognitive Level: Knowledge
Concept: Pregnancy
Reference: Lowdermilk, D. L., Perry, S. E., Cashion, K., & Alden, K. R. (2016). Maternity & women's health care. 11th ed. St. Louis, MO: Elsevier.

16. ANSWER: 2

Rationale

1. The yolk sac does not provide antibodies.
2. The yolk sac produces blood cells and plasma early in gestation until the liver can take over.
3. The yolk sac does not secrete pregnancy support hormones.
4. The yolk sac does not become the placenta.

TEST-TAKING TIP: Review embryonic and fetal development if you were unable to answer the question correctly.

Content Area: Maternal Newborn
Integrated Process: Nursing Process—Assessment
Client Need: Health Promotion and Maintenance
Cognitive Level: Knowledge
Concept: Pregnancy
Reference: Lowdermilk, D. L., Perry, S. E., Cashion, K., & Alden, K. R. (2016). Maternity & women's health care. 11th ed. St. Louis, MO: Elsevier.

17. ANSWER: 3

Rationale

1. At the time of fertilization, teratogens have less effect on congenital defects.
2. Organogenesis occurs during the embryonic period, which is day 15 to 8 weeks of gestation.
3. During the zygote period (up to day 14), teratogens have less effect on congenital defects.
4. At 20 weeks, all organs are formed.

TEST-TAKING TIP: Recall that the first 2 weeks after fertilization is a less sensitive period and weeks 3 to 8 are highly sensitive periods where teratogens can cause untoward effects.

Content Area: Maternal Newborn
Integrated Process: Nursing Process—Assessment

Client Need: Health Promotion and Maintenance
Cognitive Level: Knowledge
Concept: Pregnancy
Reference: Lowdermilk, D. L., Perry, S. E., Cashion, K., & Alden, K. R. (2016). Maternity & women's health care. 11th ed. St. Louis, MO: Elsevier.

18. ANSWER: 1
Rationale
1. The ectoderm gives rise to the nervous system, epidermis, and enamel of the teeth.
2. The mesoderm gives rise to the dermis, bone and cartilage, muscles, heart and kidney, and gonads.
3. The endoderm (entoderm) gives rise to the lining of the gastrointestinal and respiratory tracts, liver, thyroid, pancreas, and urinary bladder.
4. The endoderm and entoderm are the same germ layer.

TEST-TAKING TIP: Review the primary germ layers in embryology if you were unable to answer the question correctly.

Content Area: Maternal Newborn
Integrated Process: Nursing Process—Assessment
Client Need: Health Promotion and Maintenance
Cognitive Level: Knowledge
Concept: Pregnancy
Reference: Lowdermilk, D. L., Perry, S. E., Cashion, K., & Alden, K. R. (2016). Maternity & women's health care. 11th ed. St. Louis, MO: Elsevier.

19. ANSWER: 3
Rationale
1. Twelve weeks is too early to experience quickening.
2. Sixteen weeks is too early to experience quickening.
3. The woman experiences quickening or the first feeling of fetal movement at approximately 20 weeks of pregnancy.

4. By 24 weeks, the fetal movements are becoming more pronounced and should have been felt for weeks already.

TEST-TAKING TIP: Review benchmarks in fetal development if you were unable to answer the question correctly.

Content Area: Maternal Newborn
Integrated Process: Nursing Process—Assessment
Client Need: Health Promotion and Maintenance
Cognitive Level: Knowledge
Concept: Pregnancy
Reference: Lowdermilk, D. L., Perry, S. E., Cashion, K., & Alden, K. R. (2016). Maternity & women's health care. 11th ed. St. Louis, MO: Elsevier.

20. ANSWER: 4
Rationale
1. Twelve weeks is too early for the alveoli to be formed or fetal breathing movements to be seen.
2. Sixteen weeks is too early for the alveoli to be formed or fetal breathing movements to be seen.
3. Alveoli are formed and fetal breathing movements can be observed by ultrasound at approximately 24 weeks.
4. By 24 weeks, alveoli are formed and fetal breathing movements can be observed by ultrasound. The fetus's lungs are still too immature to function outside the womb.

TEST-TAKING TIP: Review benchmarks in fetal development if you were unable to answer the question correctly.

Content Area: Maternal Newborn
Integrated Process: Nursing Process—Assessment
Client Need: Health Promotion and Maintenance
Cognitive Level: Knowledge
Concept: Pregnancy
Reference: Lowdermilk, D. L., Perry, S. E., Cashion, K., & Alden, K. R. (2016). Maternity & women's health care. 11th ed. St. Louis, MO: Elsevier.

Care of the Woman Across the Life Span

Chapter 5

Contraception

KEY TERMS

Basal temperature chart—A daily chart of temperature obtained upon awakening

Cervical cap—A barrier contraceptive device placed over the uterine cervix designed to prevent the entry of sperm into the womb

Coitus interruptus—Coitus with withdrawal of the penis from the vagina before seminal emission occurs

Condom—A thin, flexible penile sheath made of synthetic or natural material

Diaphragm—A rubber or plastic cup that fits over the cervix uteri used for contraceptive purposes

Postcoital—Subsequent to sexual intercourse

Sexually transmitted infections (STIs)—Any disease that may be acquired as a result of sexual intercourse or other intimate contact with an infected individual

Spermicide—An agent that kills spermatozoa

Spinnbarkeit—The amount of elasticity of cervical mucus, used to determine time of ovulation. The cervical secretion can be aspirated and placed on a slide.

Toxic shock syndrome—A rare disorder similar to septic shock caused by an exotoxin produced by certain strains of *Staphylococcus aureus* and group A streptococci

Vasectomy—Removal of all or a segment of the vas deferens

I. Natural Family Planning (NFP)

NFP consists of methods that are based on the examination of naturally occurring signs and symptoms of a woman's menstrual cycle. The avoidance of pregnancy is a naturally occurring process.

A. Basal body temperature (BBT) method
1. The BBT is the body temperature immediately after rising. The woman should be instructed to take her temperature first thing each day and plot the temperature on a chart.
2. Right before the time of ovulation, the BBT decreases slightly in some women. Right after ovulation, the temperature rises and remains high until 2 to 4 days before menstruation begins (Fig. 5.1).
   a) BBT is lower during the preovulatory phase of the menstrual cycle (97–97.6 degrees). The BBT is elevated a day after ovulation and is in response to the higher levels of progesterone released by the corpus luteum. (See Chapter 2 for further discussion.) The rise in temperature varies between women, and this method of birth control is recommended only for women with normal menstrual cycles. The BBT should be used to estimate ovulation within a 3-day range.

3. The BBT will remain elevated if pregnancy has occurred and will drop if a woman's cycle begins.
4. The fertile period is defined as the first day of the temperature drop through the third consecutive day of temperature rise.
5. Nursing education
   a) The client should be instructed to take her temperature at the same time each day when she first awakens in the morning and prior to getting out of bed. To be accurate, her temperature should be taken the same way each time (orally, axillary, or rectally).
   b) The thermometer used must measure the temperature within one-tenth of a degree.
   c) The client should be instructed to use a **basal temperature chart** and to begin charting on the first day of her menstrual cycle.

B. Cervical mucus method
Leading up to ovulation, cervical mucus becomes thinner, allowing the sperm to navigate easily into the cervix. The consistency and appearance of cervical mucus in a woman's most fertile period are similar to that of raw egg whites and can be stretched an inch or

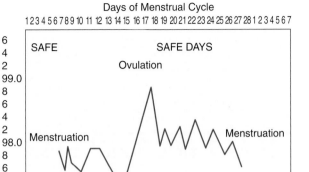

Fig 5.1 Basal body temperature chart.

two without breaking. This stretch ability is known as
spinnbarkeit.

1. To use this method of fertility awareness, a woman
must assess and understand the changes of her
cervical mucus throughout her menstrual cycle.
2. Certain types of mucus around the time of ovulation allow for greater motility and viability of the
sperm.
3. Nonfertile days begin on the fourth day following
the cessation of the wet, slippery type of cervical
mucus.
4. A woman must monitor her cervical mucus every
day for several months to learn her cycle. Every
woman is different in this manner.

C. Calendar rhythm method
1. The calendar rhythm method requires the woman
to monitor her menstrual cycle for the length of
cycle days (counting from the first day of menses)
to get an accurate determination of when ovulation occurs.
2. The beginning of the fertile period is determined
by subtracting 18 days from the end of the shortest
cycle.
3. The end of the fertile period is determined by subtracting 11 days from the end of the longest cycle.
4. This method can be difficult due to the unpre-
dictability of a woman's cycle and is recommended only in conjunction with other methods.

D. Coitus interruptus (withdrawal method) involves the
penis being withdrawn before the male ejaculates.
1. This method is only 71% effective because sperm
may be ejaculated prior to withdrawal.
2. This method requires significant control by the
male partner.
3. This method is highly discouraged as the only
form of contraception.

II. Spermicide

A. Spermicide is a chemical that decreases the motility
of the sperm and breaks down the cell membrane,
preventing it from reaching the cervical os.
B. It is available over the counter without the need for
a prescription.
C. Many products are available that use spermicides,
including condoms and intravaginal sponges,
applicators, films, creams, and gels.
D. A spermicide is recommended in conjunction with
diaphragms, condoms, and cervical caps.

III. Barrier Methods of Contraception

A. Male **condom** is a thin film sheath that's placed over
the penis. Condoms prevent pregnancy by keeping
sperm from entering a woman's body.
1. Condoms can be 80% to 90% effective if used
correctly. However, they must be used with every
intercourse and the correct size must be used to
be effective.
2. Condoms come either lubricated or nonlubricated.
The client can also add water-based lubricant to the
condom to make intercourse more comfortable.
Oil-based lubricants (e.g., petroleum jelly, massage
oil, body lotion) weaken condoms and may cause
them to break.
3. Many types of condoms are available—latex, latex-
free, spermicide, spermicide-free.
4. When used correctly during intercourse, latex
and polyurethane condoms are effective for
preventing pregnancy and **sexually transmitted
infections (STIs).**
5. No prescription is needed; they can be purchased
at drugstores.
6. Nurse education:
   a) The correct size condom should be selected to
   ensure proper fit.
   b) The condom is rolled on the erect penis before
   any sexual contact occurs.
   c) Use water-based lubricants for comfort if
   desired.
   d) A reservoir tip should be at the end of the penis
   for the collection of sperm.
   e) Pull out before the penis softens.
   f) Hold base of condom snugly against the penis
   when pulling out to ensure no spillage of
   semen.
   g) Use condom once and then throw it away.

🛑 **ALERT** Always assess for latex allergy when dispens-
ing diaphragms or male condoms. If client has hypersen-
sitivity to latex, dispense latex-free contraception
devices.

B. Female condom
 1. Female condoms can be 79% to 95% effective if used correctly with every intercourse.
 2. The female condom is a lubricated polyurethane pouch (one size fits all) that is inserted inside the vagina and secured around the cervix.
 3. The female condom contains no latex.
 4. It protects against STIs and pregnancy.
 5. No prescription is needed and it may be purchased at drugstores.
 6. Nurse education:
    a) To insert the condom, the woman should squeeze the inner ring and place it inside the vagina before any sexual contact occurs. The female condom may be inserted up to 8 hours prior to intercourse.
    b) To remove the condom, the woman should twist the outer ring and remove it carefully after intercourse.
    c) The woman should be instructed to use a new female condom with every intercourse.
C. Diaphragm
 1. **Diaphragms** can be 80% to 95% effective if used correctly with every intercourse.
 2. A diaphragm is a dome-shaped barrier covering with a flexible rim and is made of latex or silicone.
 3. Side effects include vaginal irritation and urinary tract infections.
 4. It is most effective when used with spermicide.
 5. A prescription and fitting by a health care professional is required.
 6. Nurse education:
    a) A diaphragm is used to cover the cervix, preventing sperm from reaching and fertilizing the ovum (Fig. 5.2).
    b) The diaphragm should be filled with spermicide prior to insertion.

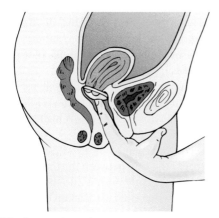

Fig 5.2 Diaphragm insertion.

   c) If the woman is allergic to latex, she should request a prescription for a diaphragm made of silicone.
   d) The diaphragm must remain in place for at least 6 hours after intercourse.
   e) Additional spermicide is needed each time the woman has intercourse.
   f) The diaphragm should be removed within 24 hours to avoid the risk of toxic shock syndrome.

🛇 ALERT Women using a diaphragm, cervical cap, or contraceptive sponge should be educated on the signs of **toxic shock syndrome** (TTS), including rash, dizziness, sore throat, fever, and vomiting.

D. Cervical caps
 1. The **cervical cap** is safe and can be inserted by a woman prior to use.
 2. The woman should place the cap prior to intercourse, and it can be worn for up to 48 hours. Some women find it hard to put in place or take out.
 3. Cervical caps require a prescription and must be fitted by a health care professional. One week after the first fitting, the woman should return to her health care provider (HCP) to check for proper placement.
 4. The cervical cap does not protect against sexually transmitted infections (STIs), including HIV, because of a high failure rate.
 5. Some women experience irritation or may have an allergic reaction to the spermicide or the cap if it is made of latex.
 6. Nurse education:
    a) Spermicide should be applied inside the cervical cap and a small amount applied to the outside.
    b) The cap should be inserted into the vagina and placed on the cervix, making sure that the entire cervix is covered.
    c) The cap may be inserted 6 hours prior to intercourse and should stay in place at least 6 hours after intercourse but no longer than 48 hours.
E. Vaginal sponge
 1. The vaginal sponge (containing spermicide) is 70% to 90% effective but must be used with every intercourse.
 2. The sponge does not protect against STIs, including HIV.
 3. Some women may experience irritation or allergic reactions with the sponge and may find it difficult to remove.
 4. The sponge needs to be removed 24 to 30 hours after insertion in order to avoid toxic shock syndrome.
 5. No prescription is needed and can be purchased at local drugstores.

6. Nursing education:
   a) The sponge should be placed inside the vagina prior to having intercourse.
   b) The sponge must be kept in place at least 6 hours after intercourse. It offers protection for up to 24 hours.
   c) The woman should be instructed that adding more spermicide each time she has intercourse is not necessary.
   d) Throw the sponge away after removal.

IV. Hormonal Contraceptives

A. Implants
   1. Are 99% effective
   2. Nexplanon
   3. Etonogestrel implant—single rod
   4. Progesterone only
   5. Long-acting and reversible
   6. Prescription and procedure required; completed in the clinic with local anesthesia
   7. Effective for 3 years
   8. Can be inserted anytime if reasonably certain a patient is not pregnant
   9. Try to insert during a woman's cycle
   10. If greater than 5 days since bleeding began, must use a backup method for 7 days
   11. Side effects include irregular bleeding

B. Combined oral contraceptives
   1. Combined pills contain two hormones, estrogen and progestin, and are taken every day. They prevent pregnancy by thickening the cervical mucus, thinning the uterus mucosa, and inhibiting the sperm from fertilizing the egg.
      a) Combined pills are packaged as 21 pills that contain hormones. One pill is taken daily for 3 weeks, followed by 1 week off. Others are packaged as 28 pills that include 21 hormone-containing pills taken daily, followed by 1 week of nonhormone pills.
   2. Progestin-only pills cause cervical mucus to thicken and the lining of the uterus to thin.
   3. Are 90% to 99% effective if used properly
   4. Does not protect against STIs, including HIV
   5. Prescription required
   6. Certain medications such as rifampin (taken to treat tuberculosis) and some supplements (e.g., St. John's wort) may make the pill less effective.
   7. Combined pills may cause nausea, changes in menstrual cycle, breast tenderness, or headaches. Medical history should be discussed with the HCP before any birth control pill is used, and the provider should be notified of any side effects.
   8. Contraindications: thrombophlebitis, severe diabetes, hypertension, smoking, cardiovascular disease, estrogen-dependent cancer, or benign or malignant liver tumors
   9. Side effects include irregular bleeding, sore breasts, nausea, vomiting, change in sex drive.
   10. Can reduce acne, cramping, and premenstrual syndrome.

(!) ALERT Women that are 35 years and older who smoke should not use estrogen-containing contraceptives as a means of birth control because of the increased risk for venous thromboembolism.

C. Transdermal Contraceptive (Patch)
   1. Small 2-in. beige square that delivers low levels of estrogen and a progestin that is absorbed through the skin
      a) Not recommended for women who weigh more than 198 pounds because of excessive adipose tissue and adequate absorption.
   2. Applied once every 3 weeks followed by one patch-free week
      a) During the week that the patch is not applied, breakthrough bleeding may occur.
   3. Side effects include skin irritation.
   4. Can be placed on the abdomen, buttock, upper outer arm, or upper torso.
      a) Should not be placed on breast.

D. Vaginal Contraceptive Ring
   1. The vaginal ring (NuvaRing) is a small, flexible plastic ring that is inserted in the vagina. The ring contains the same hormones (progestin and estrogen) found in most birth control pills.
   2. The hormones are absorbed into the bloodstream from the walls of the vagina and prevent the ovaries from releasing eggs. The hormones also cause the cervical mucus to thicken.
   3. The ring does not protect against STIs, including HIV.
   4. A visit to an HCP and a prescription are required.
   5. Certain medications such as Rifampin (taken to treat tuberculosis) and supplements (e.g., St. John's wort) may make the ring less effective.
   6. Some women experience vaginal discharge, vaginal discomfort, and mild irritation.
   7. There is a very slight increased risk of toxic shock syndrome.
   8. Like the combined birth control pill, use of the ring may increase the risk of blood clots, heart attacks, and strokes. This risk is higher in women who are very overweight.
   9. Nurse education:
      a) Squeeze the ring between the thumb and index finger and gently push it into the vagina. When first using the ring, use backup birth control (e.g., condoms) for the first 7 days after insertion of the vaginal ring.

b) The ring should be left in the vagina for 3 weeks (21 days) and then removed for 1 week. Menstrual periods will occur during the ring-free week. After the off week, a new vaginal ring should be inserted.

c) If the ring falls out and you are not able to replace it within 3 hours, another birth control method (e.g., condoms) should be used until the ring has been in place for 7 days in a row.

(!) ALERT Some medications may decrease the effectiveness of hormone-containing contraceptives. Education and a backup method are imperative for the patient to avoid pregnancy. The nurse should always closely monitor blood pressure in women taking estrogen-containing contraceptives.

E. Injectable
1. The birth control shot is an injection of progestin. The injection prevents pregnancy by keeping the ovaries from releasing eggs. It also causes cervical mucus to thicken and the lining of the uterus to thin.
2. The most commonly used injectable contraceptive is Depo-Provera (progestin only).
3. It is 95% to 99% effective if used properly.
4. It is reversible, given every 3 months.
5. A prescription is required and injection given as an intramuscular injection.
6. It is available for all ages.
7. It can be given at any time if reasonably certain that a patient is not pregnant.
8. If greater than 7 days past the start of menstrual bleeding, then a backup method should be used for 7 days.
9. This method is contraindicated in patients with diabetes.
10. Side effects include weight gain and irregular bleeding. Monitoring of body mass index (BMI)/weight is important while on this method of contraception.
11. This does not protect against STIs, including HIV.
12. It may take up to a year after stopping Depo-Provera to become pregnant, especially the longer the medication is used.
13. Some women experience side effects such as breast tenderness, spotting or bleeding between periods, weight gain, nervousness, abdominal discomfort, and/or headaches.

(!) ALERT When administering Depo-Provera, it is very important not to massage the site of the injection because this may increase the rate of absorption and decrease the effectiveness.

F. Intrauterine Devices (IUD)
1. IUDs are 99% effective in preventing pregnancy and are the most cost-effective, reversible method of birth control.
2. An IUD is a small T-shaped device that is placed in the uterus by an HCP.
3. IUDs can be taken out at any time if the woman desires to become pregnant.
4. A bimanual vaginal examination and cervical inspection are required before insertion.
5. It can be used by all ages whether the woman has had children or not.
6. STI screening is required yearly; it does not protect against STIs.
7. It is safe for use in obese women.
8. The nurse should provide counseling about the possibility of spotting or irregular bleeding.
9. Contraindications include pelvic inflammatory disease (PID), septic abortion, unexplained vaginal bleeding.
10. Nurse education:
   a) The Paragard IUD will prevent pregnancy right away. It may take a week for the Mirena or Skyla IUD to begin working, so advise the woman to use a backup birth control method, such as a condom.
   b) Once in place, Paragard IUDs are effective for 10 years or more. The Mirena IUD will last for at least 5 years and the Skyla IUD for 3 years.
   c) Common complaints after initial placement are cramping and spotting.
   d) The woman will be instructed to check for placement by making sure the IUD strings can be felt in the vagina.
   e) Seldom does the IUD come out. However, if this does occur, the woman should be instructed to call the HCP for reinsertion.
11. Types of intrauterine devices
   a) CU-IUD (copper)
      (1) Paragard
      (2) Made of plastic and a small amount of copper
      (3) 100% hormone-free
      (4) Can be inserted anytime during a woman's cycle with the reasonable certainty that she is not pregnant
      (5) Can be used within 5 days of unprotected intercourse as an emergency method
      (6) No need for backup contraceptives once it is properly inserted
      (7) Effective for 10 years
      (8) Side effects include cramping and heavy bleeding

b) LNg IUD (levonorgestrel)
  (1) Plastic
  (2) Not hormone-free because it releases a small amount of progestin to block sperm
  (3) No use of a backup method if it is inserted within 7 days of the start of the menstrual cycle
  (4) Backup method recommended if it is greater than 7 days after the start of the menstrual cycle
  (5) Effective for 5 years (Mirena)
  (6) Effective for 3 years (Skyla); smaller, good for women who have not had children

(!) ALERT Before any contraception is started, ensure that the patient is not pregnant. Take a thorough history to determine the date of her last menstrual period, last sexual intercourse, any current birth control, and birth history.

DID YOU KNOW?

In many states across America, an adolescent can be started on birth control without parental consent. This initiative was to help decrease the rate of teenage pregnancies. It is very important to be knowledgeable of the laws in the state in which a nurse is practicing in order to maintain proper confidentiality and permission standards.

V. Postcoital Emergency Contraception

A. Paragard IUD: can be used up to 5 days postintercourse
  1. Prescription and procedure required
B. Ella: 1 pill, blocks hormones needed to begin pregnancy
  1. Up to 5 days after sexual intercourse
  2. Prescription only
C. Levonorgestrel-based pills: Plan B
  1. No prescription needed
  2. High-dose birth control pills
  3. Up to 5 days postintercourse
  4. The longer after sexual intercourse, the less effective it becomes

(!) ALERT Emergency contraceptives are not a continuous form of contraception. Patient must be educated on another form of protection.

VI. Operative Sterilization

A. Vasectomy
  1. A surgical procedure consisting of ligation and severance of vas deferens. This procedure blocks sperm from entering into the semen. If all client instruction is followed, a vasectomy can be 99% effective and can result in a permanent contraceptive method.
  2. To ensure male infertility, the nurse should educate the male to use alternate forms of birth control for approximately 20 ejaculations or 1 week to several months to allow all the sperm to clear the vas deferens.
  3. Side effects include pain, infection, bleeding following surgery.
  4. Nurse education:
    a) After vasectomy, the male client should use scrotal support and only do moderate activity for a few days.
    b) Follow up with an HCP for sperm count.
B. Tubal ligation
  1. Tubal ligation is a surgical procedure consisting of severance and/or burning of fallopian tubes. This procedure results in the blocking of the fallopian tubes to prevent fertilization and is 99% effective.
  2. Side effects include pain, infection, bleeding following surgery.
  3. Tubal ligation may reverse itself in rare situations. There is a risk of ectopic pregnancy if this occurs.
  4. Nurse education
    a) The patient may have some slight vaginal bleeding.
    b) Stomach distention may be noted if a laparoscopy is performed. This should go away within a day. You may also have referred back or shoulder pain. This will go away as your body absorbs the gas.
    c) The patient may shower 24 hours after the surgery but should avoid rubbing or pulling on the incision for at least a week.
    d) Be sure to rest for a few days (or at least 24 hours) before beginning to resume normal activities. Patient should be able to resume all activities within 1 week.
    e) No backup method of birth control is needed after the surgery.
    f) A follow-up examination in 2 weeks is usually scheduled.

CASE STUDY: Putting It All Together	

Subjective Data

A 20-year-old client comes into the clinic asking to be started on birth control. She is trying to decide the best method for her. She does have a boyfriend but does not plan on getting married or have children anytime soon. She has a hard time getting up in the morning and has trouble remembering things due to her busy college academic schedule and social life.

Objective Data

Vital Signs
Blood pressure: 122/70
Pulse: 70
Temperature: 98.6°F
Respirations: 16
Height: 5'6"
Weight: 120 lb/BMI 18.5
General assessment within normal limits.
Pelvic examination and Pap smear: normal

Case Study Questions

1. What subjective assessment findings would you use to make your suggestion for a good contraceptive method?

2. What objective assessment findings would you use to make your suggestion for a good contraceptive method?

3. After analyzing the data, what would be the best contraceptive method for this client?

4. What education would be appropriate for this client?

REVIEW QUESTIONS

Be sure to read the Introduction for valuable test-taking tips.

1. A young girl comes to the OB-GYN office to begin contraception. What is the most important information the nurse should find in the history before starting a contraceptive?
   1. Do your cramps prevent you from daily activities?
   2. When was your last menstrual period?
   3. How much water do you drink?
   4. How many pads do you soak per day during your cycle?

2. A patient had unprotected sex yesterday. She is interested in emergency contraception. The nurse knows that the patient has how long to take the medication for it to be effective?
   1. 24 hr
   2. 48 hr
   3. 3 days
   4. 5 days

3. A 17-year-old patient receives emergency contraception in a clinic. What is the *priority* nursing education for this patient at this time?
   1. The need for further contraception because the emergency contraception is only temporary
   2. The need to protect herself from STIs
   3. The need to come back in for a pelvic examination 1 week after taking the medication
   4. The need to drink plenty of fluids while on this medication

4. The nurse is educating a male patient on how a vasectomy works. What is the *best* explanation for this procedure?
   1. The procedure blocks the sperm from entering into the semen and being ejaculated.
   2. The procedure removes the testicle so that sperm are not made.
   3. The tube that carries seminal fluid is blocked, causing no semen to be ejaculated.
   4. The procedure kills all sperm so they are unable to make it to the ovulated egg.

5. A 35-year-old patient comes to the clinic 2 days after a tubal ligation. She complains of abdominal pain and swelling and redness at the surgical incision. What does the nurse know is a common complication of this procedure?
   1. Ileus
   2. Liver enlargement
   3. Constipation
   4. Infection

6. A 28-year-old patient has decided to use the patch contraception. The nurse is educating her on the best site to use. Where is the *best* place to put the patch? *Select all that apply.*
   1. Buttocks
   2. Neck
   3. Breast
   4. Arm
   5. Leg

7. A patient is seen in the primary care clinic for a sinus infection and is prescribed antibiotics. The only other medication that this patient currently takes is an oral contraceptive. What is the *most* important education the nurse must give to the patient regarding her medications?
   1. If you have nausea with this combination of medication, make sure to take them with food.
   2. You must use a backup method for contraception while taking antibiotics.
   3. Oral contraceptives are contraindicated with many antibiotics.
   4. No education is necessary; these medications do not interact.

8. Which statement by the client would alert the nurse that she should not take oral contraceptives?
   1. "I drink one to two alcohol drinks a few times a week."
   2. "I am slightly overweight and have a difficult time fitting exercise into my schedule."
   3. "I am trying to limit cigarettes to one pack a week."
   4. "I try to have my boyfriend wear a condom every time we have sex."

9. Before giving a client oral combination contraceptives, which side effects should the nurse tell the patient to be aware of? *Select all that apply.*
   1. Irregular bleeding
   2. Thick vaginal discharge
   3. Nausea
   4. Breast tenderness
   5. Weight loss

10. A postpartum client is getting ready to receive a Depo-Provera injection. Which statement by the client indicates that further teaching by the nurse is necessary?
    1. "You will give this shot just like the rubella injection I received yesterday."
    2. "I will watch my weight and try to exercise daily after receiving this injection."
    3. "I will need to reschedule a follow-up appointment in 3 months."
    4. "It might take me a year to get pregnant after receiving this type of birth control."

11. The nurse is educating an adolescent patient about Depo-Provera. Which statement should be included in this teaching session?
    1. "You only need to come in every 5 months to get each injection."
    2. "You may lose weight on this medication, so make sure to maintain a well-balanced diet."
    3. "You may experience heavy bleeding or spotting monthly or none at all."
    4. "You will not be able to start this medication until you have been pregnant at least once."

12. A patient has expressed interest in receiving an implant for contraception. Which statements by the patient show that she understands the teaching given to her about her procedure and medication? *Select all that apply.*
    1. "I do not have to worry about getting pregnant for 3 years."
    2. "I will need someone to come to the office with me to drive me home the day of the procedure."
    3. "This medication could cause irregular bleeding."
    4. "I do not have to worry about STIs when I have this device placed."
    5. "The implant can only be placed the week prior to starting my menstrual cycle."

13. Which statement made by the client indicates the nurse's teaching about the IUD has been effective?
    1. "This device will keep me from getting a sexually transmitted infection."
    2. "I will need to check the attached string every month."
    3. "I will need to have my IUD placed 1 week after my period."
    4. "I will need to have the IUD replaced every year."

14. Which patient is contraindicated for the use of an intrauterine device for contraception?
    1. A patient hospitalized for PID
    2. A patient who has not had children
    3. A patient who is overweight
    4. A patient with heavy menstrual cramps

15. During a sexual history, the patient tells the nurse the only form of birth control she and her boyfriend use is the withdrawal method. What is the *best* education the nurse can give regarding this topic?
    1. "That will work for now, but as you get older you may think about getting on a prescription medication."
    2. "That method is very unreliable when used alone. You should consider using a backup method."
    3. "Withdrawal is a great method if you cannot pay for any of the other methods."
    4. "Withdrawal is just about as reliable as a male condom; however, it does not protect you from STIs."

16. A male patient comes to the clinic due to a severe inflamed rash on his penis and groin area. He says he used a condom this morning while having intercourse. What education should the nurse give the patient about his symptoms?
    1. "You will have to find a new form of contraception; you are unable to use condoms."
    2. "There are many types of condoms available. Try a latex-free version."
    3. "You will need to tell your partner not to use tampons during her cycle."
    4. "You should put hydrocortisone cream on this rash until it completely resolves."

17. A new mother is asking the nurse about birth control options. Which statement by the client is correct about breastfeeding and contraception?
    1. "As long as I only breastfeed for the first 12 months, I should be protected."
    2. "I should not supplement at all with formula if I am not using another form of contraception in the first 6 months."
    3. "I should use a combination hormone contraceptive while nursing just to be sure."
    4. "Breastfeeding is considered contraceptive before solid foods are introduced."

18. A 36-year-old female client comes into clinic to request birth control. In her history the nurse finds that she started her menses 10 days ago. What questions are important to assess in her history? *Select all that apply.*
    1. When was the last time she had sexual intercourse?
    2. When was the last time she took an antibiotic?
    3. Is she using any other form of birth control at this time?
    4. Does she smoke or drink alcohol?
    5. Does she have any chronic health problems?

19. A nurse is educating a patient on the basal body temperature method of family planning. The nurse should instruct the patient to take her temperature at what time?
    1. Immediately upon rising in the morning
    2. After she has a chance to wake up and get ready for work
    3. Immediately following lunch
    4. Once she is ready for bed at night

20. A patient using the basal body temperature method knows that she will see a temperature rise at what time in her cycle?
    1. Right before ovulation
    2. Right after ovulation
    3. Right before the start of her menses
    4. Only if a pregnancy has occurred

REVIEW QUESTION ANSWERS

1. ANSWER: 2
Rationale
1. This would be an assessment question concerning menstruation.
2. Important information for a thorough history should be date of last menstrual period, last sexual intercourse, any current birth control, and birth history.
3. This would be an assessment question concerning nutrition.
4. This would be an assessment question concerning menstruation.
TEST-TAKING TIP: It is very important to ensure that the client is not already pregnant. This initial assessment should consist of (1) having no signs or symptoms, (2) being 7 days or fewer from start of normal menses, (3) not having had sex since start of normal menses, (4) correctly and consistently using a reliable form of birth control, (5) being 7 days or fewer after a spontaneous or induced abortion, (6) being within 4 weeks postpartum, (7) fully or nearly fully breast-feeding, or (8) based on clinical judgment (consider human chorionic gonadotropin testing).
Content Area: Hormonal Contraceptives/Contraception
Integrated Process: Nursing Process—Assessment
Client Need: Physiological Integrity
Cognitive Level: Application
Concept: Sexuality
Reference: Lowdermilk, D. L., Perry, S. E., Cashion, K., & Alden, K. R. (2016). Maternity & women's health care. 11th ed. St. Louis, MO: Elsevier.

2. ANSWER: 4
Rationale
1. A woman has 5 days to take a **postcoital** emergency contraception pill to be effective.
2. A woman has 5 days to take a postcoital emergency contraception pill to be effective.
3. A woman has 5 days to take postcoital emergency contraception pill to be effective.
4. Taking any of the postcoital emergency contraception methods (Paragard, Ella, or levonorgestrel) up to 5 days after sexual intercourse will be effective.
TEST-TAKING TIP: The two methods of emergency post-coital contraception are hormonal methods and a copper-releasing IUD. Both types must be used within 5 days of unprotected intercourse.
Content Area: Postcoital Emergency Contraception/ Contraception
Integrated Process: Nursing Process—Implementation
Client Need: Safe and Effective Care Environment
Cognitive Level: Comprehension
Concept: Sexuality
Reference: Ward, S. L., & Hisley, S. M. (2016). Maternal-child nursing care. 2nd ed. Philadelphia: F.A. Davis.

3. ANSWER: 1
Rationale
1. The patient should be educated that postcoital emergency contraception will not protect her from future episodes of unprotected sex.
2. Education concerning protection should be addressed; however, this would not be the priority nursing education.

3. Following up in 1 week is not needed. The client should take a pregnancy test and/or contact her HCP if no period occurs within 3 weeks.
4. This is not necessary after postcoital emergency contraception.
TEST-TAKING TIP: Identify the word in the stem that sets a priority. The term *emergency contraception* in the stem sets a priority.
Content Area: Postcoital Emergency Contraception/ Contraception
Integrated Process: Nursing Process—Implementation
Client Need: Safe and Effective Care Environment
Cognitive Level: Application
Concept: Sexuality
Reference: Ward, S. L., & Hisley, S. M. (2016). Maternal-child nursing care. 2nd ed. Philadelphia: F.A. Davis.

4. ANSWER: 1
Rationale
1. During a **vasectomy,** the vas deferens from each testicle is clamped, cut, or otherwise sealed. This prevents sperm from mixing with the semen that is ejaculated from the penis.
2. The testicle is not removed during a vasectomy.
3. The testicles continue to produce sperm, but the sperm are reabsorbed by the body. The tubes are blocked before the seminal vesicles and prostate so the male will still ejaculate about the same amount of fluid.
4. The testicles continue to produce sperm, but the sperm are reabsorbed by the body.
TEST-TAKING TIP: Vasectomy is viewed as a permanent form of contraception and is 99% effective. Side effects should also be explained. These include infection, hematoma, excessive pain, and swelling.
Content Area: Operative Sterilization/Contraception
Integrated Process: Nursing Process—Implementation
Client Need: Physiological Integrity
Cognitive Level: Comprehensive
Concept: Male Reproduction
Reference: Murray, S. S., & McKinney, E. S. (2014). Foundations of maternal-newborn and women's health nursing. 6th ed. St. Louis, MO: Elsevier.

5. ANSWER: 4
Rationale
1. Ileus is a blockage of the intestines caused by a lack of peristalsis.
2. Liver enlargement is not a common complication of tubal ligation.
3. A woman may experience constipation after tubal ligation; however, abdominal pain, swelling, and redness at the surgical incision are not associated complications of constipation.
4. Infection is one possible complication of a tubal ligation.
TEST-TAKING TIP: Bleeding, infection, or reaction to anesthetic may occur after tubal ligation. Damage to organs, including the bowel, bladder, uterus, ovaries, blood vessels, and nerves can also occur. Abdominal pain, swelling, and redness at the surgical incision are signs of infection.
Content Area: Operative Sterilization/Contraception
Integrated Process: Nursing Process—Assessment
Client Need: Physiological Integrity

Cognitive Level: Application
Concept: Infection
Reference: Ward, S. L., & Hisley, S. M. (2016). Maternal-child nursing care. 2nd ed. Philadelphia: F.A. Davis.

6. **ANSWER: 1, 4**
   Rationale
   1. The transdermal patch may be applied to the abdomen, buttock, upper outer arm, or upper torso.
   2. The neck is not a recommended site for application of the transdermal patch.
   3. The transdermal contraception patch should not be applied to the breast.
   4. The transdermal patch may be applied to the abdomen, buttock, upper outer arm, or upper torso.
   5. The transdermal patch should be applied to the upper torso, not the lower torso.
   TEST-TAKING TIP: The transdermal contraception patch may be applied on the buttocks, upper outer arm, lower abdomen, or upper body. It should not be placed on the breasts or in a place where it will be rubbed, such as under a bra strap. Apply to skin that's clean, dry, and intact. Avoid areas of the skin that are red, irritated, or cut. Don't apply lotions, creams, powders, or makeup to the skin area where the patch is or will be placed.
   Content Area: Hormonal Contraceptives/Contraception
   Integrated Process: Nursing Process—Implementation
   Client Need: Health Promotion and Maintenance
   Cognitive Level: Application
   Concept: Sexuality
   Reference: Ward, S. L., & Hisley, S. M. (2016). Maternal-child nursing care. 2nd ed. Philadelphia: F.A. Davis.

7. **ANSWER: 2**
   Rationale
   1. Nausea and vomiting may affect the absorption of the hormones. The nurse should instruct the woman to use a contraceptive backup method for 7 days.
   2. When taking antibiotics, oral contraceptives cannot be relied upon and a second method of contraception is necessary.
   3. Oral contraceptives are not contraindicated when taking antibiotics.
   4. Education concerning the ineffective absorption of the oral hormone when taking an antibiotic must be done by the nurse.
   TEST-TAKING TIP: Antibiotics taken by mouth can potentially decrease the effectiveness of birth control pills (estrogen-containing oral contraceptives). This occurs because, in addition to killing the bacteria responsible for causing the current illness or infection, oral antibiotics also kill the normal bacteria that live in the stomach that are responsible for activating the birth control pill. As a result, the oral contraceptive may be less effective. Spotting may be the first sign that an antibiotic is interfering with the birth control pill's effectiveness. Review oral contraceptives if you missed this question.
   Content Area: Hormonal Contraceptives /Contraception
   Integrated Process: Nursing Process—Implementation
   Client Need: Physiological Integrity
   Cognitive Level: Application
   Concept: Infection
   Reference: Murray, S. S., & McKinney, E. S. (2014). Foundations of maternal-newborn and women's health nursing. 6th ed. St. Louis, MO: Elsevier.

8. **ANSWER: 3**
   Rationale
   1. Alcohol consumption is not a contraindication when taking oral contraceptives.
   2. Weighing over 198 pounds would be a contraindication with the transdermal contraceptive patch.
   3. A contraindication of taking oral contraceptives is if the client smokes cigarettes.
   4. Oral contraceptives would add protection from pregnancy for this client.
   TEST-TAKING TIP: Cigarette smoking (especially 15 or more cigarettes daily) and age (women older than 35 who are smokers or women who are older than 40 and nonsmokers) further increase the risk of stroke, blood clots, high blood pressure, and heart attacks.
   Content Area: Oral Contraceptives/Contraception
   Integrated Process: Nursing Process—Evaluation
   Client Need: Safe and Effective Care Environment
   Cognitive Level: Analysis
   Concept: Perfusion
   Reference: Lowdermilk, D. L., Perry, S. E., Cashion, K., & Alden, K. R. (2016). Maternity & women's health care. 11th ed. St. Louis, MO: Elsevier.

9. **ANSWER: 1, 3, 4**
   Rationale
   1. Vaginal bleeding between periods (spotting) or missed/irregular periods may occur, especially during the first few months of use.
   2. This is not a side effect when taking oral combination contraceptives.
   3. Nausea, vomiting, headache, bloating, breast tenderness, swelling of the ankles/feet (fluid retention), or weight change may occur when taking oral combination contraceptives.
   4. Nausea, vomiting, headache, bloating, breast tenderness, swelling of the ankles/feet (fluid retention), or weight change may occur.
   5. Weight gain from fluid retention is usually seen, not weight loss.
   TEST-TAKING TIP: Side effects are usually noted during the first 3 months after starting oral contraceptives.
   Content Area: Hormonal Contraceptives/Contraception
   Integrated Process: Nursing Process—Implementation
   Client Need: Physiological Integrity
   Cognitive Level: Application
   Concept: Female Reproduction
   Reference: Murray, S. S., & McKinney, E. S. (2014). Foundations of maternal-newborn and women's health nursing. 6th ed. St. Louis, MO: Elsevier.

10. **ANSWER: 1**
    Rationale
    1. The rubella vaccination is given subcutaneously and Depo-Provera is given intramuscularly in the deltoid or gluteus maximus muscle.
    2. Depo-Provera is associated with increased weight gain and reduction in bone mineral density.
    3. Depo-Provera is given every 3 months.
    4. If pregnancy is desired within a year, another form of contraceptive should be used.
    TEST-TAKING TIP: Depo-Provera is the brand name for medroxyprogesterone, a contraceptive injection for

women that contains the hormone progestin. Depo-Provera is given as an intramuscular injection once every 3 months. Depo-Provera typically suppresses ovulation, keeping ovaries from releasing an egg. Depo-Provera also thickens cervical mucus to keep sperm from reaching the egg. Review hormonal contraception if you missed this question.

Content Area: Hormonal Contraceptives/Contraception
Integrated Process: Nursing Process—Evaluation
Client Need: Health Promotion and Maintenance
Cognitive Level: Analysis
Concept: Family
Reference: Ward, S. L., & Hisley, S. M. (2016). Maternal-child nursing care. 2nd ed. Philadelphia: F.A. Davis.

11. **ANSWER: 3**
Rationale
1. This medication should be received every 3 months to be effective.
2. Weight gain is a side effect of Depo-Provera.
3. Irregular vaginal bleeding is a side effect of Depo-Provera.
4. This medication may be given to anyone who has not been pregnant or to anyone who has already been pregnant.
TEST-TAKING TIP: Irregular vaginal bleeding may be experienced in the first few months after starting Depo-Provera. After the second injection, the woman usually will experience amenorrhea.
Content Area: Hormonal Contraceptives/Contraception
Integrated Process: Nursing Process—Implementation
Client Need: Safe and Effective Care Environment
Cognitive Level: Application
Concept: Family
Reference: Lowdermilk, D. L., Perry, S. E., Cashion, K., & Alden, K. R. (2016). Maternity & women's health care. 11th ed. St. Louis, MO: Elsevier.

12. **ANSWER: 1, 3**
Rationale
1. Implants contain the hormone progestin and are effective for 3 years.
2. Placement of implantable contraceptives does not require sedation.
3. Irregular menstrual bleeding is the most common side effect.
4. Barrier protection must be used to prevent STIs.
5. The implant may be placed anytime during the menstrual cycle as long as the client has a negative pregnancy test.
TEST-TAKING TIP: A specific understanding of implantable contraceptives should direct you to options 1 and 3.
Content Area: Contraception
Integrated Process: Nursing Process
Client Need: Physiological Integrity
Cognitive Level: Application
Concept: Family
Reference: Lowdermilk, D. L., Perry, S. E., Cashion, K., & Alden, K. R. (2016). Maternity & women's health care. 11th ed. St. Louis, MO: Elsevier.

13. **ANSWER: 2**
Rationale
1. The IUD does not decrease the risk of contracting an STI or developing PID.
2. An IUD has a string made of plastic thread. One to 2 in. of this string hangs into the vagina. The client should be instructed to check the IUD string every 3 days for the

first 3 months after it is inserted. After that, the string should be checked monthly.
3. The IUD is usually inserted during the woman's monthly period. However, it can be inserted anytime during a woman's cycle with the reasonable certainty that she is not pregnant.
4. Depending on the type of IUD, the length of time it can stay inserted is between 5 and 10 years.
TEST-TAKING TIP: An IUD is a form of birth control that is inserted into the uterus. It is a small, flexible piece of plastic with a string on the end. IUDs prevent sperm from reaching or fertilizing an egg. They also prevent a fertilized egg from attaching to the uterus and developing into a fetus.
Content Area: Barrier Method of Contraception/Contraception
Integrated Process: Nursing Process—Implementation
Client Need: Safe and Effective Care Environment
Cognitive Level: Application
Concept: Family
Reference: Murray, S. S., & McKinney, E. S. (2014). Foundations of maternal-newborn and women's health nursing. 6th ed. St. Louis, MO: Elsevier.

14. **ANSWER: 1**
Rationale
1. A client with an active pelvic infection should not have an IUD placed.
2. IUDs are considered appropriate for the majority of women, including nulliparous women and adolescents. Both immediate postpartum insertion (within 10 minutes of placental delivery) and delayed postpartum insertion (within 4 weeks of placental delivery) are acceptable. Similarly, postabortion (spontaneous or elective) insertion is acceptable.
3. Weight is not a contraindication for IUD placement.
4. Heavy menstrual cramps are not a contraindication for IUD placement.
TEST-TAKING TIP: Ongoing pelvic infections such as PID, untreated cervicitis, puerperal sepsis, immediate postabortion or postpartum infection, endometritis, and pelvic tuberculosis are absolute contraindications for IUD placement.
Content Area: Barrier Method Contraception/Contraception
Integrated Process: Nursing Process—Planning
Client Need: Health Promotion and Maintenance
Cognitive Level: Application
Concept: Family
Reference: Lowdermilk, D. L., Perry, S. E., Cashion, K., & Alden, K. R. (2016). Maternity & women's health care. 11th ed. St. Louis, MO: Elsevier.

15. **ANSWER: 2**
Rationale
1. Using the withdrawal method for birth control requires self-control. Even then, this method isn't an especially effective form of birth control.
2. This method is only 71% effective because sperm may be ejaculated prior to withdrawal and is highly discouraged as the only form of contraception.
3. The nurse should explore with the client other forms of birth control.
4. Withdrawal is not as reliable as the male condom.

TEST-TAKING TIP: The withdrawal method of contraception, also known as *coitus interruptus,* is the practice of withdrawing the penis from the vagina prior to ejaculation. Using the withdrawal method for birth control requires self-control. Even then, the withdrawal method is not an effective form of birth control because pre-ejaculated fluid may enter the vagina. The withdrawal method doesn't offer protection from STIs.
Content Area: Natural Family Planning/Contraception
Integrated Process: Nursing Process—Implementation
Client Need: Health Promotion and Maintenance
Cognitive Level: Analysis
Concept: Family
Reference: Murray, S. S., & McKinney, E. S. (2014). Foundations of maternal-newborn and women's health nursing. 6th ed. St. Louis, MO: Elsevier.

16. **ANSWER: 2**
Rationale
1. The nurse should advise the client that he has a latex allergy from the condoms. She should instruct him to purchase the latex-free condoms next time.
2. This is the correct education concerning latex allergy and condoms.
3. Tampon use by the female partner does not have anything to do with the symptoms the male client is describing.
4. Latex allergy will disappear with discontinued use.
TEST-TAKING TIP: Latex is a milky substance produced by rubber trees. It is often found in rubber gloves, condoms, balloons, rubber bands, erasers, and toys. Latex allergies are most common in people who have regular exposure to latex products.
Content Area: Barrier Method Contraception/Contraception
Integrated Process: Nursing Process—Implementation
Client Need: Physiological Integrity
Cognitive Level: Analysis
Concept: Immunity
Reference: Lowdermilk, D. L., Perry, S. E., Cashion, K., & Alden, K. R. (2016). Maternity & women's health care. 11th ed. St. Louis, MO: Elsevier.

17. **ANSWER: 2**
Rationale
1. The client would be protected if she exclusively breastfeeds for the first 6 months and has not started menstruating.
2. Using breastfeeding as a contraceptive is acceptable if the client only breastfeeds, menstruation has not started, and her infant is less than 6 months of age.
3. Another method of contraception must be used if menstruation resumes, frequency of breastfeeding is decreased, supplementation with formula is used, or if the infant is older than 6 months.
4. Using breastfeeding as birth control can be effective for 6 months after delivery only if a woman does not substitute other foods for breast milk, feeds her infant at least every 4 hours during the day and every 6 hours at night, and has not had a period since she delivered her baby.
TEST-TAKING TIP: After 6 months, even if the woman is breastfeeding exclusively and she has not started to menstruate, she must use an additional form of birth control. If you missed this question, review Natural Family Planning.

Content Area: Natural Family Planning/Contraception
Integrated Process: Nursing Process—Evaluation
Client Need: Health Promotion and Maintenance
Cognitive Level: Analysis
Concept: Family
Reference: Ward, S. L., & Hisley, S. M. (2016). Maternal-child nursing care. 2nd ed. Philadelphia: F.A. Davis.

18. **ANSWER: 1, 3, 4, 5**
Rationale
1. Frequency of intercourse helps the nurse to determine the appropriate type of contraceptive.
2. This information would be essential only after the woman is already on oral contraceptives.
3. Before any contraception is started, ensure that the patient is not pregnant. Take a thorough history to determine the date of her last menstrual period, last sexual intercourse, any current birth control, and birth history.
4. Women who smoke and are over the age of 35 should not use estrogen-containing contraceptives as a means of birth control.
5. Some medication used for chronic health care problems such as diabetes, stroke, and so on, may be contraindicated.
TEST-TAKING TIP: When answering a "select all that apply" question, make sure you take time to understand the question before you look over the options.
Content Area: Hormonal Contraceptives/Contraception
Integrated Process: Nursing Process—Assessment
Client Need: Health Promotion and Maintenance
Cognitive Level: Analysis
Concept: Family
Reference: Ward, S. L., & Hisley, S. M. (2016). Maternal-child nursing care. 2nd ed. Philadelphia: F.A. Davis.

19. **ANSWER: 1**
Rationale
1. Basal body temperature is a person's temperature when they are fully at rest.
2. Taking temperature at this time will not give an accurate basal body temperature.
3. Taking temperature at this time will not give an accurate basal body temperature.
4. Taking temperature at this time will not give an accurate basal body temperature.
TEST-TAKING TIP: It is important to be able to accurately explain fertility-awareness-based methods in order to identify the client's fertile time and the use of abstinence. If you missed this question, review Natural Family Planning methods.
Content Area: Natural Family Planning/Contraception
Integrated Process: Nursing Process—Implementation
Client Need: Health Promotion and Maintenance
Cognitive Level: Application
Concept: Family
Reference: Lowdermilk, D. L., Perry, S. E., Cashion, K., & Alden, K. R. (2016). Maternity & women's health care. 11th ed. St. Louis, MO: Elsevier.

20. **ANSWER: 2**
Rationale
1. Ovulation occurs 1 to 2 days after an increase in basal body temperature.
2. The basal body temperature will rise after ovulation.

3. The basal body temperature will rise after ovulation and continue to stay elevated until the next cycle begins.

4. The basal body temperature will rise after ovulation and continue to stay elevated if she becomes pregnant.

TEST-TAKING TIP: Remember that before ovulation, a woman's basal body temperature is usually about 97.0° to 97.5°F. During ovulation, the body releases the hormone progesterone, which results in a slightly raised temperature—usually by 0.5°F—a day or two after ovulation. The temperature will probably stay elevated until the next cycle begins. If she becomes pregnant during that cycle, her temperature will stay elevated beyond that.

Content Area: *Natural Family Planning/Contraception*
Integrated Process: *Nursing Process—Evaluation*
Client Need: *Health Promotion and Maintenance*
Cognitive Level: *Application*
Concept: *Family*
Reference: *Lowdermilk, D. L., Perry, S. E., Cashion, K., & Alden, K. R. (2016). Maternity & women's health care. 11th ed. St. Louis, MO: Elsevier.*

Sexually Transmitted Infections

Abstinence—The practice of restraining oneself from sexual activity

Asymptomatic—Showing no symptoms

Bacterial infection—An infection caused by a microscopic single-celled organism (bacteria) allowed to enter tissues. Women may get a vaginal bacterial infection when the balance between good and bad bacteria is disrupted.

Condylomata—A wart, found on the genitals or near the anus, with a textured surface that may resemble cauliflower

Female condom—A thin rubber sheath inserted into a woman's vagina before sexual intercourse

Preterm labor—Labor that happens before 37 weeks' gestation.

Transmission—Exposure occurs through either direct or indirect contact. Direct transmission occurs when a pathogen, such as a bacterium, is transmitted directly from an infected individual to a noninfected individual.

Viral infection—An infection caused by a small infectious organism (virus) that invades cells and takes over the cell machinery. People may get a viral infection through sexual contact.

Sexually transmitted infections (STIs), also referred to as sexually transmitted diseases (STDs), are acquired through sexual contact with the penis, vagina, mouth, or anus of an infected partner. According to the 2014 fact sheet of the Centers for Disease Control and Prevention (CDC), *Sexually Transmitted Disease Surveillance* (available at www.cdc.gov/std/stats), nearly 20 million STIs occur each year, accounting for an estimated $16 billion annually in health care costs. The microorganisms that cause STIs may pass from person to person in blood, semen, or vaginal and other bodily fluids. Some STIs can also be transmitted from mother to infant during pregnancy or childbirth or through blood transfusions or shared needles. STIs can complicate pregnancies and have serious effects on the developing baby. See Figures 6.1 and 6.2 for illustrations of the female and male reproductive anatomy.

I. Types of Sexually Transmitted Infections

A. Bacterial infections
1. Chlamydia (*Chlamydia trachomatis*) is the most common reported STI in the United States. Coinfection with gonorrhea (*Neisseria gonorrhoeae*) often occurs.
   a) At-risk populations are sexually active teenagers and young adults (14 to 25 years old), men who have sex with men (MSM), and African Americans.
   b) Clinical manifestations consist of cervicitis (mucopurulent endocervical discharge) in women and urethritis (dysuria, urethral discharge) and proctitis (rectal pain, discharge, and/or bleeding) in both men and women.

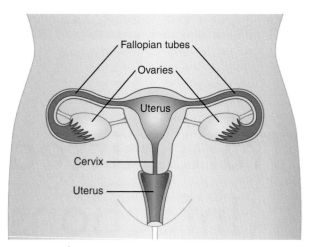

Fig 6.1 Female anatomy.

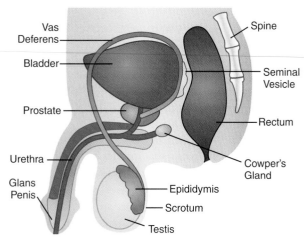

Fig 6.2 Male anatomy.

c) Diagnostic methods include urine testing or vaginal swabs. Specimens are screened using nucleic acid amplification tests (NAATs).

d) Recommended treatment is the antibiotic doxy-cycline (Adoxa) or azithromycin (Zithromax). For a complete drug and dosing regimen, refer to the CDC's *2015 Sexually Transmitted Diseases Treatment Guidelines,* available at http://cdc.gov/std/tg2015.

e) In women, pelvic inflammatory disease (PID), ectopic pregnancy, endometritis, and infertility are possible complications; in men, epididymitis is possible.

f) Untreated chlamydia in pregnant women has been associated with preterm delivery and with ophthalmia neonatorum (conjunctivitis) and blindness in the newborn.

g) Preventative measures include latex male condoms used consistently and correctly; abstinence from vaginal, anal, and oral sex;

or to be in a long-term mutually monogamous relationship with a partner who has been tested and is known to be uninfected.

h) Nursing considerations include facilitating notification of all anal, vaginal, or oral sex partners within the 60 days before the onset of symptoms or diagnosis was obtained for treatment.

i) The CDC recommends annual screening for all sexually active women younger than 25 years old, as well as older women with identified risk factors. All pregnant women should be screened for chlamydia at their first prenatal visit.

2. Gonorrhea (*Neisseria gonorrhoeae*) is the second most common reported STI in the United States with similar risk factors as chlamydia (*Chlamydia trachomatis*).

a) At-risk populations are sexually active teenagers and young adults (14 to 25 years old), MSM, and African Americans.

b) Clinical manifestations consist of cervicitis (mucopurulent endocervical discharge) in women and urethritis (dysuria, urethral dis-charge) and proctitis (rectal pain, discharge, and/or bleeding) in both men and women. Women can also present with symptoms of urinary tract infection or vaginitis. Men may complain of testicular or scrotal pain and present with creamy, yellow, sometimes bloody urethral discharge.

c) Diagnostic methods include urine testing or vaginal swabs. Specimens are screened using NAATs. The Gram stain best identifies gonor-rhea from the male urethra.

d) Recommended treatment are the antibiotics ceftriaxone (Rocephin) *and* azithromycin (Zithromax). For a complete drug and dosing regimen, refer to the CDC's *2015 Sexually Transmitted Diseases Treatment Guidelines,* available at http://cdc.gov/std/tg2015.

e) In women, PID, ectopic pregnancy, endometri-tis, and infertility are possible complications; in men, epididymitis is a possible complication. Untreated gonorrhea can lead to arthritis (painful joints) and meningitis.

f) Untreated gonorrhea in pregnant women has been associated with preterm delivery and with ophthalmia neonatorum (conjunctivitis) and blindness in the newborn.

g) Preventative measures include latex male condoms used consistently and correctly; absti-nence from vaginal, anal, and oral sex; or to be in a long-term mutually monogamous relation-ship with a partner who has been tested and is known to be uninfected.

h) Nursing considerations include facilitating notification of all anal, vaginal, or oral sex partners within 60 days before the onset of symptoms or diagnosis for treatment.

i) The CDC recommends annual screening for all sexually active women younger than 25 years old, as well as older women with identified risk factors. All pregnant women should be screened for gonorrhea at their first prenatal visit.

DID YOU KNOW?

Chlamydia trachomatis and *Neisseria gonorrhoeae* are known as "silent" infections because most infected people are asymptomatic and lack abnormal physical examination findings.

3. Syphilis (*Treponema pallidum*) (Table 6.1)
   a) At-risk populations are men and women who have unprotected sex and who are infected with other STIs. Syphilis is a major health problem, with increased cases occurring among gay, bisexual, and MSM populations.
   b) Clinical manifestations are divided into stages.
   c) Screening and diagnostic methods include two types of blood tests. Nontreponemal tests, such as the Venereal Disease Research Laboratory (VDRL) test, or the rapid plasma reagin card test (RPRCT).

d) Recommended treatment is benzathine penicillin G, 2.4 million units administered intramuscularly. For a complete drug and dosing regimen, refer to the CDC's *2015 Sexually Transmitted Diseases Treatment Guidelines,* available at http://cdc.gov/std/tg2015.

e) Preventative measures include latex male condoms used consistently and correctly to protect the infected area; abstinence from vaginal, anal, and oral sex; or to be in a long-term mutually monogamous relationship with a partner who has been tested and is known to be uninfected.

f) Nursing considerations include follow-up for identification of sexual contacts, contact notification, and contact screening. Encourage all clients with syphilis to be tested for HIV.

g) The CDC recommends that every pregnant woman be screened for syphilis at her first prenatal visit. Untreated syphilis in pregnant women results in infant death.

4. Pelvic inflammatory disease (PID)
   PID is a clinical syndrome that results from a polymicrobial infection. Microorganisms ascend from the cervix and vagina to the upper genital tract, causing an inflammatory response.
   a) At-risk populations include early age at first intercourse, multiple sex partners, frequent

Table 6.1 Stages and Manifestations of Syphilis

Stage	Clinical Manifestations	Diagnosis
Primary (2 to 3 weeks after exposure)	Chancre (firm, round, painless lesion) develops at the site where syphilis entered the body Swollen inguinal lymph nodes Untreated, resolves in 3 to 6 weeks	Direct identification of the spirochete obtained from the chancre lesion
Seconday (2 to 8 weeks later)	Fever indicating a generalized infection Maculopapular rash (flat, copper colored with small confluent bumps) involving the trunk and extremities, especially palms and soles of the feet Condyloma (large, gray or white lesions) that develop in the mouth, underarm, or groin area	Serological tests include nontreponemal tests (VDRL, RPRCT) followed by treponemal tests (FTA-ABS, MHA-TP)
Early latent (within 2 years of the initial infection)	Asymptomatic Greater chance of relapse Individual is more contagious	Positive serology
Late latent (occurs 2 years after the initial infection)	Asymptomatic	Positive serology
Tertiary (3 years after initial infection)	Damage occurs to internal organs, including the brain, spinal cord, eyes (Argyll Robertson pupils), blood vessels (aortic aneurysm), liver, bones, and joints. Symptoms include difficulty coordinating muscle movements, paralysis, numbness, gradual blindness, and dementia.	Positive serology
Congenital	Stillbirth	Mother tested positive for syphilis.

Reporting STIs

Local, state, and national agencies (e.g., county and state health departments or the CDC) require that *Chlamydia trachomatis, Neisseria gonorrhoeae,* and syphilis (*Treponema pallidum*) be reported by health care providers when they are diagnosed. Reporting of these infections allows for the collection of statistics that show how often the infection occurs. This helps researchers identify disease trends and control future outbreaks.

intercourse, intercourse without condoms, intercourse with a partner who has an STI, a history of STIs (most commonly caused by *Chlamydia trachomatis* or *Neisseria gonorrhoeae*), or previous pelvic infection. Pelvic infection can also occur just after menses, with invasive procedures such as endometrial biopsy, surgical abortion, hysteroscopy, or insertion of an intrauterine device.

b) Criteria for diagnosis consist of bilateral lower abdominal pelvic pain, adnexal tenderness, and cervical motion tenderness. Additional common clinical manifestations include increased vaginal discharge, elevated white blood cell (WBC) count, erythrocyte sedimentation rate (ESR), pain with intercourse (dyspareunia), urethritis (dysuria), and fever.

c) Diagnosis is based on physical assessment findings. The cervix is examined for abnormal cervical and vaginal discharge. An internal exam is done to assess for pelvic organ tenderness.

d) Treatment regimens must provide broad-spectrum coverage of likely pathogens, such as *Chlamydia trachomatis* and *Neisseria gonorrhoeae.* For a complete drug and dosing regimen, refer to the CDC's *2015 Sexually Transmitted Diseases Treatment Guidelines,* available at http://cdc.gov/std/tg2015.

e) Complications of PID include infertility, ectopic pregnancy, and pelvic adhesion, which can lead to chronic pelvic pain.

f) Preventive measures include abstinence, consistent use of barrier methods of birth control (condoms, diaphragms, and vaginal spermicides), and periodic screening for STIs.

g) Nursing considerations include educating women being treated for PID to abstain from sexual intercourse throughout the course of treatment. It is also essential to evaluate and treat male sex partners. Emphasis is placed on finishing all prescribed medications.

h) The CDC recommends screening of all sexually active women younger than 25 years, as well as older women with risk factors such as new or multiple sex partners or a sex partner who has an STI.

B. Viral infections
1. Human papillomavirus (HPV)
a) At-risk populations are sexually active men and women. There is an increased risk to individuals having multiple sex partners and having sex with a partner who has multiple partners.

b) Clinical manifestations result from the virus effects on the skin and mucous membranes through sexual contact. It is commonly spread during vaginal and anal sex. The most common strains of HPV cause **condylomata** (genital warts) on the female and male genitalia and can be found in the mouth. Most individuals with HPV never develop symptoms.

c) Some HPV strains affect the cervix, causing dysplasia, resulting in abnormal Papanicolaou (Pap) tests.

d) Treatment of external genital warts includes patient-applied topical application of podophyllin (Podofin 0.5% solution or gel) *or* imiquimod (Aldara 5% cream) *or* sinecatechins (Veregen 15% ointment). Electrocautery and carbon dioxide laser surgery are alternative therapies for clients with a large number or area of genital warts. Genital warts may resolve spontaneously. Podophyllin resin, interferon, and fluorouracil should not be used during pregnancy, because they can harm the fetus. For a complete drug and dosing regimen, refer to the CDC's *2015 Sexually Transmitted Diseases Treatment Guidelines,* available at http://cdc.gov/std/tg2015.

e) Complications of persistent infection can lead to cancer in both men and women.

f) Preventative measures include latex male condoms used consistently and correctly; abstinence from vaginal, anal, and oral sex; or to be in a long-term mutually monogamous relationship with a partner who has been tested and is known to be uninfected.

g) Nursing considerations include routine screening for women aged 21 to 65 years. Patient education should include the likelihood of recurrence in the first 3 months after treatment.

h) The CDC recommends vaccination of all boys and girls ages 11 or 12 years (before the onset of sexual activity), catch-up vaccines for males through age 21 and females through age 26 if they did not get vaccinated when they were younger, and men and women with compromised immune systems (HIV/AIDS).

DID YOU KNOW?

At least 40 HPV strains can infect the genitalia and perineum, including the skin of the penis, vulva, anus, and lining of the vagina, cervix, and rectum. HPV is so common that nearly all sexually active men and women get the virus at some point in their lives.

2. Herpes simplex virus

Herpes simplex virus 1 (HSV-1) is the main cause of herpes infections that occur on the mouth and lips. These include cold sores and fever blisters. HSV-1 can also be transmitted to the genitalia by oral sex. Herpes simplex virus 2 (HSV-2) is the main cause of genital herpes. Herpes simplex virus 1 (HSV-1) and HSV-2 can occur separately or together in the same individual.

a) At-risk individuals for HSV-1 are those in contact with the virus found in cold sores, saliva, and surfaces in or around the mouth and lips, and sexually active men and women participating in oral sex with someone infected with the virus. At-risk individuals for HSV-2 are sexually active men and women in contact with genital surfaces, skin, sores, or fluids of someone infected with the virus.

b) Clinical manifestations of a primary infection are localized to include bilateral painful genital lesions (that last an average of 11 to 12 days) and urethritis (dysuria, urethral discharge). Systemic symptoms peak within 3 to 4 days of onset of lesions and gradually recede over the next 3 to 4 days. Systemic symptoms include fever, malaise, headache, and myalgia (aching muscles). Asymptomatic infection is defined as infection in which serum antibody is present, but there is no known history of clinical outbreaks. Recurrent symptomatic infection is characterized by an illness lasting 5 to 10 days.

c) Treatment options include antiviral agents such as acyclovir (Zovirax), valacyclovir (Valtrex), and famciclovir (Famvir). For a complete drug and dosing regimen, refer to the CDC's *2015 Sexually Transmitted Diseases Treatment Guidelines,* available at http://cdc.gov/std/tg2015.

d) Complication of HSV-2 infection is both the acquisition and transmission of HIV infection. Even in the absence of genital herpes symptoms, HSV-2 infection increases the risk of acquiring HIV infection. Microscopic HSV-2-related ulcerations can provide a portal of entry for HIV, and HSV-2 reactivation recruits target cells for HIV to the genital skin and mucosa.

e) Preventative measures focus on proper hand washing after contact with lesions and latex male condoms used consistently and correctly to prevent the spread of genital herpes. In addition, individuals should be instructed to avoid oral contact with others and sharing objects that have contact with saliva. Abstinence from oral sex is encouraged to avoid transmitting herpes to the genitals of a sexual partner. Individuals with symptoms of genital herpes should abstain from sexual activity while experiencing any of the symptoms.

f) Nursing considerations focus on educating individuals on the clinical signs and symptoms of a symptomatic infection.

g) The CDC recommends patients with the first clinical episode of genital herpes be treated with antiviral therapy. This may have a drastic effect in initial HSV infection, especially if symptoms are less than 7 days' duration and there is no history of oral HSV.

3. Viral hepatitis B (HBV) (Table 6.2)

a) At-risk populations include men and women in contact with blood, semen, or other bodily fluids from someone infected with the virus. Transmission occurs during sexual contact

Table 6.2 Hepatitis Serology

Hepatitis B Surface Antigen (HBsAg)	Indicates the Person Is Infectious to Others
Hepatitis B surface antibody (anti-HBc)	Indicates recovery and natural immunity from HBV infection (the client has had hepatitis B)
IgM anti-HBc or anti-HBc IgM (IgM antibody to hepatitis B core antigen)	Appears at the onset of symptoms in acute hepatitis B and indicates previous or ongoing infection with HBV
Antibody to hepatitis B surface antigen (anti-HBs)	Anti-HBs is the test that should be ordered to assess whether the vaccine has been effective.
Hepatitis B e antigen (HBeAg)	Indicates the virus is replicating
Hepatitis B e antibody (HBeAb or anti-HBe)	Produced by the immune system temporarily during acute HBV infection or after a burst in viral replication

and through sharing needles, syringes, and other drug-injection equipment. Infants born to infected women are also at risk.

b) Clinical manifestations consist of fever, fatigue, loss of appetite, nausea/vomiting, abdominal pain, dark urine, clay-colored bowel movements, joint pain, and jaundice. Symptoms begin approximately 90 days after the exposure to viral hepatitis B (HBV).

c) Treatment for an acute infection includes supportive measures. Chronic HBV may result in cirrhosis of the liver or liver cancer.

d) Preventive measures for sexually transmitted hepatitis B include latex male condoms used consistently and correctly; abstinence from vaginal, anal, and oral sex; or to be in a long-term mutually monogamous relationship with a partner who has been tested and is known to be uninfected.

e) Nursing considerations focus on educating the client to the signs and symptoms of hepatitis B to prevent progression of the infection. Observe standard precautions to prevent disease transmission. Facilitate compliance to recommended vaccination to prevent the infection.

f) The CDC recommends vaccination of all infants, beginning at birth, and all children younger than age 19 years who have not been vaccinated previously.

4. HIV

a) At-risk populations include men and women in contact with blood, semen, or other bodily fluids from someone infected with the virus. Anal sex has the highest risk of transmission, with vaginal sex being the second highest. The most frequent mode of transmission is during vaginal sex.

b) Clinical manifestations of HIV vary depending on the phase of the infection. Early symptoms of HIV infection (acute HIV) consist of fever, fatigue, swollen lymph nodes, diarrhea, oral yeast (thrush), and/or shingles (herpes zoster). These symptoms may be mild and go unnoticed. **It is during this phase that the amount of virus in the bloodstream (viral load) is high and spreads more efficiently.** Clinical latent infection (chronic HIV) is characterized by persistent swelling of lymph nodes; otherwise, there are no specific signs and symptoms.

c) There are three types of HIV diagnostic tests: antibody tests, antigen/antibody tests, and nucleic acid tests (NATs). Antibody tests detect antibodies, proteins that your body makes against HIV, not HIV itself. Antigen tests and RNA tests detect HIV directly.

d) Treatment is with antiretroviral medications meant to extend the life span of an individual infected with HIV. There is no cure for HIV. For a complete drug and dosing regimen, refer to the CDC's *2015 Sexually Transmitted Diseases Treatment Guidelines,* available at http://cdc.gov/std/tg2015.

e) HIV remains in the body, and with no treatment the disease typically progresses to AIDS in about 10 years.

f) Preventive measures for HIV include latex male condoms used consistently and correctly; abstinence from vaginal, anal, and oral sex; or to be in a long-term mutually monogamous relationship with a partner who has been tested and is known to be uninfected.

g) Nursing considerations include promoting an interdisciplinary approach to care.

h) The CDC recommends HIV testing for at-risk populations to allow individuals to make better decisions about sex and health care.

C. Vaginal infections

1. Bacterial vaginosis is caused by an overgrowth of the bacteria *Gardnerella vaginalis* and a decrease or loss of *Lactobacillus acidophilus* normally found in the vagina.

a) Increased risk to women having two or more sex partners in previous 6 months and/or having sex with a new partner. Douching also contributes to an altered balance in vaginal bacteria, as does the use of antibiotics to fight an infection.

b) Clinical manifestations consist of a malodorous (fishy smelling) heavier-than-normal vaginal discharge.

c) Diagnosis is made by wet-mount microscopic detection of the causative organism. A positive whiff test is suggestive of bacterial vaginosis, as is a pH greater than 4.5 on a litmus test.

d) Treatment is with metronidazole (Flagyl). Metronidazole gel 0.75%, one full applicator (5 g) intravaginally, once a day for 5 days *or*

MAKING THE CONNECTION

Untreated STIs and HIV

Having untreated STIs such as chlamydia, gonorrhea, syphilis, and herpes simplex virus increases the individual's risk for contracting HIV. This is because a sore or break in the skin from an STI may allow HIV to more easily enter the body.

clindamycin cream 2%, one full applicator (5 g) intravaginally at bedtime for 7 days are also effective treatment options. For a complete drug and dosing regimen, refer to the CDC's *2015 Sexually Transmitted Diseases Treatment Guidelines,* available at http://cdc.gov/std/tg2015.

e) A complication in pregnant women is preterm labor due to chronic inflammation of the vaginal wall.

f) Preventative measures include latex male condoms used consistently and correctly. Wearing tight, nonabsorbent, and heat- and moisture-retaining clothing can also predispose women to bacterial vaginosis. Do not douche.

g) Nursing considerations include education on how to clean spermicide applicators and diaphragms after every use.

h) The CDC recommends treating women who are symptomatic. Treatment is not recommended for male/female sex partners of infected women.

2. Genital/vulvovaginal candidiasis (*Candidiasis albicans*)
   a) The at-risk population includes individuals with a weakened immune system.
   b) Clinical manifestations in women consist of vaginitis (itching, burning, redness, or soreness of the genitals), urethritis (dysuria), dyspareunia (painful intercourse), and a cottage-cheese-like vaginal discharge. Men with genital candidiasis may experience an itchy rash on the penis but are generally asymptomatic.
   c) Diagnosis is made by taking a sample of the vaginal secretions and looking at it under a microscope to see if an abnormal number of candida organisms are present.
   d) Several different antifungal medications are available to treat genital candidiasis.
   e) Complications include persistent, uncomfortable symptoms. There is also a chance that the infection may be passed between sex partners.
   f) Preventative measures include wearing cotton underwear to absorb moisture and keep the vagina dry. For women who experience recurrent yeast infections (more than three per year), some evidence suggests that oral or intravaginal probiotics may help to prevent frequent infections.
   g) Nursing considerations include educating women on the importance of accurately diagnosing genital/vulvovaginal candidiasis before treating themselves with over-the-counter preparations. Overuse of these medications increases the chance that the bacteria can become resistant to treatment.

h) The CDC recommends that individuals see their health care provider when experiencing symptoms of genital/vulvovaginal candidiasis, as they are similar to those of other STIs.

3. Trichomoniasis (*Trichomonas vaginalis*)
   a) At-risk populations are all sexually active men and women. During sex, the protozoan parasite is transmitted via the urogenital tract—from a penis to a vagina or from a vagina to a penis. It can also be passed from a vagina to another vagina.
   b) Clinical manifestations in women consist of vaginitis (itching, burning, redness, or soreness of the genitals), urethritis (dysuria), and dyspareunia (painful intercourse). A classic symptom in women is the presence of a yellow to yellow-green, malodorous (foul-smelling), "frothy" discharge. Men are asymptomatic carriers.
   c) Diagnosis is made by wet-mount microscopic detection of the causative organism or by a specialized vaginal culture. Inspection with a speculum often reveals vaginal and cervical redness with multiple small petechiae. A pH is greater than 4.5 on a litmus test.
   d) Treatment is with prescription antibiotic medication, either metronidazole (Flagyl) orally in a single dose or tinidazole (Tindamax) orally in a single dose. For a complete drug and dosing regimen, refer to the CDC's *2015 Sexually Transmitted Diseases Treatment Guidelines,* available at http://cdc.gov/std/tg2015.
   e) A complication in pregnant women is preterm labor due to chronic inflammation of the vaginal wall.
   f) Preventative measures include latex male condoms used consistently and correctly, abstinence from vaginal sex, or to be in a long-term mutually monogamous relationship with a partner who has been tested and is known to be uninfected.
   g) Nursing consideration includes follow-up for identification of sexual contacts, contact notification, and contact screening for treatment. Abstaining from sexual activity until both partners are treated is important.
   h) The CDC recommends that individuals infected with *Trichomoniasis vaginalis* be tested for other STIs.

DID YOU KNOW?
Individuals taking metronidazole (Flagyl) must be instructed to avoid alcohol consumption during and 24 hours after treatment to prevent significant gastrointestinal upset.

MAKING THE CONNECTION

Testing for Bacterial Vaginitis

A client who complains of vaginal discharge, itching, burning, and/or dysuria should be evaluated for vaginitis. A vaginitis test (wet mount) is done by taking a sample of vaginal discharge, placing it on a glass slide, and mixing it with a salt solution for microscopic examination. A second specimen of the vaginal discharge should be placed on a slide with a 10% KOH solution. During preparation of the KOH slide, a whiff test can be performed. The whiff test is positive if a "fishy" or amine odor is detected when KOH is added to the vaginal discharge. A positive whiff test is suggestive of bacterial vaginosis. A litmus test for pH greater than 4.5 is found in clients with trichomoniasis or bacterial vaginitis.

CASE STUDY: Putting It All Together

Subjective Data

A 22-year-old female college student presents to a community clinic seeking advice about contraception. She is shy when it comes to talking about her sexual practices and has never had a pelvic exam. She reports having two sex partners in the past 6 months and does not use condoms or any other form of contraception. Her periods have been regular until recently when she noted some "spotting between periods." Her last menstrual period was 4 weeks ago. She denies an increase in vaginal discharge, dysuria, dyspareunia, and genital lesions or sores. She has no known allergies and no current medications.

Objective Data

Vital Signs
Blood pressure: 118/68
Pulse: 74 beats per minute
Respiration: 18 breaths per minute
Temperature: 98.7°F (37.1°C)

Nursing Assessment
1. Breast, thyroid, and abdominal exam is within normal limits.
2. The genital exam reveals normal vulva and vagina.
3. The cervix appears inflamed and bleeds easily with swab insertion for diagnostic testing, and there is a purulent discharge coming from the cervical opening.
4. The bimanual exam is normal without cervical motion pain or uterine or adnexal tenderness.
5. NAAT for *Chlamydia trachomatis* is positive.
6. NAAT for *Neisseria gonorrhoeae* is negative; rapid plasma reagin is nonreactive.
7. Wet mount reveals a pH of 4.2, no clue cells or trichomonads, and numerous WBCs.
8. KOH preparation is negative for whiff test.
9. HIV antibody test is negative.
10. Pregnancy test is negative.

Case Study Questions

1. What subjective assessment findings indicate that the client is experiencing a health alteration?

2. What objective assessment findings indicate the client is experiencing a health alteration?

3. After analyzing the data that you have collected, what primary nursing diagnosis should the nurse assign to the client?

4. What interventions should the nurse plan and/or implement to meet this client's needs?

5. What client outcomes should the nurse use to evaluate the effectiveness of the nursing interventions?

REVIEW QUESTIONS

Be sure to read the Introduction for valuable test-taking tips.

1. A public health nurse is teaching a group about STIs at a local community center. Which statement made by the group demonstrates a good understanding of the disease process?
   1. "The infection can only be spread when a person is symptomatic."
   2. "I can only get the disease through vaginal intercourse."
   3. "Sexual partners of the infected person must also be treated."
   4. "Oral contraceptives are effective in protecting against STIs."

2. A nurse working in a community clinic is teaching a client about chlamydia. Which statement made by the client would indicate a need for further instruction?
   1. "Treatment is also required for individuals who are asymptomatic."
   2. "Individuals can only spread the infection if symptomatic."
   3. "All pregnant women should be screened for chlamydia."
   4. "Any sexually active individuals can be infected with chlamydia."

3. A client is being treated for gonorrhea. Which medication combination should the nurse expect to be prescribed?
   1. Ceftriaxone and azithromycin
   2. Penicillin and ceftriaxone
   3. Tetracycline and azithromycin
   4. Levofloxacin and azithromycin

4. A male client reports painful urination and a creamy yellow drainage from the urethra. During the assessment, he admits to having unprotected sex. With which STI does the nurse associate these clinical manifestations?
   1. Candidiasis
   2. HPV
   3. Trichomoniasis
   4. Gonorrhea

5. A client comes to a community clinic after being informed by a sexual partner of possible recent exposure to syphilis. The nurse will examine the client for which clinical manifestation of syphilis in the primary stage?
   1. Chancre
   2. Copper-colored rash involving the trunk and extremities
   3. Flulike symptoms
   4. Condyloma lata

6. During the physical assessment of a female client with HPV, which should the nurse expect to find?
   1. Purulent vaginal discharge
   2. Condylomata
   3. Malodorous vaginal discharge
   4. No clinical manifestation

7. A 20-year-old college student expresses concern over the recent appearance of genital warts, an assessment finding her primary care provider confirms as attributable to HPV infection. Which client education should be included?
   1. "It's important to start treatment as soon as possible, so you will receive a prescription for pills today."
   2. "There is a chance that the genital warts will clear up on their own without any treatment."
   3. "I recommend receiving an HPV vaccination today."
   4. "Unfortunately, this is going to greatly increase your chance of developing pelvic inflammatory disease."

8. A pregnant woman at 30 weeks gestation discovers she is HPV positive at her prenatal visit. Upon examination, her provider detects genital warts. Which treatment is *not* recommended in this case?
   1. Carbon dioxide laser surgery
   2. Electrocautery
   3. Surgical excision
   4. Podophyllin

9. A client comes to an outpatient clinic for evaluation. What in the client's blood sample reveals that administration of the hepatitis B vaccine has been effective?
   1. Hepatitis B surface antigen (HBsAg)
   2. anti-HBs
   3. anti-HBc IgM
   4. anti-HBc

10. An absence of what may facilitate the occurrence of bacterial vaginosis?
    1. Antibodies
    2. *Lactobacillus acidophilus*
    3. *Gardnerella vaginalis*
    4. Vaginal mucosa

11. Which best describes the signs and symptoms of trichomoniasis in women?
    1. Foul, fishy odor and thick clumpy white vaginal discharge
    2. Malodorous, frothy yellow-green vaginal discharge
    3. Dysuria and thin milky-white vaginal discharge
    4. Condition is asymptomatic in women

12. A client with a history of herpes simplex virus (HSV-2) infection asks the nurse about future sexual activity. Which response is *most* appropriate?
    1. "If the infection has healed, you do not have to use a condom."
    2. "Refrain from all sexual activity."
    3. "Use a condom during sexual activity only if the infection becomes active again."
    4. "Inform all potential sexual partners about the infection, even if it is inactive."

13. A client has an HSV-2 infection. The nurse recognizes that which of the following should be included in teaching the patient?
    1. The virus causes cold sores of the lips.
    2. Treatment is focused on relieving symptoms.
    3. The virus is cured with antibiotics.
    4. The virus is transmitted only when visible lesions are present.

14. A male client is being seen by a physician at a community clinic regarding a painless ulcer on his penis. The provider will be communicating his diagnosis of syphilis and prescribing treatment. In the primary stage of syphilis, what is the time between infection and development of symptoms?
    1. 7 days
    2. 10 days
    3. 21 days
    4. 35 days

15. A nurse is teaching a community health class of women and explains that an STI is associated with an increased risk of infertility in women. Which STIs should the nurse identify?
    1. HSV-2
    2. Syphilis
    3. Chlamydia
    4. HPV

16. A nurse is developing a plan of care for a 16-year-old female client experiencing her first outbreak of genital herpes. The client states that she contracted the disease by holding hands with someone who has syphilis. Which nursing diagnosis should the nurse identify as the *priority*?
    1. Acute pain related to the development of genital lesions
    2. Lack of knowledge about the disease and its transmission
    3. Ineffective coping related to the increased stress associated with the infection
    4. Noncompliance with treatment related to age of the client

17. When the client is started on antiretroviral drugs for HIV, what will be important for the nurse to teach the client?
    1. "This drug will cure the disease over a period of time."
    2. "This drug will not cure the disease but could extend your life expectancy."
    3. "This type of drug will be used prior to vaccines."
    4. "This drug is readily available all over the world."

18. A client who has been diagnosed with HIV develops an oral candida infection. When teaching the client, which instructions will the health care provider include?
    1. "Rinse your mouth often with a commercial mouthwash."
    2. "Include plenty of citrus juices in your diet."
    3. "Select foods that are soft or pureed."
    4. "Include hot soups and beverages with each meal."

19. How does HPV manifest in HIV-positive clients?
    1. Cough
    2. Condylomata lata
    3. Condylomata
    4. Chancre

20. The client receives zidovudine (Retrovir) for treatment of HIV infection. Which assessment data indicates an adverse reaction to the drug?
    1. Cough
    2. Enlarged lymph nodes
    3. Decreased WBC count
    4. Fever

1. ANSWER: 3
Rationale
1. Most infected people are asymptomatic and lack abnormal physical examination findings.
2. The microorganisms that cause STIs may pass from person to person in blood, semen, or vaginal and other bodily fluids.
3. Treatment extends to sexual partners of the infected person to help prevent transmission.
4. Preventative measures include latex male condoms used consistently and correctly; abstinence from vaginal, anal, and oral sex; or to be in a long-term mutually monogamous relationship with a partner who has been tested and is known to be uninfected.
TEST-TAKING TIP: Read each question to identify the correct statements about STIs. Once an incorrect statement is identified, that will be your answer.
Content Area: Sexually Transmitted Infections
Integrated Process: Nursing Process—Assessment
Client Need: Health Promotion and Maintenance
Cognitive Level: Analysis
Concept: Sexuality
Reference: Centers for Disease Control and Prevention. (2015). Sexually Transmitted Diseases. Retrieved from www.cdc.gov/std/.
Pellico, L. H. (2013). Focus on adult health medical-surgical nursing. Philadelphia: Lippincott Williams and Wilkins.

2. ANSWER: 2
Rationale
1. Most infected individuals are asymptomatic and lack abnormal physical examination findings.
2. Nursing considerations include facilitating notification of all anal, vaginal, or oral sex partners the client had in the 60 days *before* the onset of symptoms or diagnosis for treatment.
3. All pregnant women should be screened for chlamydia at their first prenatal visit.
4. Chlamydia is the most commonly reported STI, especially among sexually active teenagers and young adults (14 to 25 years old), MSM, and African Americans.
TEST-TAKING TIP: Read each answer to determine if it is a correct statement about chlamydia.
Content Area: Sexually Transmitted Infections
Integrated Process: Nursing Process—Planning
Client Need: Health Promotion and Maintenance
Cognitive Level: Application
Concept: Sexuality
Reference: Centers for Disease Control and Prevention. (2015). Sexually Transmitted Diseases. Retrieved from www.cdc.gov/std/.
Pellico, L. H. (2013). Focus on adult health medical-surgical nursing. Philadelphia: Lippincott Williams and Wilkins.

3. ANSWER: 1
Rationale
1. The CDC (2015) recommends a combination therapy using two different antimicrobials with different mechanisms of action to improve treatment efficiency. In addition, individuals infected with *Neisseria gonorrhoeae* frequently are coinfected with *Chlamydia trachomatis* and should be treated accordingly.
2. The microorganism *Neisseria gonorrhoeae* has become increasingly resistant to penicillins, tetracyclines, and fluoroquinolones (levofloxacin).
3. The microorganism *Neisseria gonorrhoeae* has become increasingly resistant to penicillins, tetracyclines, and fluoroquinolones (levofloxacin).
4. The microorganism *Neisseria gonorrhoeae* has become increasingly resistant to penicillins, tetracyclines, and fluoroquinolones (levofloxacin).
TEST-TAKING TIP: Review the pharmacodynamics of antimicrobials.
Content Area: Sexually Transmitted Infections
Integrated Process: Nursing Process—Implementation
Client Need: Treatment
Cognitive Level: Application
Concept: Sexuality
Reference: Centers for Disease Control and Prevention. (2015). 2015 Sexually Transmitted Diseases Treatment Guidelines. Retrieved from www.cdc.gov/std/tg2015.
Pellico, L. H. (2013). Focus on adult health medical-surgical nursing. Philadelphia: Lippincott Williams and Wilkins.

4. ANSWER: 4
Rationale
1. Candidiasis usually does not cause symptoms in the male partner.
2. The most common strains of HPV cause condylomata (genital warts).
3. Men are asymptomatic carriers of trichomoniasis.
4. In men, the initial symptoms of gonorrhea include urethral pain and a creamy, yellow, sometimes bloody discharge.
TEST-TAKING TIP: Read each answer to identify a clinical manifestation of gonorrhea in men. Review the clinical manifestations for bacterial infections.
Content Area: Sexually Transmitted Infections
Integrated Process: Nursing Process—Diagnosis
Client Need: Health Promotion and Maintenance
Cognitive Level: Analysis
Concept: Sexuality
Reference: Centers for Disease Control and Prevention. (2015). Sexually Transmitted Diseases. Retrieved from www.cdc.gov/std/.
Pellico, L. H. (2013). Focus on adult health medical-surgical nursing. Philadelphia: Lippincott Williams and Wilkins.

5. ANSWER: 1
Rationale
1. Appearance of a chancre at the site of exposure.
2. Copper-colored rash involving the trunk and extremities occurs in the secondary stage.
3. Flulike symptoms occur in the secondary stage.
4. Condyloma lata occur in the secondary stage.
TEST-TAKING TIP: Compare the client's complaints and physical symptoms with the phases of syphilis.
Content Area: Sexually Transmitted Infections
Integrated Process: Nursing Process—Diagnosis
Client Need: Health Promotion and Maintenance
Cognitive Level: Analysis
Concept: Sexuality
Reference: Centers for Disease Control and Prevention. (2015). Sexually Transmitted Diseases. Retrieved from www.cdc.gov/std/.
Pellico, L. H. (2013). Focus on adult health medical-surgical nursing. Philadelphia: Lippincott Williams and Wilkins.

6. **ANSWER: 2**
Rationale
1. Purulent vaginal discharge is a clinical manifestation of bacterial infections such as gonorrhea and chlamydia.
2. The most common strains of HPV cause condylomata (genital warts) on the female and male genitalia.
3. Malodorous vaginal discharge is a clinical manifestation of trichomoniasis and bacterial vaginosis.
4. The most common strains of HPV cause condylomata (genital warts) on the female and male genitalia.
TEST-TAKING TIP: Read each answer to determine if it is a correct statement about HPV.
Content Area: Sexually Transmitted Infections
Integrated Process: Nursing Process—Assessment
Client Need: Health Promotion and Maintenance
Cognitive Level: Analysis
Concept: Sexuality
Reference: Centers for Disease Control and Prevention. (2015). Sexually Transmitted Diseases. Retrieved from www.cdc.gov/std/.
Pellico, L. H. (2013). Focus on adult health medical-surgical nursing. Philadelphia: Lippincott Williams and Wilkins.

7. **ANSWER: 2**
Rationale
1. Treatment of external genital warts includes patient-applied topical application; electrocautery and carbon dioxide laser surgery are alternative therapies for clients with a large number or area of genital warts.
2. Genital warts may resolve spontaneously.
3. A vaccine is not an effective treatment of HPV but it is a recommended prevention.
4. PID develops when sexually transmitted bacteria enter the uterus and reproductive organs.
TEST-TAKING TIP: Read each answer to determine if it is a correct statement about HPV.
Content Area: Sexually Transmitted Infections
Integrated Process: Teaching/Learning
Client Need: Health Promotion and Maintenance
Cognitive Level: Knowledge
Concept: Sexuality
Reference: Centers for Disease Control and Prevention. (2015). Sexually Transmitted Diseases. Retrieved from www.cdc.gov/std/.
Pellico, L. H. (2013). Focus on adult health medical-surgical nursing. Philadelphia: Lippincott Williams and Wilkins.

8. **ANSWER: 4**
Rationale
1. Surgical choices for pregnant women with genital warts include carbon dioxide laser surgery.
2. Surgical choices for pregnant women with genital warts include electrocautery.
3. Genital warts may resolve spontaneously without treatment.
4. Podophyllin resin, interferon, and fluorouracil should not be used during pregnancy, because they can harm the fetus.
TEST-TAKING TIP: Read each answer to determine if it is a correct statement about treatment for pregnant women.
Content Area: Sexually Transmitted Infections
Integrated Process: Nursing Process—Planning
Client Need: Health Promotion and Maintenance

Cognitive Level: Knowledge
Concept: Sexuality
Reference: Centers for Disease Control and Prevention. (2015). 2015 Sexually Transmitted Diseases Treatment Guidelines. Retrieved from www.cdc.gov/std/tg2015.
Pellico, L. H. (2013). Focus on adult health medical-surgical nursing. Philadelphia: Lippincott Williams and Wilkins.

9. **ANSWER: 2**
Rationale
1. HBsAg indicates the person is infectious to others.
2. Anti-HBs is the test that should be ordered to assess whether the vaccine has been effective. The presence of anti-HBs is generally interpreted as immunity from hepatitis B virus infection.
3. Anti-HBc IgM appears at the onset of symptoms in acute hepatitis B and indicates previous or ongoing infection with HBV.
4. Anti-HBc indicates recovery and natural immunity from HBV infection (i.e., the client has had hepatitis B).
TEST-TAKING TIP: Review hepatitis serology (see Table 6.2).
Content Area: Sexually Transmitted Infections
Integrated Process: Nursing Process—Diagnosis
Client Need: Health Promotion and Maintenance
Cognitive Level: Analysis
Concept: Sexuality
Reference: Centers for Disease Control and Prevention. (2015). Sexually Transmitted Diseases. Retrieved from www.cdc.gov/std/.
Pellico, L. H. (2013). Focus on adult health medical-surgical nursing. Philadelphia: Lippincott Williams and Wilkins.

10. **ANSWER: 2**
Rationale
1. The development of antibodies occurs with hepatitis B.
2. Bacterial vaginosis is a result of a decrease or absence of *Lactobacillus acidophilus,* an acid-producing bacterium normally found in the vagina.
3. Bacterial vaginosis is a result of an overgrowth of the bacteria *Gardnerella vaginalis.*
4. Absence of vaginal mucosa is not a risk factor for bacterial vaginosis.
TEST-TAKING TIP: Read each answer to determine if it is a correct statement about bacterial vaginosis.
Content Area: Sexually Transmitted Infections
Integrated Process: Nursing Process—Diagnosis
Client Need: Health Promotion and Maintenance
Cognitive Level: Analysis
Concept: Sexuality
Reference: Centers for Disease Control and Prevention. (2015). Sexually Transmitted Diseases. Retrieved from www.cdc.gov/std/.
Pellico, L. H. (2013). Focus on adult health medical-surgical nursing. Philadelphia: Lippincott Williams and Wilkins.

11. **ANSWER: 2**
Rationale
1. A clinical manifestation of bacterial vaginosis is a fishy odor.
2. A clinical manifestation of trichomoniasis is a malodorous (foul-smelling), frothy yellow-green vaginal discharge.
3. Thin milky-white vaginal discharge is a normal finding.
4. The condition is asymptomatic in men.
TEST-TAKING TIP: Read each answer to determine if it is a correct statement about trichomoniasis.

Content Area: Sexually Transmitted Infections
Integrated Process: Nursing Process—Diagnosis
Client Need: Health Promotion and Maintenance
Cognitive Level: Analysis
Concept: Sexuality
Reference: *Centers for Disease Control and Prevention. (2015). Sexually Transmitted Diseases. Retrieved from www.cdc.gov/std/.*
Pellico, L. H. (2013). Focus on adult health medical-surgical nursing. Philadelphia: Lippincott Williams and Wilkins.

12. ANSWER: 4
Rationale
1. Recommended use of a condom during sexual activity to prevent transmission of the infection. HSV-2 is controllable, not curable.
2. Refrain from all sexual activity if the infection is active.
3. Condoms are recommended during sexual activity, even if the disease is dormant.
4. All potential sexual partners should be informed to prevent transmission of the infection.

TEST-TAKING TIP: Read each answer to determine if it is a correct statement about HSV-2.

Content Area: Sexually Transmitted Infections
Integrated Process: Teaching/Learning
Client Need: Health Promotion and Maintenance
Cognitive Level: Analysis
Concept: Sexuality
Reference: *Centers for Disease Control and Prevention. (2015). Sexually Transmitted Diseases. Retrieved from www.cdc.gov/std/.*
Pellico, L. H. (2013). Focus on adult health medical-surgical nursing. Philadelphia: Lippincott Williams and Wilkins.

13. ANSWER: 2
Rationale
1. HSV-1 causes cold sores.
2. Treatment of HSV-2 focuses on relieving symptoms.
3. HSV-2 is not curable.
4. Asymptomatic infection can be transmitted to sexual partners.

TEST-TAKING TIP: Read each answer to determine if it is a correct statement about HSV-2.

Content Area: Sexually Transmitted Infections
Integrated Process: Teaching/Learning
Client Need: Health Promotion and Maintenance
Cognitive Level: Analysis
Concept: Sexuality
Reference: *Centers for Disease Control and Prevention. (2015). Sexually Transmitted Diseases. Retrieved from www.cdc.gov/std/.*
Pellico, L. H. (2013). Focus on adult health medical-surgical nursing. Philadelphia: Lippincott Williams and Wilkins.

14. ANSWER: 3
Rationale
1. Clinical manifestations in the primary stage of syphilis develop in 2 to 3 weeks (14 to 21 days) after exposure.
2. Clinical manifestations in the primary stage of syphilis develop in 2 to 3 weeks (14 to 21 days) after exposure.
3. Clinical manifestations in the primary stage of syphilis develop in 2 to 3 weeks (14 to 21 days) after exposure.
4. Clinical manifestations in the secondary stage of syphilis develop 2 to 8 weeks after the primary stage.

TEST-TAKING TIP: Review the stages and manifestations of syphilis in (see Table 6.1).

Content Area: Sexually Transmitted Infections
Integrated Process: Nursing Process—Diagnosis
Client Need: Health Promotion and Maintenance
Cognitive Level: Analysis
Concept: Sexuality
Reference: *Centers for Disease Control and Prevention. (2015). Sexually Transmitted Diseases. Retrieved from www.cdc.gov/std/.*
Pellico, L. H. (2013). Focus on adult health medical-surgical nursing. Philadelphia: Lippincott Williams and Wilkins.

15. ANSWER: 3
Rationale
1. A complication of HSV-2 is the acquisition and transmission of HIV.
2. A complication of infection with syphilis is having a stillborn child.
3. The bacterial infections chlamydia and gonorrhea have increased risk for complications leading to infertility.
4. A complication of infection with HPV is cancer.

TEST-TAKING TIP: Review each answer to identify a complication of chlamydia.

Content Area: Sexually Transmitted Infections
Integrated Process: Nursing Process—Assessment
Client Need: Health Promotion and Maintenance
Cognitive Level: Knowledge
Concept: Sexuality
Reference: *Centers for Disease Control and Prevention. (2015). Sexually Transmitted Diseases. Retrieved from www.cdc.gov/std/.*
Pellico, L. H. (2013). Focus on adult health medical-surgical nursing. Philadelphia: Lippincott Williams and Wilkins.

16. ANSWER: 2
Rationale
1. The client is currently not complaining of pain.
2. The client displays a knowledge deficit about modes of transmission for syphilis.
3. Ineffective coping related to the increased stress associated with the infection is not the most appropriate nursing diagnosis at this time.
4. Noncompliance with treatment may not be related to the client's age.

TEST-TAKING TIP: Read each answer to identify the priority nursing diagnosis based on the information given.

Content Area: Sexually Transmitted Infections
Integrated Process: Nursing Process—Diagnosis
Client Need: Health Promotion and Maintenance
Cognitive Level: Analysis
Concept: Sexuality
Reference: *Centers for Disease Control and Prevention. (2015). Sexually Transmitted Diseases. Retrieved from www.cdc.gov/std/.*
Pellico, L. H. (2013). Focus on adult health medical-surgical nursing. Philadelphia: Lippincott Williams and Wilkins.

17. ANSWER: 2
Rationale
1. HIV is not curable.
2. HIV is not curable.
3. It is not accurate to say this type of drug will be used prior to vaccines.
4. This drug is not readily available all over the world.

TEST-TAKING TIP: Read each answer to identify the correct statement about HIV.

Content Area: Sexually Transmitted Infections
Integrated Process: Teaching/Learning
Client Need: Health Promotion and Maintenance
Cognitive Level: Knowledge
Concept: Sexuality
Reference: Centers for Disease Control and Prevention. (2015). Sexually Transmitted Diseases. *Retrieved from www.cdc.gov/std/.*
Pellico, L. H. (2013). Focus on adult health medical-surgical nursing. *Philadelphia: Lippincott Williams and Wilkins.*

18. **ANSWER: 3**
Rationale
1. These products can destroy the normal balance of microorganisms in your mouth.
2. Lesions may become painful with citrus juices in your diet.
3. Foods that are soft and pureed will not scrape the lesions.
4. Lesions may become painful with hot soups and beverages with each meal.
TEST-TAKING TIP: Read each answer to determine if it is a correct statement in the management of oral candidiasis.
Content Area: Sexually Transmitted Infections
Integrated Process: Teaching/Learning
Client Need: Health Promotion and Maintenance
Cognitive Level: Analysis
Concept: Sexuality
Reference: Centers for Disease Control and Prevention. (2015). Sexually Transmitted Diseases. *Retrieved from www.cdc.gov/std/.*
Pellico, L. H. (2013). Focus on adult health medical-surgical nursing. *Philadelphia: Lippincott Williams and Wilkins.*

19. **ANSWER: 3**
Rationale
1. Cough is not a clinical manifestation of HPV.
2. Condylomata lata appear in the secondary stage of syphilis.

3. The most common strain of HPV causes condylomata.
4. Chancres appear in the primary stage of syphilis.
TEST-TAKING TIP: Read each answer to identify the clinical manifestations of HPV.
Content Area: Sexually Transmitted Infections
Integrated Process: Nursing Process—Diagnosis
Client Need: Health Promotion and Maintenance
Cognitive Level: Analysis
Concept: Sexuality
Reference: Centers for Disease Control and Prevention. (2015). Sexually Transmitted Diseases. *Retrieved from www.cdc.gov/std/.*
Pellico, L. H. (2013). Focus on adult health medical-surgical nursing. *Philadelphia: Lippincott Williams and Wilkins.*

20. **ANSWER: 3**
Rationale
1. Cough is a symptom associated with an infection.
2. Enlarged lymph nodes are a symptom associated with an infection.
3. Retrovir (antiviral) may lower the ability of the body to fight infection, as indicated by a lowered WBC count.
4. Fever is a symptom associated with an infection.
TEST-TAKING TIP: Read each answer to identify symptoms of HIV infection versus potential adverse reactions to a medication.
Content Area: Sexually Transmitted Infections
Integrated Process: Nursing Process—Assessment
Client Need: Health Promotion and Maintenance
Cognitive Level: Analysis
Concept: Sexuality
Reference: Centers for Disease Control and Prevention. (2015). 2015 Sexually Transmitted Diseases Treatment Guidelines. *Retrieved from www.cdc.gov/std/tg2015.*
Pellico, L. H. (2013). Focus on adult health medical-surgical nursing. *Philadelphia: Lippincott Williams and Wilkins.*

Disorders of the Breast

Breast-conserving surgery—In treating breast cancer, the removal of only the tumor and not the entire breast

Breast self-examination—A technique that enables a woman to detect changes in her breasts

Ductal carcinoma in situ (DCIS)—A cluster of malignant cells in the mammary ducts that has not spread to surrounding breast tissue

Fibroadenoma (FNA)—An adenoma with fibrous tissue forming a dense stroma

Fibrocystic breast changes—A nonspecific diagnosis for a benign condition characterized by palpable lumps in the breast, usually associated with pain and tenderness

Gynecomastia—Enlargement of breast tissue in the male

Mammary glands—Compound glands of the female breast that can secrete milk

Mammography—Radiographic imaging of the breast to screen for and detect breast cancer

Many women will experience a breast disorder during their lifetime. Problems related to breast conditions cause a great deal of stress for women who have them. There are many cultural and psychological issues and beliefs that impact both men and women in today's society. One function of the breast is lactation, which plays an important role in nurturing and motherhood. Breasts are also associated with sexuality and pleasure for men and women.

These factors and others all contribute to a woman's perceptions of her body, family/social relationships, and her perceived role in society. Therefore, any threat or injury to the breast can significantly affect a woman's perception of herself. Breast disorders, and especially the threat of breast cancer, can cause significant fear and anxiety in women. When caring for these women, the nurse must be ready to assume multiple roles, including educator, counselor, and caregiver. The nurse provides education when a woman is diagnosed with a breast disorder and provides support and encouragement as the woman works through her fear and decisional conflicts related to controversies about diagnostic and treatment options for her condition.

I. Normal Breast

The primary function of the breasts (**mammary glands**) is to produce milk. Breasts are made up of fat, fibrous connective tissue, and glandular tissue that differentiates as ducts and lobules. All women, regardless of breast size,

have a similar number of lobes (approximately 15 to 25). Approximately six to ten ducts exit the nipple. Each lobe has many smaller lobules. The lobules end in dozens of tiny glands that can produce milk. Ducts and lactiferous sinuses are the tubular connections between the lobes and nipples and allow the flow of milk to exit the breast. Half of this glandular tissue is located in the upper outer quadrant. Glandular tissue and fat vary with a woman's age and weight (Fig. 7.1).

A. Breast tissue development

Breast tissue begins to develop around the sixth week in utero. Prepuberty breasts are in a resting state with ducts present but nonfunctional. At puberty, ducts elongate due to estrogen and breast buds appear but may not develop simultaneously. The young adult begins to experience ovulation, ducts elongate, and side branches of ducts and lobular tissue form, thereby influencing the progesterone effect. At maturity, the breast become pendulous after the woman has experienced many ovulatory cycles.

During pregnancy, women's breasts enlarge to twice their normal weight due to ductal growth, with branching of the mammary blood flow leading to vascular engorgement and areolar pigmentation. During lactation, the ducts and branches will dilate and become engorged with colostrum and then milk. At menopause, the lobules will recede, leaving mostly ducts, adipose tissue, and fibrous tissue. Hormone therapy can delay postmenopausal breast changes and

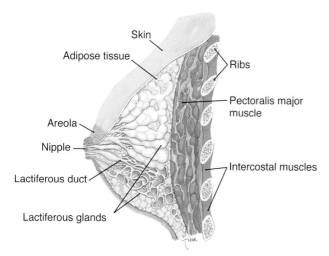

Skin

Adipose tissue

Ribs

Pectoralis major muscle

Areola

Nipple

Intercostal muscles

Lactiferous duct

Lactiferous glands

Fig 7.1 Anatomy of the breast.

mimic premenopausal states. The breasts respond to changes in levels of estrogen and progesterone during the menstrual cycle, pregnancy, breastfeeding, and menopause. Hormones can change the amount of fluid in the breasts, causing the breasts to be more sensitive or painful. Breast tissue changes can also occur when women are using hormonal contraception such as birth control pills or hormone therapy.

B. Clinical breast exam

The female breast can be assessed during any general physical or gynecological examination or whenever a woman reports or presents with an abnormality. Breast examination can be used as a screening and a diagnostic tool and includes visual inspection and palpation. Routine inspection of the breast is as follows:

1. Begin with the disrobed woman sitting in a comfortable position and facing the examiner.
2. Inspect size and symmetry.
3. A common variation noted is a slight variation from breast to breast, which is a normal finding.
4. Assess skin for color, venous pattern, thickening, and edema.
5. Nipple inversion of one or both breasts is not uncommon unless it is a recent change.
6. Redness may indicate benign local inflammation or potential superficial lymphatic invasion of a neoplasm.
7. Edema may indicate blocking of the lymphatic drainage.
8. Skin that has the appearance of an orange peel may also indicate an underlying neoplasm and is a classic sign of advanced breast cancer.
   a) Other significant observations necessitate further evaluation: ulcerations, rashes, and/or nipple discharge.
   b) Inspect and palpate the clavicular and axillary regions for swelling, discoloration, lesions, enlarged lymph nodes.

c) Palpate the entire surface of the breast and axillary tail using the flat part of the second, third, and fourth finger.
d) Use a clockwise direction with concentric circles, working from the outer areas to the nipple area.
e) Patient may be sitting or supine.
f) Palpate lymph nodes with the patient's arm abducted.
g) Examine for enlargement, noting the location, size, consistency, and mobility.
h) Adolescent breast tissue is usually firm and lobular.
i) After menopause, women's breasts are less dense because they contain less fat.
j) With pregnancy and lactation, the areola will appear darker and the breasts may feel firmer and larger with palpable lobules.

II. Breast Cancer Screening and Diagnostic Tests

A. Mammography is the most common test for screening women. Women with breast symptoms or screening abnormalities are referred for diagnostic evaluation using mammography or ultrasound and

MAKING THE CONNECTION

Recommendations for Physical Examination of the Breasts

According to the U.S. Preventive Services Task Force (2009), physical examination of the breasts can detect presymptomatic breast cancer and may find a substantial proportion of cancers in geographic areas where mammography may not always be available. However, this task force did recommend against BSE, stating that it resulted in additional imaging and biopsies with no significant decrease in breast cancer mortality. These recommendations have met with controversy and have not been adopted by the American Cancer Society (ACS), the National Comprehensive Cancer Network (NCCN), or the American Congress of Obstetricians and Gynecologists (ACOG).

The ACS still recommends BSE for women 20 and older and continues to recommend that women be taught BSE, believing that BSE has a benefit of increasing self-awareness of breast changes that leads to rapid evaluation. The Task Force updated its 2015 recommendations (Table 7.1), which continue to be somewhat controversial. Factors that can lead to variability and affect the sensitivity and specificity of CBE are age, breast density, experience of the provider, and time spent completing the exam.

Table 7.1 Current Breast Cancer Screening Recommendations for Healthy Women

Organization	BSE	CBE	Mammography
U.S. Preventative Services (USPSTF)	Against BSE	Cannot recommend for or against	Biennial, ages 50–74 Biennial, age 50 Individual choice
American Cancer Society (ACS)	BSE optional Helps with breast awareness	Every 3 years in 20s and 30s Annual age > 40	Annual age > 40, continue as long as in good health
American College of Obstetricians and Gynecologists s (ACOG)	Helps with breast awareness Consider use for high-risk patients	Every 1–3 years in ages 20–39 Annual age > 40	Annual, age 40
National Comprehensive Cancer Network (NCCN)	Helps with breast awareness	Every 13 years in ages 20–40 Annual age > 40	Annual age > 40

Source: ACS, 2014; ACOG, 2015; NCCN, 2014; USPSTF, 2009, 2015

in special cases breast magnetic resonance imaging (MRI) or breast-specific gamma imaging (BSGI) (Christinsen-Rangel, 2013). Screening mammography is used to detect breast cancer in early stages to allow for rapid evaluation and treatment. This has an overall sensitivity rate of 84.1%. However, this sensitivity rate is decreased in younger women and those with dense breast tissue. Mammography is not recommended for women under age 30 because of hormonal status, which affects breast density. Women who have had breast augmentation should still continue to be screened even though sensitivity is decreased (Christinsen-Rangel, 2013; Johnson, Thomas, & Porter, 2015).

1. Mammography is used to evaluate abnormal clinical findings (breast masses, thickening, or nipple discharge) to gather further information.
2. Schedule the mammography for the end of the menstrual cycle to decrease discomfort.

DID YOU KNOW?
The nurse should advise women not to use deodorants, body lotions, and powders that contain aluminum, calcium, or zinc prior to the test. These products may cause shadows on the mammogram (womenshealth.gov, 2013).

B. Ultrasound

Ultrasound is used to target specific areas of the breast to differentiate between cystic and solid masses. It is used in women under age 30 and in women aged 30 or older with breast symptoms.

C. Magnetic resonance imaging (MRI)

MRI is used for women who are considered high risk due to family history or genetic risk factors (*BRCA* mutations or first-degree relatives who have had breast cancer). MRI has a high sensitivity rate (71% to 100%) and high accuracy.

DID YOU KNOW?
MRI can identify the precise size of a tumor, detect the magnitude of disease, and help with assessing suitability of breast conservation.

D. Tissue analysis studies may be used to determine if breast cancer is present. Two types of tissue analysis studies include the following:

1. *Fine needle aspiration.* With this procedure, a 21- to 22-gauge needle is used to aspirate fluid from a cyst or obtain cells from a palpable solid lesion. This test provides for rapid results and causes little trauma to the tissue. The test may yield false-negative results and does not differentiate in situ from invasive cancer.
2. *Percutaneous biopsy (core needle biopsy).* This outpatient procedure, performed under local anesthesia, provides a more definitive diagnosis than fine-needle aspiration and may be used to sample both palpable and nonpalpable lesions. The biopsy of tissue, versus cells in the fine-needle aspiration, is less invasive than major breast surgery and has better cosmetic results. This test is usually performed when large tumors are close to the skin, under ultrasound guidance.

E. Surgical biopsy

This is used on areas of the breast that display as abnormal but are too small to be felt. A very thin wire is often placed in the area of a breast abnormality to guide the surgeon to the suspicious area noted on the mammogram.

1. *Excisional biopsy (lumpectomy).* This is the standard procedure for complete pathological assessment of breast masses. The entire mass, or nonpalpable lesion, and surrounding tissue margins are removed for analysis. A frozen section is performed at the time of biopsy with an immediate reading for a rapid provisional diagnosis.

Generally, this procedure is also used to confirm a diagnosis when the woman has no previous history of tissue analysis.

2. *Incisional biopsy.* Removal of a portion, or wedge, of a breast mass. Complete excision may not be possible or immediately benefit the woman. This type of biopsy is usually performed for large masses that cannot be removed without surgery. It is generally performed on women with locally advanced cancer or on women with a suspected recurrence of cancer.

3. Nursing care interventions for surgical biopsy
   a) Prior to surgery: Assess the woman's educational, physical, and psychosocial needs by reviewing the medical history. Provide support by explaining what she should expect to happen. Instruct the woman to discontinue all agents that increase the risk of bleeding, such as acetylsalicylic acid, NSAIDs, vitamin E, herbal products, and blood thinners (e.g., Coumadin). Instruct the patient to refrain from eating and drinking after midnight (depending on the type of biopsy to be performed).
   b) Postoperative care: Monitor the patient for effects of anesthesia; monitor the surgical wound for bleeding; monitor vital signs. After sedation wears off, review postsurgical care of the biopsy site, pain management techniques, and activity restrictions. Instruct the patient to remove the dressing in 48 hours, leaving Steri-Strips intact for 7 to 10 days. Instruct the patient to use a supportive bra to reduce discomfort. Patients usually return to daily activities the day after surgery. To avoid trauma to the breast, limit high-impact activities for 1 week to promote the healing process.
   c) Prior to discharge: The patient will need to demonstrate the ability to tolerate fluids, void, and ambulate. Someone must accompany the patient home. Review discharge instructions again to ensure the patient's complete understanding.

III. Benign Breast Disorders

Benign breast disorders represent a spectrum of disorders that are identified as imaging abnormalities. The disorders may be palpable on physical examination of the breast but are not cancerous. Once diagnosed and classified, the treatment goal is symptomatic relief and patient education. Some benign breast disorders may place a woman at an increased risk for developing breast cancer. Thus, women should be counseled about recommended screenings and risk-reduction behaviors and strategies.

Patients with benign breast conditions often present with breast masses or lumps, which are usually tender and bilateral. Rapid changes in the size of benign masses may occur as compared with breast malignancies. Breast malignancies usually grow slowly with an increase in mass size occurring over time. Typically, the mass or tenderness may increase before menses due to hormone changes. Therefore, masses in perimenopausal women should be reassessed in 2 to 3 weeks during different phases of the menstrual cycle.

A. Fibrocystic breast changes
   Fibrocystic breast changes are the most encountered of all benign breast conditions and include a broad grouping of disorders. Fibrocystic changes typically exhibit as breast thickness, lumpiness, or a palpable nodularity. Pain is almost always present and is the most common symptom. The exact cause is unknown but might be due to a physiological response from hormones. It has been suggested that there is an imbalance between estrogen and progestin, which produces excessive ductal stimulation and proliferation.

B. Breast cysts
   Breast cysts are small sacs filled with fluid. They can be of any size and can feel like small lumps or grapes and can be soft or firm. These often fluctuate in size during the menstrual cycle, causing pain or tenderness. Breast cysts are common in women between the ages of 30 and 50. They usually recede and disappear with menopause; however, they may continue in menopausal women who receive hormonal therapy. Patients should be educated on the importance of examining their breasts routinely even though they have breast lumps. Perimenopausal women should be reassessed 2 to 3 weeks later during a different phase of the menstrual cycle. It can be difficult to differentiate a breast cyst from cancer based on clinical findings alone. A more aggressive treatment will be required for cancer. Infection is usually ruled out first. Mammograms may be inconclusive; therefore, a breast ultrasound is more helpful in differentiating a breast cyst from a solid mass. A definitive diagnosis is made with a breast biopsy. Aspiration of the cyst fluid (fine-needle aspiration) helps to alleviate pain, especially if the cyst is very large. Treatment can include the following:
   - Use of a supportive bra both day and night (during sleep)
   - Eliminating products containing high doses of caffeine (e.g., coffee, tea, and chocolate) from the diet
   - Taking vitamin E 400 IU daily
   - Diuretics, NSAIDs, oral contraceptives, and supplemental progestin

- Danazol (Danocrine) prescription, an androgen derivative, for severe pain. Usually 100 to 200 mg twice a day, as this drug suppresses pituitary gonadotropins. Androgenic effects may include acne, edema, and hirsutism; therefore, it is wise to try a milder form of pain relief first.

C. Fibroadenoma

Fibroadenoma is the most common benign tumor of the breast and accounts for the majority of breast biopsies. The cause is unknown but these tumors usually occur between 15 and 30 years, with a peak incidence at 30 years of age. African American women tend to develop fibroadenomas more often and at an earlier age than Caucasian women. Fibroadenomas are well-defined, solid, round, movable, painless, and often rubbery masses under the skin. Though they can occur bilaterally, they are unilateral in 14% to 25% of women. Fibroadenomas usually range in size from 2 to 4 cm in diameter. These tumors usually respond to hormonal fluctuations and tend to increase in size toward the end of each menstrual cycle and during pregnancy. They can often be detected in postmenopausal women but are usually smaller after menopause (if a woman is not taking hormone therapy). Diagnostic tests to assess for fibroadenoma include the following:

- Clinical breast exam, mammogram, or ultrasound
- Fine-needle aspiration for cytological diagnosis
- Different types of biopsies, which may include open surgical, stereotactic, or ultrasound-guided biopsies. Women in their teens or early 20s may not need a biopsy if the tumor goes away on its own or if the mass does not change over a long period of time.

D. Intraductal papilloma

Intraductal papillomas are benign tumors that grow within the milk ducts of the breast. They most often occur in women ages 35 to 55 and account for more than 50% of all causes of nipple discharge. Causes and risk factors for this condition are unknown. Symptoms may include breast lumps, nipple discharge, or tissue hyperplasia. A woman may also complain about a feeling of fullness or pain beneath the areola.

Intraductal papillomas are made up of fibrous tissue, blood vessels, and glandular tissue and may be found in the large ducts near the nipple, which commonly cause clear or bloody nipple discharge. They may be felt as a small lump behind or next to the nipple but can also be found in small ducts in areas of the breast farther from the nipple. Often, there are several growths (multiple papillomas). The condition does not raise breast cancer risk unless other changes, such as atypical hyperplasia, are noted.

According to the American Cancer Association (2009), papillomatosis can also occur and is a type of hyperplasia in which there are very small areas of cell growth within the ducts. This condition is linked to a slightly increased risk of breast cancer.

1. Assessment
   a) Physical examination of the affected breast(s)
   b) Ultrasound, mammogram
   c) Breast biopsy with cytological examination of breast discharge
   d) Ductogram (x-ray with contrast dye injected into the affected duct)
   e) Surgical needle core biopsy, when nipple discharge is present. This will assist with a diagnosis. Referral to a surgeon who specializes in breast surgery should be considered. Surgery is the usual treatment for single duct discharge that has one of the following characteristics: bloody fluid, persistent cases (two times per week for 4 to 6 weeks), or masses/lumps. To rule out cancer, removal of the duct is necessary. With total duct excision, the entire ductal system of the nipple is removed using a circumareolar incision. The woman will no longer be able to breastfeed and will have reduced nipple sensitivity. Prognosis is excellent for women with one papilloma; however, women with multiple papillomas, or those at an early age, may have an increased risk of developing cancer. The risk may be higher if they have a family history of cancer or if there are abnormal cells in the biopsy.

2. Nursing role
   The nurse should provide psychological support and education on breast self-exams and awareness, screening mammography, and when to call the health care provider if they notice breast discharge or a breast lump.

E. Galactorrhea

Galactorrhea is a condition where one or both breasts make milky secretions. It may occur in women or, less common, in men. A woman who has galactorrhea produces milk even though she is not breastfeeding, and the milk production is unrelated to pregnancy. Galactorrhea is common in women of childbearing age and can occur 3 to 6 months after breastfeeding has been discontinued—usually after the first delivery—or after an abortion. Galactorrhea is caused by hyperprolactinemia, which may be a result of medications, endocrine disorders, renal disease, and breast stimulation. Breasts may leak only when the breasts are touched or with no stimulation.

1. Causes
   a) This condition is often found in women who have increased prolactin levels or an abnormal secretion of growth hormone, thyroid hormone, or corticotrophin.

b) Other causes include tumors (usually benign), especially those of the pituitary gland. Medicines (e.g., hormones, antidepressants, blood pressure medication, and certain tranquilizers), herbal supplements (e.g., nettle, fennel, blessed thistle, anise, and fenugreek seed), use of illicit substances (e.g., marijuana and opiates), pregnancy, frequent breast self-exams (daily exams), stimulation of the breast during sexual activity, oral contraceptives, or hypothyroidism may also cause galactorrhea.

2. Symptoms
   a) Milky white or yellow discharge from one or both nipples.

(!) ALERT Reddish breast discharge may be an indication of cancer. Blood in the discharge is not galactorrhea.

   b) Additional symptoms include an absence of menstrual periods (amenorrhea is commonly the primary presenting symptom), headaches, vision loss, temperature intolerance, seizures, polyuria or polydipsia (which usually indicates pituitary or hypothalamic disorders or tumors), less interest in sex, increased hair growth on chin or chest, acne, erectile dysfunction, and less interest in sex for men. Complaints of tiredness, cold intolerance, and constipation may indicate hypothyroidism. Additionally, body composition changes can be noted such as increased fat mass and decreased lean muscle mass.

3. Risks and diagnostic studies
   a) Osteoporosis and osteopenia are associated with this disorder.
   b) Laboratory blood tests to check hormone levels include serum prolactin levels, cortisol, thyroid stimulating hormone, triiodothyronine, thyroxine, and pregnancy status.

(!) ALERT Prolactin levels greater than 20 to 25 ng/mL are considered abnormal. Levels of 25 to 100 ng/mL are indicative of a tumor or functional hyperprolactinemia. Levels that are above 100 ng/mL strongly suggest a tumor. This laboratory work is best done in the morning between 8:00 a.m. and 10:00 a.m.

   c) Prolactin levels may be falsely elevated with the following activities, all of which should be avoided prior to laboratory work: manual stimulation of the breasts, breast examination, sexual activity. and exercise.
   d) When levels suggest a tumor, the patient needs to be referred for further evaluation.
   e) Thyroid studies are indicated to rule out hypothyroidism.

f) Other diagnostics may include CT scan, mammography, or MRI scans of the head to rule out pituitary tumor. If a pituitary tumor is found, bromocriptine is the primary therapy used to lower prolactin levels, as this medication assists with shrinking the tumor. An alternative long-acting dopamine agonist, cabergoline, may be used since this is often better tolerated than bromocriptine with fewer side effects.

F. Mammary duct ectasia
This is a benign condition of the lactiferous ducts behind the nipple that causes inflammation, dilation, and increased glandular secretion. The cause is unknown. The breast duct widens and its walls thicken, which can cause the duct to become blocked, leading to fluid buildup. This condition usually goes along with other benign conditions of the breast and has been associated with breast cancer. It most often occurs in women who are perimenopausal or postmenopausal (aged 45 to 55). Treatment is often not necessary, as it is a self-limiting condition. Women will require reassurance and education.

1. Symptoms
   a) Unilateral, or occasionally bilateral, thick, sticky, cheesy, viscous nipple discharge that may be white, brown, green, or purple in color
   b) Redness of the nipple or surrounding area, fever, a breast lump or a thickening near the clogged duct
   c) Complaints of burning pain or itching, nipple retraction, or a palpable mass behind the nipple
   d) Periductal mastitis or mastitis (bacterial infection), which may also develop in the inflamed area

2. Assessment
   a) Physical examination to evaluate whether the discharge can be manually expressed when the nipple is massaged systematically in quadrants
   b) Mammography, ultrasound, and aspiration with cytology screening may be required for women with infection (Christinsen-Rangel, 2013; Shockney, 2012).

3. Treatment
   While this condition may be self-limiting and often requires no treatment, there are instances when more invasive treatment may be necessary. Some women may develop a secondary infection, which will require antibiotic therapy. If an abscess occurs, it may necessitate surgical intervention with incision and drainage as well as antibiotic therapy. If surgical intervention is required, the woman is referred to a surgeon for microdochectomy or total duct excision if needed. Follow up in women who have multiple duct discharge whose

imaging and clinical examination is normal are usually treated with psychosocial reassurance and education to relieve their anxiety.

IV. Malignant Tumors of the Breast

Breast cancer is the second highest occurring cancer in women in the United States. The risk of any woman getting breast cancer is 1 in 8, and the lifetime risk of dying from breast cancer is 1 in 28. The risk increases with age, as it is low in women in their 20s and 30s but continues to rise with each decade. The median age for breast cancer diagnosis is 64 years. However, increasing age and associated risk factors account for only 50% of all cases (Johnson, Thomas, & Porter, 2015).

In 2014, the Centers for Disease Control and Prevention (CDC) reported on breast cancer rates by ethnicity and race. White women had the highest risk of getting breast cancer followed by black, Hispanic, Asian/Pacific Islander, and American Indian/Alaska Native women (CDC, 2014). The American Cancer Society's estimates for 2015 indicated that about 231,840 new cases of invasive breast cancer would be diagnosed in women, and 40,290 women would die from breast cancer.

Breast cancer is the leading cause of cancer death in women. Death rates from breast cancer have been declining since about 1989, with larger decreases in women younger than 50. These decreases are believed to be the result of earlier detection through screening and increased awareness, as well as improved treatment (American Cancer Society, 2014). Having knowledge about breast cancer rates, incidence, anatomy, and physiology, and knowing which diagnostic tests are used for diagnosing specific breast disorders are the tools that help the nurse deliver quality nursing care.

Breast cancer is the most common cancer in women, accounting for 30% of all cancers in women. In recent years, early detection has shown to decrease death rates. Hereditary breast cancer occurs when there are genetic alterations in the DNA of breast epithelial cells, resulting in overgrowth of various cells with different growth rates that tend to metastasize. While the etiology of most breast cancers is unknown, it is classified as a systemic disease that usually begins in the epithelial cells lining the mammary ducts of the breast. Metastasis occurs from seeding of the breast cancer cells into the blood or lymph system, which leads to the development of tumors in the bones, lungs, brain, and liver.

A. Breast cancer risks
   1. Female gender
   2. Increased age (older than age 50)
   3. Personal history of breast cancer
   4. Personal history of ovarian or uterine cancer
   5. Family history, especially if parent, sibling, or child
   6. Obesity and/or high-fat diet
   7. Early menarche (younger than age 12)
   8. Nulliparity
   9. First live birth at late age (older than age 30)
   10. Long-term use of postmenopausal hormone therapy
   11. Exposure to radiation
   12. Excessive alcohol consumption (two or more drinks/day)
   13. Sedentary lifestyle
   14. Cigarette smoking
   15. Exposure to carcinogens
B. Breast cancer staging
   Refers to groupings that have been developed to determine the extent of breast disease, estimate prognosis, and identify appropriate treatment plans. It is based on both clinical and pathological diagnostic findings. Cancer staging is based on tumor size and extension, node number and extent, and distant metastasis. Staging is grouped 0 through IV (Table 7.2).
C. Types of breast cancer
   1. In situ breast cancer
      a) In situ cancers are found in the ductal or lobular tissue with an overgrowth of epithelial cells confined within the borders of the ducts and lobules with no lymphatic or vesicular invasion.
   2. Lobular carcinoma in situ (LCIS)
      a) An incidental microscopic finding of abnormal tissue growth in the breast lobules
      b) Carries a 7% to 10% risk for subsequent invasive breast cancer development
      c) Recent findings suggest it may be a precursor lesion to multifocal invasive lobular or ductal carcinoma.
      d) Women diagnosed with this condition need to undergo rigorous surveillance.
      e) Annual mammography
      f) Clinical breast exams every 6 months
      g) These women should receive counseling and education that includes chemoprevention with selective estrogen receptor modulators (SERMs) such as Tamoxifen.
   3. Ductal carcinoma in situ (DCIS)
      a) Overgrowth of cells inside the milk ducts
      b) Does not invade surrounding tissue; no metastasis
      c) Women do not die from this condition unless it develops into invasive cancer.
      d) It has been estimated that 14% to 51% of untreated DCIS may progress into invasive cancer over a 10-year period.
      e) It may occur as a palpable mass or as pathological nipple discharge.
      f) Usually diagnosed on a mammogram with displaying calcifications

Table 7.2	Breast Cancer Staging				
Stage 0	**Stage 1**	**Stage 2**	**Stage 3**		**Stage 4**
		Divided into two substages, 2A and 2B	*Divided into 2 substages 3A and 3B*		
		2A	3A		
• Three types of breast cancer in situ • Abnormal cells found within cells • No tumor or invasion outside the cells	• Tumor < 2 cm, no regional lymph node metastasis, no distant metastasis	• No evidence of tumor, metastasis to lymph nodes: no distant metastasis • Tumor < 2 cm; metastasis to movable lymph nodes; no distant metastasis • Tumor > 2–5 cm; no regional lymph node metastasis; no distant metastasis	• No evidence of tumor; metastasis to lymph nodes fixed to one another or to another structure but no distant metastasis • Tumor < 2 cm; metastasis to lymph nodes fixed to one another or to another structure; no distant metastasis • Tumor > 2–5 cm; metastasis to lymph nodes fixed to one another or to other structure but no distant metastasis • Tumor > 5 cm; metastasis to lymph nodes fixed to one another or to another structure; no distant metastasis		• Any tumor status as described in this table; metastasis to internal mammary nodes; no distant metastasis • Any tumor or nodal status as described in this table; distant metastasis, including metastasis to supraclavicular lymph nodes
		2B	3B		
		• Tumor > 2–5 cm; metastasis to movable lymph nodes; no distant metastasis • Tumor > 5 cm; no regional lymph node metastasis, no distant metastasis	• Tumor any size with direct extension to chest wall (excluding pectoral muscle) and/or edema (including peau d'orange) or ulceration of the skin or satellite skin nodules confined to the same breast, or inflammatory carcinoma; any nodal status as described in this table; no distant metastasis		

Source: Taken and adapted from Johnson, J., Thomas, D. J., & Porter, B. O. (2015). Women's health problems. In L. M. Dunphy, J. E. Winward-Brown, B. O. Porter, & D. F. Thomas (Eds.). Primary care: Art and science of advanced practice nursing (p. 697). 4th ed. Philadelphia: F.A. Davis.

g) Considered to be stage 0

h) May be a precursor to invasive cancer in some women

4. Invasive carcinoma

a) Most common invasive breast cancer

b) Accounts for 80% of all cases

c) Presents as a palpable solid mass or is found on mammography

d) Arises from the duct system

e) Invades surrounding tissue in the breast

5. Infiltrating lobular carcinoma

a) Second most common type of invasive breast cancer

b) Accounts for 10% to 15% of breast cancers

c) Presents as a large, less-distinct mass or appears as an abnormal mammogram in older women.

d) Begins in the lobular epithelium

e) Displays as an ill-defined thickening of the breast

f) Very often are multifocal and bilateral

g) Metastasis with this type is more likely to occur in the peritoneum, gastrointestinal tract, and ovaries.

6. Medullary carcinoma

a) Uncommon breast cancer

b) Accounts for only 5% of invasive cancers

c) Diagnosed in women younger than age 50

d) Associated with *BRCA1* mutation

e) Usually presents in the outer quadrant of the breast as a palpable mass

f) Grows in the ducts within a capsule

g) Can become very large

h) Can be mistaken for a fibroadenoma

i) Similar in prognosis to IDC and often favorable

7. Tubular carcinoma

a) Accounts for about 2% of breast cancers

b) Axillary metastasis is uncommon.

c) Prognosis is excellent.

d) Usually discovered from an abnormal finding with mammography

8. Mucinous (colloid) carcinoma

a) Accounts for about 2% to 3% of breast cancers

b) Presents as an abnormal mammogram finding or palpable mass in older, postmenopausal women between ages 70 and 80

c) Slow growing

d) Highly favorable prognosis

9. Paget's disease

   a) Accounts for 2% of all breast cancers

   b) Associated with underlying DCIS in 95% of the cases

   c) May have an invasive component

   d) Presents as nipple cancer with eczema or ulceration of the nipple

   e) Symptoms also include red scaly pruritic lesions of the nipple.

   f) Prognosis is good if no lumps are felt in the breast tissue and the biopsy shows DCIS without invasion.

10. Inflammatory carcinomas

   a) Rare and aggressive form of breast cancer

   b) Responsible for 1% to 3% of breast cancers

   c) A variant of local advanced breast cancer with dermal lymphatic invasion

   d) Has a 5-year survival rate of 50%

   e) Higher risk is associated with African American women, women with a high body mass index, women younger in age.

   f) Nearly all women affected with this condition will have nodal involvement.

   g) Symptoms include diffuse edema and peau d'orange skin (orange peel skin), which occurs because malignant cells block the lymphatic channels in the skin.

   h) There may or not be a mass present. When a mass is present, it will be felt as an indiscrete thickening of the skin.

   i) Often confused with breast infection

   j) Spreads to other parts of the body aggressively

   k) Chemotherapy is used initially to control progression, and radiation and surgery may also be helpful

D. Protective lifestyle activities

Certain lifestyle activities may help to prevent development of breast cancer.

1. Physical activity of 30 to 60 minutes per day at a moderate intensity

2. Breastfeeding can be preventative, as it decreases the return of menstruation, resulting in decreased exposure to endogenous estrogen

3. Management of stress through the use of meditation, prayers, group support programs

E. Prevention strategies

1. Surveillance: Women at high risk benefit from additional screening. Yearly mammography beginning at age 25, clinical breast exam performed twice yearly, MRI, and ultrasound.

2. Chemoprevention is the main method used to prevent this disease.

3. Both Tamoxifen and Raloxifene (Evista) are currently used as chemopreventive agents in high-risk women.

4. The nurse's role is to provide education about the benefits and risks and side effects of these medications.

5. Prophylactic mastectomy may be used as a primary prevention strategy and has been shown to reduce breast cancer by 90%. Prophylactic mastectomy consists of a total mastectomy (removal of breast tissue only) followed by breast reconstruction if desired. Candidates for this procedure include women with a strong family history of breast cancer, women with a diagnosis of LCIS, women with atypical hyperplasia, women who have a *BRCA* gene mutation, and women with a history of breast cancer in one breast.

🛑 **ALERT** Extensive counseling that relates to the risks and benefits is extremely important prior to prophylactic mastectomy because women will have physical and psychological ramifications such as depression, anxiety, and altered body image.

   a) This procedure does not guarantee 100% protection.

   b) Women undergoing this procedure need a multidisciplinary approach and referrals to a genetic counselor, plastic surgeon, medical oncologist, and a psychiatrist to help with her decision-making process.

   c) This is considered an elective surgery.

   d) The nurse should provide information, education, clarification, and support throughout the decision-making process.

F. Treatment options—surgical and systemic management

1. Surgical management

   a) Used to gain local control of the disease

   b) Most frequent options

   c) Lumpectomy

   d) Total simple mastectomy

MAKING THE CONNECTION

Planning Treatment for Breast Cancer

When breast cancer is diagnosed after completion of biopsies and diagnostic testing, including tumor staging, an analysis of the data is reviewed to determine the best treatment options specific for each woman. Tumor size and spread will be important factors when planning treatment options. Smaller tumors and less spread will convey better outcomes.

e) Partial mastectomies done for larger tumors with tumor removal and a rim of healthy tissue

f) If cancer is invasive, a sentinel node biopsy done

2. Sentinel node evaluation
   a) Status of this node is the most important prognostic factor
   b) Highly accurate; will determine potential reoccurrence
   c) Is the first node that receives lymphatic drainage from the tumor
   d) Helps to determine the need for systematic treatment

3. Mastectomy removal of the breast, including the nipple and areola
   a) Usually recommended for women who have had:
      - radiation to the breast
      - multiple tumors in the breast in several quadrants
      - extensive DCIS that is in a large area of breast tissue
      - a large tumor compared to breast volume

4. Total simple mastectomy
   a) Removes the breast, nipple, and areola
   b) Does not remove axillary nodes
   c) Reconstruction of the breast may be performed immediately or scheduled for 1 to 2 weeks later.
   d) Outpatient or hospitalized procedure

5. Modified radical mastectomy
   a) Removes the breast, nipple, and areola, and includes node dissection
   b) Recovery period without reconstructive surgery is 2 to 3 weeks

6. Skin-sparing mastectomy
   a) Removes the breast, nipple, and areola but keeps the outer skin intact
   b) Allows good cosmetic outcome when combined with reconstruction that is done at the same time
   c) If reconstructive surgery is not done at this time, a tissue expander will be inserted for future reconstructive surgery.

7. Nipple-sparing mastectomy
   a) Done on a small number of women with tumors that are not near the nipple/areola area
   b) If reconstructive surgery is not done at this time, a tissue expander is used to hold the space for future reconstructive surgery

8. Nipple-areola-sparing mastectomy
   a) Occurs when the breast is hollowed out and reconstructive surgery is done at the same time

9. Scar-sparing breast surgery
   a) Breast is hollowed out to minimize visible surgical incisions.
   b) Done through an opening less than 2 in. in size

10. Breast reconstruction
    a) Done to promote symmetry and preserve body image
    b) Can be done immediately along with the mastectomy or later
    c) This procedure does not change survival rates or interfere with therapies or treatment of recurrent disease.
    d) It is associated with low morbidity and high patient satisfaction.
    e) Delayed reconstruction is usually done after wound healing or wound healing after radiation or adjuvant therapy.
    f) The timing of this option continues to be controversial within the medical community.
    g) The most common form of breast reconstruction involves having a tissue expander placed, followed by permanent placement of saline or silicone implants.
    h) Flap procedure can also be done by plastic reconstructive surgeons who specialize in microsurgery. With flap reconstruction, a breast is created using tissue taken from other parts of the body (abdomen, back, buttocks, or thighs). This tissue is transplanted to the chest by reconnecting blood vessels to new ones in the chest region.
    i) Nipple reconstruction uses an autologous skin graft to construct a nipple from the reaming nipple or a donor site.
    j) Tattooing of an areola can be done 4 weeks after healing has occurred.

MAKING THE CONNECTION

Breast Reconstruction—A Personal Decision

Women considering breast reconstruction should be made aware of the advantages and disadvantages of the procedure. Immediate breast reconstruction after mastectomy is a reasonable option for women with early stage breast cancer who do not anticipate radiation therapy or adjuvant chemotherapy. However, women should be counseled on the emotional effects of breast reconstruction and breast removal. Some women may not desire to replace the breasts with implants and should be supported in their decision.

11. Systemic treatment
    a) Radiation
       (1) Radiation is used for local regional control of primary breast cancer or palliation of metastatic disease.
       (2) After **breast-conserving surgery,** primary treatment can include radiation to the entire breast with or without a boost to the primary site.
       (3) After modified radical mastectomy, radiation is often done in women at risk of local recurrence.
       (4) Women with node dissection do not require radiation therapy to the axilla.
       (5) Nodes to be treated can be internal mammary lymph nodes or nodes in women with four or more positive lymph nodes, in which case supraclavicular radiation therapy is used to prevent recurrence.
       (6) Radiation therapy usually runs over a 5- to 6-week period.
       (7) Side effects can include fatigue, skin changes, lymphedema, breast pain or tenderness, breast atrophy, brachial plexopathy, radiation pneumonia, and myocardial damage.
       (8) Secondary malignancies are rare but smokers have an increased risk of lung cancer. Another issue is scarring and edema.
       (9) Skin thickening and calcification from the radiation may interfere with interpretation of subsequent mammograms, especially during the first 6 months after treatment; however, these changes resolve within 2 years.
    b) Adjuvant chemotherapy
       (1) Antineoplastic chemotherapy is used for eradication of micrometastasis disease.
       (2) The most common chemotherapeutic drugs used are antimitotic agents, anthracyclines, alkylating agents, and antimicrotubules; they are used in combination for invasive breast cancer.
       (3) They can also be used in combination with hormone therapy.
       (4) Side effects will vary with the specific agent used.
       (5) Common potential side effects include alopecia, nausea, fatigue, myelosuppression, anemia, neuropathy, and myalgia. Less common toxicities are hemorrhagic cystitis (alkylating agents), cardiomyopathy (anthracyclines), thromboembolic

events, and early menopause (in premenopausal women).
       (6) A rare complication is the development of secondary leukemia.
       (7) Pregnant women can receive antineoplastic chemotherapy during the third trimester or after delivery.
    c) Monoclonal antibodies
       (1) This is one of the newest treatment modalities.
       (2) Herceptin (a recombinant DNA–derived humanized monoclonal antibody) is used as a single agent in second-line or late therapy for women with metastatic breast cancer whose tumors overexpress HER2 protein.
       (3) Side effects may include cardiomyopathy, anemia, leukopenia, diarrhea, and infection
    d) Adjuvant hormone therapy/endocrine therapy This is the most effective systematic treatment for hormone-receptor-positive breast cancer. This type of therapy prevents cancer cells from being stimulated by endogenous estrogen by ablation of ovarian function either chemically or surgically or with aromatase inhibitors. It is also used to block the estrogen receptor (ER) pathway with SERMs. Endocrine therapy is usually started after chemotherapy and radiation therapy.
       (1) Tamoxifen is the most commonly used SERM, with a treatment period of 5 years. It has an antiestrogenic effect and is used in women whose tumors have positive hormone receptors. The greatest effect has been seen in women who have both ER-positive and progesterone-receptor (PR) positive tumors. Other favorable effects include improving a woman's blood lipid profile and providing an agonist effect on bone mineral density. However, Tamoxifen does affect the endometrium and may increase the incidence of endometrial cancer. Side effects also include mild nausea, hot flashes, menstrual irregularities, vaginal discharge, vaginal dryness and irritation, benign ovarian cysts, thromboembolic events, and ophthalmological toxicities.
       (2) Raloxifene is used to help prevent breast cancer in postmenopausal women with osteoporosis.
       (3) Nursing role
          (a) Discuss menopausal side effects and management as well as their risk for endometrial hyperplasia or cancer.

Women should be encouraged to receive yearly gynecological examinations and endometrial biopsies for any vaginal discharge or bleeding that may occur.

e) Nursing care interventions for women who receive hormonal therapy
  (1) Teach about side effects of various medications and provide suggestions for self-treatment.
  (2) Manage hot flashes by wearing layered clothing, avoiding caffeine and spicy foods, performing paced breathing exercises, using vitamin E, taking antidepressants, doing yoga, and receiving acupuncture.
  (3) Decrease vaginal dryness by using vaginal moisturizers such as Replens or vitamin E suppositories daily. The use of vaginal lubrication during intercourse such as K-Y, Astroglide, and coconut oil may also be helpful.
  (4) Manage nausea and vomiting by consuming a bland diet and taking medication in the evening.
  (5) Warm baths and nonsteroidal analgesics can help with musculoskeletal symptoms.
  (6) Women also need to be educated regarding the risks involved with hormonal therapies and must do the following:
    (a) Report any irregular bleeding to their gynecologist for evaluation.
    (b) Report any redness, swelling, or tenderness in the lower extremities or any shortness of breath to their physician as soon as possible, as this could be a sign of a thromboembolic issue.
    (c) Watch their bone health by undergoing a baseline bone density test, participating in regular weight-bearing exercise, taking calcium supplements and vitamin D, and taking bisphosphonates as needed and recommended (Calcitonin, Alendronate, etc.)

f) Nursing care interventions for women undergoing surgical treatment
  (1) Preoperative nursing care interventions
    (a) Assessment includes performing a thorough history as discussed earlier with biopsy
    (b) General preop teaching and care
    (c) Expectations regarding physical appearance, pain management, equipment that will be used (e.g., IVs, drains etc.), and postoperative care and teaching should be discussed and reviewed.

    (d) Emotional support, as fear and anxiety are very common
    (e) Referral to organization such as Reach to Recovery
    (f) Inform her that when she awakes, her arm on the affected side will feel tight.
    (g) Remind her that she can no longer have her blood pressure taken, have blood drawn, or receive injections in the affected arm.
  (2) Postoperative care precautions must be taken to prevent or minimize lymphedema in the affected arm.
    (a) Positioning and teaching
      i) Elevate the affected arm with pillows above the level of the right atrium to promote comfort and lymphatic channel return.
      ii) This arm cannot be used for intravenous therapy or any injection, and blood is never drawn from this arm.
      iii) Encourage early movement of this arm.
      iv) Any increase in size of this arm should be reported immediately.
      v) Explain that there is a need to avoid trauma or irritation to the affected arm. She may also experience alterations in sensation, and the removal of some lymph nodes may impact her ability to sense irritation or prevent her being aware of infection.
    (b) Monitor for signs of shock and infection
      i) Assess vital signs but do not use the affected arm for blood pressure measurement.
      ii) Monitor parenteral fluids until adequate oral intake is established.
      iii) Assess wound site and drain sites, looking for redness, swelling, localized heat, fever, increasing pain, and foul-smelling discharge.
      iv) Wound care involves monitoring for hemorrhage noting drainage on dressing and in drainage tubes.
      v) Reinforce dressings as needed.
      vi) Demonstrate the procedure for emptying and recording the amount of drainage.

vii) Drains should be emptied every 8 hours, or more frequently if needed.

viii) Drains are usually removed when drainage is less than 30 mL in 24 hours.

ix) To prevent pneumonia and complications, turn the woman every 4 hours, alternating between the unaffected side and affected side. Have the woman cough and take deep breaths every 2 hours, while nurse applies support to the chest.

(c) Pain

i) Provide pain management as needed. Monitor pain level using a pain scale to identify the intensity.

ii) Administer analgesics as ordered to relieve the patient's discomfort.

iii) Teach and reinforce the use of relaxation techniques to help reduce anxiety and provide distraction.

iv) Auscultate breath sounds every 2 hours. Encourage active range of motion (ROM) exercises for her legs.

(d) Body image

i) Provide opportunities for the patient to express her feelings and concerns regarding body image changes using therapeutic communication techniques.

ii) Facilitate verbalization of her feelings and concerns.

iii) Refer her to support groups and established programs.

iv) Provide emotional support and encouragement.

(e) Mobility

i) Mobility and early ambulation are key to improving circulation, ventilation, and the prevention of bone loss. Teach the patient to do exercises slowly and gently to prevent injury and pain.

ii) Encourage hand, arm, and wrist exercises in the immediate postoperative period. This enhances fluid return and prevents muscle atrophy. Initially the patient should exercise only by clenching and extending her fingers with progression to the wrists and elbow. She will then progress to gradually abducting her arm and raising it to and over her head.

iii) Teach the patient the other exercises to be performed after the drains are removed to promote ROM in the arm and axillary area. Arm exercise should be encouraged four times a day and increased as tolerated or stopped at the point of pain.

iv) Caution the patient not to lift anything heavier than 10 pounds for 4 to 6 weeks to avoid straining the arm on the affected side.

v) Encourage the resumption of mobility and self-care activities of daily living. This will help the patient gain control of her life and will provide psychosocial benefits. Activities of daily living should be encouraged by assisting with washing her face, brushing her hair, and so on, with her hand and arm on the affected side.

vi) The patient will also need information about being fitted for a permanent breast prosthesis 6 to 7 weeks after surgery. This fitting is done by a prosthesis fitter.

vii) Make a referral to home nursing care if the patient needs assistance caring for the incision.

viii) Patient will see her surgeon within 5 to 7 days after surgery. Physical therapy will be prescribed to assist with improving her mobility and strength in the affected arm.

ix) Women having only sentinel node surgery should have full ROM back within a few days. Women with axillary node dissection have to work much harder at restoring ROM but should be back at baseline ROM on by the fourth postoperative week.

(f) Discharge teaching

i) Women undergoing mastectomy with an expander are usually in the hospital for 24 hours. Women having mastectomy and reconstruction will be in the hospital for 3 to 5 days. Teaching is of the utmost importance and should begin preoperatively.

ii) When this is not possible, teaching needs to be done with the patient when her caregiver is present. Printed information needs to be used, as the patient may be experiencing stress and may be recovering from anesthesia, which may cause her to be forgetful.

(g) Mastectomy without reconstruction teaching

  i) The patient should always wash hands before and after touching the incision site.

  ii) The patient should empty surgical drains twice daily and as needed. Keep a record of the date, time, drain site, and amount of drainage. This record should be brought to her doctor visit.

  iii) The patient should avoid driving, lifting more than 10 pounds, or reaching above her head until the physician gives permission.

  iv) The patient should take medication for pain as soon as pain begins.

  v) The patient should perform arm exercises as directed.

  vi) Advise her to call the physician if inflammation at the site or swelling occurs at the incision site or in the arm.

  vii) She should avoid tight-fitting clothing, jewelry, and anything that can decrease circulation in the affected arm.

  viii) Until the drains are removed, the patient should wear loose-fitting underwear or camisole and pin the drains inside the clothing.

  ix) The patient will be given a surgical bra that will hold a temporary breast form; this is until she can be fitted for a mastectomy bra and breast prosthesis. After drains are removed and surgical sites are still healing, a mastectomy bra or camisole with a cotton-filled muslin temporary prosthesis can be worn.

  x) Advise the patient to avoid depilatory creams, strong deodorants, and shaving of the affected chest area, axilla, and arm.

  xi) She should sponge bathe for the first 48 hours, then shower. Thoroughly dry afterward and reapply fresh dressings.

  xii) The patient should see the surgeon's office for incision checks, drain inspection, and possible drain and staple removal as directed at discharge.

  xiii) The patient may contact Reach to Recovery or a breast center staff person for assistance with obtaining an external prosthesis and lingerie once the dressings and staples are removed and the incisional site is healed and nontender. She can contact the insurance company for information about coverage of prosthesis and wig if needed. She should obtain prescriptions for the prosthesis and wig to submit with receipts to the insurance company. If insurance does not pay for this, she should contact the agency social worker or American Cancer Society for assistance.

  xiv) The patient should practice BSE on the unaffected side and affected surgical side and axilla, keep all follow-up appointments for examination mammography and testing to detect recurrent breast cancer.

  xvi) The patient should expect decreased sensation and tingling in the incision site and in the affected arm for weeks or months postsurgery.

  xvii) The patient may resume sexual activities as desired.

  xviii) The patient should be encouraged to participate in breast cancer survivor support groups.

  xix) The nurse should encourage mothers, daughters, and sisters to learn about and practice BSE and to receive annual professional examinations and mammograms as recommended.

(h) Women who underwent mastectomy and reconstructive surgery
Much of the above teaching for mastectomy will also be applicable here, but there is additional information that these patients will need:

(i) There should be no tight compression of the reconstructed breasts until approved by the patient's plastic surgeon.

(ii) The patient will need to wear loosely fitting garments for the first 3 to 4 weeks.

(iii) Remind the patient that her surgery is a work in progress and final cosmetic results of reconstruction take many weeks.

(iv) The patient should assess/observe skin for potential of poor peripheral circulation that can cause skin necrosis. She should notify the physician of any skin changes immediately.

(v) Reinforce dressings as needed.

(vi) Patient should empty the drain and record the amount of drainage, the date, and the time.

(vii) Drains should be emptied every 8 hours, or more frequently if needed.

(viii) Drains are usually removed when drainage is less than 30 mL over 24 hours.

(ix) Explain that there is a need to avoid trauma or irritation to the affected arm.

(x) Explain that the patient may experience alterations in sensation and that the removal of some lymph nodes may impact her ability to sense irritation or prevent her being aware of infection.

(xi) Reinforce that the patient needs to protect the affected arm from injury and infection. She should avoid having blood drawn, receiving injections, and having blood pressure taken on the affected side.

CASE STUDY: Putting It All Together

Subjective Data

Judy is a 40-year-old white female in good health. She presents with a chief complaint of a small lump in the left breast that has been there for the last month. She has a family history that includes her mother being diagnosed 10 years ago with breast cancer at age 60. She underwent a mastectomy with radiation and chemotherapy. Her mother is currently 70 years and doing well. She also had an aunt diagnosed with ovarian cancer at age 46 who succumbed to the disease. Her menstrual periods started at age 11. She is widowed and a single parent of three children aged 8, 10, and 15. She works full time as a manager of a grocery store. She is anxious and states, "I am worried and unsure of what this is." She has had a mammogram done the past 2 years with normal findings. She has a history of a fibrocystic lump that was diagnosed after fine-needle aspiration when she was 28 years old.

Objective Data

• Physical exam reveals the following:
• Temperature: 98.6°F
• Blood pressure: 124/80 mm Hg
• Pulse: 80 bpm
• Respirations: 18 bpm
• Weight: 185 lb
• Height: 5'4"

   Breast exam reveals no nipple inversion, redness, ulceration, discharge, or swelling. Skin does not feel warm and is clear with no visible redness or veining on either breast. Clinical breast examination reveals a thickening and a small mass, 2 cm, in the left breast that feels soft and fluid filled. There is no swelling or node enlargement in the axilla of either breast. Judy appears anxious and fearful.

Case Study Questions

A. What are Judy's breast cancer risk factors?

_____

_____

_____

Continued

CASE STUDY: Putting It All Together (Continued)

Case Study Questions

B. What test would you anticipate the physician to order?

_____

_____

_____

C. Judy's mass was found to be benign. She is considered at a high risk for developing breast cancer. What prevention strategies can be offered to her?

_____

_____

_____

_____

_____

_____

_____

_____

_____

_____

REVIEW QUESTIONS

1. A nurse is performing a gynecological health history interview on a 17-year-old Caucasian adolescent. The girl appears anxious and states, "I found a lump in my left breast, and I am worried that it may be cancer." What factors should the nurse be aware of prior to responding to this patient? *Select all that apply.*
   1. Breast fibroadenomas are the most common breast tumor in women after puberty and between the ages of 15 and 30.
   2. African American women tend to develop fibroadenomas more often and at an earlier age than Caucasian women.
   3. Young women are at increased risk for breast cancer.
   4. The cause of fibroadenoma is a cancerous condition.

2. Which are major risk factors for breast cancer? *Select all that apply.*
   1. Female gender
   2. Increasing age over 50 years
   3. Personal history of breast cancer (in situ or invasive), family history of breast cancer in first-degree relatives (parent, sibling, child)
   4. High-fat diet
   5. Alcohol consumption (two or more drinks/day)

3. Which factors contribute to a woman's perception of her body? *Select all that apply.*
   1. Role of motherhood
   2. Sexuality
   3. Relationships at work
   4. Family and social relationships

4. A 40-year-old woman has just been diagnosed with stage 2 breast cancer. Which of the following are common reactions? *Select all that apply.*
   1. Anxiety regarding changes in family reactions, body image, disability, and pain
   2. Concern about disruptions related to treatment
   3. Fear of death
   4. Decisional conflict related to controversies about treatment options
   5. Readiness for preoperative and postoperative education

5. According to the standard staging classification for breast cancer, which criteria reflects stage 2 breast cancer?
   1. Tumor smaller than 2 cm, no regional lymph node metastasis, no distant metastasis
   2. No evidence of tumor; metastasis to lymph nodes fixed to one another or to other structure but no distant metastasis
   3. Tumor larger than 5 cm; metastasis to lymph nodes fixed to one another or to other structure; no distant metastasis
   4. Tumor larger than 2 to 5 cm; no regional lymph node metastasis; no distant metastasis

6. Which statement is *not* true regarding breast reconstruction?
   1. It promotes symmetry and preserves body image.
   2. It is always done immediately along with the mastectomy.
   3. It does not change survival rates or interfere with therapies or treatment of recurrent disease.
   4. It is associated with low morbidity and high patient satisfaction.

7. Mastectomy is usually recommended for which women?
   1. Those who have not had radiation to the breast
   2. Those who have multiple tumors in the breast in several quadrants
   3. Those with no extensive DCIS
   4. Those with a small tumor compared to breast volume

8. The nurse is teaching a woman receiving adjuvant hormonal therapy on how she can manage her side effects and symptoms. Which education and teaching will the nurse include? *Select all that apply.*
   1. Wear layered clothing and avoid caffeine and spicy foods to help relieve hot flashes
   2. Decrease vaginal dryness by using vaginal moisturizers such as Replens or vitamin E suppositories daily
   3. Manage nausea and vomiting by consuming a bland diet and taking medication first thing in the morning.
   4. Ease musculoskeletal symptoms with warm baths and nonsteroidal analgesics

9. A woman has been diagnosed with galactorrhea. Which signs and symptoms should the nurse expect to see? *Select all that apply.*
   1. Milky white discharge from one or both nipples
   2. Absence of menstrual periods
   3. Temperature intolerance
   4. Less interest in sex
   5. Bleeding nipple discharge

10. Which statement by the woman indicates that she does not understand the teaching provided about postmastectomy breast reconstruction home care?
    1. "I will avoid trauma to my breasts."
    2. "I will need to wear a tight bra immediately."
    3. "I have to empty my drains every 8 hours."
    4. "I must notify the doctor if I notice any skin ulceration or changes in breast color such as redness."
    5. "I will reinforce my dressing as needed."

11. A nurse is providing preoperative teaching for a woman who is undergoing a total mastectomy. Which will this teaching include? *Select all that apply.*
    1. Explain that she will have an IV, a drain, and a dressing in place on awakening. Tell her about expectations she may have regarding physical appearance, pain management, equipment that will be used (IVs, drains, etc.).
    2. Explain that she will be provided pain management as needed; monitor and review the pain scale to be used to identify level of intensity.
    3. Have her elevate the affected arm with pillows.
    4. Turn the woman every 4 hours, alternating between the unaffected side and affected side. To prevent pneumonia and complications, have her cough and take deep breaths every 2 hours, while nurse applies support to the chest.

12. List in order of priority the immediate postoperative mastectomy nursing actions.
    1. Elevate the affected arm with pillows above the level of the right atrium to promote comfort and lymphatic channel return.
    2. Assess vital signs, being careful not to use the affected arm for blood pressure measurement, and monitor parenteral fluids.
    3. Monitor for hemorrhage by assessing drainage from dressing and drainage tubes.
    4. Teach and reinforce the use of relaxation techniques to help reduce anxiety and provide distraction.
    5. Turn the woman every 4 hours, alternating between the unaffected side and affected side. To prevent pneumonia and complications, have the woman cough and take deep breaths every 2 hours, while nurse applies support to the chest.

13. When performing a breast assessment, the nurse is inspecting the woman's skin for which of the following? *Select all that apply.*
    1. Color
    2. Thickening
    3. Size and symmetry
    4. Venous pattern
    5. Edema

14. A woman has been diagnosed with single intraductal papilloma and has nipple discharge. Which diagnostic tests will *most* likely be required?
    1. MRI
    2. Mammogram
    3. Core needle biopsy
    4. Ductogram

15. The nurse is providing a 20-year-old woman diagnosed with fibrocystic disease with education about her condition. Which information should be included? *Select all that apply.*
    1. Pain or tenderness is never present with fibrocystic disease.
    2. The cysts are thought to be hormone related.
    3. The cysts can be of any size, can feel like small lumps or grapes, and can be soft or firm.
    4. It is not a common finding in women between the ages of 30 and 50.
    5. The cysts usually recede and disappear with menopause.

REVIEW QUESTION ANSWERS

1. ANSWER: 1, 2, 3
Rationale
1. Benign fibroadenoma is the most common breast tumor in adolescent populations (women after puberty and between the ages of 15 and 30).
2. African American women tend to develop fibroadenomas more often and at an earlier age than Caucasian women.
3. Age is a nonmodifiable risk factor, as older women are at increased risk for breast cancer. The risk increases with age, as it is low in women in their 20s and 30s but continues to rise with each decade.
4. Fibroadenoma is a common benign condition of the breast.
TEST-TAKING TIP: To answer a "select all that apply" question, consider each answer option as a true or false. Determine if the answer is either a yes or a no or if it applies or does not apply to the stem.
Content Area: Fibroadenoma (FNA)/Disorders of the Breast
Integrated Process: Nursing Process—Teaching/Learning
Client Need: Psychosocial Integrity; Physiological Integrity; Health Promotion and Maintenance; Safe and Effective Care Environment
Cognitive Level: Application/Analysis
Concept: Critical Thinking
Reference: Christinsen-Rangel, L. C. (2013). Breast health. In E. Q. Youngkin, M. S. Davis, M. S. Schadewald, & C. Juve (Eds.). Women's health: A primary care clinical guide. 4th ed. Boston: Pearson.
Galactorrhea Overview. (2014). Retrieved from http://familydoctor.org/familydoctor/en/diseases-conditions/galactorrhea.html.
Shockney, L. D. (2012). Problems of the breast. In D. L. Lowdermilk, S. E. Perry, K. Cashion, & K. R. Alden (Eds.). Maternity & women's health care. 10th ed. St. Louis, MO: Elsevier.
U.S. National Library Medline Plus Encyclopedia. (2013). Intraductal papilloma. Retrieved from www.nlm.nih.gov/medlineplus/ency/article/001238.htm.

2. ANSWER: 1, 2, 3
Rationale
1. Female gender is a major risk factor for the development of breast cancer and is nonmodifiable.
2. Increasing age is considered to be a major risk factor for the development of breast cancer and is nonmodifiable.
3. Personal history of breast cancer (in situ or invasive) and family history of breast cancer in first-degree relatives (parent, sibling, child) are considered to be major genetic risk factors for the development of breast cancer and are nonmodifiable.
4. A high-fat diet is considered to be a possible risk factor for the development of breast cancer.
5. Alcohol consumption (two or more drinks/day) is considered to be a possible risk factor for the development of breast cancer.
TEST-TAKING TIP: Review information and statistics regarding breast cancer rates for ethnicity, race, and death rates.
Content Area: Breast Cancer Incidence and Statistics for Women/Disorders of the Breast
Integrated Process: Nursing Process—Caring; Teaching/Learning; Communication and Documentation; Clinical Problem Solving
Client Need: Reduction of Risk Potential; Health Promotion and Maintenance

Cognitive Level: Application
Concept: Promoting Health
Reference: Johnson, J., Thomas, D. J., & Porter, B. O. (2015). Women's health problems. In L. M. Dunphy, J. E. Winward-Brown, B. O. Porter, & D. F. Thomas (Eds.). Primary care: Art and science of advanced practice nursing. Philadelphia: F.A. Davis.

3. ANSWER: 1, 2, 4
Rationale
1. One function of the breast is lactation, which is a source of infant nourishment and plays an important role in nurturing and motherhood.
2. The breasts are associated with sexuality and pleasure for both men and women.
3. A woman's perception of her work environment response is important, as she may be concerned about her loss of income or job security, as well as health benefits/insurance.
4. A woman's perception of her relationships with family and social networks impacts her identification of her gender role and functioning.
TEST-TAKING TIP: There are many cultural and psychological issues and beliefs that can impact both men and women in American society.
Content Area: Breast Development/Disorders of the Breast
Integrated Process: Nursing Process—Planning
Client Need: Health Promotion and Maintenance; Physiological Integrity; Reduction of Risk Potential; Physiological Adaption
Cognitive Level: Comprehension
Concept: Sexuality
Reference: Johnson, J., Thomas, D. J., & Porter, B. O. (2015). Women's health problems. In L. M. Dunphy, J. E. Winward-Brown, B. O. Porter, & D. F. Thomas, D.F. (Eds.). Primary care: Art and science of advanced practice nursing. 4th ed. Philadelphia: F.A. Davis.
National Cancer Institute. (2016). Breast cancer treatment. Retrieved from www.cancer.gov/types/breast/patient/breast-trestment-pdq.

4. ANSWER: 1, 2, 3, 4
Rationale
1. Women diagnosed with breast cancer will often show intense emotional reactions regarding family response, body image, sexual functioning, disability, and pain.
2. Women diagnosed with breast cancer will be concerned about the disease disrupting her life and family processes.
3. Women with breast cancer often experience fear of death.
4. Women will experience decisional conflict as they are presented with choices as well as risks and benefits of specific treatment options.
5. Women will be anxious and not ready for specific education regarding the preoperative and postoperative education, as the emotional reaction to the diagnosis is typically intense.
TEST-TAKING TIP: Remember the nurse should always provide opportunities for the woman to express her feelings and concerns regarding body image changes using therapeutic communication techniques. The nurse should facilitate verbalization of her feelings and concerns, refer her to support groups and established programs, and provide emotional support and encouragement.
Content Area: Breast Cancer Diagnosis, Prognosis, Treatment/Disorders of the Breast

Integrated Process: Nursing Process—Clinical Problem Solving; Caring; Communication and Documentation; Teaching/Learning
Client Need: Safe and Effective Care Environment; Health Promotion and Maintenance; Psychosocial Integrity; Physiological Integrity
Cognitive Level: Application
Concept: Grief and Loss
Reference: Branch, L. G. (2004). Breast health. In E. Q. Youngkin & M. S. Davis (Eds.). Women's health: A primary care clinical guide. 3rd ed. Boston: Pearson.
Christinsen-Rangel, L. C. (2013). Breast health. In E. Q. Youngkin, M. S. Davis, M. S. Schadewald, & C. Juve. (Eds.). Women's health: A primary care clinical guide. 4th ed. Boston: Pearson.

5. ANSWER: 4
Rationale
1. A tumor smaller than 2 cm, with no regional lymph node metastasis and no distant metastasis is classified as stage 1.
2. A stage 1 classification is no evidence of tumor; metastasis to lymph nodes is fixed to one another or to another structure but no distant metastasis.
3. Tumor smaller than 2 cm, metastasis to lymph nodes fixed to one another or to another structure, and no distant metastasis is classified as stage 3A.
4. A tumor larger than 2 to 5 cm, with no regional lymph node metastasis and no distant metastasis is classified as stage 2B.
TEST-TAKING TIP: Determination of breast cancer is the first step in evaluating the client. Staging the cancer is necessary to understand the severity and to plan for the best medical therapy.
Content Area: Breast Cancer Staging/Contraception
Integrated Process: Nursing Process—Clinical Problem Solving; Caring; Communication and Documentation; Teaching/Learning
Client Need: Safe and Effective Care Environment; Reduction Risk Potential; Physiological Integrity; Psychological Integrity
Cognitive Level: Application
Concept: Cellular Regulation
Reference: Johnson, J., Thomas, D. J., & Porter, B. O. (2015). Women's health problems. In L. M. Dunphy, J. E. Winward-Brown, B. O. Porter, & D. F. Thomas (Eds.). Primary care: Art and science of advanced practice nursing (p. 697). 4th ed. Philadelphia: F.A. Davis.
National Cancer Institute. (2016). Breast cancer treatment. Retrieved from www.cancer.gov/types/breast/patient/breast-trestment-pdq.
Christinsen-Rangel, L. C. (2013). Breast health. In E. Q. Youngkin, M. S. Davis, M. S. Schadewald, & C. Juve. (2013). Women's health: A primary care clinical guide. 4th ed. Boston: Pearson.

6. ANSWER: 2
Rationale
1. Breast reconstruction promotes symmetry and preserves the woman's body image.
2. Breast reconstruction can be done immediately along with the mastectomy or it can be done later.
3. Breast reconstruction does not change survival rates or interfere with therapies or treatment for recurrent breast cancer.
4. A breast reconstruction procedure is associated with low morbidity and high patient satisfaction.
TEST-TAKING TIP: Immediate breast reconstruction after mastectomy is a reasonable option for women with early

stage breast cancer who do not anticipate radiation therapy or adjuvant chemotherapy.
Content Area: Breast Cancer Diagnosis, Prognosis, Treatment/Disorders of the Breast
Integrated Process: Nursing Process—Clinical Problem Solving; Caring; Communication and Documentation; Teaching/Learning
Client Need: Safe and Effective Care Environment; Health Promotion and Maintenance; Psychosocial Integrity; Physiological Integrity
Cognitive Level: Application
Concept: Self
Reference: Christinsen-Rangel, L. C. (2013). Breast health. In E. Q. Youngkin, M. S. Davis, M. S. Schadewald, & C. Juve (Eds.). Women's health: A primary care clinical guide. 4th ed. Boston: Pearson.
Hinkle, J. L., & Cheever, K. H. (2014). Brunner and Sudarth's textbook of medical and surgical nursing (Vol. 2). 13th ed. Philadelphia: Wolters Kluwer/Lippincott Williams & Wilkins.
Johnson, J., Thomas, D. J., & Porter, B.O. (2015). Women's health problems. In L. M. Dunphy, J. E. Winward-Brown, B. O. Porter, & D. F. Thomas (Eds.). Primary care: Art and science of advanced practice nursing (pp. 679-754). 4th ed. Philadelphia: F.A. Davis.
Shockney, L. D. (2012). Problems of the breast. In D. L. Lowdermilk, S. E. Perry, K. Cashion, & K. R. Alden (Eds.). Maternity & women's health care. 10th ed. St. Louis, MO: Elsevier.

7. ANSWER: 2
Rationale
1. Mastectomy is done for women who have had radiation.
2. Mastectomy is done for women who have multiple tumors in the breast in several quadrants.
3. Mastectomy is done for women who have extensive DCIS.
4. Mastectomy is done for women who have a large area of breast tissue or large tumors.
TEST-TAKING TIP: The type of mastectomy usually depends on the type, stage, and location of the cancer. The different types of surgery are total simple mastectomy, modified radical mastectomy, skin-sparing mastectomy, nipple-sparing mastectomy, and nipple-areola sparing mastectomy.
Content Area: Breast Cancer Diagnosis, Prognosis, Treatment/Disorders of the Breast
Integrated Process: Nursing Process—Clinical Problem Solving; Caring; Communication and Documentation; Teaching/Learning
Client Need: Safe and Effective Care Environment; Health Promotion and Maintenance; Psychosocial Integrity; Physiological Integrity
Cognitive Level: Application
Concept: Critical Thinking
Reference: Christinsen-Rangel, L. C. (2013). Breast health. In E. Q. Youngkin, M. S. Davis, M. S. Schadewald, & C. Juve (Eds.). Women's health: A primary care clinical guide. 4th ed. Boston: Pearson.
Hinkle, J. L., & Cheever, K. H. (2014). Brunner and Sudarth's textbook of medical and surgical nursing (Vol. 2). 13th ed. Philadelphia: Wolters Kluwer/Lippincott Williams & Wilkins.
Johnson, J., Thomas, D. J., & Porter, B. O. (2015). Women's health problems. In L. M. Dunphy, J. E. Winward-Brown, B. O. Porter, & D. F. Thomas (Eds.). Primary care: Art and science of advanced practice nursing (pp. 679-754). 4th ed. Philadelphia: F.A. Davis.
Shockney, L. D. (2012). Problems of the breast. In D. L. Lowdermilk, S. E. Perry, K. Cashion, & K. R. Alden (Eds.). Maternity & women's health care. 10th ed. St. Louis, MO: Elsevier.

8. ANSWER: 1, 2, 4
Rationale
1. Wearing layered clothing and avoiding caffeine and spicy foods helps to relieve hot flashes.

2. Vaginal dryness can be decreased by using vaginal moisturizers such as Replens or vitamin E suppositories daily.
3. Nausea and vomiting should be managed by consuming a bland diet and taking medication in the evening.
4. Warm baths and nonsteroidal analgesics can help with the musculoskeletal symptoms.

TEST-TAKING TIP: This type of therapy prevents cancer cells from being stimulated by endogenous estrogen by ablation of ovarian function either chemically or surgically and by aromatase inhibitors. It is also used to block the ER pathway with SERMs. Endocrine therapy is usually started after chemotherapy and radiation therapy.

Content Area: Breast Cancer Diagnosis, Prognosis, Treatment/ Disorders of the Breast
Integrated Process: Nursing Process—Clinical Problem Solving; Caring; Communication and Documentation; Teaching/Learning
Client Need: Safe and Effective Care Environment; Health Promotion and Maintenance; Psychosocial Integrity; Physiological Integrity
Cognitive Level: Application
Concept: Comfort
Reference: Christinsen-Rangel, L. C. (2013). Breast health. In E. Q. Youngkin, M. S. Davis, M. S. Schadewald, & C. Juve (Eds.). Women's health: A primary care clinical guide. 4th ed. Boston: Pearson
Hinkle, J. L., & Cheever, K. H. (2014). Brunner and Sudarth's textbook of medical and surgical nursing (Vol. 2). 13th ed. Philadelphia: Wolters Kluwer/Lippincott Williams & Wilkins.
Johnson, J., Thomas, D. J., & Porter, B. O. (2015). Women's health problems. In L. M. Dunphy, J. E. Winward-Brown, B. O. Porter, & D. F. Thomas (Eds.). Primary care: Art and science of advanced practice nursing (pp. 679-754). 4th ed. Philadelphia: F.A. Davis.
Shockney, L. D. (2012). Problems of the breast. In D. L. Lowdermilk, S. E. Perry, K. Cashion, & K. R. Alden (Eds.). Maternity & women's health care. 10th ed. St. Louis, MO: Elsevier.

9. **ANSWER: 1, 2, 3, 4**
Rationale
1. Milky white discharge from one or both nipples (discharge may also be yellow or greenish in color) is a symptom of galactorrhea.
2. An absence of menstrual periods (amenorrhea is a primary symptom of galactorrhea).
3. Temperature intolerance is a symptom of galactorrhea and may be associated with a hypothyroid disorder.
4. Less interest in sex is a symptom of galactorrhea.
5. Blood in the discharge is not galactorrhea. If the fluid is reddish, this may be an indication of cancer.

TEST-TAKING TIP: Galactorrhea is caused by hyperpro-lactinemia, which may be a result of certain medications, endocrine disorders, renal disease, and breast stimulation. Breasts may leak only when the breasts are touched or with no stimulation.

Content Area: Galactorrhea/Disorders of the Breast
Integrated Process: Nursing Process—Clinical Problem Solving; Caring; Communication and Documentation; Teaching/Learning
Client Need: Psychosocial Integrity; Physiological Integrity; Health Promotion and Maintenance; Safe and Effective Care Environment
Cognitive Level: Application
Concept: Female Reproduction

Reference: Christinsen-Rangel, L. C. (2013). Breast health. In E. Q. Youngkin, M. S. Davis, M. S. Schadewald, & C. Juve (Eds.). Women's health: A primary care clinical guide. 4th Ed. Boston: Pearson.
Shockney, L. D. (2012). Problems of the breast. In D. L. Lowdermilk, S. E. Perry, K. Cashion, & K. R. Alden (Eds.). Maternity & women's health care. 10th ed. St. Louis, MO: Elsevier.

10. **ANSWER: 2**
Rationale
1. There is a need to avoid trauma or irritation to the affected arm and to protect the affected arm from injury and infection. She should avoid blood draws, injections, and blood pressure measurements on that arm.
2. There should be no tight compression of the recon-structed breasts until approved by her plastic surgeon. She will need to wear loose-fitting garments for the first 3 to 4 weeks.
3. She should empty the drain and record the amount of drainage, date, and time. Drains should be emptied every 8 hours, or more frequently if needed. Drains are usually removed when drainage is less than 30 mL over 24 hours.
4. She should assess/observe skin for potential of poor pe-ripheral circulation that can cause skin necrosis. She should immediately notify the physician of any skin changes.
5. She should reinforce her dressing as needed.

TEST-TAKING TIP: Postoperative care precautions must be used to prevent or minimize lymphedema in the affected arm. Additional teaching should include elevating the affected arm, not allowing intravenous therapy or blood to be drawn from the affected arm, and encouraging early movement.

Content Area: Breast Cancer Diagnosis, Prognosis, Treatment/ Disorders of the Breast
Integrated Process: Nursing Process—Clinical Problem Solving; Caring; Communication and Documentation; Teaching/Learning
Client Need: Safe and Effective Care Environment; Health Promotion and Maintenance; Psychosocial Integrity; Physiological Integrity
Cognitive Level: Analysis
Concept: Perioperative
Reference: Christinsen-Rangel, L. C. (2013). Breast health. In E. Q. Youngkin, M. S. Davis, M. S. Schadewald, & C. Juve (Eds.). Women's health: A primary care clinical guide. 4th ed. Boston: Pearson.
Hinkle, J. L., & Cheever, K. H. (2014). Brunner and Sudarth's textbook of medical and surgical nursing (Vol. 2). 13th ed. Philadelphia: Wolters Kluwer/Lippincott Williams & Wilkins.
Johnson, J., Thomas, D. J., & Porter, B. O. (2015). Women's health problems. In L. M. Dunphy, J. E. Winward-Brown, B. O. Porter, & D. F. Thomas (Eds.). Primary care: Art and science of advanced practice nursing (pp. 679-754). 4th ed. Philadelphia: F.A. Davis.
Shockney, L. D. (2012). Problems of the breast. In D. L. Lowdermilk, S. E. Perry, K. Cashion, & K. R. Alden (Eds.). Maternity & women's health care. 10th ed. St. Louis, MO: Elsevier.

11. **ANSWER: 1, 2, 3, 4**
Rationale
1. Expectations regarding physical appearance, pain man-agement equipment that will be used (IVs, drains, etc.), and postoperative care and teaching should be discussed and reviewed.
2. Pain management will be provided as needed, and pain level will be measured using a pain scale to identify type and intensity. Analgesics as ordered to relieve the patient's discomfort as needed.

3. Postoperative care special precautions must be used to prevent or minimize lymphedema in the affected arm. Elevate the affected arm with pillows above the level of the right atrium to promote comfort and lymphatic channel return. Patient will be encouraged to move her arm early.

4. The patient will be turned every 4 hours, alternating between the unaffected side and affected side. To prevent pneumonia and complications, the nurse will encourage the patient to cough and take deep breaths every 2 hours, while the nurse supports the chest.

TEST-TAKING TIP: Clients who have a clear understanding of the surgical procedure and postoperative care often experience a decrease in anxiety.

Content Area: Breast Cancer Diagnosis, Prognosis, Treatment/ Disorders of the Breast

Integrated Process: Nursing Process—Clinical Problem Solving; Caring; Communication and Documentation; Teaching/Learning

Client Need: Safe and Effective Care Environment; Health Promotion and Maintenance; Psychosocial Integrity; Physiological Integrity

Cognitive Level: Application

Concept: Perioperative

Reference: Christinsen-Rangel, L. C. (2013). Breast health. In E. Q. Youngkin, M. S. Davis, M. S. Schadewald, & C. Juve (Eds.). Women's health: A primary care clinical guide. 4th ed. Boston: Pearson.

Hinkle, J. L., & Cheever, K. H. (2014). Brunner and Sudarth's textbook of medical and surgical nursing (Vol. 2). 13th ed. Philadelphia: Wolters Kluwer/Lippincott Williams & Wilkins.

Johnson, J., Thomas, D. J., & Porter, B. O. (2015). Women's health problems. In L. M. Dunphy, J. E. Winward-Brown, B. O. Porter, & D. F. Thomas (Eds.). Primary care: Art and science of advanced practice nursing (pp. 679-754). 4th ed. Philadelphia: F.A. Davis.

Shockney, L. D. (2012). Problems of the breast. In D. L. Lowdermilk, S. E. Perry, K. Cashion, & K. R. Alden (Eds.). Maternity & women's health care. 10th ed. St. Louis, MO: Elsevier.

12. **ANSWER: 1, 2, 3, 4, 5**

Rationale

1. Postoperative care precautions must be used to prevent or minimize lymphedema in the affected arm. Elevate the affected arm with pillows above the level of the right atrium to promote comfort and lymphatic channel return. Any in-crease in size of this arm should be reported immediately.

2. Monitoring for signs of shock and infection includes assessing vital signs. Do not use the affected arm for blood pressure measurement and use parenteral fluids until adequate oral intake is established.

3. Wound care involves monitoring for hemorrhage (dressing, drainage tubes, or Jackson-Pratt drains with dressings reinforced as needed).

4. Teaching and encouraging relaxation techniques begin postoperatively, when the woman is awake and responsive.

5. Turn the woman every 4 hours, alternating between the unaffected side and affected side. To prevent pneumonia and complications, have the woman cough and take deep breaths every 2 hours, while nurse applies support to the chest.

TEST-TAKING TIP: When prioritizing care, always refer to Maslow's hierarchy of needs.

Content Area: Breast Cancer Diagnosis, Prognosis, Treatment/ Disorders of the Breast

Integrated Process: Nursing Process—Clinical Problem Solving; Caring; Communication and Documentation; Teaching/Learning

Client Need: Safe and Effective Care Environment; Health Promotion and Maintenance; Psychosocial Integrity; Physiological Integrity

Cognitive Level: Application

Concept: Perioperative

Reference: Christinsen-Rangel, L. C. (2013). Breast health. In E. Q. Youngkin, M. S. Davis, M.S. Schadewald, & C. Juve (Eds.). Women's health: A primary care clinical guide. 4th ed. Boston: Pearson.

Hinkle, J. L., & Cheever, K. H. (2014). Brunner and Sudarth's textbook of medical and surgical nursing (Vol. 2). 13th ed. Philadelphia: Wolters Kluwer/Lippincott Williams & Wilkins.

Johnson, J., Thomas, D. J., & Porter, B. O. (2015). Women's health problems. In L. M. Dunphy, J. E. Winward-Brown, B. O. Porter, & D. F. Thomas (Eds.). Primary care: Art and science of advanced practice nursing (pp. 679-754). 4th ed. Philadelphia: F.A. Davis.

Shockney, L. D. (2012). Problems of the breast. In D. L. Lowdermilk, S. E. Perry, K. Cashion, & K. R. Alden (Eds.). Maternity & women's health care. 10th ed. St. Louis, MO: Elsevier.

13. **ANSWER: 1, 2, 4, 5**

Rationale

1. The skin is inspected for color. Redness may indicate benign local inflammation or infection. Skin with the appearance of an orange peel may also indicate an underlying neoplasm.

2. The skin is inspected for thickening, which may indicate a potential superficial lymphatic invasion of a neoplasm.

3. A routine inspection of the breast begins with the disrobed woman sitting in a comfortable position facing the examiner, who checks breast size and symmetry.

4. The skin is inspected for venous pattern, indicating blood supply to the area.

5. The skin is inspected for edema, which may indicate a blockage of lymphatic drainage.

TEST-TAKING TIP: Breast examination can be used both as a screening and a diagnostic tool and includes visual inspection and palpation.

Content Area: Clinical Breast Exam/Breast Disorder

Integrated Process: Nursing Process—Clinical Problem Solving; Teaching/Learning; Communication and Documentation

Client Need: Health Promotion and Maintenance; Physiological Integrity; Reduction of Risk Potential

Cognitive Level: Application/Evaluation

Concept: Critical Thinking

Reference: Christinsen-Rangel, L. C. (2013). Breast health. In E. Q. Youngkin, M. S. Davis, M. S. Schadewald, & C. Juve (Eds.). Women's health a primary care clinical guide. 4th ed. Boston: Pearson.

Hinkle, J. L., & Cheever, K. H. (2014). Brunner and Sudarth's textbook of medical and surgical nursing (Vol. 2). 13th ed. Philadelphia: Wolters Kluwer/Lippincott Williams & Wilkins.

Johnson, J., Thomas, D. J., & Porter, B. O. (2015). Women's health problems. In L. M. Dunphy, J. E. Winward-Brown, B. O. Porter, & D. F. Thomas (Eds.). Primary care: Art and science of advanced practice nursing (pp. 679-754). 4th ed. Philadelphia: F.A. Davis.

Weber, J., & Kelly, J. (2009). Health assessment in nursing. 4th ed. Philadelphia: Lippincott Williams & Wilkins.

14. **ANSWER: 3**

Rationale

1. An MRI would not be performed as an initial diagnostic test due to cost.

2. A mammogram is usually done for screening since the patient has nipple discharge. She will need an ultrasound study.

3. When there is nipple discharge, a surgical needle core biopsy is performed to assist with a diagnosis. The usual treatment is removal of the duct with biopsy to rule out cancer.

4. Ductograms are no longer used, as x-ray with contrast dye injected into the affected duct (ductogram) has been replaced by ultrasound, ductoscopy, and ductal lavage.

TEST-TAKING TIP: Intraductal papilloma is a benign tumor that grows within the milk ducts of the breast. Symptoms may include breast lumps, nipple discharge, or tissue hyperplasia. The client may also complain of a feeling of fullness or pain beneath the areola.

Content Area: Intraductal Papilloma/Breast Disorders
Integrated Process: Nursing Process—Clinical Problem Solving; Caring; Communication and Documentation; Teaching/Learning
Client Need: Psychosocial Integrity; Physiological Integrity; Health Promotion and Maintenance; Safe and Effective Care Environment
Cognitive Level: Application
Concept: Critical Thinking

Reference: Christinsen-Rangel, L. C. (2013). Breast health. In E. Q. Youngkin, M. S. Davis, M. S. Schadewald, & C. Juve (Eds.). Women's health: A primary care clinical guide. 4th ed. Boston: Pearson.
Galactorrhea Overview. (2014). Retrieved from http://familydoctor.org/familydoctor/en/diseases-conditions/galactorrhea.export.html.
Shockney, L. D. (2012). Problems of the breast. In D. L. Lowdermilk, S. E. Perry, K. Cashion, & K. R. Alden (Eds.). Maternity & women's health care. 10th ed. St. Louis, MO: Elsevier.
U.S. National Library Medline Plus Encyclopedia. (2013). Intraductal papilloma. Retrieved from www.nlm.nih.gov/medlineplus/ency/article/001238.htm.

15. **ANSWER: 2, 3, 5**
Rationale
1. Pain is almost always present and is the most common symptom.
2. Exact cause is unknown but is often thought to be due to a physiological response from hormones. It has been suggested that there is an imbalance between estrogen and progestin, which produces excessive ductal stimulation and proliferation.
3. Breast cysts are small sacs filled with fluid. They can be of any size and can feel like small lumps or grapes and can be soft or firm. Breast cysts increase in size just before the menstrual cycle.
4. It is common in women between the ages of 30 and 50.
5. They usually recede and disappear with menopause. However, they may continue in menopausal women who receive hormonal therapy for menopausal symptoms.

TEST-TAKING TIP: Fibrocystic changes typically exhibit as breast thickness, lumpiness, or a palpable nodularity. Pain is almost always present and is the most common symptom.

Content Area: Benign Breast Conditions/Breast Disorders
Integrated Process: Nursing Process—Teaching/Learning; Communication and Documentation
Client Need: Health Promotion and Maintenance; Psychosocial Integrity
Cognitive Level: Application
Concept: Cellular Regulation

Reference: Johnson, J., Thomas, D. J., & Porter, B. O. (2015). Women's health problems. In L. M. Dunphy, J. E. Winward-Brown, B. O. Porter, & D. F. Thomas (Eds.). Primary care: Art and science of advanced practice nursing (pp. 679-754). 4th ed. Philadelphia: F.A. Davis

Gynecological Disorders

I. Menstrual Disorders

There are a variety of menstrual disorders that affect women mostly during the reproductive years. These include menstrual cramps, **dysmenorrhea, premenstrual syndrome (PMS),** and **amenorrhea** (Table 8.1). Menstrual cramps are due to cramping in the uterus from myometrial contractions induced by prostaglandins during the second phase of the menstrual cycle and are usually mild. Dysmenorrhea is a more intense form of menstrual cramps that result from an increase in the level of prostaglandin production.

DID YOU KNOW?
Prostaglandins are chemical mediators that cause pain due to inflammatory response.

A. Dysmenorrhea
  1. Painful menstrual cramps that begin 1 to 2 days prior to the start of menstrual bleeding and resolve by the end of menses
  2. Associated symptoms include nausea, vomiting, headache, pain in back and inner thighs, and loose stools

  3. Nursing role
     a) Teach relaxation and breathing techniques
     b) Heat reduces uterine contractions and increases the blood flow to uterine tissues
     c) Encourage exercise
     d) Dietary modifications include decreasing sodium and caffeine intake
  4. Treatment
     a) NSAIDs to inhibit the synthesis of prostaglandins
     b) Oral contraceptive pills (OCPs) suppress luteinizing hormone (LH) and follicle-stimulating hormone (FSH), inhibiting ovulation and altering the **endometrium.**

DID YOU KNOW?
Dysmenorrhea may affect a woman's ability to perform daily activities for 2 or more days each month. Severe pain can indicate other conditions such as **endometriosis,** pelvic inflammatory disease, fibroids, or pelvic adhesions. Women with severe pain should be seen by a health care provider (HCP) for further evaluation.

Table 8.1 **Menstrual Disorders**

Menstrual Disorder	Signs and Symptoms	Etiology	Management/Nursing Role
Dysmenorrhea	Painful menstrual cramps Occur 1–2 days prior to start of menstrual cycle Associated symptoms: headache, vomiting, nausea	Increased levels of prostaglandins are released during the second phase of the menstrual cycle, causing painful cramping of the uterus	NSAIDs for pain Oral contraceptives Instruct client on relaxation techniques, use of heat, and exercise
Amenorrhea (primary/secondary)	Absences of menses Primary: Menses has not occurred by age 15. Secondary: A woman who has had normal menstrual cycles stops having them for 3 months or more.	**Primary:** Genetic disorders Body build (low body fat, low levels of estrogen) Congenital disorders **Secondary:** Pregnancy Hormonal factors: lack of ovarian production, PCOS Excessive exercise leads to lower body fat Excessively low body weight: interrupts hormones potentially leading to anovulation (eating disorders)	**Primary:** 90% have unknown cause; provide emotional support if needed Treatment of underlying cause/hormone therapy if indicated **Secondary:** Identify and treat underlying cause Provide information on cause (excessive exercise/athletic activity) Treatment for those with eating disorders (anorexia/bulimia)
Abnormal uterine bleeding	Change in the normal menstrual bleeding pattern Includes: Heavier bleeding with menstrual cycle Bleeding between cycles Bleeding for longer period of time or more frequent cycles	Uterine fibroids Endometrial polyps or hyperplasia Endometrial cancer Pregnancy complications Anovulatory cycle with continuous estrogen production Infection of the cervix, vaginitis, sexually transmitted infection, or cervical dysplasia	Treat underlying cause Antibiotics if infection Treatment with hormone therapy for anovulatory cycles Surgical treatment as needed for fibroids, hyperplasia, cancer
Premenstrual syndrome (PMS)	Occurs during the last week of the luteal phase of the menstrual cycle Occurs regularly with each cycle Symptoms: irritability, bloating or fluid retention, heart palpitations, mood swings	Exact cause unknown Fluctuation in estrogen and progesterone levels Excessive production of aldosterone (leads to water retention) Alteration in carbohydrate metabolism and hypoglycemia	Provide emotional support Encourage exercise and healthy diet Diuretics (decrease fluid retention) Antidepressants OCPs to prevent hormone fluctuations (inhibits ovulation)
Premenstrual dysphoric disorder (PMDD)	*DSM-V* diagnosis Exhibits marked depression, anxiety, affective lability, decreased interest in activities, excessive sleep or inability to sleep, fatigue, breast tenderness/bloating, lack of concentration, alteration in appetite, anger or irritability, or feeling overwhelmed Occurs regularly and symptoms are absent the last week of the menstrual cycle	Exact cause unknown Fluctuation in estrogen and progesterone levels Excessive production of aldosterone (leads to water retention) Alteration in carbohydrate metabolism and hypoglycemia	Provide emotional support OCPs Antidepressants or CNS depressants Refer for counseling if needed

B. Amenorrhea
1. Amenorrhea is the absence of menstruation. This disorder can be further divided into two categories: primary and secondary amenorrhea.
   a) Primary amenorrhea: the absence of the start of menses (menarche) by age 15
   b) Secondary amenorrhea: the absence of menstruation for more than 3 consecutive months in a female who has previously had normal menstrual cycles
2. Etiologies of amenorrhea
   a) Genetic disorders (Turner's syndrome)
   b) Congenital obstruction
   c) Congenital absence of the uterus, ovaries, or vagina
   d) Hormonal factors: **polycystic ovary syndrome** or thyroid malfunction
   e) Excessively low body weight (at least 10% under normal weight). Decreased body weight interrupts normal hormone production and can result in amenorrhea. This can be a problem in women with eating disorders.
   f) Excessive exercise: occurs in athletes with rigorous training. A decrease in body fat leads to a decrease in estrogen production, leading to a cessation in menstruation.
3. Treatment
   a) Treatment of amenorrhea is guided by the underlying cause (see Table 8.1).

🛑 **ALERT** The primary cause for secondary amenorrhea is pregnancy. Women who present with amenorrhea should have a pregnancy test.

C. Premenstrual syndrome
1. Premenstrual syndrome
   a) A constellation of symptoms that occur regularly during the last week of the luteal phase (2 weeks before the onset of menses)
   b) Symptoms range from irritability and mood changes to fluid retention, nausea, constipation, acne, and visual disturbances or migraine headaches.
   c) Although an exact cause for PMS has not been found, it is thought the fluctuation of estrogen and progesterone levels during the menstrual cycle play a large role. The symptoms of PMS are usually milder than what manifests in **premenstrual dysphoric disorder (PMDD).** Diagnostic criteria for PMDD is outlined in the *DSM-V.*
2. PMDD
   a) Symptoms of PMDD are characterized by marked depression, anxiety, affective lability, and decreased interest in activities.

   b) There are 11 symptoms listed in the *DSM-V* for a PMDD diagnosis. The client must exhibit five of these in order to be diagnosed with this disorder.
   c) Symptoms of PMS/PMDD are always absent the week following menses. If a client is experiencing symptoms such as depression or anxiety that are continuous, she needs evaluation by an HCP to determine if there are other causes for her symptoms.

DID YOU KNOW?
A woman with PMDD may exhibit not only psychological symptoms but also physical symptoms. These may include breast tenderness and swelling, headaches, and joint or muscle pain. The symptoms may be accompanied by suicidal thoughts. The nurse's role is to assess the client for any suicidal thoughts or plans and ensure treatment is obtained if needed.

3. Other potential causes of PMS
   a) Alterations in carbohydrate metabolism and hypoglycemia
   b) Excessive production of aldosterone, causing sodium and water retention that result in bloating
   c) Excessive prostaglandin production, causing inflammation and pain
4. Nursing role
   a) Encourage exercise five to six times a week.
   b) Ensure client is eating a well-balanced diet, including a decrease in salt, sugar, and caffeine intake and an increase in vegetables and whole grains.
   c) Encourage adequate rest/sleep.
5. Treatment of symptoms
   a) Diuretics to reduce fluid retention
   b) Oral contraceptives to suppress LH and FSH to inhibit ovulation and control the levels of estrogen and progesterone
   c) Central nervous system (CNS) depressants to promote relaxation
   d) Antidepressants
   e) NSAIDs to inhibit the synthesis of prostaglandins to reduce pain and inflammation
D. Endometriosis
1. Endometriosis (Fig. 8.1)
   a) A benign disorder of the reproductive tract with the presence and growth of endometrial tissue outside the uterus
   b) Although an exact cause has not been found, it is hypothesized that endometrial tissue refluxes through the fallopian tubes and into the peritoneal cavity, implanting on the ovaries and surrounding organs. This is called *retrograde*

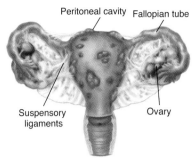

Peritoneal cavity Fallopian tube
Suspensory ligaments Ovary

Fig 8.1 Sites of occurrence of endometriosis.

menstruation. This tissue bleeds in a cyclic fashion with the menstrual cycle. The bleeding leads to severe inflammation, which causes scarring, fibrosis, and adhesions.

c) It has been found that the severity of symptoms a woman experiences does not correlate with the amount of endometriosis.

ALERT Women with a first-degree relative (mother or sister) with endometriosis are six times more likely to develop the disorder than women without a family history.

2. Symptoms of endometriosis
   a) Cyclic pain ranging from mild to severe. Pain may be located in the back, pelvis, or lower abdomen.
   b) Heavy bleeding during menstruation
   c) Episodes of diarrhea and constipation and possible pain during defecation
   d) **Dyspareunia** (pain with intercourse)
   e) Infertility due to adhesions, scar tissue, and fibrosis

DID YOU KNOW?
Endometriosis is most likely to develop in women aged 30 to 40. It can cause adhesions that bind organs together, increasing the risk of infertility. This is a concern for women who have delayed childbearing. Treatment for endometriosis is dependent on the woman's desire for fertility.

3. Nursing role
   a) Provide emotional support for those with infertility
   b) Education on endometriosis symptoms and management
   c) Explore options for symptom relief: NSAIDs, heat, relaxation
   d) Provide education on treatment plan: surgical or pharmacological
4. Treatment options
   a) NSAIDs for pain relief
   b) Oral contraceptives or medroxyprogesterone to suppress ovulation and menstruation,

which stops or decreases cyclic pelvic pain and bleeding

c) Danazol, gonadotropin-releasing hormone, and leuprolide (Lupron) are used to suppress the release of FSH and LH, prohibiting the release of estrogen, which stimulates endometrial production.

d) Surgical options: laparoscopy for the lysis of endometrial tissue growths, indicated for those women who desire fertility. A hysterectomy, removal of ovaries and fallopian tubes, and lysis of adhesions can be used for those who do not desire fertility.

DID YOU KNOW?
Symptoms of endometriosis usually return 1 to 5 years after medications for symptoms are stopped. To ensure safe and effective care, it is important for nurses to provide education to clients about medications and diagnoses.

E. Abnormal uterine bleeding
   1. **Abnormal uterine bleeding (AUB)** is a change in the menstrual cycle from the normal bleeding pattern.
      a) AUB can include a cadre of changes, including heavy bleeding with the menstrual cycle, frequent menses, bleeding between periods, or bleeding for a longer period of time than normal.
      b) Abnormal bleeding can also include too little bleeding or amenorrhea. Normal menstrual cycles usually last 4 to 8 days and occur every 24 to 38 days (Table 8.2).
   2. Causes of abnormal uterine bleeding
      a) Uterine fibroids: fibroid tumors that develop in the uterine muscle
      b) Endometrial polyps
      c) Endometrial or cervical cancer
      d) Complications of pregnancy
      e) Cervicitis: inflammation of the cervix that can be caused by infection or inflammation

DID YOU KNOW?
Women with abnormal uterine bleeding should be referred to an HCP for an evaluation. All patients should have a pregnancy test. Other tests for AUB evaluation may include Pap smear, endometrial biopsy, or pelvic ultrasound.

Table 8.2 **Normal Menstrual Cycle**

Menstrual Cycle	Average 28 days 21–35 days in adults 21–45 days in young teens
Days of Menstruation	Bleeding average: 3–5 days Range: 2–7 days

3. Treatment of AUB is specific to the cause of the bleeding.
   a) OCPs may be used to regulate the menstrual cycle.
   b) NSAIDs may be used to decrease the amount of blood loss.
   c) Invasive or surgical treatments may be indicated for cancer, uterine fibroids, and polyps.

F. Ovarian cysts

An ovarian cyst is a benign fluid-filled sac that develops inside or on the surface of the ovaries. These cysts can be painful at times and cause bleeding. Most ovarian cysts are often found during routine pelvic examinations. The two most common types of cysts are follicular cysts and corpus luteum cysts.

1. Follicular cysts
   a) These occur during the first half of the menstrual cycle (follicular phase).
   b) They form when the ovarian follicle fails to rupture and release an oocyte. Fluid remains in the follicle and forms a cyst.
   c) They are usually asymptomatic and shrink after two to three menstrual cycles.
   d) Follicular cysts occur unilaterally.
   e) If symptoms do occur, the client will present with pain and the sensation of heaviness or an achy feeling in the pelvis.
2. Corpus luteum cysts
   a) These occur during the second half of the menstrual cycle (luteal phase).
   b) Typically, if fertilization does not occur, the corpus luteum shrinks and disappears. A corpus luteum cyst develops when it remains in the ovary and fills with fluid or blood.
   c) Symptoms that occur are acute lower abdominal pain, ovarian tenderness, and delayed or irregular menses.
   d) A hemorrhagic cyst is when bleeding occurs within the cyst.
   e) Corpus luteum cysts typically resolve within one to two menstrual cycles or they may rupture.
   f) A cyst that ruptures may cause acute and severe pain. This may require surgical intervention.
3. Treatment of ovarian cysts
   a) NSAIDs for mild pain
   b) Oral contraceptives to prevent ovulation. OCPs will decrease the risk of developing additional cysts.
   c) If a cyst persists for more than 3 months or causes severe pain, surgical removal may be indicated.

🛑 **ALERT** A CA-125 blood test is often performed on women with ovarian cysts who are at high risk for ovarian cancer. CA-125 is a biomarker for ovarian cancer, but it is not always elevated in women with ovarian cancer or it may be elevated in women who do not have ovarian cancer. Because of this, it is not recommended for women with average risk for ovarian cancer and should be used with caution.

4. Polycystic ovary syndrome
   a) Polycystic ovary syndrome (PCOS) is an endocrine disorder whose cause is not fully understood. There is a possible genetic component to the etiology due to the occurrence in family history.
   b) Women with PCOS have a constellation of manifestations and hormone imbalances that can lead to multiple health problems.
5. Manifestations of PCOS (Table 8.3)
   a) Increased levels of testosterone, estrogen, and LH
      (1) Increase in testosterone can lead to **hirsutism,** acne, and oily skin
      (2) Increase in estrogen can lead to high levels of unopposed estrogen, increasing the risk of breast, ovarian, and uterine cancer
      (3) Increase in LH and testosterone can contribute to infertility
   b) Decrease in the secretion of FSH, which in combination with increased LH and testosterone contributes to infertility
   c) Polycystic ovaries adding to increasing estrogen levels
6. Long-term sequelae of PCOS
   a) Obesity: half of all women with PCOS are obese, which can increase the risk for type 2 diabetes.
   b) Hyperinsulinemia: insulin resistance places women at risk for impaired glucose intolerance, which may lead to type 2 diabetes.
   c) Cancer: endometrial, ovarian, breast
      (1) Due to high levels of estrogen in the body from the multiple cysts on the ovaries
   d) Infertility: due to high testosterone and LH levels and low FSH, causing anovulation

Table 8.3 Key Points of PCOS

- Anovulation resulting in infertility
- Abnormal uterine bleeding
  - Irregular, infrequent, or absent
- Physical changes
  - Hirsutism, oily skin, severe acne, obesity
- Multiple cysts on ovaries
- High risk for type 2 diabetes due to hyperinsulinemia

e) Cardiovascular disease, hypertension, and dyslipidemia: related to obesity, hormonal changes, increased glucose intolerance, and insulin resistance

DID YOU KNOW?

PCOS is the most common cause of female infertility. The combination of high testosterone and LH levels with a decrease in FSH inhibits ovulation in most women with PCOS. Weight loss is key to helping women with PCOS improve fertility. Weight reduction, through a healthy diet and exercise, can increase fertility by decreasing testosterone and increasing glucose metabolism, causing an increase in the frequency of ovulation and menstruation.

7. Signs and symptoms of PCOS
   a) Infertility
   b) Abnormal uterine bleeding
   c) Hirsutism
   d) Ovarian cysts
   e) Obesity
   f) Oily skin and acne
   g) Pelvic pain
   h) Male-pattern baldness
8. Treatment of PCOS
   a) Oral contraceptives can decrease testosterone levels and inhibit LH production; this assists with regulating menses and decreasing acne and hirsutism.
   b) Diabetic medications such as metformin (Glucophage) have been used to decrease glucose levels and lower testosterone.
   c) Clomiphene citrate (Clomid), a fertility drug, may be used to induce ovulation in those women who desire fertility.
9. Nursing role
   a) Encourage weight reduction through diet and exercise.
   b) Educate the client on the physical manifestations of PCOS and the risk factors of possible long-term complications.
   c) Explain benefits and risks of medications prescribed by the HCP.
   d) Assess for signs of depression or anxiety related to body changes or infertility due to PCOS.

II. Pelvic Floor Dysfunctions

Pelvic floor dysfunction occurs when the pelvic muscles are unable to adequately support the pelvic organs and result in pelvic organ prolapse. The pelvic organs that may prolapse include the bladder, uterus, rectum, and small intestine. Multiple reasons for the muscle weakness exist. After menopause, pelvic muscles atrophy or lose their elasticity. Also, muscle weakness can occur from damage

---

MAKING THE CONNECTION

Nursing Care for Women with PCOS

PCOS is a multidimensional disorder affecting physical and emotional aspects of a woman's life. The nurse can play a critical role in the identification, evaluation, and follow-up of these women. A key role for the nurse is to provide open communication about body image related to PCOS changes. In addition, coaching the client about healthy dietary habits and weight loss is paramount to improving her symptoms. Ensuring continued follow-up in the woman with PCOS facing long-term complications can be a challenge and is an essential part of nursing care.

during a vaginal birth of a large baby or difficult delivery, obesity, chronic cough, chronic constipation, or strenuous exercise. Pelvic organ prolapse can lead to dyspareunia, urinary incontinence, and bowel dysfunction. Common disorders related to pelvic organ prolapse include **cystocele, rectocele,** enterocele, and uterine prolapse (Fig. 8.2).

A. Cystocele
   Occurs when the muscle of the anterior vaginal wall weakens and the bladder herniates into the vagina.
B. Associated symptoms (Table 8.4)
   • Urinary stress incontinence with sneezing, laughing, and coughing
   • Feeling of vaginal fullness
   • Dyspareunia
   • Difficulty voiding, which may lead to increase in bladder infections
C. Rectocele/enterocele
   1. Rectocele is when the posterior wall of the vagina weakens and the rectum protrudes or balloons into the vagina.
   2. Enterocele is when muscle damage occurs higher in the colon and the small intestine bulges into the vagina.
   3. Constipation results from both a rectocele and enterocele.
D. Uterine prolapse
   1. A protrusion of the uterus into the vagina. The degree of the prolapse is determined by the location of the cervix in the vagina. It could protrude outside the vagina.
   2. Symptoms include backache, heaviness in the vagina, and dyspareunia.
E. Treatment for pelvic floor dysfunction depends on the degree of prolapse.
   1. Kegel exercises can strengthen the pelvic floor muscles.
   2. Estrogen replacement may benefit postmenopausal women to reverse atrophy of vaginal tissues and improve tone. This can be given orally or vaginally.

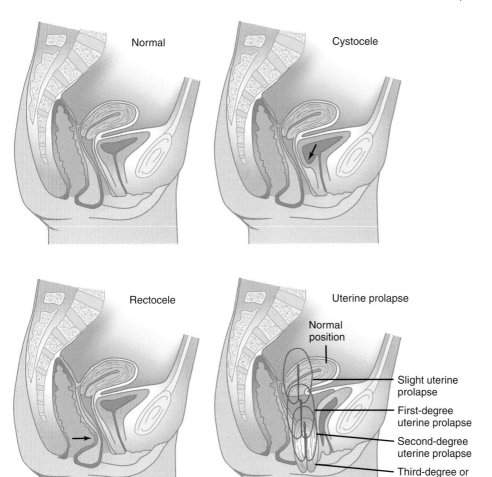

Fig 8.2 Cystocele, rectocele, and uterine prolapse.

Labels in figure: Normal; Cystocele; Rectocele; Uterine prolapse; Normal position; Slight uterine prolapse; First-degree uterine prolapse; Second-degree uterine prolapse; Third-degree or complete uterine prolapse

Table 8.4	Symptoms Associated With Pelvic Relaxation

- Pelvic pressure or heaviness
- Dyspareunia
- Urinary difficulties
  - Difficulty voiding
  - Incomplete bladder emptying
  - Frequent bladder infections
  - Urinary incontinence
- Constipation or incomplete defecation
- Back pain

3. A vaginal **pessary** is a rubber or silicone ring or disc that is inserted in the vagina to provide support for the prolapsed uterus or bladder (Fig. 8.3).
4. Surgical interventions may be required for symptomatic women who have not been helped by other methods or if the pelvic relaxation results in the structure protruding beyond the vaginal opening.

F. Nursing role
1. Instruct on Kegel exercises to improve pelvic floor musculature.
2. Encourage a high-fiber diet and increased water intake to prevent constipation.
3. Educate on the relationship between obesity and the increased risk for a cystocele or rectocele due to more pressure on pelvic muscles. Develop a weight-reduction plan with the client.

III.   Malignant Gynecological Disorders

A. Cervical cancer
1. Cervical cancer is the fourth most common cancer in women worldwide.[1] It is a slow-growing cancer that can be detected in early stages of precancerous cellular changes called *dysplasia*. Through routine screening with a Papanicolaou (Pap) test and treatment of dysplasia, most cases of cervical cancer are preventable.
   a) Most women who develop cervical cancer have not had regular Pap tests or may live in regions with inadequate screening.

[1]National Cancer Institute. (2015). Cervical cancer treatment (PDQ®)–Health professional version. Retrieved from http://www.cancer.gov/types/cervical/hp/cervical-treatment-pdq.

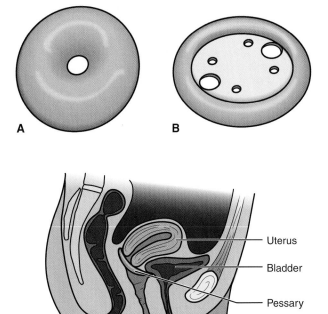

C

Fig 8.3 Vaginal pessary and inserted pessary.

b) Human papillomavirus (HPV) is the primary risk factor for cervical cancer. Table 8.5 shows other risk factors.

c) HPV is divided into low-risk and high-risk groups. Low-risk HPV is responsible for condyloma (skin warts) and do not cause cancer. High-risk HPV causes cancer, with types 16 and 18 being responsible for most cervical cancers.

d) More than 90% of cervical cancers can be detected early with the combination of a Pap test and HPV screening.

e) More than 80% of women will be infected with one type of HPV during their lifetime (National Cancer Institute, 2015).

f) Most HPV infections resolve on their own within 1 to 2 years and do not cause cancer. Persistent infections of high-risk HPV may progress to cancer.

Table 8.5	**Risk Factors of Cervical Cancer**

High-risk HPV—types 16 and 18 most common cause
Smoking tobacco
Multiple sexual partners
Sexually transmitted infections
High parity
Long-term use of oral contraceptives (greater than 5 years)
Early onset of sexual activity (before 16 years)

2. Signs and symptoms of cervical cancer
   Women with early cervical cancer may not present with symptoms. Possible early signs and symptoms may include the following:
   a) Vaginal bleeding between periods
   b) Unusual vaginal discharge (pink, bloody, brown, foul-smelling)
   c) Dyspareunia
   d) Postcoital bleeding
   e) Heavier bleeding with periods or bleeding that lasts longer (AUB)

3. Advanced signs of cervical cancer
   a) Loss of appetite (anorexia)
   b) Unexplained weight loss
   c) Fatigue
   d) Pelvic, back, and/or leg pain
   e) Leaking of urine or feces from vagina
   f) Abnormal uterine bleeding

4. Prevention of HPV infection
   a) There are currently three FDA-approved vaccines for the prevention of HPV infections. These vaccines do not treat established HPV infections or diseases caused by HPV. The vaccines available for females aged 9 to 26 include:
      • Gardasil (4 valent vaccine).
      • Gardasil 9 (9 valent vaccine).
      • Cervarix (2 valent vaccine).
   HPV vaccines should be administered in a three-dose schedule, with the second dose administered 1 to 2 months after the first dose and the third dose administered 6 months after the first dose. The minimum interval between the first and second doses of vaccine is 4 weeks.

5. Treatment of cervical cancer
   Prior to treatment of cervical cancer, women have a biopsy of the cervical tissue so it can be pathologically examined to determine the presence and extent of cancer. Colposcopy is a type of cervical biopsy that can be performed in the HCP's office,

MAKING THE CONNECTION

HPV Vaccines

Understanding the purpose and the targeted HPV types of the various vaccines allows the nurse to give clients accurate information about preventing genital warts and educating them on vaginal, cervical, and anal cancers. Both the Gardasil quadrivalent and Gardasil 9 target low-risk and high-risk HPV types. The Cervarix vaccine prevents cervical cancer caused by high-risk HPV types 16 and 18. Low-risk HPV causes genital warts and high-risk HPV causes cervical, vaginal, vulvar, and anal cancers.

as well as an endocervical curettage (ECC). Other methods of biopsy and treatment include:

a) Loop electrosurgical excision procedure (LEEP) is used to obtain cells for pathological examination and removal of abnormal cells.

b) Surgical conization is used to remove abnormal cells for biopsy and can be the treatment if all abnormal cells are obtained in the biopsy. This is determined by the pathologist. Conization involves removing a cone-shaped piece of tissue from the cervix and cervical canal.

c) Cryosurgery is used to destroy the abnormal cells by freezing the tissue.

d) Laser vaporization conization is the use of a laser to destroy cervical tissue containing abnormal cells.

Once the biopsies have been examined by the pathologist and it is determined that the cancer has moved beyond the cervix, further treatment may include chemotherapy, radiation, or surgery.

6. Nursing role

a) Encourage Pap tests as recommended for age and previous history.

b) Educate on effectiveness of HPV vaccine in preventing high-risk HPV infection, and encourage females aged 9 to 26 to be vaccinated.

c) Teach clients pre- and postcare if biopsies are required:

• No tampons or sexual intercourse for 4 weeks after the procedure to help prevent infection

• Vaginal discharge expected for approximately 3 weeks

• Use NSAIDs for pain

B. Uterine cancer

1. Uterine cancer is also referred to as *endometrial cancer* and is the most common malignancy in the reproductive tract. Cancer forms in the lining (endometrium) of the uterus. Histological examination of the endometrial tissue is used to establish a diagnosis.

DID YOU KNOW?

The Pap test is not a reliable screening test for diagnosing uterine cancer. A procedure that directly samples the endometrial tissue must be used. An endometrial biopsy is most commonly performed and is done in the HCP's office.

2. Risk factors

a) Postmenopausal estrogen therapy, which is the use of unopposed estrogen, or estrogen without the use of progesterone, can cause endometrial hyperplasia.

b) Unopposed estrogen exposure that is produced by the body (endogenous):

• Nulliparity or low parity

• Obesity: estrogen levels are increased through production in the fatty tissue

• Chronic anovulation

• Menopause after 52

• Tamoxifen (drug used to treat breast cancer)

• Hereditary nonpolyposis colorectal cancer syndrome

c) Other risk factors include:

• Diabetes mellitus

• Hypertension

• Family history of uterine cancer

• Personal history of breast or ovarian cancer

3. Signs and symptoms

Uterine cancer is most commonly found in women aged 60 to 70 years. Because this is a slow-growing cancer, early detection can lead to effective treatment. Signs and symptoms include the following:

a) Postmenopausal bleeding, which occurs when a woman who has entered menopause begins to experience bleeding

b) Heavy or prolonged bleeding or bleeding between periods in premenopausal women

c) Pelvic pain

d) Dyspareunia

ALERT The most common symptom of uterine cancer is irregular vaginal bleeding. This includes postmenopausal bleeding, bleeding between periods, or changes in the normal bleeding pattern.

4. Treatment

Treatment of uterine cancer is based on cancer staging. Most women will undergo surgery to remove the cancer. If the woman is in poor health, surgery may not be an option and she may receive radiation therapy only. Treatment options include:

• Hysterectomy

• Removal of the fallopian tubes and ovaries (bilateral salpingo-oophorectomy)

• Chemotherapy

• Radiation

5. Nursing role

a) Provide education to women about risk factors for uterine cancer.

b) Ensure women are aware of early signs and symptoms of uterine cancer.

c) Provide emotional support to the client during diagnosis and treatment.

C. Ovarian cancer

1. Ovarian cancer is the eighth most common cancer among women in the United States. Although ovarian cancer is not the most

The Nurse and Malignant Gynecological Disorders

Malignant gynecological disorders present with many similar signs and symptoms. It is important for nurses to be aware of the various risk factors for gynecological cancers, the specific target ages for these cancers, and the presenting signs and symptoms. This knowledge helps the nurse be a better client advocate and ensure that information provided is relevant to the client's needs. For example, a 28-year-old female calls the nurse with complaints of vaginal bleeding that is occurring between her periods and bleeding after intercourse. The client tells the nurse she is in a monogamous relationship. Review of her chart reveals that her last Pap test was abnormal with a positive screen for high-risk HPV. It is documented that the client did not follow up for cervical biopsies as scheduled. The prudent nurse recognizes that the age of the patient, the history of intermenstrual and postcoital bleeding, and history of an abnormal Pap with high-risk HPV are risk factors for cervical cancer. The nurse should recommend an appointment with the HCP for an examination and Pap test.

common form of cancer, it causes more deaths than any other cancer in the female reproductive tract (National Cancer Institute, 2015). The high mortality can be attributed to difficulty in detecting the cancer and often it having spread throughout the pelvis once it has been discovered.

2. Risk factors
   a) Family history of ovarian cancer in a first-degree relative
   b) Nulliparity
   c) Talcum powder use on the perineum—in the past, talcum powder sometimes contained asbestos.
   d) High-fat diet
   e) Personal history of breast cancer and/or tested positive for *BRCA1* or *BRCA2*
   f) Women age 55 or older; mostly develops in women after menopause

ALERT Women at the highest risk for ovarian cancer are those with a family history (first-degree relative) of the disease.

3. Signs and symptoms
   a) Early stages of ovarian cancer usually are asymptomatic.
   b) Subtle early warning signs:
      - Bloating or abdominal swelling—may feel clothes are tighter around the waist
      - Pressure in the pelvis or lower abdomen
      - Feeling full after eating only a small amount
      - Urinary frequency or dysuria
      - A solid, fixed pelvic mass on examination
      - CA-125 serum biomarker
4. Treatment is surgical
   a) Hysterectomy and bilateral salpingo-oophorectomy
   b) Chemotherapy
   c) Radiation
5. Nursing role
   a) Provide women with information regarding risk factors for ovarian cancer and early signs and symptoms.
   b) Provide emotional support for women during diagnoses and treatment of cancer.
   c) Ensure women understand their treatment plan and the side effects of chemotherapy and radiation.

CASE STUDY: Putting It All Together

Subjective Data

Mary is a 28-year-old female who has been married for 3 years and wants to conceive her first child. She states that she and her husband have been trying for 2 years and she is getting frustrated. She states her periods are not regular and occur about once every 3 months. You notice that Mary is becoming tearful as she talks with you. She tells you that her family HCP told her she had polycystic ovary syndrome a few years ago and admits that she really does not know what that means. Mary denies taking any medications.

Objective Data

Nursing Assessment
Gender: white female
Age: 28 years old
Education: high school graduate with some college
Occupation: works as a receptionist at a law firm

Social: lives with her husband, denies tobacco, occasional alcohol use
Blood pressure: 140/90
Heart rate: 102
Respiratory rate: 20
Weight: 196 lb
Height: 5'5"
BMI: 32 (Obese)
Her physical examination is normal other than skin is pale and dry. Hirsutism and acne are noted on face.

Laboratory Results
CBC: normal
Fasting glucose: 210
Lipids: elevated triglycerides 190 (norm < 150); LDL and HDL normal

Case Study Questions

1. What are significant subjective findings in the above scenario of MW?

2. The HCP has seen Mary and a pelvic ultrasound has been completed. It was noted that Mary has multiple cysts on her bilateral ovaries. The HCP explains to Mary that she has polycystic ovary syndrome (PCOS). She is visibly upset. Glucophage is prescribed and weight loss is encouraged. What are the significant objective findings?

3. As the nurse caring for Mary, what are three priority problems that should be addressed before Mary leaves the office today? What are the associated nursing interventions?

4. Name four outcomes that occur with weight loss in a woman with PCOS.

REVIEW QUESTIONS

Be sure to read the Introduction for valuable test-taking tips.

1. A 17-year-old client presents to the clinic with concerns that she has not begun menstruating. She states that she is a gymnast and has been competing since she was 9 years old. Based on this history, what does the nurse know the client is most likely experiencing?
   1. Secondary amenorrhea
   2. Polycystic ovary syndrome
   3. Primary amenorrhea
   4. Dysmenorrhea

2. The nurse is counseling a client on dietary recommendations for dysmenorrhea. Which statement by the client indicates understanding of the recommendations?
   1. "I should adopt a vegan diet."
   2. "I should avoid pretzels and potato chips."
   3. "I should increase my intake of cranberry juice."
   4. "I should avoid dairy."

3. The client calls the nurse and states she has not had a menstrual cycle in 3 months. What does the nurse know is the most common cause of secondary amenorrhea?
   1. Weight loss
   2. Pregnancy
   3. Cancer
   4. Menopause

4. Which pharmacological preparation is the least effective in relieving symptoms of dysmenorrhea?
   1. Ibuprofen
   2. Acetaminophen
   3. Oral contraceptive pills
   4. Naproxen sodium

5. Which should the nurse recommend to the client to relieve premenstrual syndrome (PMS) symptoms? *Select all that apply.*
   1. NSAIDs to decrease pain
   2. Exercise 5 to 6 times a week
   3. Decrease caffeine
   4. Decrease fiber

6. A woman is noted to have multiple soft warts on her perineum and rectal areas. The nurse suspects that this client has which type of infection?
   1. HIV
   2. HPV
   3. Syphilis
   4. Herpes simplex virus

7. The nurse is discussing risk factors for endometriosis with a new nurse. Which client would the nurse identify as being at the *highest* risk for developing endometriosis?
   1. One who smokes one pack per day
   2. One who states her menstrual cycles are irregular
   3. One who states her mother had endometriosis
   4. One who had a previous cesarean section

8. The client has been taking danazol for endometriosis for 3 years. She tells you that she would like to have a baby and wants to stop taking this medication. She wants to know what will happen when she stops. Which is the nurse's *best* response?
   1. "Nothing, your endometriosis will not return."
   2. "If you stop taking danazol, it could increase your blood pressure."
   3. "Once you stop any medication for endometriosis, your symptoms may return in 1 to 5 years."
   4. "Once you stop the medication, the growths from endometriosis will return in 2 to 3 months."

9. The nurse is reviewing the chart of a client who is complaining of heavy bleeding with her menstrual cycles. The nurse is aware that which of the following is a possible cause?
   1. Uterine fibroids
   2. Excessive exercise
   3. Normal finding in pregnancy
   4. Diet high in fat

10. A 60-year-old client with a palpable mass to the right adnexa and family history of ovarian cancer is seen by the HCP. The nurse anticipates the order for which of the following laboratory results?
    1. CBC
    2. Blood glucose
    3. CA-125
    4. FSH and LH

11. The nurse is meeting with a client who was newly diagnosed with polycystic ovary syndrome. She knows that the client has the potential for which diagnoses? *Select all that apply.*
    1. Knowledge deficit
    2. Disturbed body image
    3. Risk for type 2 diabetes
    4. Impaired mobility

12. Which is a constellation of physical and psychological symptoms beginning in the luteal phase of the menstrual cycle and followed by a symptom-free period?
    1. Endometriosis
    2. Abnormal uterine bleeding
    3. Premenstrual syndrome
    4. Depression

13. A 58-year-old woman tells the nurse that she has started to experience pain during intercourse. The nurse should document that this woman is experiencing which of the following?
    1. Dyspnea
    2. Dyspareunia
    3. Dyspepsia
    4. Dysmenorrhea

14. The nurse is preparing a 51-year-old client for a vaginal examination. The nurse should place the client in which position?
    1. Prone
    2. Lateral Sims'
    3. Lithotomy
    4. High Fowler's

15. The nurse is assessing a client who has a suspected cystocele. Which signs and symptoms should the nurse expect? *Select all that apply.*
    1. Frequent bladder infections
    2. Sense of fullness in the vaginal area
    3. Leaking of urine
    4. Irregular vaginal bleeding

16. The nurse has completed instructions on ways to improve the client's symptoms related to her rectocele. Which statement by the client indicates a need for further education?
    1. "Weight loss will decrease pressure on the pelvic floor."
    2. "Increasing fiber and water in my diet will help prevent constipation."
    3. "Heavy lifting will not affect my rectocele."
    4. "Kegel exercises will help with pelvic floor strength."

17. The nurse is teaching a sex education class to teenage girls. The nurse informs them that which age group should receive a vaccination to prevent HPV infection?
    1. 13–29
    2. 12–26
    3. 9–26
    4. 7–20

18. The nurse taught a class on HPV and cervical cancer. Which statement by the student indicates a need for further teaching?
    1. "Most HPV infections resolve on their own within 1 to 2 years."
    2. "I can get the HPV vaccination to prevent the most common types of HPV that could cause cervical cancer."
    3. "Genital warts cause cervical cancer."
    4. "A persistent infection of HPV type 16 or 18 can lead to cervical cancer."

19. Which statement by the client indicates further teaching is needed about uterine cancer?
    1. "A Pap test is used to diagnose uterine cancer."
    2. "Uterine cancer is the most common cancer of the reproductive tract."
    3. "I used estrogen for 2 years without progesterone. This puts me at risk for developing uterine cancer."
    4. "Postmenopausal bleeding could indicate uterine cancer."

20. Which are risk factors for ovarian cancer? *Select all that apply.*
    1. Talc use on the perineum
    2. First-degree relative with ovarian cancer
    3. Three or more children
    4. High-fat diet

REVIEW QUESTION ANSWERS

1. ANSWER: 3
Rationale
1. *Secondary* refers to menstruation that has occurred at least once but has stopped, typically for 6 months or longer.
2. Polycystic ovary syndrome is a condition in which the ovaries stop functioning normally in women who are younger than 40 years.
3. The definition of primary amenorrhea is the absence of a menstrual cycle in a female aged 15 years or older who has never had a menstrual cycle. The most likely cause of her amenorrhea is excessive athletic activity as a competing gymnast for the past 8 years. Excessive exercise can decrease body fat, which in turn will decrease estrogen and result in the absence of the menstrual cycle.
4. *Dysmenorrhea* refers to the symptom of painful menstruation.
TEST-TAKING TIP: Excessive exercise can be a cause for both primary and secondary amenorrhea. Recall that secondary amenorrhea occurs in a female who has an absence of the menstrual cycle for 3 or more consecutive months after having regular cycles.
Content Area: Menstrual Disorders; Care of the Woman Across the Life Span
Integrated Process: Nursing Process—Assessment
Client Need: Physiological Adaptation; Health Promotion and Maintenance
Cognitive Level: Comprehension
Concept: Female Reproduction
Reference: Ward, S. L., & Hisley, S. M. (2009). Maternal-child nursing care: Optimizing outcomes for mothers, children & families. *Philadelphia: F.A. Davis.*

2. ANSWER: 2
Rationale
1. There is no reason for the client to adopt a vegan diet.
2. This client has the best understanding of dietary recommendations for dysmenorrhea symptoms, which include avoiding salty foods and caffeine.
3. There is no reason for the client to increase intake of cranberry juice.
4. There is no reason for the client to avoid dairy.
TEST-TAKING TIP: Foods that are high in sodium can increase water retention and cause bloating. The intake of caffeine may cause vasoconstriction. Both water retention and vasoconstriction can increase menstrual cramping.
Content Area: Menstrual Disorders; Care of the Woman Across the Life Span
Integrated Process: Nursing Process—Implementation
Client Need: Physiological Integrity; Health Promotion and Maintenance
Cognitive Level: Evaluation
Concept: Female Reproduction
Reference: Durham, R. F., & Chapman, L. (2014). Maternal-newborn nursing: The critical components of nursing care. 2nd ed. *Philadelphia: F.A. Davis.*

3. ANSWER: 2
Rationale
1. Weight loss is not a cause of secondary amenorrhea.
2. Secondary amenorrhea is the absence of the menstrual cycle for more than 3 consecutive months in a female with a previous history of normal cycles. The most common cause of secondary amenorrhea is pregnancy.
3. Cancer is not a cause of secondary amenorrhea.
4. Menopause is not a cause of secondary amenorrhea.
TEST-TAKING TIP: There are multiple causes for amenorrhea. These include pregnancy, congenital, genetic, and hormonal. The most common of these is pregnancy.
Content Area: Menstrual Disorders; Care of the Woman Across the Life Span
Integrated Process: Nursing Process—Assessment
Client Need: Physiological Adaptation
Cognitive Level: Comprehension
Concept: Female Reproduction
Reference: Durham, R. F., & Chapman, L. (2014). Maternal-newborn nursing: The critical components of nursing care. 2nd ed. *Philadelphia: F.A. Davis.*

4. ANSWER: 2
Rationale
1. Ibuprofen is an NSAID, which decreases pain by blocking the synthesis of prostaglandins, which cause contractions of the myometrium of the uterus.
2. Acetaminophen is the least effective in relieving symptoms of dysmenorrhea.
3. Oral contraceptives are also an alternative pharmacological preparation that is used to decrease symptoms of dysmenorrhea.
4. Naproxen sodium is an NSAID, which decreases pain by blocking the synthesis of prostaglandins, which cause contractions of the myometrium of the uterus.
TEST-TAKING TIP: Understanding the pathophysiology behind dysmenorrhea will guide the selection of the best medication to treat this disorder.
Content Area: Menstrual Disorders; Care of the Woman Across the Life Span
Integrated Process: Nursing Process—Planning
Client Need: Physiological Integrity; Pharmacology
Cognitive Level: Comprehension
Concept: Female Reproduction
Reference: Durham, R. F., & Chapman, L. (2014). Maternal-newborn nursing: The critical components of nursing care. 2nd ed. *Philadelphia: F.A. Davis.*

5. ANSWER: 1, 2, 3
Rationale
1. PMS can result in bloating, headaches, joint pain, and irritability. The recommendations of exercising 5 to 6 times a week, taking NSAIDs, and decreasing caffeine can help reduce these symptoms.
2. PMS can result in bloating, headaches, joint pain, and irritability. The recommendations of exercising 5 to 6 times a week, taking NSAIDs, and decreasing caffeine can help reduce these symptoms.
3. PMS can result in bloating, headaches, joint pain, and irritability. The recommendations of exercising 5 to 6 times a week, taking NSAIDs, and decreasing caffeine can help reduce these symptoms.
4. Decreasing fiber does not provide any benefit.
TEST-TAKING TIP: The use of NSAIDs can help with menstrual cramping, joint pain, and headaches. Exercise and/or antidepressant or antianxiety medications can improve irritability. Decreasing caffeine and foods high in sodium can reduce bloating.

Content Area: Menstrual Disorders; Care of the Woman Across the Life Span
Integrated Process: Nursing Process—Planning
Client Need: Health Promotion and Maintenance; Pharmacology
Cognitive Level: Application
Concept: Female Reproduction
Reference: Ladewig, P. A., London, M. L., & Davidson, M. R. (2010). Contemporary maternal-newborn nursing care. 7th ed. New York: Pearson.

6. **ANSWER: 2**
Rationale
1. HIV has symptoms that are systemic, such as weight loss and fatigue.
2. Low-risk HPV can cause soft warts on the perineum and rectal areas.
3. Syphilis (primary) presents with a nonpainful chancre.
4. Herpes simplex virus is characterized with multiple painful vesicle type lesions.
TEST-TAKING TIP: The nurse should know how various sexually transmitted diseases present and be able to educate the client regarding symptoms.
Content Area: Menstrual Disorders; Care of the Woman Across the Life Span
Integrated Process: Nursing Process—Assessment
Client Need: Pathophysiology; Health Promotion and Maintenance
Cognitive Level: Comprehension
Concept: Female Reproduction
Reference: Ladewig, P. A., London, M. L., & Davidson, M. R. (2010). Contemporary maternal-newborn nursing care. 7th ed. New York: Pearson. National Cancer Institute. (2015). Cervical cancer treatment (PDQ)—health professional version. Retrieved from www.cancer.gov/types/cervical/hp/cervical-treatment-pdq.

7. **ANSWER: 3**
Rationale
1. Smoking is not a risk factor for developing endometriosis.
2. Irregular periods are not risk factors for developing endometriosis.
3. Women with a first-degree relative with endometriosis are six times more likely to develop the disorder than women without a family history.
4. Previous cesarean section is not a risk factor for developing endometriosis.
TEST-TAKING TIP: Understanding risk factors and presenting symptoms for various disorders helps the nurse provide education to clients based on specific needs. Some symptoms that you would expect to see are cyclic pain, heavy bleeding during menstruation, and dyspareunia.
Content Area: Endometriosis; Care of the Woman Across the Life Span
Integrated Process: Nursing Process—Assessment
Client Need: Safe, Effective Care Environment; Establishing Priorities; Health Promotion and Maintenance
Cognitive Level: Synthesis
Concept: Female Reproduction
Reference: Ward, S. L., & Hisley, S. M. (2009). Maternal-child nursing care: Optimizing outcomes for mothers, children & families. Philadelphia: F.A. Davis.

8. **ANSWER: 3**
Rationale
1. This is an incorrect statement. Once any medication for endometriosis is discontinued, the symptoms usually return within 1 to 5 years.
2. Danazol is used to treat endometriosis, a disease that causes infertility, pain before and during menstrual periods, pain during and after sexual activity, and heavy or irregular bleeding. Stopping this drug will not cause an increase in blood pressure. However, after stopping this drug, symptoms of endometriosis may return within 1 to 5 years.
3. Once any medications for endometriosis are discontinued, the symptoms usually return within 1 to 5 years.
4. Growths may return within 1 to 5 years.
TEST-TAKING TIP: Recall that endometriosis is caused by reflux menstruation. Once the medication that is being used to control hormone levels is discontinued, the body may resume producing the ectopic endometrium that results in endometriosis.
Content Area: Endometriosis; Care of the Woman Across the Life Span
Integrated Process: Nursing Process—Implementation
Client Need: Physiological Integrity: Pharmacological and Parenteral Therapies; Safe and Effective Care Environment
Cognitive Level: Application
Concept: Female Reproduction
Reference: Ward, S. L., & Hisley, S. M. (2009). Maternal-child nursing care: Optimizing outcomes for mothers, children & families. Philadelphia: F.A. Davis.

9. **ANSWER: 1**
Rationale
1. Uterine fibroids are one cause of abnormal uterine bleeding. Others include endometrial polyps, infection, cancer, and complications of pregnancy.
2. Excessive exercise does not have a role in heavy bleeding during the menstrual cycle.
3. Heavy bleeding is not a normal finding in pregnancy.
4. A high-fat diet does not have a role in heavy bleeding during the menstrual cycle.
TEST-TAKING TIP: Remember that heavy bleeding is considered abnormal uterine bleeding. Recall causes of this disorder and eliminate those factors that you know are normal findings.
Content Area: Uterine Fibroids; Care of the Woman Across the Life Span
Integrated Process: Nursing Process—Assessment
Client Need: Physiological Adaptation; Pathophysiology
Cognitive Level: Analysis
Concept: Female Reproduction
Reference: Ladewig, P. A., London, M. L., & Davidson, M. R. (2010). Contemporary maternal-newborn nursing care. 7th ed. New York: Pearson.

10. **ANSWER: 3**
Rationale
1. A CBC will not give information concerning ovarian cancer.
2. A blood glucose would not give any information concerning ovarian cancer.
3. The nurse is preparing ahead to perform the procedure that will most likely be ordered by the HCP in a 60-year-old

female with a palpable adnexal mass and a family history of ovarian cancer. The nurse is aware that the client's age, family history of ovarian cancer, and a palpable adnexal mass are all risk factors for ovarian cancer. The family history makes her high risk for ovarian cancer and one that a CA-125 is usually performed on.
4. An FSH and LH would not give any information concerning ovarian cancer.

TEST-TAKING TIP: The CA-125 is not used as a screening test. This cancer antigen test is reserved for women who present with symptoms that are highly suggestive of ovarian cancer and have a family history. CA-125 is often elevated in women with ovarian cancer, but it may be elevated in women who do not have ovarian cancer.
Content Area: Ovarian Cancer; Care of the Woman Across the Life Span
Integrated Process: Nursing Process—Planning
Client Need: Physiological Integrity; Safe and Effective Care Environment
Cognitive Level: Synthesis
Concept: Cellular Regulation
Reference: Perry, S. E., Hockenberry, M. F., Lowdermilk, D. L., & Wilson, D. (2014). Maternal child nursing care. 5th ed. St. Louis, MO: Elsevier.

11. ANSWER: 1, 2, 3
Rationale
1. PCOS is a syndrome with a multitude of manifestations affecting the client's physical appearance and psychosocial integrity. Knowledge deficit, disturbed body image, and the risk for type 2 diabetes are all appropriate diagnoses for the nurse to address.
2. PCOS is a syndrome with a multitude of manifestations affecting the client's physical appearance and psychosocial integrity. Knowledge deficit, disturbed body image, and the risk for type 2 diabetes are all appropriate diagnoses for the nurse to address.
3. PCOS is a syndrome with a multitude of manifestations affecting the client's physical appearance and psychosocial integrity. Knowledge deficit, disturbed body image, and the risk for type 2 diabetes are all appropriate diagnoses for the nurse to address.
4. Impaired mobility is not a factor in PCOS.

TEST-TAKING TIP: Recall that PCOS is multifactorial, and the manifestations can result in many long-term consequences. The newly diagnosed patient will most often have a knowledge deficit.
Content Area: Polycystic Ovary Syndrome; Care of the Woman Across the Life Span
Integrated Process: Nursing Process—Planning
Client Need: Health Promotion and Maintenance; Psychosocial Integrity; Physiological Integrity
Cognitive Level: Evaluation
Concept: Female Reproduction
Reference: Ladewig, P. A., London, M. L., & Davidson, M. R. (2010). Contemporary maternal-newborn nursing care. 7th ed. New York: Pearson.

12. ANSWER: 3
Rationale
1. Endometriosis is an often painful disorder in which tissue that normally lines the inside of the uterus (the endometrium) grows outside the uterus (endometrial

implant). Endometriosis most commonly involves your ovaries, bowel, or the tissue lining your pelvis.
2. Abnormal uterine bleeding is any bleeding from the uterus (through your vagina) other than normal monthly menstruation.
3. This is the definition of premenstrual syndrome.
4. Depression is a mood disorder that causes a persistent feeling of sadness and loss of interest.

TEST-TAKING TIP: PMS has multiple symptoms that occur at the beginning of the menstrual cycle but always includes a symptom-free period during the week following menses. If a client is experiencing PMS symptoms throughout the entire month, she needs further evaluation.
Content Area: Menstrual Disorders; Care of the Woman Across the Life Span
Integrated Process: Nursing Process—Assessment
Client Need: Physiological Integrity; Health Promotion and Maintenance
Cognitive Level: Knowledge
Concept: Female Reproduction
Reference: Durham, R. F., & Chapman, L. (2014). Maternal-newborn nursing: The critical components of nursing care. 2nd ed. *Philadelphia: F.A. Davis.*

13. ANSWER: 2
Rationale
1. Difficult or labored breathing, shortness of breath.
2. This is the definition of dyspareunia, which is defined as persistent or recurrent genital pain that occurs just before, during, or after intercourse.
3. Dyspepsia can be defined as painful, difficult, or disturbed digestion, which may be accompanied by symptoms such as nausea and vomiting, heartburn, bloating, and stomach discomfort.
4. *Dysmenorrhea* is the medical term for the painful cramps that may occur immediately before or during the menstrual period. There are two types of dysmenorrhea: primary dysmenorrhea and secondary dysmenorrhea.

TEST-TAKING TIP: It is important to know the medical terms of many patient complaints for proper documentation.
Content Area: Menstrual Disorders; Care of the Woman Across the Life Span
Integrated Process: Nursing Process—Assessment
Client Need: Physiological Integrity; Health Promotion and Maintenance
Cognitive Level: Knowledge
Concept: Female Reproduction
Reference: Durham, R. F., & Chapman, L. (2014). Maternal-newborn nursing: The critical components of nursing care. 2nd ed. *Philadelphia: F.A. Davis.*

14. ANSWER: 3
Rationale
1. Prone position is when one lies flat with the chest down and back up (dorsal side is up, and the ventral side is down).
2. Lateral position is a body position in which one is in the side-lying position, pillow under head, underarm at stomach and under calf.
3. The lithotomy position is a common position for surgical procedures and medical examinations involving the pelvis and lower abdomen, as well as a common position for childbirth. In this position, the individual's feet are

above or at the same level as the hips (often in stirrups), with the perineum positioned at the edge of the examination table. Lithotomy is the appropriate position for the client undergoing a pelvic examination.

4. The high Fowler's position is when a patient is placed with the head of the bed elevated as high as possible. The upper half of the patient's body is between 60 degrees and 90 degrees in relation to the lower half of the body.

TEST-TAKING TIP: Recall the multiple patient positions.
Content Area: Vaginal Examination; Care of the Woman Across the Life Span
Integrated Process: Nursing Process—Implementation
Client Need: Safe and Effective Care Environment
Cognitive Level: Comprehension
Concept: Assessment
Reference: Durham, R. F., & Chapman, L. (2014). Maternal-newborn nursing: The critical components of nursing care. 2nd ed. Philadelphia: F.A. Davis.

15. ANSWER: 1, 2, 3
Rationale
1. Women with a cystocele may complain of frequent bladder infections, a sense of fullness in the vaginal area, leaking urine, and dyspareunia.
2. Women with a cystocele may complain of frequent bladder infections, a sense of fullness in the vaginal area, leaking urine, and dyspareunia.
3. Women with a cystocele may complain of frequent bladder infections, a sense of fullness in the vaginal area, leaking urine, and dyspareunia.
4. Irregular vaginal bleeding is not associated with a cystocele.

TEST-TAKING TIP: A cystocele is the bulging of the bladder through the anterior vaginal wall. This can cause an incomplete emptying of the bladder, resulting in frequent bladder infections or leaking of urine.
Content Area: Cystocele; Care of the Woman Across the Life Span
Integrated Process: Nursing Process—Assessment
Client Need: Health Promotion and Maintenance; Physiological Integrity; Pathophysiology
Cognitive Level: Synthesis
Concept: Urinary Elimination
Reference: Perry, S. E., Hockenberry, M. F., Lowdermilk, D. L., & Wilson, D. (2014). Maternal child nursing care. 5th ed. St. Louis, MO: Elsevier.

16. ANSWER: 3
Rationale
1. Heavy lifting and obesity put increased pressure on the pelvic floor muscles, adding to the already weakened musculature in women with a rectocele.
2. Relieving constipation will not improve the client's symptoms related to her rectocele.
3. This client needs further education.
4. Strengthening the muscles of the vagina and pelvis with Kegel exercises often improves pelvic muscle tone and uterine support.

TEST-TAKING TIP: Education for women with pelvic floor dysfunction is necessary to help prevent further weakening of the pelvic muscles.
Content Area: Rectocele; Care of the Woman Across the Life Span

Integrated Process: Nursing Process—Evaluation
Client Need: Safe and Effective Care Environment; Health Promotion and Maintenance
Cognitive Level: Evaluation
Concept: Bowel Elimination
Reference: Durham, R. F., & Chapman, L. (2014). Maternal-newborn nursing: The critical components of nursing care. 2nd ed. Philadelphia: F.A. Davis.

17. ANSWER: 3
Rationale
1. This is not the age recommendation for receiving HPV prevention.
2. This is not the age recommendation for receiving HPV prevention.
3. The three FDA-approved vaccines for HPV prevention are recommended for females aged 9 to 26, regardless of sexual activity or previous HPV infections.
4. This is not the age recommendation for receiving HPV prevention.

TEST-TAKING TIP: Currently there are three FDA-approved vaccines for HPV prevention. The vaccines do not cure previous infections. These vaccines are given in a three-dose schedule. The second dose should be administered 1 to 2 months after the first dose and the third dose administered 6 months after the first dose. The minimum interval between the first and second doses of vaccine is 4 weeks. It is imperative that the nurse is aware of the vaccination schedule for all routine vaccinations.
Content Area: Cervical Cancer; Care of the Woman Across the Life Span
Integrated Process: Nursing Process—Implementation
Client Need: Health Promotion and Maintenance; Safe and Effective Care Environment
Cognitive Level: Synthesis
Concept: Infection
Reference: National Cancer Institute. (2015). Cervical cancer treatment (PDQ)—health professional version. Retrieved from www.cancer.gov/types/cervical/hp/cervical-treatment-pdq.

18. ANSWER: 3
Rationale
1. Most HPV infections resolve on their own within 1 to 2 years.
2. Low-risk HPV types cause genital warts and do not develop into cervical cancer.
3. Not all types of genital warts cause cervical cancer.
4. HPV type 16 or 18 can lead to cervical cancer.

TEST-TAKING TIP: Low-risk HPV infections are the cause of genital warts. The low-risk HPV types are not causes of cervical cancer. The high-risk HPV infections that are persistent are the most common cause of cervical cancer.
Content Area: Cervical Cancer; Care of the Woman Across the Life Span
Integrated Process: Nursing Process—Evaluation
Client Need: Safe and Effective Care Environment; Health Promotion and Maintenance; Physiological Integrity
Cognitive Level: Evaluation
Concept: Infection
Reference: National Cancer Institute. (2015). HPV and cancer. Retrieved from www.cancer.gov/about-cancer/causes-prevention/risk/infectious-agents/hpv-fact-sheet.

19. ANSWER: 1

Rationale

1. Direct histological examination of the uterine lining is needed to diagnose uterine cancer. A Pap test is an evaluation of cervical cells. The client who stated, "A Pap test is used to diagnose uterine cancer" needs further teaching.
2. This is a correct response. Uterine cancer is the most common cancer of the reproductive tract.
3. Using estrogen for 2 years without progesterone is a risk factor for developing uterine cancer.
4. Postmenopausal bleeding could be an indication of uterine cancer.

TEST-TAKING TIP: Uterine cancer involves the endometrium. An endometrial biopsy, dilation and curettage, or other methods that take a direct sampling of the endometrium are used to diagnose uterine cancer.

Content Area: Uterine Cancer; Care of the Woman Across the Life Span
Integrated Process: Nursing Process—Evaluation
Client Need: Health Promotion and Maintenance; Physiological Integrity; Pharmacology
Cognitive Level: Evaluation
Concept: Cellular Regulation
Reference: *Ward, S. L., & Hisley, S. M. (2009).* Maternal-child nursing care: Optimizing outcomes for mothers, children & families. *Philadelphia: F.A. Davis.*

20. ANSWER: 1, 2, 4

Rationale

1. Using talcum powder on the perineum, having a first-degree relative with ovarian cancer, and eating a high-fat diet are all risk factors for ovarian cancer.
2. Using talcum powder on the perineum, having a first-degree relative with ovarian cancer, and eating a high-fat diet are all risk factors for ovarian cancer.
3. Nulliparity is a risk factor, not having three or more children.
4. Using talcum powder on the perineum, having a first-degree relative with ovarian cancer, and eating a high-fat diet are all risk factors for ovarian cancer.

TEST-TAKING TIP: Having a first-degree relative with ovarian cancer yields the highest potential for ovarian cancer. Nulliparity is a risk factor because the woman without children did not have the interruption of estrogen that occurs during pregnancy. Unopposed estrogen is a risk factor for ovarian cancer.

Content Area: Ovarian Cancer; Care of the Woman Across the Life Span
Integrated Process: Nursing Process—Assessment
Client Need: Safe and Effective Care Environment; Health Promotion and Maintenance; Physiological Integrity
Cognitive Level: Analysis
Concept: Cellular Regulation
Reference: *Ladewig, P. A., London, M. L., & Davidson, M. R. (2010).* Contemporary maternal-newborn nursing care. *7th ed. New York: Pearson.*

Antepartum

Anatomy and Physiology of Pregnancy

Ballottement—In the pregnant woman, during a vaginal examination, the examiner pushes against the cervix and the presenting part of the fetus. The fetus floats away from the examiner's finger and then "bounces" back. This is one of the fetal, or positive, signs of pregnancy.

Braxton Hicks contractions—Intermittent, painless contractions that may be noticed by the pregnant woman after second trimester as the uterus rises into the abdominal cavity. Occurring more often in the last weeks of pregnancy, they are often associated with "false" labor.

Chadwick's sign—The increased vascularity of the uterus and cervix during pregnancy causes the cervix to have a bluish-purple color, as opposed to its usual pinkish tones. This is another presumptive/probable sign of pregnancy.

Diastasis recti—In some pregnant women, the abdominis recti muscles separate at the midline in the last months of pregnancy. Multigravid women and women carrying multiple fetuses or one larger fetus are more likely to experience this. The muscles repair over a period of recovery following delivery.

Glycosuria—An abnormal amount of sugar detected (measured) in the urine. It is a result of excess glucose in the blood, which is filtered out in the kidneys.

Goodell's sign—During the fifth to eighth week of pregnancy, the cervix softens. This is also a presumptive/probable sign of pregnancy.

Hegar's sign—During the fifth to twelfth weeks of pregnancy, the lower uterine segment softens. This can be palpated by an examiner. It is another presumptive sign of pregnancy.

Human chorionic gonadotropin (hCG)—The hormone produced by the placenta during pregnancy. It maintains the corpus luteum in the ovary, part of the suppression of ovulation during pregnancy. It can be detected in the urine as early as before the first missed menses and is the basis for home pregnancy tests.

Human placental lactogen (hPL)—Another hormone produced by the placenta, it helps to break down maternal fats to make them useful for nourishing the fetus. It also seems to play a role in gestational diabetes because it alters maternal metabolism, increases insulin resistance, and decreases carbohydrate absorption in the pregnant woman.

Hyperemia—Literally meaning "increased blood," this refers to the increase in blood flow to the uterus during pregnancy. It is supported by an overall increase in the volume of blood in the pregnant woman's body and the relaxation of the associated arterioles.

Hyperemesis gravidarum—Some women experience repeated and prolonged vomiting (lasting beyond the first trimester of pregnancy). In some cases, it leads to dehydration, weight loss, and electrolyte imbalance.

Kegel exercises—These exercises involve tightening and relaxing the levator ani and coccygeal muscles (the pelvic diaphragm). These muscles support the female pelvic floor and are stretched during vaginal childbirth. Recovery following pregnancy and maintaining urinary continence in later life will be improved by performing regular Kegel exercises.

Leukorrhea—A whitish, odorless mucus discharge from the vagina. It is often a normal occurrence during pregnancy but may be pathological if it changes in amount, appearance, or odor.

Linea nigra—A change in the skin pigment that appears as a line from the umbilicus (sometimes from the xyphoid process) to the pubis symphysis. It occurs in

Continued

50% to 75% of pregnant women, though it is more obvious in light-skinned women.

Melasma (chloasma) gravidarum—Sometimes referred to as the "mask of pregnancy," this pigment darkening occurs over the nose bridge and the cheeks during pregnancy. It is thought to be caused by the hormones that stimulate melanin production during pregnancy. Some women experience this while taking oral contraceptives.

Palmar erythema—Reddened skin over the palms of the hands that is associated with a number of physical conditions, including pregnancy. It is another condition thought to be associated with hormonal changes.

Progesterone—The female hormone secreted from the adrenal cortex, corpus luteum, and the placenta (during pregnancy). Before implantation of the fertilized ovum, progesterone stimulates endometrial thickening. Following implantation, it supports embryonic development.

Prolactin—This is an anterior pituitary hormone that stimulates and supports human milk production.

Proteinuria—The appearance of protein in the urine. This is not normal and the detection of increasing amounts is an indicator of worsening pregnancy-induced hypertension.

Quickening—Typically, between the sixteenth and twentieth week of pregnancy, a woman first feels fetal movement.

Relaxin—Produced by the corpus luteum, the breast, and the placenta during pregnancy, this hormone relaxes the pelvis floor and the symphysis pubis and softens the cervix. Relaxin has a role in hemodynamic changes of pregnancy, increased cardiac output, and renal blood flow.

Striae gravidarum—These reddish stretch marks may form on the pregnant woman's abdomen, breasts, thighs, and buttocks. Following pregnancy and subsequent weight loss, these marks fade to a silvery, less visible appearance.

Trimester—The weeks of pregnancy are divided into three trimesters of 12 to 14 weeks, or 3 months each; first trimester, weeks 1 to 14; second trimester, weeks 15 to 28; and the final trimester, weeks 28 to date of delivery.

Uterine ligaments—These ligaments include the ovarian, infundibulopelvic, round, broad, cardinal, and uterosacral ligaments. They provide support for the female reproductive organs and promote fetal positioning during labor. Though they grow and stretch during pregnancy, they are also responsible for some of the pelvic discomforts of pregnancy.

During the antepartum period, changes occur in every body system to facilitate the pregnancy and the growing fetus and to prepare for delivery and birth. To ensure a good outcome, the client must be provided with education concerning the following maternal physiological adaptation and anticipatory guidance pertaining to the common discomforts associated with these changes.

I. Endocrine System

Just as the hormones of the endocrine system drive the reproductive cycle, the endocrine system changes in response to implantation of the embryo to support the continuation of a pregnancy. As the placenta grows, it becomes a temporary "gland," producing additional hormones that promote the growth of the fetus and help facilitate the physiological changes in the pregnant woman's body.

A. Pituitary gland
1. Prior to pregnancy, the pituitary gland secretes follicle-stimulating hormone (FSH) and luteinizing hormone (LH), which are responsible for changes in the ovaries during the ovarian cycle.
2. After conception, the pituitary gland grows slightly larger and secretes hormones that

stimulate lactation, produce pigmentation changes, stimulate uterine muscle contractions, and alter metabolism.
3. The anterior pituitary increases the production of prolactin, especially during the third trimester.
4. Production of oxytocin by the posterior pituitary gland increases during labor, inducing contractions. Following delivery, oxytocin maintains uterine tone, which prevents hemorrhage. Oxytocin also stimulates the ejection of the milk produced in the mammary glands of the breasts.

MAKING THE CONNECTION

Exogenous Oxytocin
Oxytocin produced as an exogenous medication can be helpful in eliciting effective contractions during labor, when the woman's body is not able to provide effective uterine activity. It can also be administered routinely following delivery of the placenta to ensure uterine tone. For women who have a delayed letdown reflex during breastfeeding, intranasal oxytocin spray may be prescribed to aid in releasing milk for the suckling infant.

B. Adrenal glands
 1. Responding to increased estrogen levels and adrenocorticotropic hormone, the adrenal cortex increases production of cortisol. Increased cortisol affects the metabolism of carbohydrates and proteins necessary for the growth of the developing fetus.
 2. Unfortunately, increased levels of cortisol also predispose the pregnant woman to insulin resistance, which promotes hyperglycemia that may contribute to the development of gestational diabetes.
 3. An increase in aldosterone production early in the second trimester may be a response to the body's increased secretion of sodium due to increased progesterone.

C. Thyroid gland
 1. Alteration of the production of thyroid hormone supports other changes in maternal metabolism.
 2. An increase in production and secretion of thyroxine (T4) causes an increase in the size of the thyroid gland. Levels of T3 and T4 rise until the end of the first trimester, where they remain at elevated levels until the end of the pregnancy. The increase in size can often be felt by an experienced examiner.
 3. Treatment of hypothyroidism during pregnancy is critical to maintain the pregnancy and healthy fetal brain development. Since T3 and T4 should be somewhat elevated during normal pregnancy, the laboratory finding of low levels should trigger further thyroid investigation for possible hormone replacement.

ALERT The symptoms of hyperthyroidism unrelated to pregnancy can be masked by normal signs and symptoms of pregnancy, such as heat intolerance, tachycardia, nausea, and vomiting. Laboratory tests of thyroid function must be interpreted by a practitioner based on expected values during pregnancy. Adequate amounts of iodine to support increased thyroid production are needed in the maternal diet.

D. The pancreas
 1. Due to the growing fetus's need for nutrients from the mother, the islets of Langerhans in the pancreas are stimulated to increase insulin production.
 2. It is possible that inadequate insulin production in concert with other pregnancy hormones (see the placenta) can contribute to a woman developing gestational diabetes.
 3. All pregnant women should undergo a glucose challenge test during the 28th week of pregnancy in order to identify hyperglycemia, which may require treatment.
  a) Gestational hyperglycemia is usually initially treated with a counted card diet and mild exercise. This will be determined based on the data collected from blood glucose levels measured throughout the day before and after meals.

E. The placenta
 Taking on the role of an endocrine gland, the placenta produces hormones specifically involved in altering the physiological environment for fetal growth and development.
 1. Progesterone
  a) The placenta takes over progesterone production from the corpus luteum. Adequate amounts of this hormone are critical to sustaining the pregnancy.
  b) Progesterone relaxes the uterus, maintains the endometrial foundation, and suppresses uterine contractions (by interfering with prostaglandin production).
  c) In concert with estrogen, progesterone prepares the milk-producing structures in the breasts.
  d) Progesterone influences the maternal immune system, preventing the mother from identifying the fetus as a foreign substance, which would lead to rejection.
   (1) Women who have had spontaneous abortions, especially toward the end of the first trimester, should have progesterone levels measured prior to becoming pregnant again.
  e) This hormone also slows gastrointestinal motility, leading to some of the symptoms of gastrointestinal distress in pregnancy.
  f) Progesterone contributes to the daytime tiredness experienced by most women in the first trimester. If possible, women should take a short nap during the day and plan a regular nighttime sleep schedule.
 2. Estrogens
  a) By the seventh week of pregnancy, the placenta takes over the production of estrogen, previously performed by the corpus luteum.
  b) As the pregnancy continues, estrogen stimulates an increase in vascularity, enabling the uterus to provide adequate circulation for the growing fetus.
  c) Estrogen during pregnancy causes the development of the ductal system necessary for milk production. However, high estrogen levels throughout pregnancy inhibit milk production.
  d) It is also responsible for hyperpigmentation that is evident in the linea nigra and melisma gravidarum, or "mask of pregnancy" (Fig. 9.1).
 3. Human chorionic gonadotropin (hCG)
  a) During the implantation process, the trophoblast that develops into the placenta secretes hCG. The role of hCG is to stimulate the corpus luteum to

**Reproductive System Effects
of the Major Pregnancy Hormones**

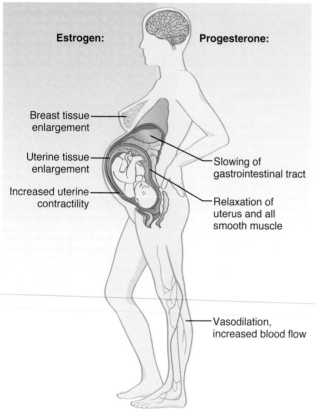

Estrogen:

Breast tissue enlargement

Uterine tissue enlargement

Increased uterine contractility

Progesterone:

Slowing of gastrointestinal tract

Relaxation of uterus and all smooth muscle

Vasodilation, increased blood flow

Fig 9.1 Reproductive system effects of the major pregnancy hormones.

continue estrogen and progesterone production until the placenta is developed enough to perform that function.

b) It is possible to detect small amounts of hCG in a pregnant woman's urine within 3 weeks after the last menstrual period. This is the substance measured in the various over-the-counter urine tests for pregnancy.

4. Human placental somatomammotropin (**human placental lactogen [hPL]**)

a) This hormone, produced by the placenta, alters the mother's metabolism, aiding in carbohydrate, protein, and fat availability for the growing fetus.

b) However, hPL is also an insulin antagonist that decreases maternal glucose metabolism in order to increase its availability to the growing fetus.

c) It acts as growth hormone contributing to breast development.

5. Relaxin

a) The primary source of relaxin is initially from the corpus luteum; however, it seems that the placenta also has some part in its production.

b) Relaxin also limits uterine contractions by relaxing smooth muscle and aiding in softening of the cervix.

c) It aids in changes in cartilage and ligaments that support the uterus and cervix, allowing for growth and accommodation of the uterus and fetus as they grow.

F. Prostaglandins

1. Prostaglandins are lipids that are produced in many different organs. Their function in pregnancy is not well understood, but they have a purpose related to the specific organs where they are found.

2. Historically, the application of prostaglandin E was used to soften the cervix and induce labor, so function has been understood in the reproductive system. It is believed to be involved in the initiation of labor.

3. Decreased vascular levels are thought to contribute to hypertension and the development of pre-eclampsia (hypertension of pregnancy).

II. Reproductive System

The reproductive system is the system that most profoundly changes during pregnancy. Initially stimulated by the hormones of reproduction, the reproductive organs and structures begin to alter their functions and structures to adapt to the needs of the developing embryo and then the fetus.

A. Uterus

1. The uterus increases from approximately 50 g to over 1,100 g at term due to hypertrophy of the muscle cells in the uterine wall. In the first months of pregnancy, the walls thicken but become thinner as the uterus rises out of the pelvis and expands in the abdomen. The cells do not appreciably increase in number.

2. Following implantation, the endometrium becomes the "decidua." There are three layers that persist to support the forming placenta and cover the fetus as the fetal membranes develop.

3. The volume or capacity of the uterus increases from 10 to 20 mL to 5 liters or more. Assessment of the growth of the uterus is accomplished by measuring the height of the fundus from the top of the symphysis pubis to the palpated top of the uterus (see Chapter 10 for further discussion) (Fig. 9.2).

4. Until late in a normal pregnancy, the contractility of the uterine muscles is greatly decreased under the influence of progesterone and relaxin.

5. Uteroplacental blood flow increases throughout pregnancy to over 500 mL per minute, or about one-sixth of the volume of maternal blood. The majority of this blood flows to the placental bed.

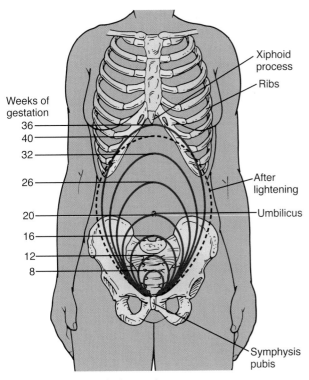

Weeks of gestation
36
40
32
26
20
16
12
8

Xiphoid process
Ribs
After lightening
Umbilicus
Symphysis pubis

Fig 9.2 Uterine height by weeks.

6. The supportive/connective tissues stretch and relax to allow for uterine growth but increase in size to continue to support the enlarging uterus and its contents.
   a) Women who experience pain from the stretching of the broad and round ligaments may find relief by:
      • Performing pelvic rocking (either while standing or on hands and knees).
      • Taking a warm shower or bath and changing positions frequently.
      • Not standing or sitting in one place for an extended period of time.
7. The softening of the lower uterine segment by the end of the first month of pregnancy, or **Hegar's sign,** is a probable sign of pregnancy.
8. **Braxton Hicks contractions** begin around the fourth month. These intermittent contractions may not be felt by the mother until the last months of pregnancy. They may become more uncomfortable in the last weeks of pregnancy, leading the woman to wonder if she is in labor.
   a) These "false" contractions may be relieved if the woman walks for a bit, empties her bladder if it is full, or consumes several glasses of water if she has not had her daily recommended amount of four to six glasses per day.

ALERT Women should be educated to be alert for signs of preterm labor, including experiencing painful, regular contractions or lower back pains that persist whether lying down or when walking, prior to the 37th week of pregnancy. Some women notice increased pressure in the pelvic region and do not feel the contractions, though cervical thinning or dilation is occurring. In any case, she should notify the health care provider and proceed to the hospital for evaluation.

B. Cervix
   1. Changes in the cervix begin with increased vascularity that results in softening (**Goodell's sign**) and a bluish tint (**Chadwick's sign**).
   2. The mucus glands of the cervix, stimulated by estrogen, increase and secrete increased amounts of mucus.
      a) A "mucus plug" seals the endocervical canal, preventing the entrance of bacteria into the uterus.
      b) This plug is released when the cervix begins to dilate shortly before or at the onset of labor.
   3. The increased amounts of mucus contribute to the common discharge during pregnancy.
      a) At the start of labor, as the cervix dilates, the discharge may become blood-tinged.
C. Vagina and vulva
   1. The tissues of the vagina experience changes similar to the changes seen in the cervix, hyperplasia and increased blood flow caused by increased estrogen levels.
   2. Epithelial mucosa of the vaginal walls thicken and add to the increase in vaginal secretions. This **leukorrhea** is thicker than the secretions produced by nulliparous women and has a more acidic pH to discourage bacterial growth; staining of undergarments may be prevented by use of a panty liner.
   3. The glycogen content of the thick secretions can feed a common vaginal yeast, *Candida albicans.* Daily cleansing of the external labia and vulva and wearing cotton underwear can help to prevent the overgrowth of candida. If candida multiplies, secretions may take on a lumpy appearance and cause intense itching of the vulva. Topical antiyeast creams may be purchased over the counter, but a woman should consult her health care provider before using these medications.
   4. In the last weeks of pregnancy, the walls of the vagina relax, preparing to expand for delivery.
   5. Engorgement of vaginal and pelvic tissues through the second and third trimesters may contribute to increased sexual desire and orgasmic response for some pregnant women.
      a) Sexual expression during pregnancy is unique for each couple. Intercourse during pregnancy is safe except in the presence of preterm labor, vaginal bleeding, or the premature rupture of membranes.

b) Intercourse may be more relaxed in the absence of concern for birth control.

c) Sore breasts or engorged female organs will require good communication between partners for what is pleasurable and what is not.

(1) Alternative positions for intercourse should be considered, especially in late pregnancy when the supine position for the woman is both uncomfortable and discouraged for hemodynamic reasons.

(2) Alternative forms of sexual intimacy should be explored, especially if pelvic rest (no intercourse) or prohibition of stimulation to female orgasm is prescribed by the health care provider.

D. Ovaries

1. Ovulation stops due to the increased levels of estrogen and progesterone; negative feedback to the pituitary gland ceases secretion of FSH and LH.

2. The prolonged existence of the progesterone-producing corpus luteal cyst is associated with an increased size of the cyst within the ovary. This continues until the placenta begins producing progesterone in good amounts toward the end of the first trimester.

3. The ovaries remain inactive until hormone levels return to prepregnant levels.

(!) ALERT Ovulation can be suppressed during the first 6 months of exclusively breastfeeding under very specific conditions (see Chapter 5 for further discussion). Otherwise, fertility/ovulation can return at any time and contraception should be used.

E. Breasts

1. In the early weeks of pregnancy, most women experience increased tingling and sensitivity of the breasts.

MAKING THE CONNECTION

Education Prevention

The nurse should instruct pregnant women not to insert artificial objects into the vagina during pregnancy. This includes tampons, douches, or other cleansing agents. If changes in the amount, color, texture, or odor of vaginal secretions occur, the client should call her health care provider because it could indicate a vaginal infection. If the mucus plug is expelled prior to 36 weeks, health care provider advice should also be sought. Any cramping or pain in the uterus that is unrelenting should be reported to the health care provider as soon as possible. Any bleeding or gush of fluid from the vagina should prompt the client to go to the hospital for evaluation.

---

2. The consistency of the breast may become firmer with palpable nodules.

3. Increased circulation to breast tissues causes breast enlargement, usually requiring a woman to utilize a larger bra cup size. As the uterus expands the abdomen and chest cavity, a larger bra circumference will be needed also.

a) An undergarment specialist or pregnancy garment specialty shop can assist women in obtaining a bra that will be adjustable throughout pregnancy and in the first weeks following delivery.

b) A soft supportive bra may be worn during sleep to help alleviate early sensitivity and discomfort.

4. Areolar pigment will darken and appear larger as the breast size increases. The appearance of superficial veins may become more visible, and **striae** may appear.

5. Sebaceous glands (known as *Montgomery tubercles*) in the areola increase activity to moisturize the tissues.

6. During the second trimester, small amounts of precolostrum may be secreted from the nipples as a thin, clear fluid. In the last trimester, the fluid will become the more yellow and thicker colostrum.

a) Absorbent breast pads may be inserted in the bra to absorb leakage.

7. Nurses may suggest that women with flat or inverted nipples use physical nipple eversion to help prepare for breastfeeding.

(!) ALERT If the health care provider prescribes pelvic rest (avoiding sexual intercourse or stimulation), the client should be cautioned against nipple stimulation. The release of increased oxytocin may be associated with nipple stimulation. If a risk of preterm labor exists, nipple stroking, pulling, or rolling may induce contractions.

III. Cardiovascular System

In general, the changes in the cardiovascular system associated with pregnancy occur to meet the needs of the growing fetus (or fetuses), yet still meet the needs of the pregnant woman. Women with cardiovascular disorders or risk must consult with their health care provider before attempting pregnancy. Their pregnancies are considered high risk due to the demands pregnancy places on the cardiovascular system.

A. Blood pressure

1. Early in pregnancy, there is a decrease in peripheral vascular resistance (20% to 30%). This results in an overall decrease of 10 to 20 mm Hg in

diastolic blood pressure between the 24th and 32nd weeks of pregnancy. The pregnant woman may experience orthostatic hypotension; teach her to get up from a flat or sitting position slowly.

2. As the fetus grows, resting or sleeping in the supine position places excessive pressure on the vena cava, resulting in decreased blood return to the heart and cardiac output (Fig. 9.3).
   a) This may decrease blood pressure enough to interrupt optimal blood flow and perfusion through the placenta to the fetus.
   b) Instruct the pregnant woman to avoid lying flat on her back. Side-lying and semi-side-lying positions can be comfortably accomplished with the use of extra pillows behind the back, cradling the abdomen, and between the knees.
3. Over time, the increase in total blood volume aids in preventing symptoms of low blood pressure.
4. An increase of blood pressure with a systolic level at or above 140 mm Hg, or a diastolic reading equal to or greater than 90 mm Hg, is indicative of a hypertensive disorder.
   a) After the 20th week of pregnancy, instruct pregnant woman to be alert to the onset of pounding headaches or sudden swelling of the hands and/or face. These should be reported to the health care provider immediately.

B. Blood volume
1. Overall blood volume (red blood cell, plasma, white blood cell, coagulation factors) increases by 30% to 50% during pregnancy.
   a) This accounts for approximately 4 pounds of pregnancy weight gain.
      (1) Increased blood volume leads to increased vascular congestion responsible for Chadwick's sign, the bluish mucosa evident in the cervix, vagina, and vulva.
   b) Uterine blood flow is 500 to 600 mL per minute by the end of pregnancy.

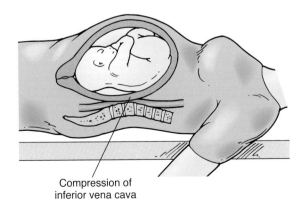

Compression of inferior vena cava

Fig 9.3 Supine hypotension.

2. Red blood cells
   a) Although the red blood cell (RBC) count will increase by approximately 30% (20% to 30% increase in RBC volume) during pregnancy, the plasma volume also increases by about 50%.
   b) This results in a physiological "anemia" of pregnancy, characterized by lower hemoglobin and hematocrit measurement.
   c) All pregnant women should be instructed in adjusted dietary practices to meet their needs and the needs of the fetus, including iron-rich and iron-enriched foods. They may want to get a plan just for their dietary needs and preferences from https://www.choosemyplate.gov/ (see Chapter 11 for further discussion).
      (1) The gastrointestinal tract increases iron absorption during pregnancy.
      (2) Maintaining maternal iron stores can be difficult in spite of increased iron absorption by the digestive tract.
      (3) Although most women will be prescribed a pregnancy multivitamin and mineral product, some women will require an additional vitamin supplement.
      (4) Iron is best absorbed when taken with vitamin C or a citrus juice.
      (5) The pregnant woman needs to increase fluid intake to at least 10 glasses of fluids per day; 4 to 6 of these should be plain water. Warm environmental conditions or exercise will require an additional increase in fluid needs.
3. White blood cells (WBCs)
   a) During pregnancy, normal (not indicating infection) counts may rise to 16,000 mm³.
4. Coagulation factors
   a) A general increase in some clotting factors and a decrease in coagulation inhibiting factors.
   b) Fibrin in the plasma increases by 40%.
   c) Fibrinogen increases by up to 50%.
   d) Platelets (thrombocytes) should remain at prepregnant levels through pregnancy.
      (1) Significant decreases in platelets are associated with possible liver dysfunction, most notably occurring with worsening pre-eclampsia.

ALERT Coagulation changes predispose pregnant women to hypercoagulopathy, or an increased risk of blood clots. The client should inform the health care provider if she develops soreness in the lower extremities that is accompanied by redness, warmth, and localized swelling. Based on the presence of a deep vein thrombosis in a prior pregnancy, some women may be at high risk for recurrence.

C. Heart
1. The heart rate increases by 10 to 20 beats per minute to accommodate circulation of the increased blood volume.
   a) Cardiac output increases progressively by an average of 40% until the third trimester, with a corresponding increase in stroke volume of 25% to 30%.
      (1) Cardiac output increases during exercise. The pregnant woman should exercise but should be aware of the corresponding increases in heart rate during exercise and perform moderate exercise to maintain safe rates.
D. Circulation
1. Progesterone leads to the relaxation of arterioles; this reduces blood pressure but also decreases efficient venous return.
2. Venous stasis and pressure cause localized edema and promote the development of venous varicosities in the legs ("spider" or varicose veins), vulva, or anus (see Gastrointestinal System section below).
   a) Moderate exercise and frequent position changes, including periodic horizontal rest, help to prevent the development of varicosities.
   b) Encourage the pregnant woman to avoid crossing her legs.
   c) Discourage the wearing of tight, restrictive undergarments, clothing, or stockings.
   d) Pregnant women who must travel long distances or have a long commute must plan to promote peripheral circulation.
      (1) Check with the health care provider for any specific concerns.
      (2) Plan ambulation hourly if possible.
      (3) Wear nonbinding moderate pressure stockings (15–20 mm Hg) during the trip.
3. A sudden increase in weekly weight gain and swelling or edema in the last trimester of pregnancy is not normal and should be reported to the health care provider.

IV. Respiratory System

The respiratory system is affected by hormonal changes of pregnancy, especially **progesterone** and **prostaglandins.** The system must be able to provide adequate amounts of oxygen for mother and fetus and remove carbon dioxide efficiently. The growing uterus gradually forces repositioning of the lungs and makes the work of breathing more uncomfortable, especially in late pregnancy when lying down.

A. Upper airway
1. Vascular congestion and smooth muscle relaxation may lead to complaints of dyspnea, nasal congestion, and nose bleeds.
   a) Maintaining a moist environment through the use of a humidifier and/or saline nasal sprays (*not* decongestant sprays) will be helpful.
   b) Protect the mouth and nose from cold air.
B. Lungs
1. The lungs are displaced upward and outward by the expanding uterus; the diaphragm elevates by up to 4 cm as the thoracic cage expands outward by about 2 cm.
   a) The ligaments of the rib cage are relaxed by **estrogen.**
   b) In addition to a larger bra cup size, the pregnant woman will require a larger chest size; the entire circumference increases by 5 to 7 cm.
   c) Though the breathing work of the abdomen decreases, the diaphragm continues to do the primary work of breathing.
   d) Elevating the head and chest on pillows or sleeping in a recliner in semi-Fowler's position (30° elevation) may help to alleviate both upper airway congestion and dyspnea.
C. Lung volume
1. The respiratory rate increases slightly but may be more noticeable during exertion.
2. The tidal volume, or volume of air inspired and expired during normal breathing, increases by 30% to 50% (500–700 L per minute), helping to compensate for a reduced expiratory volume.
D. Ventilation
1. The efficiency of gas exchange increases because the tidal volume has increased, though the respiratory rate has only increased slightly or not at all.
2. From the end of the first trimester through the remaining pregnancy, the amount of air taken into the lungs in 1 minute ("minute ventilation") increases by 30% to 50%.
3. The respiratory sensors become more sensitive to a rise in arterial CO_2 levels, improving the removal of CO_2 from the system.
4. Respiratory and metabolic compensatory factors in the pregnant woman reveal an arterial acid-base "picture" of compensated respiratory alkalosis.

ALERT Pregnant women who smoke or have underlying respiratory disorders such as asthma are at risk for having reduced optimal respiratory function during pregnancy. Smoking cessation programs should be readily available to pregnant women. Women with asthma should consult with their health care providers on the appropriate types and administration of antiasthma medications. Over-the-counter bronchodilators and oral or intranasal decongestants should be avoided due to the potential to increase blood pressure and raise the heart rate.

V. Gastrointestinal System

Changes in the gastrointestinal (GI) system during pregnancy are both anatomic and physiological. As with other systems, the hormonal changes, the demands of the growing fetus, and the increasing space required by the uterus account for the majority of change. Many of the most common complaints associated with pregnancy arise from changes in the GI tract, from the mouth and esophagus all the way down to the anus.

A. Mouth
   1. Hyperemia of the gums is due to vascular congestion and may lead to gingival bleeding during brushing or flossing.
      a) Good oral hygiene is important; brushing with a soft toothbrush and flossing with a soft floss may help avoid bleeding.
      b) Poor oral hygiene may lead to oral inflammation and exacerbate gum disease.
         (1) A dental checkup prior to or early in pregnancy can identify any work that needs to be done at a time when reclining in the dental chair is more comfortable.
         (2) Major dental work requiring prolonged or general anesthetic should be accomplished prior to pregnancy or delayed until after.
   2. Excessive saliva (ptyalism) may occur during pregnancy and may produce a bitter taste.
      a) Chewing gum, sucking on lozenges, eating small frequent meals, and avoiding starchy food often help.

B. Esophagus
   1. The lower esophageal sphincter (cardiac sphincter) relaxes due to hormonal influences, leading to acid reflux or "heartburn."
      a) Heartburn is not related to the amount of hair the fetus has; this is an old wives' tale.
      b) Eating more frequent, smaller meals and taking solids and liquids at staggered times may help.
      c) Sitting up after meals will also help, as will elevating the head of the bed at night for sleep. (The same preventions that aid breathing.)

(!) ALERT Ingesting antacid medications, including H2 blockers, proton-pump inhibitors, and products containing alkalizing agents should only be done under the advice of the health care provider. Some may be prohibited during pregnancy while others, such as simple baking soda preparations, may lead to electrolyte imbalances.

C. Gallbladder
   1. The gallbladder enlarges and becomes hypotonic under the influence of progesterone.
   2. An emptying of bile slows after the first trimester, potentially trapping cholesterol.
      a) Though not common, this places some women at risk for gallstones.
      b) Avoiding fried or other greasy foods may prevent the bloated or gassy feeling related to gallbladder changes.

D. Stomach and intestines
   1. The smooth muscle of the stomach and intestines relaxes, causing delayed stomach emptying and slowed peristalsis.
      a) Delayed gastric emptying contributes to reflux and heartburn.
      b) Slowed digestion leads to complaints of bloating and flatulence (gas).
         (1) Avoid spicy or gas-producing foods such as baked beans or cucumbers.
      c) Near term, intake of small meals may alleviate these symptoms. Avoidance of meals within several hours of sleep may also help.
   2. The enlarging uterus pushes the intestine and stomach upward and outward, further interfering with digestion.
   3. Nutrient absorption is more efficient, increasing the uptake of minerals, carbohydrates, and proteins.
      a) The colon reabsorbs water so well that the remaining stool becomes more formed and may be difficult to pass (constipation).
         (1) The woman experiencing constipation may benefit from increased water intake.
         (2) Dietary fiber in fruits, vegetables, and whole grains will add bulk and promote retaining more fluid for a softer stool. Dietary fiber additives are safe as long as laxative ingredients are not added.

(!) ALERT As with antacid remedies, over-the-counter or herbal laxatives should not be used without the advice of the health care provider. Some stool softeners may be recommended by the health care provider, especially if the client is on an iron supplement, which may contribute to constipation. The client at risk for preterm labor should avoid undue stimulation of the intestines because intestinal irritation with increased peristalsis may stimulate uterine activity.

E. Anus
   1. The combination of venous congestion and the weight of the uterine contents often lead to anal varices, more commonly known as *hemorrhoids.*
      a) Loose-fitting lower garments avoid impeding venous return from the pelvis.

b) Changing positions and lying down in a lateral position as often as possible will promote circulation.
2. Straining and stretching the anal sphincter with hard stools may cause bleeding of the hemorrhoids.
   a) While uncomfortable, most hemorrhoids are not a serious problem.
   b) Following the recommendations to relieve constipation will help.
   c) Applying hemorrhoid cream aids in cooling, moisturizing, and shrinking.
   d) Pads soaked with witch hazel, a plant-based astringent that relieves inflammation, can help shrink the tissues.
F. Nausea and vomiting
1. Nausea, sometimes accompanied by vomiting, is common in the first trimester of pregnancy. It affects 70% to 90% of all pregnant women.
   a) Although they are gastrointestinal symptoms, the cause or causes are not well understood.
   b) Because the patterns of estrogen and hCG levels during pregnancy occur at the time of the appearance and subsequent cessation of the symptoms, it is thought that they are primarily responsible. The changes in metabolism may also explain some of the experience.
   c) Some weight loss may be experienced in the first trimester but should stop when appetite and intake increase.
   d) Not all women experience nausea or vomiting in the same way.
      (1) Some have nausea that begins upon rising in the morning but dissipates through the day, while others are more affected at night.
      (2) For some women, the symptoms begin between the 4th and 6th week, while others begin even earlier.
      (3) For most women the symptoms subside by the 8th to 12th week, while some do not get relief until closer to mid-pregnancy.
      (4) Some women vomit once or twice per day, yet others only experience nausea.
      (5) Many women are repelled by certain foods or odors that seem to stimulate the nausea centers in the brain.
   e) Routine suggestions for relief include:
      • Eating dry crackers or toast before rising in the morning
      • Avoiding ingestion of foods and liquids at the same time
      • Eating small, more frequent meals to keep blood sugar levels more consistent
      • Preparing favorite "comfort foods" that appeal to the individual
      • Taking vitamin and mineral supplements at the time of day that nausea is less of a problem
      • Sipping cool lemon-lime soda or ginger ale (not diet drinks)
      • Sucking on hard candy
      • Sniffing aromatherapy natural oils such as ginger, citrus, or lavender, known to calm or interrupt the nausea center in the brain
   f) Nausea and vomiting that is severe enough to prevent tolerance of any fluids or solid food may lead to fluid and electrolyte imbalance.
      (1) Prolonged and persistent nausea and vomiting is known as *hyperemesis gravidarum.*
      (2) There is more danger to the woman than to the fetus in this situation.
      (3) Antiemetic drugs may be prescribed by the health care provider but often do little to stem severe vomiting.
      (4) IV fluids, electrolytes, and total parenteral nutrition may be required to maintain homeostasis.
      (5) The goal of IV therapy and other interventions is to help the client maintain her daily activities as much as possible—work, school, or care for other children.

V. Urinary System

The maternal urinary system undergoes both functional changes and structural adaptation. It must excrete waste products for the mother and for those sent by the fetus into the maternal circulation. Increased blood volume requires the kidneys to increase their filtration rate accordingly.
A. Kidneys
1. The kidneys respond to an increase in renal plasma flow of 50% to 80% by elongating about 1 cm during pregnancy. The volume of the kidney increases by about 30%.
   a) Renal plasma flow benefits from a lateral lying position rather than the supine position.
   b) Glomerular filtration rates (GFR) increase early in the first trimester and reach maximum rates by the end of the trimester, an average of 110 to 180 mL/min.
2. The renal calyces and pelvis dilate, probably due to relaxation caused by progesterone.
3. Substances such as amino acids, water-soluble vitamins, and minerals are filtered and excreted in larger amounts than in the nonpregnant woman. The increase in calcium absorption by the intestines

(due to increased systemic vitamin D or calciferol) counters a loss in the kidneys.

  a) Potassium retention during the filtration process is offset by the maternal and fetal tissues' use of potassium from the plasma.

  b) Although increased GFR encourages increased sodium excretion, electrolyte balance is maintained by increases in tubular reabsorption of sodium.

    (1) Aldosterone levels also promote sodium and fluid retention.

    (2) Sodium excretion is associated with increased urination. This is also influenced by an increased fluid intake.

  c) Glucose excretion increases.

    (1) Glycosuria does not indicate abnormal glucose metabolism.

    (2) The glucose challenge test measures serum glucose levels, not urine glucose.

  d) Protein is also excreted at levels above those prior to pregnancy.

    (1) Proteinuria over 300 mg of protein (albumin) in a 24-hour urine specimen may indicate renal failure, pre-eclampsia, or a urinary tract infection.

4. Angiotensin II levels are increased during pregnancy. However, a potential increase in blood pressure is averted because angiotensin II receptors seem to be less responsive in pregnant women.

  a) The pregnant woman whose body cannot maintain this balance of angiotensin II production and decreased sensitivity is likely to develop increases in blood pressure any time after the 20th week of pregnancy, known as pre-eclampsia.

MAKING THE CONNECTION

Decreased Venous Return

Changes in both the cardiovascular and urinary system are often evidenced by swelling, especially in the lower extremities in later pregnancy. This is aggravated by several factors, including the retention of sodium and water and increasing uterine size and weight that impedes venous return from the lower extremities. Women who are working on their feet for long periods or who are overweight may have increased dependent swelling. All pregnant women should attempt to rest during the day. This rest should be with legs and feet elevated above the level of the heart if possible. Sodium intake should be limited by avoiding preserved meats, salty snacks, or added table salt. Water intake should not be reduced. Exercise that increases circulation and balances metabolism should be part of the pregnant woman's daily routine.

B. Ureters

1. A combination of smooth muscle relaxation and pressure from the expanding uterus cause the ureters to elongate and dilate.

  a) If urine does not empty completely from the ureters, the risk for urinary tract infection (UTI) increases.

C. Bladder and urethra

1. In early pregnancy, the growing uterus remains in the pelvic cavity, lying directly over the bladder.

  a) Most women experience urinary frequency in the first trimester.

    (1) **Kegel exercises** of the pelvic floor muscles may help to control bladder leakage (see Chapter 17 for further discussion).

  b) Decreasing fluid intake is not beneficial.

  c) Avoiding fluids that may irritate the bladder, such as caffeinated drinks or acidic juices, should decrease urgency.

  d) Teach the client to empty her bladder immediately following intercourse to help prevent a UTI.

2. As the pregnancy progresses, pressure is relieved and frequency abates.

3. In the third trimester, the weight and position of the uterus push the bladder forward and up, stretching the urethra.

  a) Frequency returns, and if the bladder cannot be emptied completely, the risk of infection increases.

  b) Frequency associated with bladder pain and possibly blood-tinged urine may indicate a UTI.

ALERT UTIs may stimulate uterine contractions in addition to other symptoms. Any pregnant woman with a UTI should be assessed for contractions and a woman with preterm contractions should be assessed for a possible UTI.

VI. Integumentary System

A. Skin

1. During pregnancy, blood flow to the skin increases up to four times due to peripheral blood vessel dilation.

  a) This change may result in small angiomas or spider veins appearing on the face, neck, chest, or arms.

  b) Palmar erythema is another change in the appearance of skin related to peripheral blood flow.

  c) Facial flushing and surface warmth often accompanied by increased perspiration are also possible changes. Some people refer to this as the "glow" of pregnancy.

2. Hormonal influence increases melanocyte activity, causing changes in skin pigmentation in several areas (see the "Endocrine System" section).
   a) The **linea nigra,** a vertical line extending from the umbilicus to the mons pubis, becomes darker.
   b) **Melasma (chloasma)** is a hyperpigmentation that occurs across the nose and cheeks in a masklike shape.
   c) Darkening of the areolas and nipples, anal and vulvar skin, and other darkened skin such as moles occurs.
      (1) Skin exposed to the sun should be protected by a 30 to 45 SPF sunscreen.
3. Striae gravidarum appear on skin that has been stretched over structures that increase in size, such as the abdomen, breast, thighs, and buttocks.
   a) Some women develop many of these reddened lines, but others have few, if any, marks. Striae gravidarum tend to be familial.
   b) Keeping the skin moist and massaging it may keep it supple, but there are no apparent "cures" for striae.
      (1) Avoiding excessive weight gain will help to limit skin stretching.
   c) Following the pregnancy, when the skin tissues return to prepregnant shape and size, the striae thin and fade to a silvery tone.
4. Some women experience an increase in sebaceous oil production related to the increase in estrogens. This may cause acne that develops on the face or back.
   a) Women with dry skin may find that their skin normalizes during pregnancy.
   b) Tell pregnant women that keeping the skin clean and moisturized and getting the ideal amounts of nutrients and fluids is the best way to keep skin healthy during pregnancy.

B. Hair and nails
1. In the last weeks of pregnancy, the hair follicles that are in a stage of growth increase in number. This limits the number of hairs that are shed, making hair appear more full.
   a) Hair is shed at an increased rate following delivery. Women should be reassured that they are not balding.
2. Nail growth and appearance may change, becoming more brittle or soft, grooved across the nail, or curved.

🚫 **ALERT** Chemical hair processing, such as perm waves or coloring with professional dyes, may be contraindicated during pregnancy. The hair may not respond to the treatment in the expected manner due to the other changes of pregnancy. For safety concerns, pregnant women should consult with the primary health care provider before proceeding.

VII. Musculoskeletal System

A. Bone tissue
1. The old wives' tale of losing "a tooth for every baby" is not true, but care of the teeth is important.
   a) The growing fetus needs calcium. However, the mother's stores will be adequate to meet both her and the fetus's needs.
      (1) Care of the teeth is still important (see the "Gastrointestinal System" section).
   b) The bones in the remainder of the system do not change in structure.

B. Muscles and connective tissues
1. Muscle symptoms during pregnancy may be related to the balance or increase of minerals and electrolytes.
   a) Leg cramps, often occurring at night, may be caused by the increased amounts of calcium in the system.
      (1) Reduce dairy intake for a short time.
      (2) Apply counter stretch by slowly dorsiflexing at the ankle.
   b) Other muscle discomfort may be due to overexercising or not warming up enough before more exercise.
   c) For women carrying one very large or multiple fetuses, the stretching of the abdominus rectus muscles may eventually cause them to separate along the abdominal midline (**diastasis recti).**
      (1) This is not painful, nor is its occurrence under the control of the pregnant woman.
      (2) After delivery, an abdominal binder may be offered to the client with a diastasis.
      (3) Teach the client to avoid sit-ups or other abdominal crunches until the muscle has rejoined.
2. Most of the changes to the musculoskeletal system occur in the joints and ligaments.
3. Softening of the connective tissues in the joints in general also produces changes in the joints in the pelvis. This is in preparation for the stretching of the pelvis that will be needed for a vaginal delivery.
   a) Pelvic relaxation contributes to a gait change, or the pregnancy "waddle."
4. Slight swelling in the joints of the hands may make wedding bands difficult to remove.
   a) Advise the client to remove rings and store safely or place on a chain necklace to avoid having to cut the ring off to promote circulation to the finger.
   b) Joints in the feet relax. When combined with carrying increased weight and edema, the woman's feet become wider.
      (1) Footwear should be measured for the correct size, width, and support.

(2) Instruct client to avoid exercise that requires good balance during the last month of pregnancy.

c) The stretching of the round ligaments may cause lower back discomfort.

  (1) The client can try massage and warmth or conscious relaxation techniques.

  (2) Suggest that she lie down in a lateral position and flex her knees toward the abdomen.

  (3) Try pelvic rocking or a similar exercise.

  (4) Instruct the client to try bending toward the pain.

5. Increasing weight of the uterus causes a change in the woman's center of gravity.

a) Lordosis, or sway back, is the body's attempt to balance the heavy load.

b) Backaches can be treated with a nondrug topical pain reliever.

  (1) Teach the client good posture for pregnancy and how to pick up heavy objects and employ lifting equipment when available.

  (2) A pregnancy support belt helps to lift the abdomen and alter the center of gravity, doing some of the work of the abdominal muscles and taking some strain off the back.

  (3) Explain the importance of sitting in chairs that have good seat, back, and arm support.

  (4) Suggest the client sleep on a supportive mattress and use extra pillows for positioning.

  (5) Consider walking or swimming for safe exercise in the last trimester.

MAKING THE CONNECTION

Providing Prenatal Care

Pregnancy is a time when most women have regular contact with the health care system. This is an ideal time to reinforce healthy habits and provide information. The nurse often has a willing audience in the client who is eager to learn all that she can about self-care and preparing to care for her infant. Written client materials should back up what is said in the clinic, but the primary therapeutic communication and relationship is often between the nurse and the client.

CASE STUDY: Putting It All Together

Subjective Data

Ms. Chang is pregnant for the first time. She is a 34-year-old college-educated career woman who travels around the United States for business on a monthly basis. She chose to conceive because she wanted to have a child before her mid-30s, fearing that conceiving might be increasingly difficult. She is in for her first prenatal visit. During this visit, her history reveals the following:

• She and her partner have been a couple for 6 years. They have no known family genetic disorders.

• She has used hormonal birth control and had been off the pill for 6 months when she conceived. Her last menstrual period puts her at 8 weeks.

• She has had all recommended childhood and adult vaccinations and denies any past sexually transmitted infections.

• She reports her diet is varied, including all food groups. She has experienced nausea and some loss of appetite for fish and eggs.

• She has never smoked, and she last consumed alcohol over 3 months ago.

She has a list of questions and concerns about her pregnancy experience so far. She says she has been surprised by the extreme fatigue and daylong nausea and wonders if it is like this for every pregnant woman or if it is because of her age. She explains that she can only tolerate small meals and that her nausea does subside somewhat after a half sandwich, bowl of oatmeal, or small serving of oriental noodles.

She belongs to a local health club/gym but has been too tired to exercise for several weeks. She canceled a business trip with a 2-hour flight because she was afraid of getting sick on the plane. She says she is safe in her current relationship, having had only one other serious relationship due to the time she has invested in her education and career.

She describes increased thirst and more frequent trips to the bathroom than usual, and she has a mucous vaginal discharge. She has started reading about pregnancy on the many websites available for pregnant women. She thinks that her symptoms are common but wonders when they will improve.

Objective Data

Nursing Assessment

> **Vital Signs**
> Blood pressure: 108/64
> Pulse: 86 bpm
> Respiration: 14 bpm
> Temperature: 98°F
> She is alert and able to give a thorough health history.
> Her BMI is 23; she explains that she has lost 4 to 5 pounds over the past few weeks.
> Her skin is clear but appears slightly flushed, her hair is clean and styled, and her nails are manicured.
> A urine sample is collected and several tubes of blood are drawn in the laboratory.

Continued

CASE STUDY: Putting It All Together (Continued)

Case Study Questions

The nurse should be prepared to answer the patient's questions:

1. How long will Ms. Chang be able to travel for her job?

2. When will she get her energy back?

3. What types of exercise are safe?

4. How much fluid should she drink? ("I feel like I am always running to the bathroom.")

5. What are her risks, if any?

6. Is there anything else she can do for the nausea?

7. Will she feel like eating a balanced diet?

8. What information can you share with her about her pregnancy and recommendations for her personal situation?

REVIEW QUESTIONS

Be sure to read the Introduction for valuable test-taking tips.

1. A client is complaining of heartburn. The nurse understands this is caused by which change of pregnancy?
   1. An increase in water reabsorption by the colon
   2. The relaxation of the lower esophageal ("cardiac") sphincter
   3. A decrease in the capacity of the stomach
   4. An increase in stomach acid production

2. A nurse is educating a pregnant client about ways to prevent UTIs. Which statement by the client indicates that she understands the information from the nurse?
   1. "I should decrease my fluid intake."
   2. "Drinking Coke will prevent me from getting a UTI."
   3. "I should always empty my bladder right after I have intercourse."
   4. "I should drink orange juice every morning."

3. The decrease in systemic vascular resistance aids in decreasing which physiological measure?
   1. Cardiac output
   2. Pulse rate
   3. Renal blood flow
   4. Blood pressure

4. The nurse is educating a pregnant client about common discomforts during the third trimester. Which statement by the nurse is appropriate?
   1. "Perform pelvic-tilt exercises."
   2. "Eat crackers prior to getting out of bed in the morning."
   3. "Use humidifiers or saline nose drops."
   4. "Wear a supportive bra."

5. The nurse is educating a client at her first prenatal visit about hormone changes. The nurse explains that which of the following is the purpose of progesterone?
   1. Stimulates uterine development
   2. Relaxes pelvic ligaments and joints
   3. Prepares breasts for lactation
   4. Relaxes smooth muscles

6. A nurse is reviewing the laboratory results for a prenatal client. She notices that her hemoglobin is 10.5. The nurse realizes this laboratory result indicates which of the following?
   1. Low vitamin intake has resulted in a decrease in red blood cell production.
   2. Plasma volume increase is greater than red blood cell production and has resulted in a decrease in hemoglobin.
   3. This is a serious problem that might harm the fetus.
   4. A repeat blood test should be done immediately to confirm that the client has anemia.

7. After receiving information on the signs and symptoms of potential complications during pregnancy, the prenatal client knows to immediately report which of the following to her health care provider? *Select all that apply.*
   1. Backache and flank pain
   2. Burning on urination
   3. Enlargement of breasts and tenderness
   4. Abdominal cramping and vaginal bleeding
   5. Urinary frequency

8. A client is 8 weeks pregnant and has been eating more times during the day but ingesting smaller amounts of food at each meal or snack. What is her *most* likely goal?
   1. Weight loss
   2. Managing waves of nausea
   3. Preventing gastric reflux
   4. Managing daytime fatigue

9. Now in her second trimester of pregnancy, the client, who was a marathon runner before nausea and overwhelming tiredness kept her from exercising regularly, is wondering whether she can run now. What is the nurse's *best* response?
   1. "Certainly, if you feel up to it."
   2. "Your level of exercise will be somewhat modified by the changes occurring in your body."
   3. "Your primary health care provider will need to give you permission."
   4. "Because your body is meeting the needs of two people now, you should avoid too much exercise."

10. Jose's wife, Camilla, is 5 months pregnant and seems more interested in sex than during the first trimester. However, he has told her he is worried about having normal "relations," fearing it will hurt the baby. What information can the nurse provide to assist in their decision about sexual activity?
    1. "The baby is well protected and will not be injured during intercourse as long as the membranes remain intact and there are no symptoms of preterm labor."
    2. "Your husband is correct to be concerned. It would be best if you avoid female orgasm during intercourse."
    3. "Intercourse is okay, but avoid experimenting with different partner positions."
    4. "Enjoy intimate relations while you can. Things will change after the baby is born."

11. A client at 20 weeks gestation has just been examined during a prenatal visit. Which assessment should the nurse recognize as an abnormal finding and the need for further testing?
    1. Fundal height of 26 cm
    2. Pulse rate 15 bpm higher than her prepregnancy pulse
    3. Blood pressure of 128/68
    4. Deep tendon reflexes +2

12. A physician has just documented on a prenatal client. The nurse notices that the physician notes the presence of Goodell's sign. The nurse understands that this sign indicates which of the following?
    1. Changes in the cervix
    2. Changes in the uterus
    3. Passive movement of an unengaged fetus
    4. Fetus that has begun to descend and engage in the pelvis

13. A woman who is primigravida is complaining of leg cramps. Which statement by the nurse best describes how to provide relief from this discomfort?
    1. "Extend both of your legs and touch your toes to stretch your calf muscle."
    2. "Dorsiflex the foot to relieve the cramping."
    3. "Elevate the leg above your heart until the cramp has subsided."
    4. "Plantar flex the foot to relieve the cramping."

14. The nurse is educating a client about varicosities during pregnancy. Which statement by the client indicates effective teaching?
    1. "I need to wear knee-high hose every day to increase my leg circulation."
    2. "When I sit at my desk, both of my feet should be resting on the floor."
    3. "I should perform Kegel exercises twice a day."
    4. "I should call the physician if I do not feel my baby move."

15. A client in her third trimester reports increased perineal pressure. Which is the clinical cause for this complaint?
    1. Fundal height
    2. Urinary infection
    3. Constipation
    4. Hydramnios

16. A client at 26 weeks gestation is in the office after being discharged from the hospital for preterm contractions. She states that she no longer is having contractions but is really having trouble with heart-burn and reflux. Which is the nurse's best response?
    1. "Mix 1 teaspoon of baking soda in a glass of water and drink before eating your meal."
    2. "Use a laxative when your reflux is bad and this will help to empty your stomach."
    3. "Always drink plenty of fluids with your meals to help dilute the food."
    4. "Avoid foods that contain a lot of fat."

17. A client at 10 weeks gestation is being seen by the nurse. The client reports that she has nausea and vomiting each morning. Which is the nurse's best response?
    1. "Drink a large glass of milk before you get out of bed."
    2. "Eat crackers before you get out of bed."
    3. "Eat dinner before 6:00 p.m. every night."
    4. "Eat small meals during the day."

18. A young woman comes to the neighborhood clinic explaining that she had a negative urine pregnancy test last week but a positive test today. What is the best explanation?
    1. "It is probable that the hCG levels were not high enough to be detected last week."
    2. "It is likely that you may not be pregnant, so wait to see if you get your period."
    3. "Don't worry, this happens sometimes. You should perform another test in a few days."
    4. "Shall we set up a complete examination to see if you are really pregnant?"

19. The woman who is primigravida is in the clinic for her first prenatal visit. She states that she has experienced dizziness when she gets out of bed and sometimes when she stands up from a sitting position. What is the reason for this?
    1. She is experiencing hypoglycemia from being diabetic.
    2. She is standing up too quickly and must be careful to avoid injury.
    3. She needs to drink more fluids to prevent orthostatic hypotension and it will clear up soon.
    4. She is not getting enough exercise, so circulation to the head and upper extremities is less than optimal.

20. During the third trimester, which new symptom might be reported by the pregnant woman?
    1. Dyspnea
    2. Stuffy nose and sinuses
    3. Nausea and vomiting
    4. Fatigue

21. A nurse is discussing quickening with a client. Which statement by the client indicates effective understanding?
    1. "Quickening is when I first feel my baby move."
    2. "Quickening is an irregular contraction that I may feel."
    3. "Quickening is when my baby will drop into my pelvis."
    4. "Quickening is when the palms of my hands become pink and have blotches."

22. When might pelvic rest in the second or third trimester be prescribed? *Select all that apply.*
    1. When the patient has preterm contractions
    2. When the patient has a prior history of preterm delivery
    3. When the patient finds intercourse uncomfortable
    4. When the patient has vaginal bleeding
    5. When the patient experiences sore back muscles

23. Janice is in her last month of pregnancy. She is preparing to breastfeed and notices that her bra is sticking to her nipples and leaves a crusty residue when she removes her clothes at the end of the day. What is the *priority* intervention the nurse should recommend?
    1. "Stop preparing your nipples so that the discharge will stop."
    2. "Try inserting a nipple shield in your bra."
    3. "Insert a soft breast pad into your bra when you dress."
    4. "Try to express more fluid and massage it onto the nipple and areola."

24. Susan is in her 34th week of pregnancy. She is distressed that stretch marks have begun to appear on her breasts, abdomen, and inner thighs. Which information is *most* accurate?
    1. Less than 10 pounds of weight gain during pregnancy will decrease the chance of developing stretch marks.
    2. Applying natural oils and vitamin preparations to the skin will minimize their formation.
    3. Losing weight after pregnancy will make them disappear.
    4. The appearance of the skin will always look this way, so there is no reason to focus on their appearance.

25. An OB clinical client has phoned, concerned that her gums have bled after brushing her teeth this week. What is the pregnancy change behind this symptom?
    1. An infection of the gums related to a change in oral pH
    2. Improper brushing technique for more sensitive gums
    3. Hyperemia of the gums due to increased venous congestion
    4. The effects of prostaglandins on mucus membranes

REVIEW QUESTION ANSWERS

1. ANSWER: 2

Rationales

1. An increase in water reabsorption by the colon is not a common change in pregnancy.

2. The relaxation of the lower esophageal ("cardiac") sphincter is causing heartburn.

3. Heartburn is not caused by a decrease in the capacity of the stomach.

4. Pregnancy does not cause an increase in stomach acid production.

TEST-TAKING TIP: Increased progesterone production during pregnancy causes decreased tone and motility of the smooth muscles; this triggers esophageal reflux and slows emptying of the stomach.

Content Area: Gastrointestinal System; Anatomy and Physiology of Pregnancy

Integrated Process: Nursing Process—Assessment

Client Need: Physiological Integrity—Physiological Adaptation

Cognitive Level: Application

Concept: Digestion

Reference: Ward, S. L., & Hisley, S. M. (2016). Maternal-child nursing care. *2nd ed. Philadelphia: F.A. Davis.*

2. ANSWER: 3

Rationales

1. Decreasing fluids can cause dehydration and put the woman at high risk for preterm contractions.

2. Carbonated drinks should be avoided because they increase urine alkalinity.

3. Emptying the bladder right after intercourse will help to decrease the risk for developing a UTI.

4. Acidic juices may irritate the bladder and decrease the urge to void.

TEST-TAKING TIP: Review measures to prevent UTIs if you had difficulty with this question.

Content Area: Urinary System; Anatomy and Physiology of Pregnancy

Integrated Process: Nursing Process; Teaching/Learning

Client Need: Physiological Integrity—Reduction of Risk Potential

Cognitive Level: Application

Concept: Infection

Reference: Lowdermilk, D. L., Perry, S. E., Cashion, K., & Alden, K. R. (2016). Maternity & women's health care. *11th ed. St. Louis, MO: Elsevier.*

3. ANSWER: 4

Rationales

1. Cardiac output increases as a result of the increase in blood volume.

2. Heart rate increases by 10 to 20 beats per minute to accommodate the increase in blood volume.

3. The kidneys respond to an increase in renal plasma flow of 50% to 80% by elongating about 1 cm during pregnancy.

4. Blood pressure is maintained by a decrease in peripheral vascular resistance (20% to 30%).

TEST-TAKING TIP: Review cardiac changes in pregnancy if you missed this question.

Content Area: Cardiovascular; Anatomy and Physiology of Pregnancy

Integrated Process: Nursing Process—Assessment

Client Need: Physiological Integrity—Physiological Adaptation

Cognitive Level: Comprehension

Concept: Pregnancy

Reference: Durham, R. F., & Chapman, L. (2016). Maternal-child nursing care. *2nd ed. Philadelphia: F.A. Davis.*

4. ANSWER: 1

Rationales

1. Joint pain, backache, and hypermobility of joints are common discomforts expressed by the pregnant client during the third trimester.

2. This education would be discussed during the first trimester. Nausea and vomiting during the first trimester is caused by the hormone hCG.

3. Nasal stuffiness and epistaxis (nosebleeds) are a common complaint during the first trimester and are caused by the increase in circulating estrogen.

4. Hypertrophy of mammary gland tissue begins in the first trimester.

TEST-TAKING TIP: It is important for the nurse to be able to anticipate important teaching information in the appropriate trimester.

Content Area: Musculoskeletal System; Anatomy and Physiology of Pregnancy

Integrated Process: Nursing Process—Assessment

Client Need: Health Promotion and Maintenance

Cognitive Level: Application

Concept: Pregnancy

Reference: London, M. L., Ladewig, P. A., Davidson, M. R., Ball, J. W., Bindler, R. C., & Cowen, K. J. (2014). Maternal & child nursing care. *4th ed. New Jersey: Pearson.*

5. ANSWER: 4

Rationales

1. Estrogen stimulates uterine development.

2. Estrogen relaxes pelvic ligaments and joints.

3. Prolactin prepares breasts for lactation.

4. Progesterone relaxes smooth muscles.

TEST-TAKING TIP: If you missed this question, review all the physiological effects and hormone changes that occur during pregnancy.

Content Area: Reproductive System; Anatomy and Physiology of Pregnancy

Integrated Process: Nursing Process Teaching/Learning

Client Need: Health Promotion and Maintenance

Cognitive Level: Application

Concept: Pregnancy

Reference: London, M. L., Ladewig, P. A., Davidson, M. R., Ball, J. W., Bindler, R. C., & Cowen, K. J. (2014). Maternal & child nursing care. *4th ed. New Jersey: Pearson.*

6. ANSWER: 2

Rationales

1. Vitamin intake does not impact red blood cell production.

2. Plasma volume increase is greater than red blood cell production and has resulted in a decrease in hemoglobin.

3. This is a normal occurrence in pregnancy.

4. This is an expected laboratory result and does not have to be repeated at this time.

TEST-TAKING TIP: Physiological anemia of pregnancy results because the blood volume increases to a greater extent than red cell mass, resulting in a reduction in blood viscosity and hemodilution anemia.

Content Area: Cardiovascular System; Anatomy and Physiology of Pregnancy
Integrated Process: Nursing Process—Assessment
Client Need: Physiological Integrity—Physiological Adaptation
Cognitive Level: Application
Concept: Pregnancy
Reference: London, M. L., Ladewig, P. A., Davidson, M. R., Ball, J. W., Bindler, R. C., & Cowen, K. J. (2014). Maternal & child nursing care. 4th ed. New Jersey: Pearson.

7. ANSWERS: 1, 2, 4
Rationales
1. Backache and flank pain are signs of a kidney infection or preterm labor.
2. Burning on urination is a sign of a bladder infection.
3. Enlargement of the breasts and breast tenderness are normal physiological changes in pregnancy.
4. Abdominal cramping and vaginal bleeding are signs of a miscarriage or ectopic pregnancy.
5. Urinary frequency is a normal physiological symptom of pregnancy, especially in the first and third trimesters.
TEST-TAKING TIP: Review the potential signs of complications during pregnancy.
Content Area: Reproductive System; Anatomy and Physiology of Pregnancy
Integrated Process: Nursing Process—Teaching/Learning
Client Need: Physiological Integrity—Reduction of Risk Potential
Cognitive Level: Application
Concept: Pregnancy
Reference: Ward, S. L., & Hisley, S. M. (2016). Maternal-child nursing care. 2nd ed. Philadelphia: F.A. Davis.

8. ANSWER: 2
Rationales
1. The question does not indicate that the client is taking in reduced calories for weight loss.
2. To help with nausea, the client should eat five to six small meals per day.
3. Gastric reflux is a common discomfort in the second trimester. The client should avoid gas-producing and fried foods.
4. A change in eating will not help with fatigue.
TEST-TAKING TIP: This question states that the client is 8 weeks pregnant, so she is in her first trimester. Nausea is a common discomfort during this time period. Review the common discomforts associated with each trimester.
Content Area: Gastrointestinal; Anatomy and Physiology of Pregnancy
Integrated Process: Nursing Process—Planning
Client Need: Physiological Integrity—Basic Care and Comfort
Cognitive Level: Analysis
Concept: Pregnancy
Reference: London, M. L., Ladewig, P. A., Davidson, M. R., Ball, J. W., Bindler, R. C., & Cowen, K. J. (2014). Maternal & child nursing care. 4th ed. New Jersey: Pearson.

9. ANSWER: 2
Rationales
1. As pregnancy progresses, the client may experience decreased cardiac reserve and increased respiratory effort, which may result in physiological stress, especially if the exercise is strenuous and lasts a long time.

2. As pregnancy progresses, the client should be advised to decrease her exercise level.
3. This answer does not provide any information to the client.
4. The client should be advised to exercise at least three times per week.
TEST-TAKING TIP: Pregnant clients should be advised to exercise for 10 to 15 minutes, rest for 2 to 3 minutes, and then exercise for another 10 to 15 minutes.
Content Area: Musculoskeletal System; Anatomy and Physiology of Pregnancy
Integrated Process: Nursing Process—Teaching/Learning
Client Need: Physiological Integrity—Basic Care and Comfort
Cognitive Level: Application
Concept: Pregnancy
Reference: Ward, S. L., & Hisley, S. M. (2016). Maternal-child nursing care. 2nd ed. Philadelphia: F.A. Davis.

10. ANSWER: 1
Rationales
1. Sexual activity during pregnancy is safe unless risk factors have been identified.
2. This is not a contraindication during pregnancy.
3. Experimenting with different partner positions may have to be implemented due to the weight gain and gravida uterus during pregnancy.
4. This statement does not answer the client's question.
TEST-TAKING TIP: Health care providers should always address client's concerns in an open manner and provide information that will encourage communication.
Content Area: Reproductive System; Anatomy and Physiology of Pregnancy
Integrated Process: Nursing Process—Teaching/Learning
Client Need: Safe and Effective Care Environment—Management of Care
Cognitive Level: Application
Concept: Pregnancy
Reference: Durham, R. F., & Chapman, L. (2016). Maternal-child nursing care. 2nd ed. Philadelphia: F.A. Davis.

11. ANSWER: 1
Rationales
1. Measurements should be 2 cm between 20 weeks and 36 weeks of gestation.
2. This is a normal assessment finding.
3. This is a normal assessment finding.
4. This is a normal assessment finding.
TEST-TAKING TIP: At 12 weeks and 14 weeks, fundal height measurement should be done at each prenatal visit to monitor the fetus's growth. This involves measuring the distance from the top of the pelvic bone (symphysis pubis) to the top of the uterus (fundus).
Content Area: Reproductive System; Anatomy and Physiology of Pregnancy
Integrated Process: Nursing Process—Assessment
Client Need: Physiological Integrity—Reduction of Risk Potential
Cognitive Level: Application
Concept: Pregnancy
Reference: Lowdermilk, D. L., Perry, S. E., Cashion, K., & Alden, K. R. (2016). Maternity & women's health care. 11th ed. St. Louis, MO: Elsevier.

---

12. ANSWER: 1

Rationales

1. Changes in the cervix is called *Goodell's sign*.
2. Changes in uterus would be recorded as fundal height.
3. Ballottement is the passive movement of an unengaged fetus.
4. Lightening involves the descend of the fetus into the pelvis.

TEST-TAKING TIP: Goodell's sign may be noted from the beginning of the sixth week of pregnancy. This cervical change is a result of increased vascularity, slight hypertrophy, and hyperplasia of cells.

Content Area: Reproductive System; Anatomy and Physiology of Pregnancy
Integrated Process: Nursing Process—Assessment
Client Need: Physiological Integrity—Physiological Adaptation
Cognitive Level: Application
Concept: Pregnancy
Reference: Murray, S. S., & McKinney, E. S. (2014). Foundations of maternal-newborn and women's health nursing. 6th ed. St. Louis, MO: Elsevier.

13. ANSWER: 2

Rationales

1. This will not relieve leg cramping.
2. This is the correct maneuver to relieve leg cramping.
3. Elevating the legs several times a day may help to prevent leg cramps.
4. This may make the leg cramps worse.

TEST-TAKING TIP: Leg cramps (gastrocnemius spasm) is a result of compression of the nerves that supply the lower extremities because of the growing uterus. Several factors may play a part in developing leg cramps: having reduced serum calcium or increased serum phosphorus, pointing toes when stretching, or drinking more than 1 L of milk per day.

Content Area: Musculoskeletal System; Anatomy and Physiology of Pregnancy
Integrated Process: Nursing Process—Implementation
Client Need: Physiological Integrity—Basic Care and Comfort
Cognitive Level: Application
Concept: Pregnancy
Reference: Lowdermilk, D. L., Perry, S. E., Cashion, K., & Alden, K. R. (2016). Maternity & women's health care. 11th ed. St. Louis, MO: Elsevier.

14. ANSWER: 2

Rationales

1. Constrictive clothing such as knee-high hose should be avoided during pregnancy.
2. The client should be advised that when sitting, she should not cross her legs.
3. Kegel exercise is advised to help with pelvic floor tone.
4. Decreased fetal movement is related to increased uteroplacental insufficiency.

TEST-TAKING TIP: Varicosities during pregnancy are a result of vascular relaxations resulting from the increase in progesterone and impaired venous return from the enlarged uterus.

Content Area: Cardiovascular System; Anatomy and Physiology of Pregnancy
Integrated Process: Nursing Process—Evaluation
Client Need: Physiological Integrity—Basic Care and Comfort

Cognitive Level: Analysis
Concept: Pregnancy
Reference: Ward, S. L., & Hisley, S. M. (2016). Maternal-child nursing care. 2nd ed. Philadelphia: F.A. Davis

15. ANSWER: 3

Rationales

1. A fundal height complaint would be dyspnea.
2. A urinary infection complaint would be burning when urinating and frequency.
3. Lightening occurs at the end of the third trimester and is the fetus descending into the pelvis.
4. The question did not indicate that the client had been diagnosed with hydramnios.

Content Area: Reproductive System; Anatomy and Physiology of Pregnancy
Integrated Process: Nursing Process—Assessment
Client Need: Health Promotion and Maintenance
Cognitive Level: Application
Concept: Pregnancy
Reference: Durham, R. F., & Chapman, L. (2016). Maternal-child nursing care. 2nd ed. Philadelphia: F.A. Davis.

16. ANSWER: 4

Rationales

1. Simple baking soda preparations may lead to electrolyte imbalances.
2. The woman at risk for preterm labor should avoid undue stimulation of the intestines because intestinal irritation with increased peristalsis may stimulate uterine activity.
3. Consuming beverages with meals will overload the stomach, making reflux worse.
4. Avoiding greasy and fatty food will help to reduce heartburn and reflux.

TEST-TAKING TIP: Review relief measures for dyspepsia if you missed this question.

Content Area: Gastrointestinal System; Anatomy and Physiology of Pregnancy
Integrated Process: Nursing Process—Implementation
Client Need: Physiological Integrity—Basic Care and Comfort
Cognitive Level: Application
Concept: Pregnancy
Reference: Ward, S. L., & Hisley, S. M. (2016). Maternal-child nursing care. 2nd ed. Philadelphia: F.A. Davis.

17. ANSWER: 2

Rationales

1. Milk will not help her nausea.
2. Eating crackers or dry toast 1/2 to 1 hour prior to getting out of bed will help with nausea.
3. The client should be instructed to avoid an empty stomach.
4. Eating small meals during the day will help with nausea during the day but does not address her morning sickness.

TEST-TAKING TIP: Review nursing education for pregnancy discomforts.

Content Area: Gastrointestinal System; Anatomy and Physiology of Pregnancy
Integrated Process: Nursing Process—Implementation
Client Need: Physiological Integrity—Basic Care and Comfort

Cognitive Level: Application
Concept: Pregnancy
Reference: Lowdermilk, D. L., Perry, S. E., Cashion, K., & Alden, K. R. (2016). Maternity & women's health care. 11th ed. St. Louis, MO: Elsevier.

18. **ANSWER: 1**
Rationales
1. Small amounts of hCG can be detected in a pregnant woman's urine within 3 weeks after the last menstrual period.
2. The client may be pregnant. It may have been too soon to be detected by an over-the-counter pregnancy test.
3. This statement does not address the client's question.
4. This statement does not address the client's question concerning why she had a negative test last week and a positive test this week.
TEST-TAKING TIP: Read the question carefully. This client was asking about the pregnancy test.
Content Area: Endocrine System; Anatomy and Physiology of Pregnancy
Integrated Process: Nursing Process—Teaching/Learning
Client Need: Physiological Integrity—Physiological Adaptation
Cognitive Level: Analysis
Concept: Pregnancy
Reference: Lowdermilk, D. L., Perry, S. E., Cashion, K., & Alden, K. R. (2016). Maternity & women's health care. 11th ed. St. Louis, MO: Elsevier.

19. **ANSWER: 2**
Rationales
1. Low blood sugar should not be a problem in the first trimester unless the client is diabetic.
2. Decreased peripheral arterial resistance can cause orthostatic hypotension in the first months of pregnancy.
3. Drinking more fluids will not prevent the client from experiencing orthostatic hypotension.
4. Exercise is not the reason why the client is experiencing the dizziness.
TEST-TAKING TIP: Review the common cardiovascular changes of pregnancy if you missed this question.
Content Area: Cardiovascular System; Anatomy and Physiology of Pregnancy
Integrated Process: Nursing Process—Teaching/Learning
Client Need: Physiological Integrity—Physiological Adaptation
Cognitive Level: Analysis
Concept: Pregnancy
Reference: Lowdermilk, D. L., Perry, S. E., Cashion, K., & Alden, K. R. (2016). Maternity & women's health care. 11th ed. St. Louis, MO: Elsevier.

20. **ANSWER: 1**
Rationales
1. The growing fetus put an upward pressure on the diaphragm, creating shortness of breath.
2. Stuffy nose and sinuses would be a common complaint expressed by the client in her first or second trimester.
3. Nausea and vomiting would be a common complaint expressed by the client in the first trimester.
4. Fatigue would be a common complaint expressed by the client in the first trimester.
TEST-TAKING TIP: Review common complaints and which trimester they occur if you missed this question.

Content Area: Respiratory System; Anatomy and Physiology of Pregnancy
Integrated Process: Nursing Process—Assessment
Client Need: Physiological Integrity
Cognitive Level: Application
Concept: Pregnancy
Reference: Durham, R. F., & Chapman, L. (2016). Maternal-child nursing care. 2nd ed. Philadelphia: F.A. Davis.

21. **ANSWER: 1**
Rationales
1. First recognition of fetal movement is called *quickening.*
2. Braxton Hicks contractions are irregular contractions.
3. Lightening is the descent of the fetus into the pelvis.
4. Palmar erythema is when the client's hands become pink and develop blotches.
TEST-TAKING TIP: Quickening can usually be detected by the multiparous client as early as 14 to 16 weeks. It is usually around the 18th to 20th week for a nulliparous client. Clients usually describe it as a flutter.
Content Area: Reproductive System; Anatomy and Physiology of Pregnancy
Integrated Process: Nursing Process—Implementation
Client Need: Physiological Integrity—Physiological Adaptation
Cognitive Level: Application
Concept: Pregnancy
Reference: Durham, R. F., & Chapman, L. (2016). Maternal-child nursing care. 2nd ed. Philadelphia: F.A. Davis.

22. **ANSWER: 1, 2, 4**
Rationales
1. Pelvic rest (avoiding sexual intercourse or stimulation) may be prescribed if the client experiences preterm contractions.
2. Pelvic rest (avoiding sexual intercourse or stimulation) may be prescribed if the client has a prior history of preterm labor.
3. Changing partner position should be discussed if the client finds intercourse uncomfortable.
4. Pelvic risk (avoiding sexual intercourse or stimulation) may be prescribed if the client experiences vaginal bleeding.
5. If the client experiences sore back muscles, pelvic exercises may be prescribed.
TEST-TAKING TIP: Review preterm education if you missed this question.
Content Area: Reproductive System; Anatomy and Physiology of Pregnancy
Integrated Process: Nursing Process—Teaching/Learning
Client Need: Physiological Integrity—Reduction of Risk Potential
Cognitive Level: Application
Concept: Pregnancy
Reference: Durham, R. F., & Chapman, L. (2016). Maternal-child nursing care. 2nd ed. Philadelphia: F.A. Davis.

23. **ANSWER: 3**
Rationales
During the second trimester, small amounts of precolostrum may be secreted from the nipples as a thin, clear fluid. In the

last trimester, the fluid will become the more yellowish and thicker colostrum.

1. This discharge is a natural occurrence in the last trimester.

2. A nipple shield would be suggested if the client had inverted nipples and was trying to breastfeed.

3. Absorbent breast pads may be inserted in the bra to absorb leakage.

4. This would be advised to a breastfeeding postpartum client who developed cracked nipples.

TEST-TAKING TIP: Review care of the breasts during the antepartum period if you missed this question.

Content Area: Reproductive System; Anatomy and Physiology of Pregnancy

Integrated Process: Nursing Process—Teaching/Learning

Client Need: Physiological Integrity—Basic Care and Comfort

Cognitive Level: Application

Concept: Pregnancy

Reference: Ward, S. L., & Hisley, S. M. (2016). Maternal-child nursing care. *2nd ed. Philadelphia: F.A. Davis.*

24. **ANSWER: 2**

Rationales

1. Pregnant women should gain weight according to their prepregnancy weight. Striae gravidarum have a tendency to be familial.

2. Keeping the skin moist and massaging it may keep it supple, but there are no apparent "cures" for striae.

3. Losing weight after pregnancy will not make striae disappear.

4. After pregnancy, the striae become thinner and fade to a silvery tone.

TEST-TAKING TIP: Important to understand the normal integumentary changes during pregnancy. Review these changes if you missed this question.

Content Area: Integumentary; Anatomy and Physiology of Pregnancy

Integrated Process: Nursing Process—Teaching/Learning

Client Need: Physiological Integrity—Physiological Adaptation

Cognitive Level: Application

Concept: Pregnancy

Reference: Durham, R. F., & Chapman, L. (2016). Maternal-child nursing care. *2nd ed. Philadelphia: F.A. Davis.*

25. **ANSWER: 3**

Rationales

1. The oral pH during pregnancy does not change.

2. Improper brushing technique is not the cause for the bleeding gums.

3. Inflammation of the gums occurs because of the increased blood supply and increased estrogen.

4. Prostaglandin changes during pregnancy do not have an effect on the gums.

TEST-TAKING TIP: Gingivitis can develop during pregnancy because of hypertrophy and edema. The pregnant client's gums may bleed during regular brushing. The nurse should advise the client to use a soft toothbrush during this time.

Content Area: Gastrointestinal System; Anatomy and Physiology of Pregnancy

Integrated Process: Nursing Process—Teaching/Learning

Client Need: Physiological Integrity—Basic Care and Comfort

Cognitive Level: Application

Concept: Pregnancy

Reference: Lowdermilk, D. L., Perry, S. E., Cashion, K., & Alden, K. R. (2016). Maternity & women's health care. *11th ed. St. Louis, MO: Elsevier.*

Chapter 10

Prenatal Care

KEY TERMS

Abortion—Birth that occurs prior to 20 weeks gestation or the birth of a fetus weighing less than 500 grams

Antepartum—The time between conception and onset of labor (prenatal)

Gestation—The number of weeks since the first day of the last menstrual period

Gravida—The number of times a woman has been pregnant, regardless of the number of infants delivered at term and the number of fetuses with each pregnancy. Also included in this number is the woman's current pregnancy.

Multigravida—A woman who is currently in her second pregnancy or any successive pregnancies

Multipara—A woman who has had two or more births past 20 weeks gestation

Naegele's rule—A system to estimate the day in the year labor will begin

Nulligravida—A woman who has never been pregnant

Para—The number of times a woman has carried a fetus past 20 weeks gestation regardless of the number of infants delivered alive or the number of fetuses with each pregnancy

Post-term—Birth that occurs after 42 weeks gestation

Primigravida—A woman who is pregnant for the first time

Primipara—A woman who has had one birth past 20 weeks gestation regardless if born alive or dead or the number of fetuses

Preterm—Birth that occurs after 20 weeks but before 37 completed weeks

Pseudocyesis—False pregnancy caused by changes in the endocrine system, resulting in secretions of hormones that lead to the appearance of some signs and symptoms associated with pregnancy

Stillbirth—An infant born dead after 20 weeks gestation

Term—Birth that occurs between 39 weeks and 41 completed weeks

I. Prenatal Care

Prenatal care is a series of visits conducted from the time of conception to the onset of labor. This time is also known as the **antepartum** period. Prenatal care is both beneficial and cost-effective and is usually provided by an obstetrician or midwife. Services include prepregnancy health, medical/surgical history, screening of risk profiles, emotional status, dietary and lifestyle advice, weighing to ensure proper weight gain, and examination for problems of pregnancy.

II. Birth History

A. The terms *gravida* and *para* (G/P) are used in the obstetrical history to indicate the number of pregnancies. Consequently, twins, triplets, and so on, count as one pregnancy and one birth.

1. **Gravida** refers to the number of times a woman has been pregnant, regardless of the number of infants delivered at term and the number of fetuses with each pregnancy. Also included in this number is the woman's current pregnancy.

2. **Para** refers to the number of times a woman has carried a fetus past 20 weeks **gestation** regardless of the number of infants delivered alive or the number of fetuses with each pregnancy.

B. The term *gravida, term, preterm, abortion, living* (GTPAL) is used to quickly determine how many times someone has given birth or how far they've gotten before losing a pregnancy. GTPAL is a clearer way of providing an obstetrical history. As in the G/P, twins, triplets, and so on, count as one pregnancy and one birth except when counting the number of living children.

G: gravida is the number of times a woman has been pregnant, regardless of the number of infants delivered at term and the number of fetuses with each pregnancy. Also included in this number is the woman's current pregnancy.

T: **term** refers to any term delivery, live or still birth, after 37 completed weeks.

P: **preterm** refers to any delivery, live or still birth, before 37 completed weeks.

A: **abortion** refers to any delivery before 20 weeks gestation (spontaneous abortion or induced abortion).

L: *living* refers to the number of currently living children.

III. Determination of Due Date

A. Estimated date of delivery (EDD), estimated date of confinement (EDC), or estimated date of birth (EDB) This is calculated from the menstrual history. Estimation of the due date *cannot* be viewed as a completely accurate prediction; however:

- It does give physicians and midwives a basis to monitor the development of the pregnancy.

MAKING THE CONNECTION

The G/P and the GTPAL Approach

Mary Smith presents to her nurse midwife for her first prenatal care visit. She is currently 8 weeks pregnant. When asked about her past pregnancies, Ms. Smith states, "I have four living children. I delivered a little girl at 24 weeks, twin boys at 37 weeks, and a boy at 38 weeks." Using the G/P system, how would you document Ms. Smith's obstetrical history? Using the GTPAL system, how would you document Ms. Smith's obstetrical history?

Answer: Ms. Smith is a G4/P3 or G4T1P2A0L4

- It allows physicians/midwives the ability to track the growth of the baby, and schedule diagnostic and screening tests.
- It permits the health care provider to better handle the complication of premature birth.

The most common method to determine the EDB is **Naegele's rule.** To use this method, begin with the first day of the last menstrual period (LMP), subtract 3 months, and add 7 days.

DID YOU KNOW?

Naegele's rule is an accurate way to determine the EDB. However, this method is reliable only if the woman's menses begins approximately every 28 days (because if her cycle is irregular, the time of ovulation may not be accurate), and she must know the first day of her last menstrual period.

IV. Signs of Pregnancy

Diagnosis of pregnancy is determined by pregnancy-related physical and hormonal changes and are classified by presumptive, probable, or positive signs of pregnancy.

A. Presumptive or subjective changes

These are symptoms the woman experiences and reports to the physician or midwife. These symptoms may be caused by other conditions and cannot be considered confirmation of pregnancy. However, presumptive symptoms may serve as diagnostic clues (Table 10.1).

Table 10.1 Presumptive (Subjective) Changes of Pregnancy

Presumptive (Subjective) Changes	Causes	Other Causes
Amenorrhea—one of the earliest symptoms	Absence of menses is one of the earliest symptoms a woman reports when pregnant.	Also may be caused by: • *Endocrine problems: thyroid, pituitary, adrenal, ovarian, early menopause, **pseudocyesis*** • *Metabolic problems: anemia, diabetes mellitus, malnutrition* • *Psychological factors: intense desire to become pregnant, emotional shock* • *Chronic illness: malignancy*
Nausea and vomiting—often called morning sickness and occurs frequently during first trimester	Caused by hormonal changes due to pregnancy	Emotional problems, gastrointestinal disorders, infections, pseudocyesis
Frequent urination—common during first and third trimester	Caused by pressure on bladder from enlarging uterus	UTIs, cystocele, pelvic tumors, urethral diverticula
Breast tenderness	Caused by hormonal changes due to pregnancy	Premenstrual syndrome, mastitis, pseudocyesis
Quickening—perception of fetal movement. Occurs during second trimester	Stage of pregnancy at which movements of the fetus can be felt by uterine muscles	Flatus, peristalsis, abdominal muscle contractions
Leukorrhea—white milky odorless discharge	Increase of hormones, especially estrogen. Causes an increase in vaginal discharge	Vaginal infection
Fatigue	Hormonal changes due to pregnancy	Illness, stress, lifestyle changes

B. Probable or objective changes

These are signs that are observed by the examiner. However, because these changes can have other causes, a positive diagnosis of pregnancy cannot be confirmed (Table 10.2).

C. Positive or diagnostic signs

These are objective signs of pregnancy that cannot be caused by a pathological state and are definite confirmation of a pregnancy:

- Fetal heartbeat can be detected by eighth week with Doppler device.
- Fetal movement can be palpated by the examiner after 20 weeks gestation.
- Fetus can be visualized by ultrasound.

V. First Prenatal Visit

The first prenatal visit occurs during the first **trimester**, which is from the first day of the last menstrual period through 14 completed weeks. A thorough history and physical help the health care provider to determine the status of the woman's prepregnancy health and if any high-risk conditions exist and to form a basis for comparison of data collected with subsequent visits. The first visit is usually when the woman suspects she is pregnant, frequently after her first missed period around 6 to 8 weeks gestation. The optimal timing for the initial prenatal visit is at or before 10 weeks gestation, as several of the recommended screening tests may be performed during this period. Each woman planning to become pregnant or each prenatal visit should be visit-specific, such as screening tests, education, immunizations, and/or chemoprophylaxis as described in the American Congress of Obstetricians and Gynecologists' schedule of prenatal visits (*Guidelines for Perinatal Care,* 7th edition, October 2012).

A. Assessment

1. Menstrual history, which includes menarche, regularity, frequency, duration of menses, and date of last menstrual period

Table 10.2 Probable (Objective) Changes of Pregnancy

Probable (Objective) Changes	Causes	Other Causes
Goodell's sign	Softening of the tip of the cervix	Pelvic congestion, infection, or hormonal imbalance
Chadwick's sign	Violet-bluish color of the vaginal mucosa and cervix	Pelvic congestion, infection, or hormonal imbalance
Hegar's sign	Softening of the lower uterine segment	Pelvic congestion
Uterine enlargement	Enlargement due to hypertrophy, hyperplasia, and stretching of muscle fibers	Uterine or abdominal tumors
Braxton Hicks contractions	Intermittent uterine contractions caused by increase in hormones, especially estrogen	Uterine fibroids (leiomyomas) or tumor
Uterine souffle	A blowing sound, synchronous with the cardiac systole of the mother, heard on auscultation over the pregnant uterus	Conditions that vastly increase uterine blood flow (large uterine or ovarian tumors)
Skin changes—increased pigmentation of: • *Nipples/areolae* • *Chloasma (mask of pregnancy), which are brownish or yellowish patches that are seen most commonly on the forehead, upper cheeks, nose, and chin*	Increased pigmentation stimulated by higher levels of estrogen and progesterone occurring during pregnancy and increased melanocyte-stimulating hormone made by the placenta	Oral contraceptive pills
• *Linea nigra, which are dark vertical lines that appear on the abdomen during pregnancy* • *Striae gravidarum (stretch marks)*	Results from decreased connective tissue strength because of elevated adrenal steroid levels	Weight gain, pelvic tumor
Ballottement	Palpation of the fetus floating within the uterus by tapping it gently and feeling it rebound	Uterine tumors, ascites
Positive pregnancy test	Results from the presence of hCG	Choriocarcinoma, hydatidiform mole, increased pituitary gonadotropins at menopause
Fetal outline palpation	Usually can be palpated after 24 weeks	Uterine myomas

2. Obstetrical history, which should include all pregnancies, complications, outcomes, contraceptive use, and sexual history
   a) Specific medical terms are used when discussing the client's obstetrical history:
      - **Primipara** is a woman who has had one birth past 20 weeks gestation, regardless if the baby was born alive or dead or the number of fetuses.
      - **Primigravida** is a woman who is pregnant for the first time.
      - **Multipara** is a woman who has had two or more births past 20 weeks gestation.
      - **Multigravida** is a woman who is currently in her second pregnancy or any successive pregnancies.
      - **Nulligravida** is a woman who has never been pregnant.
      - **Preterm** is a birth that occurs after 20 weeks but before 37 completed weeks.
      - Term is a birth that occurs between 38 and 41 completed weeks.
      - Post-term is a birth that occurs after 42 weeks gestation.
      - **Stillbirth** is an infant born dead after 20 weeks gestation.
3. Medical history, which should include past illnesses, surgeries, and current medications

(I) ALERT When taking a health history, it is crucial to list all prescribed medications and over-the-counter (OTC) medications the patient is taking now and prior to becoming pregnant. Some medications and OTC medications may pose a risk to the fetus if taken during pregnancy.

4. Family history
5. Genetic history
6. Domestic violence screening
7. Assess for tobacco, alcohol, drug use
8. Screen for depression using a standardized screening tool
9. Prescriptions: prenatal vitamins and iron supplementation as necessary

B. Physical assessment

During the initial prenatal visit, the physical examination should include a complete head-to-toe assessment. The purpose of a comprehensive examination is to gather baseline data about the woman's health status as well as to identify any nonpregnancy-related preexisting condition. Although most pregnant women are healthy, many high-risk conditions can affect women during their childbearing years and during pregnancy. Therefore, a careful physical examination with clear documentation of findings is an important part of the initial prenatal visit.

1. Vital signs are taken to establish reference values for subsequent visits. Included should be temperature,

pulse, respiration, and blood pressure. Fetal heart tones may be assessed at the initial visit, depending on gestational age.

2. Evaluation of height, weight, and calculation of body mass index (BMI).
3. Examination of breasts and nipples for inverted nipples, which might interfere with breastfeeding.
4. Pelvic examination to confirm the pregnancy and to determine gestation. An examiner will look for signs of pregnancy, which include Chadwick's sign (color of cervix), Goodell's sign (softening of the tip of the cervix), and Hegar's sign (softening of the region between the body of the uterus and the cervix). Evaluation of the uterine size and the fundal height will also be performed at this time. Palpation of pelvic contents is done to identify any abnormal masses or tumors.
   a) Nursing responsibilities during the pelvic examination include assembling necessary equipment, such as a speculum, lubricant, spatula for cervical scraping, glass slide, culture tube with sterile cotton-tipped applicator, examination gloves, and examination light. The nurse should instruct the patient to empty her bladder. This will make the examination more comfortable for the client and make it easier for the examiner to evaluate the size of the uterus. Have the patient remove her clothing and put on a patient gown. The nurse must always remember to provide privacy for the client. The patient should be positioned on the examination table in the lithotomy position with a drape to cover her.

(I) ALERT Gloves should be worn for procedures that involve contact with body fluids, such as drawing blood, handling urine specimens, and conducting pelvic examinations. It is important to inquire about latex allergies with any patient before beginning an examination.

C. Education and counseling
   1. Scope of care provided in the office and anticipated schedule of visits. Routine prenatal care is determined by individual needs and assessment of risk factors. For a woman who is considered low risk, this schedule is followed:
      a) Every 4 weeks for the first 28 weeks
      b) Every 2 weeks until 36 weeks gestation
      c) Every week after 36 weeks gestation
   2. Counsel the patient regarding specific complications identified in the initial health history and/or physical assessment.
   3. Discuss routine laboratory studies/testing that will be done during the initial visit and subsequent visits
   4. Discuss genetic counseling and available prenatal diagnostic testing (invasive and noninvasive).

5. Provide information about prenatal classes, nutrition, exercise, working, travel, routine dental care, tobacco use and smoke exposure, alcohol/drug consumption, over-the-counter medications, and pets.
6. Assess barriers to care (e.g., transportation, child care issues, work schedule).
7. Encourage and provide influenza vaccination, regardless of the stage of pregnancy, during influenza season.

ALERT Only the inactive form of the influenza vaccine should be given during pregnancy. Vaccines for human papillomavirus, influenza in live attenuated form, measles, mumps, rubella, varicella, or the tuberculosis given for travel are contraindicated during pregnancy.

D. Routine laboratory/diagnostic studies
See Table 10.3 for routine laboratory/diagnostic studies to be performed at the first prenatal visit.

DID YOU KNOW?

When taking a health history, it is important to interview the patient in a quiet, private environment so you can establish the client's trust. This environment is important in order to obtain a complete and honest health and social history.

VI. Subsequent Prenatal Visits

A. Every visit
The following should be checked during each visit:
- Vital signs: blood pressure, pulse, temperature
- Weight (height/weight/BMI, taken during the initial visit only). Assessment of fetal heart tones with amplification starting at the 10th week.
- Uterine size for progressive growth and consistency with EDD (see Chapter 9)
- Domestic violence screening
- Assessment of tobacco use and smoke exposure
- Urine dip for protein and glucose (see Chapter 16)

B. 11 to 14 weeks gestation
1. Perform pelvic examination if fetal heart tones not heard with amplification
2. Encourage breastfeeding as the best choice for feeding. Women should be offered breastfeeding classes during the prenatal period.

Table 10.3 Laboratory/Diagnostic Studies

Routine Laboratory/Diagnostic Studies and Normal Findings	Indication and Schedule for Screening/Testing
Complete blood count	
White blood cell count (WBC): 5,000–12,000/µL	Evaluation for infection
Red blood cell count (RBC): 4.2–5.4 million/µL	Anemia
Hematocrit (HCT): 38%–47%	Measures the amount of volume red blood cells take up in the blood. The value is given as a percentage of red blood cells in a volume of blood.
Hemoglobin (Hgb): 12–16 g/dL (areas of higher altitude may have higher levels of hemoglobin)	Measure of the blood's ability to carry oxygen throughout the body. Screened at preconception and/or early in the first trimester; repeated in third trimester. Values less than 11 g/dL in the first trimester, less than 10.5 g/dL in the second trimester, and less than 11 g/dL in the third trimester indicate anemia. Hgb less than 12 g/dL requires nutritional counseling and less than 11 g/dL requires iron supplementation (American College of Obstetricians and Gynecologist [ACOG], 2010).
Platelet count: 150,000 and 450,000 per µL of blood (150–450 × 109/L).	Important in blood clotting
Blood type (A, B, AB, O)	Determines blood type
Rh and antibody screen (Rh+/−)	Determines if the Rh antigen is in blood. Also helps to identify if a fetus is at risk for developing erythroblastosis fetalis or hyperbilirubinemia during the neonatal period.
Urinalysis followed by urine culture for positive results	Detect bacterial infection in the urinary tract, which can lead to kidney infection or increased risk of preterm delivery and low birth weight.
Rubella titer: 1:10 or above indicates immunity	Determines immunity to rubella. If patient is nonimmune, vaccination can be given during postpartum periods before discharge from the hospital and patient should be told to avoid children who have rubella.
Syphilis test Venereal Disease Research Laboratory (VDRL) Rapid Reagan	Serological test for syphilis

Continued

Table 10.3 Laboratory/Diagnostic Studies (Continued)

Gonorrhea/chlamydia	Detection for sexually transmitted infections, which can cause miscarriage or infect the neonate during delivery. Obtained from cervical cells. If positive, a test of cure should be offered to the patient 4 weeks after completing treatment and counseling provided to decrease risk of reinfection and refer partner for testing and treatment. Those women who are 25 years of age or younger or who are at risk should be screened again during the third trimester.
HIV antibody test	Testing is offered to all women, especially those at high risk, so management can begin to reduce transmission to fetus. Offered at preconception or first trimester; may be repeated in third trimester if at high risk.
Hepatitis B screen	A negative test for the virus means either that there is no current infection or there is not yet a sufficient amount of the antigen to be detected. If a woman participates in high-risk activities that may transmit the hepatitis B virus (such as unprotected sexual contact or intravenous drug use), retesting later in the pregnancy is generally advised.
Hepatitis B surface antigen (HBsAg)	Screening should be offered to all couples regardless of ethnicity. Genetic counseling is recommended for individuals with a family history of cystic fibrosis or those found to be carriers.
Cystic fibrosis	Screening should be offered to individuals of African, Southeast Asian, and Mediterranean descent. Couples at risk for having a child with sickle cell or thalassemia should be offered genetic counseling to review prenatal testing and reproduction options.
Hemoglobinopathy screening	Women with the following risk factors should be screened for gestational diabetes at the first prenatal visit: • *Prepregnancy BMI ≥ 30 kg/m²* • *Personal history of GDM* • *Known impaired glucose metabolism*
Gestational diabetes screen Ultrasound	Recommended at the initial visit in order to determine gestational age and identify multiple gestations.

3. Review laboratory data. Offer iron supplementation for patients with anemia.
4. Offer screening test for aneuploidy.
   a) All pregnant women, regardless of age, should be counseled and offered noninvasive and invasive prenatal diagnostic testing for aneuploidy with a discussion of the risks and benefits (see Chapter 3).
   b) Women found to have increased risk for aneuploidy with noninvasive screening should be offered genetic counseling and the option of chorionic villus sampling or second-trimester amniocentesis.
5. Discuss the risks, benefits, and alternatives to labor after cesarean, if previous low transverse cesarean delivery, and cover the risks and benefits of repeat cesarean delivery.

C. 15 to 20 weeks gestation
   This begins the second trimester, which lasts through 28 completed weeks.
   1. Offer anatomic survey ultrasound to be completed at 18 to 20 weeks.

2. Offer multiple marker screen test if the patient did not have first-trimester screening (invasive or noninvasive) for aneuploidy (see Chapter 12).
3. Offer maternal serum alpha-fetoprotein test to women who elect first-trimester screening or invasive testing for aneuploidy (see Chapter 12).
4. Review signs and symptoms of preterm labor (PTL).

D. 24 to 28 weeks gestation
   1. Screening for gestational diabetes (See Chapter 16.)
   2. Select baby's medical provider.
   3. Discuss normal fetal movement and fetal kick counts.
   4. Discuss prenatal classes.
   5. Discuss postpartum contraception.

E. 27 to 36 weeks gestation
   1. Tdap should be administered during each pregnancy, regardless of patient's prior history of receiving. Optimal timing is between 27 and 36 weeks gestation to maximize maternal antibody response and passive antibody transfer levels in the newborn. Discuss with the patient that other adults who will be around the newborn, such as

partners, grandparents, older siblings, and babysitters, should also be vaccinated.

F. 28 weeks gestation

This begins the third trimester, which goes through 40 completed weeks.

1. Repeat type and screen if Rh negative, and repeat hemoglobin (Hb) and hematocrit (HCT).

2. Administer Rh-immune globulin if mother is Rh-negative and her indirect Coombs test is negative (–).

3. Confirm and document name of baby's medical provider.

4. Discuss cord blood banking so pregnant woman can make an informed decision on whether to participate in a public or private umbilical cord blood banking program.

G. 32 to 34 weeks gestation

1. Repeat testing for women at risk for sexually transmitted disease, including rapid plasma reagin, HIV, gonorrhea, and chlamydia.

2. Discuss group B strep (GBS) screening and management protocol.

H. 36 weeks gestation

1. Determine fetal position by ultrasound or Leopold's maneuver.

2. Screen for GBS. Vaginal and rectal swab cultures to determine presence of GBS bacterial colonization before onset of labor. Screening is not needed if treatment in labor is indicated based on other risk factors such as GBS bacteria during any trimester of the current pregnancy or previous infant with invasive GBS disease.

3. Discuss the risks and benefits of herpes simplex prophylaxis in women with a history of genital herpes.

4. Educate on latent phase of labor, rupture of membranes, active labor management, analgesia in labor.

I. 38 weeks gestation

1. Review labor education; discuss contraception, with an emphasis on the benefits of long-acting reversible contraception such as intrauterine devices and implants.

J. > 41 weeks gestation

1. Baseline nonstress test or contraction stress test, ultrasonography, biophysical profile, or a combination of these tests (see Chapter 14)

2. Discuss labor induction after 41 weeks.

VII. Danger Signs During Pregnancy

A. First-trimester danger signs
- Abdominal pain/cramping: possible indication of threatened abortion, urinary tract infection (UTI)
- Vaginal spotting or bleeding: possible indication of abortion
- Persistent vomiting and nausea: possible indication of hyperemesis gravidarum
- Dysuria, frequency, urgency: possible indication of UTI
- Fever and chills: possible indication of infection

B. Second-trimester danger signs
- Vaginal bleeding: possible indication of infection, preterm labor, placenta previa, or abruption
- Pelvic or abdominal pain/cramping: possible indication of PTL, urinary tract infection, pyelonephritis, or appendicitis
- Fever and chills: possible indication of infection
- Dysuria, frequency, and urgency: possible indication of UTI
- Absence of fetal movement: possible fetal distress or demise
- Persistent nausea and vomiting: possible indication of hyperemesis gravidarum

C. Third-trimester danger signs
- Pelvic or abdominal pain/cramping, low backache, pelvic pressure, leaking of amniotic fluid, increase in vaginal discharge: possible indication of PTL, UTI, pyelonephritis, or appendicitis
- Vaginal bleeding: possible indication of infection, PTL, placenta previa, or abruption
- Persistent nausea and vomiting: possible indication of hyperemesis gravidarum
- Decreased or absence of movement: possible fetal distress or demise
- Fever and chills: possible indication of infection
- Severe headache that does not respond to usual relief measures or is accompanied by visual changes: possible indication of hypertensive disorder

CASE STUDY: Putting It All Together

Stephanie is a 25-year-old who presents to her first prenatal office visit on August 11. When asked by the nurse about her past pregnancies, Stephanie states that she has a 3-year-old boy delivered vaginally at 38 weeks and a 1-year-old girl delivered by cesarean section at 41 weeks plus 5 days. She states that she had a miscarriage between the birth of her son and daughter. Stephanie also added that she is not sure about her last menstrual period but thinks that it was June 1 because she missed her period last month. She was not trying to get pregnant, so she wasn't keeping a good record of her menstrual periods. When asked why she thinks she is pregnant, Stephanie states that she has been feeling extremely tired and her breasts are very tender. When she wakes up in the morning, the smell of coffee makes her nauseated and she loves her coffee in the morning. Upon inspection, the examiner notes a bluish color of the vaginal mucosa and cervical softening when palpated.

Case Study Questions

1. Calculate Stephanie's G/P and GTPAL.

2. Calculate Stephanie EDD using Naegele's rule.

3. Approximately how many weeks gestation is Stephanie at her first prenatal visit?

4. What would the nurse document as the presumptive signs of Stephanie's case history?

5. What would the nurse document as the probable signs of pregnancy?

6. What other questions would be important to ask Stephanie during this initial interview?

7. As the nurse, how would you prepare Stephanie for her pelvic examination?

8. What routine laboratory tests/screens would be done during the initial prenatal visit? As the nurse, how would you educate Stephanie regarding these tests/screenings?

9. When should Stephanie return for her next prenatal visit?

REVIEW QUESTIONS

Be sure to read the Introduction for valuable test-taking tips.

1. The nurse documents a prenatal patient's GTPAL as G5T2P1A1L4. Which obstetric history is consistent with this assessment?
   1. The woman is currently pregnant, has five living children.
   2. The woman is currently pregnant and had two preterm pregnancies.
   3. The woman is not currently pregnant and has had one abortion.
   4. The woman is currently pregnant and had one set of twins.

2. A new client is seen at the prenatal clinic and says she thinks she is pregnant. The first day of her last menstrual period was April 1, 2014. What is her EDB?
   1. December 30, 2014
   2. January 1, 2015
   3. January 8, 2015
   4. December 8, 2014

3. When assessing a prenatal client at follow-up prenatal visits during the second trimester, the nurse should anticipate which assessments to be performed at each visit? *Select all that apply.*
   1. Cervical examination
   2. Weight, height, BMI
   3. Fetal ultrasound
   4. Fundal height
   5. Blood pressure

4. The nurse is educating a primigravida patient during her first prenatal clinic appointment about follow-up prenatal care. How often will follow-up prenatal clinic visits be scheduled if the patient has a low-risk pregnancy and develops no complications? *Select all that apply.*
   1. Every 2 weeks for the first 28 weeks
   2. Every 4 weeks until 30 weeks
   3. Every 4 weeks until 28 weeks
   4. Every 2 weeks after 28 completed weeks until 36 weeks gestation
   5. Every week after 31 completed weeks until 36 weeks gestation

5. The nurse is educating a primigravida patient about prenatal testing/screening. She inquires why she needs to be tested for HIV. Which of the following is the nurse's *best* response?
   1. "It is a recommended screening for all women, regardless of risk factors."
   2. "It is a recommended screening for a woman who is not married."
   3. "It is a recommended screening for a woman who has had gonorrhea."
   4. "It is a recommended screening for a woman who has had more than one sexual partner."

6. A multigravida patient comes into the clinic for one of her second-trimester prenatal visits. The nurse reviews her laboratories that were drawn prior to the visit. Which laboratories results should concern the nurse *most*?
   1. Platelet count of 200,000 per μL (microliter) of blood
   2. Hemoglobin 9.5 g/dL
   3. White blood cell count of 11,000/μL
   4. Rubella titer ratio of 1:10

7. A 20-year-old gravida 1 para 0 presents to the prenatal clinic with a chief complaint that she feels like she is pregnant. Which are presumptive signs of pregnancy? *Select all that apply.*
   1. Linea nigra
   2. Breast tenderness
   3. Leukorrhea
   4. Chadwick's sign
   5. Positive pregnancy test

8. Which statement by the patient indicates to the nurse that the patient understands danger signs during the second trimester?
   1. "I should contact the doctor if I experience heartburn."
   2. "I should contact the doctor if I experience constipation."
   3. "I should contact the doctor if I experience hurting when I urinate."
   4. "I should contact the doctor if I experience leg cramps."

9. A pregnant woman is being seen at her first prenatal visit. The RN should correct which action of a student nurse who is preparing the client for a pelvic examination?
   1. Asking the client if she needs something to drink
   2. Assembling the necessary equipment for the pelvic examination
   3. Positioning the client in the lithotomy position
   4. Explaining the procedure prior to the pelvic examination

10. A gravida 1 para 0 who is 10 weeks pregnant has her first prenatal visit. After performing a history and physical, which test ordered by the physician should the nurse verify with the examiner?
    1. Serological test for syphilis
    2. Rubella vaccine
    3. Clean-catch urinalysis
    4. Abdominal ultrasound

11. A nurse is reviewing the record of a woman who has just been told that she is pregnant. The physician has documented the presence of Goodell's sign. The nurse determines this sign refers to which of the following?
    1. A softening of the tip of the cervix
    2. A soft blowing sound that corresponds to the maternal pulse
    3. Enlargement of the uterus
    4. A softening of the lower uterine segment

12. A primigravida patient asks the nurse to explain the term *quickening.* Which statement by the nurse is correct?
    1. "It is intermittent uterine contractions caused by the increase in hormones, especially estrogen."
    2. "It is the absence of menses and is one of the earliest symptoms a woman reports when she is pregnant."
    3. "It is when the mother can first feel the movements of the fetus."
    4. "It is an increase in vaginal discharge caused by the increase in estrogen."

13. The nurse is assessing the client for the presence of ballottement. Which should the nurse perform to test for the presence of ballottement?
    1. Palpate the uterus for contractions
    2. Assess the skin for increased pigmentation
    3. Initiate a gentle upward tap on the cervix
    4. Palpate the abdomen for fetal outline

14. A 26-year-old multigravida patient is 14 weeks pregnant and is scheduled for a maternal serum alpha-fetoprotein test. She asks the nurse, "What does this test indicate?" The nurse explains that this test can detect which of the following?
    1. Leg defects
    2. Gastrointestinal defects
    3. Neural tube defects
    4. Renal defects

15. The nurse is educating a gravida 1 para 0 who is 28 weeks pregnant. Which educational topics are appropriate for the nurse to discuss with the patient at this prenatal visit? *Select all that apply.*
    1. Discussion of prenatal classes
    2. Discussion of alcohol use
    3. Discussion of family history for pregnancy-induced hypertension
    4. Discussion of signs and symptom of preterm labor
    5. Discussion of fetal movement and kick counts

16. A woman comes to the prenatal clinic because she thinks she is pregnant. Which of the following are probable signs of pregnancy? *Select all that apply.*
    1. Amenorrhea
    2. Uterine enlargement
    3. Positive pregnancy test
    4. Breast tenderness
    5. Brownish patches on the forehead, cheeks, nose, and chin

17. A nurse is examining a G1P0 who is 10 weeks gestation. The nurse notes a bluish coloration of her cervix. The nurse should document this finding as which positive sign?
    1. Quickening
    2. Goodell's sign
    3. Chadwick's sign
    4. Hegar's sign

18. A nurse is taking a birth history assessment on a client who is 8 weeks gestation and has one child who was born at 38 weeks. Which is consistent with this birth history?
    1. Primipara
    2. Primigravida
    3. Nulligravida
    4. Multipara

19. A nurse is performing an initial assessment of a multigravida patient who is 10 weeks gestation. Which assessment finding would necessitate further testing?
    1. Rubella titer ratio of 1:10
    2. Blood type A+
    3. White blood cell count of 5,000
    4. Previous history of gestational diabetes

20. A primipara patient who is 12 weeks gestation is being scheduled for an abdominal ultrasound. The client asks the nurse why she needs this test. What is the nurse's *best* response?
    1. "This test is to determine the position of the fetus."
    2. "This test is to determine if there is enough amniotic fluid."
    3. "This test is to determine how many weeks gestation you are."
    4. "This test is to determine fetal breathing movements."

REVIEW QUESTION ANSWERS

1. ANSWER: 4

Rationale

1. The woman is currently pregnant and has four living children.
2. The woman is currently pregnant and had one preterm pregnancy.
3. The woman is currently pregnant and has had one abortion.
4. The woman is currently pregnant and had one set of twins.

TEST-TAKING TIP: *Gravida* refers to the number of times a woman has been pregnant regardless of the outcome of the pregnancy. Remember, if the woman is currently pregnant, then the pregnancy should be counted. The results of the pregnancy are documented in the GTPAL. The client has been pregnant five times (G5) and has had two term deliveries, one preterm delivery, one abortion, and is currently pregnant. If all of her deliveries were still living, she should have three living children. However, she has four living children, so one of her pregnancies must have been twins. Twins, triplets, and so on, count as one pregnancy and one birth except when counting the number of living children.

Content Area: Birth History/Prenatal Care
Integrated Process: Nursing Process—Assessment
Client Need: Management of Care
Cognitive Level: Analysis
Concept: Prenatal
Reference: London, M. L., Ladewig, P. A., Davidson, M. R., Ball, J. W., Bindler, R. C., & Cowen, K. J. (2014). Maternal & child nursing care. 4th ed. New Jersey: Pearson.

2. ANSWER: 3

Rationale

1. This is an incorrect estimated date.
2. This is an incorrect estimated date.
3. January 1, 2014, is the correct expected date of birth.
4. This is an incorrect estimated date.

TEST-TAKING TIP: Naegele's rule is an accurate and the most common method to determine the EDD, EDC, or EDB, calculated from the menstrual history. To use this method, subtract 3 months from the first day of the last menstrual period (LMP) and add 7 days. Adjust the year if needed.
Example:
LMP: 4 – 1 – 2014
Minus 3 months plus 7 days:
Adjust the year: January 8, 2015

Content Area: Determination of Due Date/Prenatal Care
Integrated Process: Nursing Process—Assessment
Client Need: Management of Care
Cognitive Level: Analysis
Concept: Prenatal
Reference: Perry, S. E., Hockenberry, M. F., Lowdermilk, D. L., & Wilson, D. (2014). Maternal child nursing care. 5th ed. St. Louis, MO: Elsevier.

3. ANSWER: 4, 5

Rationale

1. A cervical examination is recommended at the first prenatal visit in the first trimester and again in the third trimester for cervical readiness for labor.
2. Weight, height, and BMI should be recorded on the first initial visit to determine the recommended weight gain during the pregnancy. The patient should then be weighed at each prenatal visit until labor begins.
3. Second-trimester ultrasound is done to detect structural or fetal abnormalities. However, this screening is not done routinely at each prenatal visit.
4. Fundal height is used as an indicator of uterine size and correlates with the weeks of gestation between 22 and 34 weeks. For accuracy, fundal height should be measured by the same examiner at each prenatal visit. A decrease or sudden increase may indicate a possible complication.
5. Blood pressure should be recorded at each prenatal visit. High blood pressure may indicate possible complications.

TEST-TAKING TIP: Be aware of what is asked in the stem of the question. For this question, your answer will be focused on the second trimester and at each visit.

Content Area: Prenatal Care/Second Trimester
Integrated Process: Nursing Process—Assessment
Client Need: Physiological Integrity
Cognitive Level: Analysis
Concept: Prenatal
Reference: Lowdermilk, D. L., Perry, S. E., Cashion, K., & Alden, K. R. (2016). Maternity & women's health care. 11th ed. St. Louis, MO: Elsevier.

4. ANSWER: 3, 4

Rationale

1. Every 4 weeks for the first 28 weeks
2. Every 4 weeks until the first 28 weeks
3. This answer is correct.
4. This answer is correct.
5. Every week 30 completed weeks until 36 weeks gestation

TEST-TAKING TIP: Rule out incorrect options in questions that require "Select all that apply."

Content Area: Subsequent Prenatal Visits/Prenatal Care
Integrated Process: Nursing Process—Implementation
Client Need: Management of Care
Cognitive Level: Comprehension
Concept: Prenatal
Reference: Durham, R. F., & Chapman, L. (2014). Maternal-newborn nursing: The critical components of nursing care. 2nd ed. Philadelphia: F.A. Davis.

5. ANSWER: 1

Rationale

1. All women should be tested, regardless of risk factors.
2. A woman who is not married is the incorrect answer.
3. A woman who has had gonorrhea is the incorrect answer.
4. A woman who has had more than one sexual partner is the incorrect answer.

TEST-TAKING TIP: The Centers for Disease Control recommends HIV screening for all women as a standard part of prenatal care in order to identify and treat HIV and to prevent transmission of HIV to infants. The opt-out option for testing is offered to all women. For women who decline, the health care provider should address objections and encourage HIV screenings.

Content Area: Laboratory; Diagnostic Studies; Prenatal Care
Integrated Process: Nursing Process—Implementation
Client Need: Safety and Infection Control
Cognitive Level: Comprehensive
Concept: Prenatal

Reference: Akkerman, D., Cleland, L., Croft, G., Eskuchen, K., Heim C., Levine, A., & Westby, E. (2012). Routine prenatal care. Bloomingtom, MN: Institute for Clinical Systems Improvement (ICSI). Available at: http://www.icsi.org/_asset/13n9y4/Prenatal.pdf.

6. ANSWER: 2

Rationale

1. Platelet count of 200,000 per μL of blood is within the normal limits.
2. Hemoglobin 9.5 g/dL indicates anemia in a pregnant woman. Values less than 11 g/dL in the first trimester, less than 10.5 g/dL in the second trimester, and less than 11 g/dL in the third trimester indicate would need further intervention.
3. White blood cell count of 11,000/μL is within the normal limits
4. Rubella titer ratio of 1:10 shows immunity.

TEST-TAKING TIP: Be familiar with the normal laboratories of pregnancy and indications for further intervention.
Content Area: Laboratory; Diagnostic Studies; Prenatal Care
Integrated Process: Nursing Process—Assessment
Client Need: Physiological Integrity
Cognitive Level: Analysis
Concept: Prenatal
Reference: Perry, S. E., Hockenberry, M. F., Lowdermilk, D. L., & Wilson, D. (2014). Maternal child nursing care. 5th ed. St. Louis, MO: Elsevier.

7. ANSWER: 2, 3

Rationale

1. Incorrect answer. Linea nigra is a probable sign.
2. Correct answer. Breast tenderness is a presumptive sign.
3. Correct answer. Leukorrhea is a presumptive sign.
4. Incorrect answer. Chadwick's sign is a probable sign.
5. Incorrect answer. Positive pregnancy test is a probable sign.

TEST-TAKING TIP: Presumptive signs are subjective symptoms that a woman reports to the health care provider. Probable or objective signs can be observed by the health care provider.
Content Area: Signs of Pregnancy; Prenatal Care—Signs of Pregnancy
Integrated Process: Nursing Process—Assessment
Client Need: Physiological Integrity
Cognitive Level: Comprehension
Concept: Prenatal
Reference: Perry, S. E., Hockenberry, M. F., Lowdermilk, D. L., & Wilson, D. (2014). Maternal child nursing care. 5th ed. St. Louis, MO: Elsevier.

8. ANSWER: 3

Rationale

1. Heartburn is a common discomfort of pregnancy. It usually appears during the second and third trimesters and is a result of increased production of progesterone and displacement of the stomach related to the enlargement of the uterus.
2. Constipation is a common discomfort of pregnancy. Increased progesterone during pregnancy causes bowel sluggishness, resulting in constipation. Other causes of constipation are the displacement of intestines resulting with the increased growth of the fetus and iron supplementation prescribed to a woman during pregnancy.

3. Urinary frequency is a common occurrence, especially during the first and third trimesters. However, pain, burning when voiding, or blood in the urine are signs of a bladder infection, which could lead to preterm labor. These complaints must be reported to the physician or midwife.
4. Leg cramps are a common occurrence, especially during the night but may occur during other times of the day.

TEST-TAKING TIP: It is important to know the discomforts of pregnancy and what complaints need to be reported to the physician.
Content Area: Danger Signs of Pregnancy; Prenatal Care
Integrated Process: Nursing Process—Evaluation
Client Need: Safety and Infection Control
Cognitive Level: Analysis
Concept: Prenatal
Reference: London, M. L., Ladewig, P. A., Davidson, M. R., Ball, J. W., Bindler, R. C., & Cowen, K. J. (2014). Maternal & child nursing care. 4th ed. New Jersey: Pearson.

9. ANSWER: 1

Rationale

1. The nurse should ask the woman if she needs to empty her bladder prior to the pelvic examination.
2. The nurse should assemble the necessary equipment for the pelvic examination.
3. This is the correct position for the pelvic examination.
4. Explanation for a procedure should always be done prior to the procedure.

TEST-TAKING TIP: It is easier for the examiner to evaluate the size of the uterus when the bladder is empty. Also, by emptying the bladder, the patient will have decreased pelvic pressure and discomfort during the examination.
Content Area: Physical Assessment; Prenatal Care
Integrated Process: Nursing Process—Implementation
Client Need: Basic Care and Comfort
Cognitive Level: Application
Concept: Prenatal
Reference: Durham, R. F., & Chapman, L. (2014). Maternal-newborn nursing: The critical components of nursing care. 2nd ed. Philadelphia: F.A. Davis.

10. ANSWER: 2

Rationale

1. Serological testing for syphilis would be performed at the first prenatal visit and would be considered a routine order for a pregnant woman.
2. The nurse would need to clarify this order with the physician because the rubella vaccine is contraindicated during pregnancy. A rubella titer would be performed to determine immunity. If the patient is nonimmune, then vaccination would be given after birth during the postpartum period and prior to discharge from the hospital. The patient should be educated to avoid children who have rubella.
3. Urinalysis would be performed to identify women with infection or metabolic problems and would be considered a routine order for a pregnant woman.
4. Abdominal ultrasound would be considered a routine order for a pregnant woman.

TEST-TAKING TIP: Live virus vaccines are contraindicated during pregnancy because viral infection is easily transmitted to the fetus.

Content Area: Testing and Screening; Prenatal Care
Integrated Process: Nursing Process—Implementation
Client Need: Safety and Infection Control
Cognitive Level: Analysis
Concept: Prenatal
Reference: Perry, S. E., Hockenberry, M. F., Lowdermilk, D. L., & Wilson, D. (2014). Maternal child nursing care. 5th ed. St. Louis, MO: Elsevier.

11. ANSWER: 4
Rationale
1. Hegar's sign is the softening of the lower uterine segment.
2. Uterine souffle is the soft blowing sound that corresponds to the maternal pulse.
3. Enlargement of the uterus
4. Goodell's sign is the softening of the tip of the cervix.
TEST-TAKING TIP: Read each option carefully and use the process of elimination to rule out incorrect responses.
Content Area: Signs of Pregnancy/Prenatal Care
Integrated Process: Nursing Process—Assessment
Client Need: Physiological Integrity
Cognitive Level: Comprehensive
Concept: Prenatal
Reference: London, M. L., Ladewig, P. A., Davidson, M. R., Ball, J. W., Bindler, R. C., & Cowen, K. J. (2014). Maternal & child nursing care. 4th ed. New Jersey: Pearson.

12. ANSWER: 3
Rationale
1. Braxton Hicks contractions are intermittent uterine contractions caused by an increase in hormones, especially estrogen.
2. Amenorrhea is the absence of menses and is one of the earliest symptoms a woman reports when pregnant.
3. Quickening is when the mother can first feel the movements of the fetus.
4. Leukorrhea is a white milky odorless discharge caused by the increase in estrogen.
TEST-TAKING TIP: It is important to know what the medical terms mean. Read each option carefully and use the process of elimination to rule out incorrect responses.
Content Area: Signs of Pregnancy/Prenatal Care
Integrated Process: Nursing Process—Evaluation
Client Need: Physiological Adaptation
Cognitive Level: Comprehensive
Concept: Prenatal
Reference: Durham, R. F., & Chapman, L. (2014). Maternal-newborn nursing: The critical components of nursing care. 2nd ed. Philadelphia: F.A. Davis.

13. ANSWER: 3
Rationale
1. Palpating the uterus for contractions is not ballottement.
2. Incorrect answer.
3. Initiating a gentle upward tap on the cervix will make the fetus float upward. A rebound of the fetus can be felt by the examiner.
4. Palpating the abdomen for the fetal outline is called Leopold's maneuver.

TEST-TAKING TIP: It is important to understand how to perform prenatal assessments.
Content Area: Signs of Pregnancy/Prenatal Care
Integrated Process: Nursing Process—Assessment
Client Need: Physiological Adaptation
Cognitive Level: Application
Concept: Prenatal
Reference: Durham, R. F., & Chapman, L. (2014). Maternal-newborn nursing: The critical components of nursing care. 2nd ed. Philadelphia: F.A. Davis.

14. ANSWER: 3
Rationale
1. Leg defects is an incorrect answer.
2. Cardiac defects is an incorrect answer.
3. Neural tube defects is the correct answer.
4. Renal defects is an incorrect answer.
TEST-TAKING TIP: The level of alpha-fetoprotein (AFP) in the blood is used in a maternal serum triple or quadruple screening test. Generally done between 15 and 20 weeks, these tests check the levels of three or four substances in a pregnant woman's blood. The triple screen checks AFP, human chorionic gonadotropin (hCG), and a type of estrogen called *unconjugated estriol*, or uE3. The quad screen checks these substances and the level of the hormone inhibin A. The levels of these substances—along with a woman's age and other factors—help the doctor estimate the chance that the baby may have certain problems or birth defects.
Content Area: Testing; Screening; Prenatal Care
Integrated Process: Nursing Process—Implementation
Client Need: Physiological Adaptation
Cognitive Level: Comprehensive
Concept: Prenatal
Reference: Perry, S. E., Hockenberry, M. F., Lowdermilk, D. L., & Wilson, D. (2014). Maternal child nursing care. 5th ed. St. Louis, MO: Elsevier.

15. ANSWER: 1, 4, 5
Rationale
1. Discussion of the various prenatal classes should begin during this trimester. This will give the expectant woman and her partner time to make an appointment and attend before the birth of their infant.
2. Alcohol, tobacco, and drugs should have been discussed at the first prenatal visit.
3. Family health history should have been discussed at the first prenatal visit. A thorough history and physical helps the health care provider determine the status of the woman's prepregnancy health or if there is any high-risk potential, such as women who are at risk for developing pregnancy-induced hypertension, women in their first pregnancy, women whose sisters and mother had pregnancy-induced hypertension, women carrying multiple babies, women younger than age 20 or older that age 40, and women who had high blood pressure or kidney disease prior to pregnancy (see Chapter 13).
4. Discussion of signs and symptoms of preterm labor is appropriate for this visit.
5. Discussion of fetal movement and kick counts is appropriate for this visit.

TEST-TAKING TIP: Think about why the nurse would need to educate the patient about each topic. You will need to consider fetal development, weeks of gestation and trimester, and danger signs. Use the process of elimination to determine which information is important during this trimester.
Content Area: Education; Prenatal Care
Integrated Process: Nursing Process—Implementation
Client Need: Health Promotion and Maintenance
Cognitive Level: Analysis
Concept: Prenatal
Reference: Akkerman, D., Cleland, L., Croft, G., Eskuchen, K., Heim, C., Levine, A., & Westby, E. (2012). Routine prenatal care. Bloomingtom (MN): Institute for Clinical Systems Improvement (ICSI). Available at: http://www.icsi.org/_asset/13n9y4/Prenatal.pdf.

16. **ANSWERS: 2, 3, 5**
Rationale
1. Amenorrhea is a presumptive or subjective change provided by the woman.
2. This is a probable sign of pregnancy observed by the examiner.
3. This is a probable sign of pregnancy observed by the examiner.
4. Breast tenderness is a presumptive or subjective change noticed by the woman.
5. This is a probable sign of pregnancy observed by the examiner.
TEST-TAKING STRATEGY: Probable signs of pregnancy are observed findings by the examiner but may be manifested from other causes.
Content Area: Signs of Pregnancy; Prenatal Care
Integrated Process: Nursing Process—Assessment
Client Needs: Health Promotion and Maintenance—Ante/Intra/Postpartum and Newborn Care
Cognitive Level: Application
Concept: Prenatal
Reference: Ward, S. L., & Hisley, S. M. (2016). Maternal-child nursing care. 2nd ed. Philadelphia: F.A. Davis.

17. **ANSWER: 3**
Rationale
1. This is the first indication of the woman feeling fetal movement.
2. Goodell's sign refers to the softening of the cervix.
3. Chadwick's sign refers to the change in the vascularity of the cervix that makes it a blue-violet color.
4. Hegar's sign is the softening of the tissue between the body of the uterus and cervix.
TEST-TAKING STRATEGY: Many changes occur as a result in the increase of progesterone and estrogen during pregnancy. It is important to know and understand these changes in order to assess, implement, and evaluate nursing interventions.
Content Area: Signs of Pregnancy; Prenatal Care
Integrated Process: Nursing Process—Assessment
Client Needs: Health Promotion and Maintenance:
Ante/Intra/Postpartum and Newborn Care
Cognitive Level: Application
Concept: Prenatal
Reference: Ward, S. L., & Hisley, S. M. (2016). Maternal-child nursing care. 2nd ed. Philadelphia: F.A. Davis.

18. **ANSWER: 1**
Rationale
1. Primipara is a woman who has had one birth past 20 weeks gestation, regardless if the baby was born alive or dead or the number of fetuses.
2. Primigravida is a woman who is pregnant for the first time. This client is pregnant for the second time.
3. Nulligravida is a woman who has never been pregnant.
4. Multipara is a woman who has had two or more births past 20 weeks gestation.
TEST-TAKING STRATEGY: In obstetrics, it is important to understand and be able to describe a client's obstetrical history using common terms. These terms may be used in test items and the definitions of these terms may determine the correct answer.
Content Area: Birth History; Prenatal Care
Integrated Process: Nursing Process—Assessment
Client Needs: Health Promotion and Maintenance: Ante/Intra/Postpartum and Newborn Care
Cognitive Level: Comprehension
Concept: Prenatal
Reference: Durham, R. F., & Chapman, L. (2016). Maternal-child nursing care. 2nd ed. Philadelphia: F.A. Davis.

19. **ANSWER: 4**
Rationale
1. A ratio of 1:10 indicates immunity to rubella.
2. RhoGAM is indicated only if woman is Rh−.
3. This is a normal laboratory.
4. Women with the following risk factors should be screened for gestational diabetes at the first prenatal visit: prepregnancy BMI greater than 30 kg/m, personal history of gestational diabetes mellitus (GDM), or known impaired glucose metabolism.
TEST-TAKING STRATEGY: This question tests your ability to interpret important data. Options 1, 2, and 3 are all normal findings and no further testing is needed. The key word in the stem is *multigravida,* meaning that this client has had previous pregnancies.
Content Area: Routine Laboratory; Diagnostic Studies; Prenatal Care
Integrated Process: Nursing Process—Assessment
Client Needs: Health Promotion and Maintenance: Ante/Intra/Postpartum and Newborn Care
Cognitive Level: Application
Concept: Prenatal
Reference: Durham, R. F., & Chapman, L. (2016). Maternal-child nursing care. 2nd ed. Philadelphia: F.A. Davis.

20. **ANSWER: 3**
1. Abdominal ultrasound would be performed in the third trimester to determine the position of the fetus for delivery. This client is in the first trimester.
2. Abdominal ultrasound would be performed in the late second and third trimesters to determine amniotic fluid index.
3. This would be an indication for the scheduling of an abdominal ultrasound.
4. Abdominal ultrasound is a component of a biophysical profile in which fetal breathing movements are assessed.

However, this test would not be ordered until later in the pregnancy.

TEST-TAKING STRATEGY: Abdominal ultrasound can establish gestational age during the first 20 weeks because fetal growth is consistent during this time.

Content Area: Routine Laboratory; Diagnostic Studies; Prenatal Care

Integrated Process: Nursing Process—Assessment
Client Needs: Health Promotion and Maintenance: Ante/Intra/Postpartum and Newborn Care
Cognitive Level: Application
Concept: Prenatal

Reference: Durham, R. F., & Chapman, L. (2016). Maternal-child nursing care. 2nd ed. Philadelphia: F.A. Davis.

Maternal Nutrition

Anorexia nervosa—An eating disorder involving starvation of the body based on the fear of gaining weight

Body mass index (BMI)—An estimate of body fat that is calculated based upon the patient's height and weight values

Bulimia nervosa—An eating disorder characterized by compulsive consumption and purging of food

Calories—A unit of heat used to convert food into energy

Folic acid—A B vitamin (also known as *folate*). Adequate supplementation in pregnancy can help to prevent birth defects of the baby's brain, specifically, neural tube defects.

Listeriosis—A gram-positive bacillus found readily in the environment that is related to foodborne illnesses

Mercury—A metallic element found in some fish and shellfish. Excessive consumption of mercury-containing foods can lead to pregnancy complications.

Pica—A craving for unusual substances such as dirt, clay, chalk, ice

Vegan—A diet without the consumption or utilization of animal products, such as eggs, meat, or dairy

Vegetarian—A diet without meat or meat products

I. Maternal Nutrition Description

Maternal nutrition includes consumption of a variety of foods in appropriate amounts to allow adequate maternal weight gain, including vitamin and mineral supplementation during pregnancy. By using the MyPlate program offered through the United States Department of Agriculture, pregnant women can learn more about nutrition and how to plan healthy meals during pregnancy. Health care professionals can also utilize this site to educate patients on healthy eating and exercise. The website www.choosemyplate.gov also helps pregnant women learn how to make healthy food choices at each mealtime and how to incorporate safe exercise routines into their daily schedules.[1]

A. Weight gain
1. At a pregnant woman's initial prenatal visit, her weight and current **body mass index (BMI)** should be ascertained and documented.
2. During this initial visit, the patient should receive counseling about appropriate weight gain during her pregnancy based on her current weight and BMI (Table 11.1).

DID YOU KNOW?

Obese women are at a greater risk for having a large-for-gestational-age infant and a post-term birth.[2] Babies born to obese women are also at a greater risk for childhood obesity.

ALERT Maternal obesity increases the risk for gestational diabetes, maternal hypertension, pre-eclampsia, and delivery complications, including increased rate of cesarean delivery. Babies born to obese mothers are more likely to suffer from macrosomia, or large for gestational age, which can place them at greater risk for birth injuries and other neonatal complications, including stillbirth.

B. Calories
1. **Calories** are the single most important nutritional factor affecting a neonate and determining birth weight.
2. In pregnancy, it is recommended that women increase their daily caloric intake to include a total of 1,800 calories daily during the first trimester,

[1]United States Department of Agriculture. (2015). Health and nutrition information. Retrieved from https://www.choosemyplate.gov/moms-pregnancy-breastfeeding.

[2]Gillen-Goldstein, J., Funai, E. F., Roque, H., & Ruvel, J. M. (2015). Nutrition in pregnancy. Retrieved from http://enjoypregnancyclub.com/wp-content/uploads/2016/05/Nutrition-in-pregnancy.pdf.

Table 11.1 Weight Gain Recommendations for Pregnancy (IOM, 2009)

Prepregnancy Weight Category	Body Mass Index	Recommended Range of Total Weight (lb)	Recommended Rates of Weight Gain in the Second and Third Trimesters (lb) (Mean Range [lb/wk])
Underweight	Less than 18.5	28–40	1 (1–1.3)
Normal weight	18.5–24.9	25–35	1 (0.8–1)
Overweight	25–29.9	15–25	0.6 (0.5–0.7)
Obese	30 and greater	11–20	0.5 (0.4–0.6)

2,200 calories daily during the second trimester, and about 2,400 calories daily during the third trimester.

C. Protein
  1. Proteins are a part of the five food groups and are an essential part of a pregnant woman's dietary intake.
  2. Proteins can be found in foods like lean meat, poultry, seafood, beans, eggs, nuts, legumes, and seeds.
     a) Complete protein: Growth and repair of the body require the availability and utilization of amino acids. The body needs a combination of 21 amino acids to stay healthy. While the body can manufacture some of the amino acids it needs, diet must supply others, which are classified as essential amino acids. A complete protein contains all nine of the essential amino acids. All animal products contain every essential amino acid, while plant products generally lack one or more.
     b) Incomplete protein: When a protein lacks one or more of the nine essential amino acids, it is known as an incomplete protein. Peanut butter lacks the essential amino acid methionine but is high in lysine. All plant-based proteins are incomplete protein sources except for soy and quinoa. A client can obtain all the essential amino acids even if they do not consume complete proteins by consuming more than one plant-based protein within a 24-hour period. Pregnant women need approximately 70 grams of protein intake per day to promote fetal growth and development.
D. Water and hydration
  1. During pregnancy, the demands for hydration increase as the body must prepare to support fetal circulation, amniotic fluid development, and increased circulatory volume; thus the amount of oral intake of fluids must be adequate.
  2. The amount of hydration must be enough to equalize the decreased motility of the gut, which can cause constipation, and increased fluids are needed to aid in the absorption of essential vitamins and nutrients throughout the gastrointestinal system.
  3. It is recommended that pregnant women consume eight to ten 8-ounce glasses of water daily.
     a) Water intake can include fruit juice or vegetables but at least four to six glasses of fluid should be water.
     b) Clients should be cautioned about drinking diet sodas because they are high in sodium, contain artificial sweeteners, and promote diuresis.
E. Minerals and vitamins
  1. Calcium is very important to pregnant women, as it helps to build the fetus's bones and teeth.
     a) All women of childbearing age should get about 1,000 to 1,300 mg of calcium daily.
     b) The best sources of calcium are milk, cheese, yogurt, and vegetables such as broccoli and dark leafy greens like kale.
     c) Calcium can even be found in large amounts in sardines or pregnant women can take a calcium supplement.
  2. Iron is extremely important in pregnancy, as it helps to carry oxygen to organs and tissues. During pregnancy, women need additional levels to support the fetus.
     a) The daily recommended dose of iron during pregnancy is 27 mg, which is found in most prenatal vitamin supplements.
     b) In pregnancy it is recommended that women eat iron-rich foods, which include lean red meat, poultry, fish, dried beans, iron-fortified cereals, green leafy vegetables.
     c) Iron is also absorbed more easily if it is eaten with vitamin C–rich foods, such as citrus fruits or orange juice.
  3. **Folic acid,** or folate, is a B vitamin that is very important for pregnant women.
     a) Women should begin taking this vitamin before they start trying to conceive, as it can help

to prevent birth defects of the baby's brain, specifically neural tube defects.

b) Current dietary guidelines recommend pregnant women take 600 micrograms (mcg) of folic acid daily.

DID YOU KNOW?

Although the recommended dose of folic acid is 600 mcg, most health care providers order 1 mg of folic acid, which is the prescriptive strength and requires the patient to obtain the vitamins through a pharmacist.

4. Pregnant women should take about 85 milligrams of vitamin C per day, as it helps with tissue growth, healing, and repair and acts as an antioxidant while protecting the body from infection.
   a) No supplementation is required, as most women are able to meet the required daily allowance from their dietary intake.
   b) Vitamin C is found in citrus fruits, leafy greens, strawberries, fruit juices, and fortified cereals.
5. All pregnant women need 600 units of vitamin D daily, as it works with calcium to help build bones and teeth.
   a) It also helps to support strong eyesight and healthy skin.
   b) Vitamin D can be found in fortified milk and fish such as salmon. Exposure to sunlight can provide a healthy dose of vitamin D, though women must be cautious of prolonged exposure to harmful rays.

II. Eating Disorders Affecting Pregnancy

A. Pica

Pica is defined as a craving for unusual substances, such as dirt, clay, and chalk, and has been reported in the literature.

1. It is thought to impact about one-fifth of all pregnant women who are considered high risk.[3]
2. It often goes unreported and can lead to serious pregnancy complications, including nutrient deficiencies, constipation, electrolyte imbalance, lead poisoning, dental complications, weight gain, and metabolic disturbances.[4]

MAKING THE CONNECTION

Pica

Eating clay or soil can result in iron deficiency anemia or hypokalemia secondary to clay binding to potassium in the intestines and increase in excretion. Ingestion of contaminated soil can result in toxoplasmosis and hookworm in the intestines, causing gastrointestinal disturbances. Ingestion of lead-laden substances can cause neonatal complications and childhood developmental delays. Ingestion of freezer ice or ice chips may result in broken or sensitive teeth.

3. There are several theories of why women are susceptible to pica.
   a) Nutritional theory proposes there is a deficiency of certain nutrients in the female body.
   b) Sensory theory relates to the individual feeling satisfied and enjoying the texture or smell of the substance they ingest.
   c) Cultural theory relates to certain cultural roots that suggest ingesting certain substances is a ritual or practice and considered normal.
   d) Psychological theory relates to a response to stressful situations or a manifestation of an oral fixation.[5]
4. Treatment of pica will depend on what caused the disorder and the type of substances being ingested.
   a) Conduct a thorough health history of the patient at the onset of care.
   b) Counsel the patient of the disorder and provide positive reinforcement if they are found to have this eating disorder.
   c) Try supplements and dietary counseling to correct any nutritional deficiencies.
   d) Follow-up of CBC and chemistry levels for anemia and electrolyte imbalance are important.
   e) Educate and continue to evaluate the patient as part of your plan of care.
5. Alternative considerations for cravings
   a) Consider potential substitutes for the cravings such as chewing sugarless gum.
   b) Replace ice with frozen fruit juices.
   c) Replace mud and dirt cravings with stone ground flour.
   d) Replace detergent and washing powder with powdery foods or flour or mouthwash.

[3]Mills, M. E. (2007). Craving more than food: The implications of pica in pregnancy. *Nursing for Women's Health, 11*(3): 266–273.
[4]Mills, M. E. (2007). Craving more than food: The implications of pica in pregnancy. *Nursing for Women's Health, 11*(3): 266–273.
[5]Mills, M. E. (2007). Craving more than food: The implications of pica in pregnancy. *Nursing for Women's Health, 11*(3): 266–273.

DID YOU KNOW?

The PICA Assessment and Counseling Mnemonic is helpful with identifying pica in the clinical setting: P—be patient-centered; I—ice is the most common ingested substance; C— monitor nonverbal communication; A—assess patient for anemia.

B. Eating disorders

Eating disorders are defined as psychiatric disorders that are characterized by the diminished desire to eat or to gain weight.

1. About 1 in 20 pregnant females will experience some form of an eating disorder.
2. There are several types of eating disorders, including anorexia nervosa, bulimia nervosa, binge–purge disorder.
   a) Anorexia nervosa is an eating disorder in which the person has little to no desire to eat and gain weight. It is related to obsessive-compulsive disorder.
      (1) Severe anxiety can result in pregnant women with a history of **anorexia nervosa,** related to the fear of a changing body habitus and consistently gaining weight.
   b) **Bulimia nervosa** is defined as recurrent episodes of purging after binge eating. It is usually related to anxiety and depressive symptomology.
      (1) The uncontrolled binge eating involves ingesting a large amount of calories. These calories usually consist of simple carbohydrates.
      (2) Clients with bulimia may present with erosion of tooth enamel (from the excessive vomiting), mouth sores, dry skin, thin hair, and/or lack of energy.

⊗ ALERT Pregnancy risks related to eating disorders include maternal risk for anemia, miscarriages, premature or preterm labor, cesarean sections, and postpartum depression. Neonatal risks include low birth weight, microcephaly, and small for gestational age.

3. Identification is key to a healthy outcome by using simple questionnaires or screening tools. Counseling and positive reinforcement should be incorporated in the plan of care. Referral to psych and a registered dietitian should be incorporated in your plan of care. Objectives of care for the anorectic patient after identification should include:
   - Restoring lean body mass
   - Preserving immune function
   - Preventing metabolic complications
   - Reversing cellular injury
   - Preventing cardio and respiratory failure

C. Mercury exposure

During pregnancy, **mercury** can result in health hazards to the fetus if consumed in large amounts. Mercury can be found in both fish and shellfish products.

1. Fish that contain high levels of mercury include shark, swordfish, king mackerel, tilefish.
2. Fetal exposure to mercury can result in physical and mental deficits, including brain, vision, and hearing damage.
3. Fish that contain low levels of mercury include salmon, shrimp, pollock, tuna (light canned), tilapia, catfish, and cod.
4. It is recommended that women eat 8 to 12 ounces of a variety of fish every week and pay attention to any advisories related to the body of water it was caught from.

D. Listeriosis

Listeriosis is an illness caused by a gram-positive bacillus that is found readily in the environment and causes foodborne illnesses with sporadic and outbreak-related cases.[6]

DID YOU KNOW?

Maternal infections may be asymptomatic at times; however, symptoms can be flu-like, such as myalgia, backache, headache, and gastrointestinal.

1. Fetal and neonatal exposure to an exposed mother results in fetal loss, premature labor and delivery, neonatal sepsis, meningitis, and possible neonatal death.[7]
2. Foods considered high risk for listeriosis include hot dogs, luncheon meats, meat spreads, smoked seafood, raw or unpasteurized products, soft cheeses, and unwashed raw vegetables.
3. Prevention of listeriosis
   a) Avoid hot dogs, luncheon meats, or deli meats unless reheated until steaming.
   b) Avoid getting fluid from hot dog packages on other foods, utensils, and food-preparation surfaces.
   c) Wash hands after handling all uncooked meat.
   d) Avoid soft cheeses such as feta, Brie, and Camembert or blue-veined cheeses and Mexican-style cheeses such as queso blanco, queso fresco, and panela, unless they have

[6]American College of Obstetricians and Gynecologists (ACOG). (2015). ACOG issues guidelines for managing listeriosis during pregnancy. Retrieved from http://www.mdedge.com/obgmanagement/article/87675/obstetrics/acog-issues-guidelines-managing-listeriosis-during-pregnancy.
[7]American College of Obstetricians and Gynecologists (ACOG). (2015). ACOG issues guidelines for managing listeriosis during pregnancy. Retrieved from http://www.mdedge.com/obgmanagement/article/87675/obstetrics/acog-issues-guidelines-managing-listeriosis-during-pregnancy.

labels that clearly state they are made from pasteurized milk. It is safe to eat hard cheeses, semisoft cheeses such as mozzarella, pasteurized processed cheese slices and spreads, cream cheese, and cottage cheese.

e) Avoid refrigerated pâté or meat spreads.

f) Avoid refrigerated smoked seafood unless it is an ingredient in a cooked dish such as a casserole.

g) Do not drink raw (unpasteurized) milk or eat foods that contain unpasteurized milk.

h) Use all refrigerated perishable items that are precooked or ready-to-eat as soon as possible.

i) Clean your refrigerator regularly.

j) Use a refrigerator thermometer to make sure that the refrigerator always stays at 40°F or below.

4. Management of symptomatic patients with diagnosed listeriosis and who are febrile involves hospital admission, blood cultures, and treatment with IV antibiotics (ampicillin). If delivery results, the placenta is also cultured for microorganisms.[8] The neonate should be admitted to the NICU for further evaluation and treatment.

E. Herbal supplements
Herbal supplements are a part of a whole plant whose effects during pregnancy after ingestion may result in adverse consequences.

1. Some herbs are considered safe during pregnancy in that they may have potential benefits to both the mother and the fetus.

ALERT Black haw has been known to prevent miscarriages, relax uterine muscles, and ease tension. Herbs to avoid during pregnancy include aloe vera, black and blue cohosh, and caraway, which have all been linked to stimulating uterine contractions.

a) Ginger has been used to ease morning sickness and nausea symptoms during the first trimester.

Milk thistle has been used to stimulate blood flow to the breast glands and stimulate milk production and enrich milk flow.

2. Counseling and education of herbal use and supplementation during pregnancy should be considered early on. Inquiry into both prescription and over-the-counter supplements should be addressed during the health history intake.

F. Vegetarian diet
A **vegetarian** diet is a diet without meat or meat products. The **vegan** diet is a strict diet in which no animal products are consumed, such as meat, dairy, or eggs. Many turn to this form of diet as a healthier way of life.

1. There are several different types of vegetarian diets:
   • Lacto-vegetarians diets include milk products.
   • Lacto-ovo vegetarians diets include egg and dairy products in addition to plant-based foods.
   • Vegan diets include only plant-based foods.

2. Veganism during pregnancy can be safe as long as the pregnant woman is well nourished and consuming foods with adequate amounts of calcium and protein.

3. Nutritional considerations with a vegan pregnant woman should include adequate caloric intake within her suggested BMI.

4. Reinforcement of protein supplementation should come from nuts, grains, legumes, and tofu.

5. Dietary iron can come from soy, beans, lentils, spinach, molasses, dried apricots, prunes, and raisins.

6. Dietary intake of calcium and vitamin D includes tofu and dark-green, leafy vegetables, along with tablet-form supplementations if inadequate.

7. Folic acid and vitamin B12 are needed to reduce the incidence of neural tube defects in the growing fetus and should come from oral supplements.

[8]American College of Obstetricians and Gynecologists (ACOG). (2015). ACOG issues guidelines for managing listeriosis during pregnancy. Retrieved from http://www.mdedge.com/obgmanagement/article/87675/obstetrics/acog-issues-guidelines-managing-listeriosis-during-pregnancy.

CASE STUDY: Putting It All Together

Amanda is a 24-year-old G1 P0000 who presents to your prenatal clinical for her first prenatal visit. She has a good relationship with her significant other, and this pregnancy was not planned. She took a pregnancy test at home and believes she is 10 weeks pregnant. Amanda offers a history of anxiety and worries that she will "gain a lot of weight during the pregnancy." As you collect her health history, you document a history of mild depression as a teenager treated with therapy and medication. She currently denies being on any medication except for prenatal vitamins. She offers a history of iron deficiency anemia as a child and recalls taking iron tablets daily. Socially, she works full-time as an administrative assistant and runs about 4 miles daily as her form of exercise. She denies smoking, drinking, or using drugs. Her family history is unremarkable. She has tried a number of diets in the past to keep her weight down and has succeeded.

Review of Systems

• She has been struggling to maintain her current weight of 105 pounds. She says her significant other does not want her to gain weight.
• She drinks an "adequate" amount of water.

• She occasionally feels out of breath and tired during running but pushes herself to continue her goal.

Vital Signs
Temp: 98.7°F
Pulse: 50
Respiration: 16
Blood pressure: 90/60
Height: 5'4"
Weight: 107 lb
BMI: 18.4
Pain scale: 0/10
General appearance: appropriate affect and responsive to questions
Integumentary: skin is cool to touch, no apparent lesions or aberrations, decreased skin turgor, lips and mucous membranes pink, nail beds pallor
HEENT: hair thinning and short
Cardiac: no murmurs auscultated
Pulmonary: CTA bilaterally
Extremities: Moves all extremities without incidence; grossly intact neurological assessment
Abdomen: soft and nontender to palpation, FHT + LLQ at 155

Case Study Questions

1. What subjective assessment findings indicate that Amanda is experiencing a health alteration?

2. What objective assessment findings indicate that she is experiencing a health alteration?

3. After analyzing the data, what nursing diagnoses should the nurse give Amanda?

4. What interventions should the nurse implement to meet Amanda's needs?

5. What outcomes should the nurse use to evaluate the effectiveness of nursing interventions and to make sure Amanda is meeting her needs?

REVIEW QUESTIONS

Be sure to read the Introduction for valuable test-taking tips.

1. A nurse is assessing the weight gain of a client who is 16 weeks pregnant. The nurse understands that inadequate weight gain is associated with a high risk for which complication?
   1. Delivering an infant with macrosomia
   2. Delivering an infant that has a low birth weight
   3. Delivering an infant with congenital anomalies
   4. Delivering an infant that will have to be transferred to the intensive care unit

2. Which report made by a client indicates to the nurse that she may have pica?
   1. She craves unusual substances such as dirt, clay, and chalk.
   2. She abstains from meat-derived food sources (vegetarian).
   3. She has an unusual craving for fish that contain high levels of mercury.
   4. She has an infectious disease that can cause central nervous system disorders.

3. A client has been diagnosed with iron-deficiency anemia. The nurse understands that the client needs to avoid consuming which of the following while taking iron supplements?
   1. Milk
   2. Meat
   3. Orange juice
   4. Water

4. A nurse is teaching a client about adequate protein intake. Which teaching by the nurse indicates a meal composed of adequate protein?
   1. Grilled cheese sandwich, tomato-basil soup, and soda
   2. Bacon, lettuce, and egg sandwich; grits; and orange juice
   3. Peanut butter sandwich, potato chips, and lemonade
   4. Eggplant, avocado, and tomato sandwich; carrot sticks; water

5. Which fish should a pregnant client be advised to avoid?
   1. Shark, salmon, and tilefish
   2. Catfish, red snapper, and light tuna
   3. Salmon, light tuna, and tilefish
   4. Tilefish, shark, mackerel

6. The nurse is assessing the dietary habits of a pregnant client. The client states that her usual lunch consists of a sandwich of lunch meat, white bread, mayonnaise, mustard, and tomato. For what fetal complication is her fetus at risk?
   1. Meningitis
   2. Retinopathy
   3. Necrotizing enterocolitis
   4. Postmaturity

7. Which of the food choices of a pregnant client should indicate to the nurse that further teaching is needed? *Select all that apply.*
   1. Grilled salmon sandwich with potato chips
   2. Leftover turkey and dressing with cranberry sauce
   3. Grilled chicken salad with ranch dressing
   4. Pizza with bread sticks
   5. Unwashed broccoli

8. A pregnant client is complaining of morning sickness. Which of the following herbs should the nurse recommend?
   1. Ginger
   2. Black cohosh
   3. Black haw
   4. Aloe vera

9. A pregnant client tells the nurse that she only eats a plant-based diet. How should the nurse counsel this client?
   1. "It is important that you incorporate meat products into your diet for protein during your pregnancy."
   2. "It is important that we refer you to a therapist to discuss your eating disorder."
   3. "Your newborn is at a high risk for developing complications."
   4. "Let's discuss how we can ensure adequate caloric intake and proper nutrients during your pregnancy with your plant-based diet."

10. Your 27-week-gestation client tells you that her mother made some cookies with caraway seeds and she suddenly feels abdominal tightening. How would you *best* respond to this patient?
    1. Instruct your client that the abdominal pain may be related to uterine contractions from the caraway.
    2. Instruct your client that she may have food poisoning and may need to be admitted for treatment.
    3. Advise your client to continue eating the cookies, as the tightening may be related to fatigue and dehydration.
    4. Counsel her to monitor fetal kick counts daily and advise if the pains are more intense.

11. You are conducting a physical examination on an 18-year-old primipara and notice she has a dry scaling tongue with eroded teeth. Which complications should you consider as you further assess this patient?
    1. Anorexia nervosa
    2. Bulimia nervosa
    3. Dehydration
    4. Dental caries

12. A new prenatal client is receiving nutrition education. Which should the nurse advise the client to avoid?
    1. Greek yogurt
    2. Grilled cheese sandwich
    3. Bagel with cream cheese
    4. Greek salad with feta cheese

13. A nurse is counseling a client in her third trimester about recommended caloric intake. What is the daily caloric intake that the nurse should recommend?
    1. 1,800 calories
    2. 2,000 calories
    3. 2,200 calories
    4. 2, 400 calories

14. The nurse is teaching a pregnant client about food safety. Which client statement is *most* important for the nurse to discuss?
    1. Platters used for uncooked meats should be washed properly prior to using again.
    2. Sandwiches should be sealed properly prior to serving.
    3. Thaw frozen foods at room temperature before cooking.
    4. Leftovers must be refrigerated within at least 3 hours after serving.

15. An overweight pregnant client is being counseled for obesity. Which statement of the client's indicates that she understands the rationale for reducing her high caloric intake?
    1. "If I don't watch my weight, my baby might develop high blood pressure after he is born."
    2. "Instead of eating so much, I need to take extra vitamins."
    3. "I need to watch my weight so my baby will not be born by cesarean section."
    4. "My being overweight will make my newborn have high blood sugars."

16. The nurse is assessing the hydration status of a 24-week primigravida. The client states that she drinks at least eight glasses of fruit juice per day. Which statement should be made by the nurse?
    1. "Fruit juices are good sources of folic acid."
    2. "To get good hydration, you need to consume eight to ten 8-ounce glasses of water daily."
    3. "You can also drink tea and coffee to get your required water content per day."
    4. "Fruit juice is a good source of water but you need to increase the amount you drink to 10 glasses per day."

17. Infants born to overweight or obese mothers are at greater risk for which complication?
    1. Pica
    2. Childhood obesity
    3. Autism
    4. Anemia

18. What are the *best* nondairy sources of calcium in the diet?
    1. Sardines
    2. Peas
    3. Strawberries
    4. Poultry

19. A client is on a lacto-ovo vegetarian diet. What type of foods would the nurse recommend to the client?
    1. Oysters, yogurt, and turkey
    2. Fish, milk, and poached eggs
    3. Chicken, cheese, and grilled eggplant
    4. Boiled eggs and chocolate milk

20. Which herbs would you counsel a lactating client to use to stimulate blood flow to the breast glands, stimulate milk production, and enrich milk flow?
    1. Milk thistle
    2. Cabbage juice
    3. Lanolin
    4. Aloe vera

REVIEW QUESTION ANSWERS

1. ANSWER: 2
Rationale
1. Macrosomia is associated with an increase in weight gain and gestational diabetes.
2. Inadequate weight gain is associated with an increased risk for giving birth to a low-birth-weight infant.
3. Congenital anomalies are associated with high maternal weight gain early in pregnancy.
4. Giving birth to a low-birth-weight infant does not automatically cause the infant to be admitted to the intensive care unit.

TEST-TAKING TIP: Weight gain is important to ensure normal fetal growth and development, development of maternal organs, and lactation. Adequate weight gain should be approximately 0.5 kg per week in the second and third trimesters for underweight women.
Content Area: Weight Gain During Pregnancy; Maternal Nutrition
Integrated Process: Nursing Process—Assessment
Client Need: Health Promotion and Maintenance—Lifestyle Choices
Cognitive Level: Comprehension
Concept: Nutrition
Reference: Lowdermilk, D. L., Perry, S. E., Cashion, K., & Alden, K. R. (2016). Maternity & women's health care. 11th ed. St. Louis, MO: Elsevier.

2. ANSWER: 1
Rationale
1. Pica is a craving for unusual substances, such as dirt, clay, and chalk.
2. This is the definition of vegetarianism.
3. An unusual craving for fish that contain high levels of mercury is not pica.
4. Pica is not an infectious disease that can cause central nervous system disorders.

TEST-TAKING TIP: Eating nonfood substances is potentially harmful to both client and fetus. Other nonfood substances may be cigarette ashes, baking soda, plaster, coffee grounds, mothballs, toothpaste, and soap.
Content Area: Eating Disorders Affecting Pregnancy; Maternal Nutrition
Integrated Process: Nursing Process—Assessment
Client Need: Health Promotion and Maintenance—High-Risk Behaviors
Cognitive Level: Comprehension
Concept: Diversity
Reference: Lowdermilk, D. L., Perry, S. E., Cashion, K., & Alden, K. R. (2016). Maternity & women's health care. 11th ed. St. Louis, MO: Elsevier.

3. ANSWER: 1
Rationale
1. The client should avoid taking iron with milk or antacids because of decreased absorption.
2. Meats, fish, and poultry contain natural sources of iron.
3. Absorption is increased when taking iron supplements with vitamin C or with orange juice.
4. Fiber and fluids help to prevent constipation, which is a side effect of taking iron supplements.

TEST-TAKING TIP: Iron supplements should be taken 1 hour before or 2 hours after meals with water on an empty stomach. Coffee, tea, milk, dietary fiber, supplemental calcium may interfere with the absorption of iron.
Content Area: Iron; Maternal Nutrition
Integrated Process: Nursing Process—Teaching/Learning
Client Need: Physiological Integrity—Pharmacological and Parenteral Therapies: Medication Administration
Cognitive Level: Application
Concept: Nutrition
Reference: Durham, R. F., & Chapman, L. (2016). Maternal-child nursing care. 2nd ed. Philadelphia: F.A. Davis.

4. ANSWER: 2
Rationale
1. Low or nonfat mozzarella and cottage cheese provide the most protein per calorie; full-fat cheeses typically provide only 1gram protein per 20 calories and are less optimal sources of protein.
2. The bacon and egg sandwich contains the highest amount of protein at about 16 grams.
3. When a protein lacks one or more of the nine essential amino acids, it is known as an incomplete protein. Peanut butter lacks the essential amino acid methionine but is high in lysine. All plant-based proteins are incomplete protein sources except for soy and quinoa.
4. This sandwich is not a good source of protein.

TEST-TAKING TIP: Protein is an essential nutrient. The body is constantly breaking down proteins in cells, organs, and tissues. Protein from the food is broken down into amino acids that replace proteins in your body. A complete protein contains all the essential amino acids the body needs to stay healthy. Review foods containing complete and incomplete protein.
Content Area: Protein; Maternal Nutrition
Integrated Process: Nursing Process—Teaching/Learning
Client Need: Physiological Integrity; Basic Care and Comfort; Nutrition and Oral Hydration
Cognitive Level: Analysis
Concept: Nutrition
Reference: Ward, S. L., & Hisley, S. M. (2016). Maternal-child nursing care. 2nd ed. Philadelphia: F.A. Davis.

5. ANSWER: 4
Rationale
1. Salmon is low in mercury.
2. Catfish, shrimp, and light tuna are good sources of protein and low in mercury.
3. Salmon, light tuna, and cod are good sources of protein and are low in mercury.
4. Species of fish that are long-lived and high on the food chain, such as marlin, tuna, shark, swordfish, king mackerel, tilefish (Gulf of Mexico), and northern pike, contain higher concentrations of mercury than others.

TEST-TAKING TIP: When answers have options that contain two or more facts, identify a fact that is incorrect and eliminate that answer. By deleting distractors, you increase your chance of selecting the correct answer.
Content Area: Mercury; Maternal Nutrition
Integrated Process: Nursing Process—Teaching/Learning

Client Need: Health Promotion and Maintenance—Health Promotion/Disease Prevention
Cognitive Level: Analysis
Reference: Ward, S. L., & Hisley, S. M. (2016). Maternal-child nursing care. 2nd ed. Philadelphia: F.A. Davis.

6. ANSWER: 1
Rationale
1. Listeriosis is a serious infection that a person can get by eating food contaminated with the bacterium *Listeria monocytogenes.* Pregnant women and their developing fetus are particularly susceptible to *Listeria,* which can cause a blood infection, meningitis, and other serious and potentially life-threatening complications.
2. Listeriosis does not cause retinopathy in a newborn.
3. Necrotizing enterocolitis is not caused by listeriosis.
4. Postmaturity is not a result of a pregnant client contacting *Listeria.*

TEST-TAKING TIP: Remember pregnant women should not eat foods with a high risk of *Listeria* contamination. These include hot dogs, lunch meats, or cold cuts served cold or heated to less than 165 degrees; refrigerated pâté and meat spreads; refrigerated smoked seafood; raw (unpasteurized) milk; unpasteurized soft cheeses, such as feta, queso blanco, Brie, and blue-veined cheeses; and unwashed raw produce (when eating raw fruits and vegetables, skin should be washed thoroughly in running tap water, even if it will be peeled or cut).
Content Area: Listeria; Maternal Nutrition
Integrated Process: Nursing Process—Assessment
Client Need: Health Promotion and Maintenance—Lifestyle Choices
Cognitive Level: Analysis
Concept: Nutrition
Reference: Ward, S. L., & Hisley, S. M. (2016). Maternal-child nursing care. 2nd ed. Philadelphia: F.A. Davis.

7. ANSWER: 2, 5
Rationale
1. Pregnant women should eat up to 8 to 12 ounces (two average meals) a week of a variety of fish and shellfish that are lower in mercury. Five of the most commonly eaten fish that are low in mercury are shrimp, canned light tuna, salmon, pollock, and catfish.
2. Because *Listeria* contamination can also occur after food has already been cooked or processed, and the bacteria can survive—and continue to grow—in the refrigerator, heat all previously cooked leftovers to 165°F or until they're steaming hot.
3. Grilled chicken salad with ranch dressing would be an adequate meal for a pregnant client.
4. Pizza with bread sticks would be an adequate meal for a pregnant client.
5. Washing hands, kitchen surfaces, utensils, and fruits and vegetables reduces the risk of bacterial growth.

TEST-TAKING TIP: Remember to educate the client about using a clean food thermometer to make sure the reheated food has reached 165 degrees.
Content Area: Listeria; Maternal Nutrition
Integrated Process: Nursing Process—Teaching/Learning
Client Need: Health Promotion and Maintenance—Health Promotion/Disease Prevention

Cognitive Level: Analysis
Concept: Nutrition
Reference: Lowdermilk, D. L., Perry, S. E., Cashion, K., & Alden, K. R. (2016). Maternity & women's health care. 11th ed. St. Louis, MO: Elsevier.

8. ANSWER: 1
Rationale
1. Ginger helps relieve nausea and vomiting and is safe to take while pregnant.
2. Black cohosh should be avoided during pregnancy.
3. Black haw should be avoided during pregnancy.
4. Aloe vera should be avoided during pregnancy.

TEST-TAKING TIP: Although herbs are natural, not all herbs are safe to take during pregnancy. The FDA urges pregnant women not to take any herbal products without talking to their health care provider first.
Content Area: Herb Supplements; Maternal Nutrition
Integrated Process: Nursing Process—Teaching/Learning
Client Need: Health Promotion and Maintenance—Health Promotion/Disease Prevention
Cognitive Level: Application
Concept: Diversity
Reference: Lowdermilk, D. L., Perry, S. E., Cashion, K., & Alden, K. R. (2016). Maternity & women's health care. 11th ed. St. Louis, MO: Elsevier.

9. ANSWER: 4
Rationale
1. The nurse should not overlook the client's dietary choices.
2. This is not considered a disorder but is a patient choice.
3. Infants of mothers who are strict vegans are at risk for failure to thrive; however, some vegans know how to incorporate the proper supplements into their diet without harming their fetus. It is not the best answer.
4. This response is more accepting of her dietary choice and shows how you can help her maintain a healthy pregnancy with this choice.

TEST-TAKING TIP: The vegan diet includes fruits, vegetables, beans, grains, seeds, and nuts. All animal sources of protein—including meat, poultry, fish, eggs, milk, cheese, and other dairy products—are excluded from the diet.
Content Area: Vegetarian Diets; Maternal Nutrition
Integrated Process: Nursing Process—Planning
Client Need: Health Promotion and Maintenance—Lifestyle Choices
Cognitive Level: Application
Concept: Diversity
Reference: Lowdermilk, D. L., Perry, S. E., Cashion, K., & Alden, K. R. (2016). Maternity & women's health care. 11th ed. St. Louis, MO: Elsevier.

10. ANSWER: 1
Rationale
1. Caraway can cause uterine contractions.
2. This would not be a symptom of food poisoning.
3. This is an inappropriate response by the nurse. The nurse should always assess further if the patient complains of abdominal tightening.
4. This is an inappropriate response.

TEST-TAKING TIP: Herbs are natural substances; however, not all herbs are safe to take during pregnancy. The FDA urges pregnant women to talk to their health care provider before taking any herbal product. Some herbal

products may contain substances that are contraindicated in pregnancy.
Content Area: Herbal Supplements; Maternal Nutrition
Integrated Process: Nursing Process—Assessment
Client Need: Health Promotion and Maintenance—Health Promotion/Disease Prevention
Cognitive Level: Application
Concept: Diversity
Reference: Lowdermilk, D. L., Perry, S. E., Cashion, K., & Alden, K. R. (2016). Maternity & women's health care. 11th ed. St. Louis, MO: Elsevier.

11. **ANSWER: 2**
Rationale
1. Assessment findings of anorexia nervosa would include eating less than needed to maintain a body weight that's at or above the minimum normal weight for age and height, an intense fear of gaining weight or becoming fat, a persistent behavior that interferes with weight gain, and denying the seriousness of having a low body weight.
2. Clients with bulimia nervosa binge eat and then perform self-induced vomiting and diarrhea. The vomiting can lead to a dry scaly tongue with eroded teeth.
3. Dehydration does not cause a dry scaly tongue or eroded teeth.
4. Dental caries is not a clinical finding associated with bulimia nervosa.
TEST-TAKING TIP: Focus on what the question is asking. Think about the clinical manifestation of bulimia nervosa and the induced vomiting, which will cause a dry scaly tongue and eroded teeth.
Content Area: Bulimia Nervosa/Maternal Nutrition
Integrated Process: Nursing Process—Assessment
Client Need: Health Promotion and Maintenance—High-Risk Behaviors
Cognitive Level: Analysis
Concept: Nutrition
Reference: Lowdermilk, D. L., Perry, S. E., Cashion, K., & Alden, K. R. (2016). Maternity & women's health care. 11th ed. St. Louis, MO: Elsevier.

12. **ANSWER: 3**
Rationale
1. Yogurt is an excellent dairy source and can be safely consumed.
2. Hard cheeses such as cheddar and semisoft cheeses such as mozzarella are safe to consume.
3. Pasteurized processed cheese slices and spreads such as cream cheese and cottage cheese can also be safely consumed.
4. The CDC has recommended that pregnant women avoid soft cheeses such as feta, Brie, Camembert, and blue-veined cheeses and Mexican-style cheeses such as queso fresco, queso blanco, and panela that do not state they are pasteurized.
TEST-TAKING TIP: *Listeria monocytogenes* is a type of bacteria that is found in water and soil. Vegetables can become contaminated from the soil, and animals can also be carriers. *Listeria* has been found in uncooked meats, uncooked vegetables, unpasteurized milk, foods made from unpasteurized milk, and processed foods. Listeria is killed by pasteurization and cooking. There is a chance that contamination may occur in ready-to-eat foods such as

hot dogs and deli meats because contamination may occur after cooking and before packaging.
Content Area: Listeria; Maternal Nutrition
Integrated Process: Nursing Process—Teaching/Learning
Client Need: Health Promotion and Maintenance—Health Promotion/Disease Prevention
Cognitive Level: Application
Concept: Nutrition
Reference: Lowdermilk, D. L., Perry, S. E., Cashion, K., & Alden, K. R. (2016). Maternity & women's health care. 11th ed. St. Louis, MO: Elsevier.

13. **ANSWER: 4**
Rationale
1. This is the recommended caloric intake during the first trimester.
2. The client should increase her caloric intake between the first and second trimesters from 1,800 to 2,200 calories daily.
3. This is the recommended caloric intake during the second trimester.
4. This is the recommended caloric intake during the third trimester.
TEST-TAKING TIP: In pregnancy, it is recommended that women increase their daily caloric intake to include a total of 1,800 calories daily during the first trimester, 2,200 calories daily during the second trimester, and about 2,400 calories daily during the third trimester. Review caloric intake for each trimester.
Content Area: Weight Gain During Pregnancy; Maternal Nutrition
Integrated Process: Nursing Process—Teaching/Learning
Client Need: Health Promotion and Maintenance—Health Promotion/Disease Prevention
Cognitive Level: Comprehension
Concept: Nutrition
Reference: Lowdermilk, D. L., Perry, S. E., Cashion, K., & Alden, K. R. (2016). Maternity & women's health care. 11th ed. St. Louis, MO: Elsevier.

14. **ANSWER: 1**
Rationale
1. Dishes that held uncooked meat must be washed properly before cooked foods are placed on them.
2. Sandwiches should be sealed; however, more importantly the nurse should advise the client to reheat until steaming hot prior to eating.
3. Foods should be cooked from the frozen state or thawed in the refrigerator.
4. Leftovers must be refrigerated as soon as the meal is finished.
TEST-TAKING TIP: This question tests the students' ability to provide correct information that needs to be taught to the client. It is very important that the student understands the information so that the client can maintain health and wellness.
Content Area: Listeria; Maternal Nutrition
Integrated Process: Nursing Process—Implementation
Client Need: Health Promotion and Maintenance—Health Promotion/Disease Prevention
Cognitive Level: Application
Concept: Promoting Health
Reference: Durham, R. F., & Chapman, L. (2016). Maternal-child nursing care. 2nd ed. Philadelphia: F.A. Davis.

15. ANSWER: 3

Rationale

1. The pregnant client is at risk for developing high blood pressure.

2. Extra vitamin supplementation will not reduce weight.

3. Babies born to obese mothers are more likely to suffer from macrosomia, or large for gestational age, which can place them at greater risk for birth injuries and other neonatal complications, including stillbirth.

4. Delivering a large for gestational age neonate will put the neonate at risk for hypoglycemia.

TEST-TAKING TIP: This test question is designed to evaluate your ability to identify if teaching was successful regarding obesity and the need for reducing caloric intake. It is important to understand the consequences of improper nutrition and obesity during pregnancy.

Content Area: Weight Gain During Pregnancy; Maternal Nutrition

Integrated Process: Nursing Process—Evaluation

Client Need: Health Promotion and Maintenance—Lifestyle Choices

Cognitive Level: Application

Concept: Nutrition

Reference: Durham, R. F., & Chapman, L. (2016). Maternal-child nursing care. 2nd ed. Philadelphia: F.A. Davis.

16. ANSWER: 1

Rationale

1. Although this is an accurate statement, this is not the appropriate intake for water.

2. Adequate water intake consists of consuming eight to ten 8-ounce glasses of water daily.

3. High levels of caffeine during pregnancy can result in the neonate having a low birth weight. Caffeine should be limited to no more than 200 mg a day.

4. Fruit juice is not an appropriate substitute for water.

TEST-TAKING TIP: General fluid needs increase during pregnancy in order to support fetal circulation, amniotic fluid, and a higher blood volume. The current recommendation for water intake is drinking 8 to 10 glasses of water each day.

Content Area: Water/Maternal Nutrition

Integrated Process: Nursing Process—Teaching/Learning

Client Need: Health Promotion and Maintenance—Health Promotion/Disease Prevention

Cognitive Level: Application

Concept: Promoting Health

Reference: Lowdermilk, D. L., Perry, S. E., Cashion, K., & Alden, K. R. (2016). Maternity & women's health care. 11th ed. St. Louis, MO: Elsevier.

17. ANSWER: 2

Rationale

1. Pica during pregnancy can lead to nutritional deficiencies resulting in preterm birth.

2. Infants born to obese women are also at a greater risk for childhood obesity.

3. Autism is not a risk associated with maternal overweight or obesity.

4. Anemia is not a risk associated with maternal overweight or obesity.

TEST-TAKING TIP: The key term in this question is *at greater risk*. The stem is asking you to identify which option is more important to discuss with the client. Important to know fetal and neonatal risk factors when discussing maternal problems.

Content Area: Weight Gain During Pregnancy; Maternal Nutrition

Integrated Process: Nursing Process—Teaching/Learning

Client Need: Health Promotion and Maintenance—Health Promotion/Disease Prevention

Cognitive Level: Comprehension

Concept: Promoting Health

Reference: Lowdermilk, D. L., Perry, S. E., Cashion, K., & Alden, K. R. (2016). Maternity & women's health care. 11th ed. St. Louis, MO: Elsevier.

18. ANSWER: 1

Rationale

1. Sardines deliver more calcium per serving than virtually any other food, largely because they're full of soft, edible bones. A 3-ounce serving of oil-packed Atlantic sardines provides 175 calories and just over 320 milligrams of calcium.

2. Green peas contain 25 milligrams of calcium per 100 grams. They are not a good source of calcium.

3. Strawberries are not a good source of calcium.

4. Poultry is not as good a source of calcium as sardines.

TEST-TAKING TIP: The daily recommended amount of calcium for a pregnant woman aged 19 or older is 1,000 mg and 1,300 mg for an adolescent. This amount provides adequate calcium for fetal growth while maintaining adequate calcium for the pregnant woman.

Content Area: Calcium/Maternal Nutrition

Integrated Process: Nursing Process—Planning

Client Need: Health Promotion and Maintenance—Health Promotion/Disease Prevention

Cognitive Level: Application

Concept: Pregnancy

Reference: Ward, S. L., & Hisley, S. M. (2016). Maternal-child nursing care. 2nd ed. Philadelphia: F.A. Davis.

19. ANSWER: 4

Rationale

1. Lacto-ovo vegetarianism is the practice of avoiding meat, fish, and poultry while allowing the consumption of dairy and some other animal-based products.

2. Lacto-ovo vegetarianism is the practice of avoiding meat, fish, and poultry while allowing the consumption of dairy and some other animal-based products.

3. Lacto-ovo vegetarianism is the practice of avoiding meat, fish, and poultry while allowing the consumption of dairy and some other animal-based products.

4. Clients on a lacto-ovo vegetarian diet should eat eggs and dairy products but avoid meat, poultry, and seafood.

TEST-TAKING TIP: This question is testing the student's knowledge about the diet of a lacto-ovo vegetarian. Use the process of elimination and knowledge of the diet of a lacto-ovo vegetarian. Answers 1, 2, and 3 can be disregarded because meat, poultry, and seafood can be eliminated.

Content Area: Vegetarian/Maternal Nutrition
Integrated Process: Nursing Process—Planning
Client Need: Health Promotion and Maintenance—Lifestyle Choices
Cognitive Level: Application
Concept: Diversity
Reference: Lowdermilk, D. L., Perry, S. E., Cashion, K., & Alden, K. R. (2016). Maternity & women's health care. 11th ed. St. Louis, MO: Elsevier.

20. **ANSWER: 1**
Rationale
1. Milk thistle has been used to stimulate blood flow to the breast glands and stimulate milk production and enrich milk flow.
2. Cabbage juice does not have any effect on lactation.
3. Lanolin is used by breastfeeding moms experiencing nipple soreness.

4. Aloe vera should be avoided during pregnancy because it has been linked to stimulation of uterine contractions.
TEST-TAKING TIP: Herbs to avoid during pregnancy include aloe vera, black and blue cohosh, and caraway, which have all been linked to stimulating uterine contractions.
Content Area: Herbs During Pregnancy; Maternal Nutrition
Integrated Process: Nursing Process—Teaching/Learning
Client Need: Health Promotion and Maintenance—Health Promotion/Disease Prevention
Cognitive Level: Comprehension
Concept: Diversity
Reference: Lowdermilk, D. L., Perry, S. E., Cashion, K., & Alden, K. R. (2016). Maternity & women's health care. 11th ed. St. Louis, MO: Elsevier.

Chapter 12

Assessment of Fetal Well-Being

KEY TERMS

Acceleration—An abrupt increase in the fetal heart rate (FHR) of at least 15 beats per minute (bpm) and lasting 15 seconds or more above the baseline FHR. If the fetus is 32 weeks or less, an increase of at least 10 bpm for 10 seconds or more is an acceleration.

Amniocentesis—Transabdominal puncture and aspiration of the amniotic sac by ultrasound to remove amniotic fluid

Baseline fetal heart rate—The mean fetal heart rate rounded to 5 bpm observed between contractions over a 10-minute period, excluding accelerations and decelerations. The baseline FHR segment must be greater than 2 minutes of tracing in 10 minutes or it is considered indeterminate.

Biophysical profile—An evaluation of the current fetal status using five variables by ultrasonography and nonstress testing. A specific value (normal = 2, abnormal = 0) is assigned to fetal breathing movements, gross body movement, fetal tone, amniotic fluid volume, and fetal heart rate reactivity.

Bradycardia—A baseline FHR of less than 110 bpm

Contraction stress test (CST)—Assessment of the FHR in response to uterine contractions. A CST is negative if the fetus demonstrates no late or significant **variable decelerations** with uterine contractions. A CST is positive if 50% or more of contractions within the 10-minute tracing produce late decelerations, even if less than three contractions occur.

Deceleration—Decrease in the FHR described as abrupt or gradual in nature. Decelerations may be recurrent (occurring with more than 50% of contractions in a 20-minute period) or intermittent (occurring with less than 50% of contractions in a 20-minute period).

Doppler ultrasound blood flow studies—Using ultrasound to measure blood flow in the uterine artery, umbilical arteries, and fetal middle cerebral artery; indicates vascular status and fetal compensatory responses

Early deceleration—A gradual decrease in the FHR, at least 30 seconds to the nadir (lowest point of the deceleration), that occurs with a uterine contraction. The deceleration begins and ends with the contraction, including the nadir occurring at the peak of the contraction.

Electronic fetal monitoring—An assessment of the FHR and uterine activity that includes an auditory and visual assessment generated by a fetal monitor

Fetal heart rate variability—Irregular fluctuations of the FHR, evaluated over a 10-minute period, excluding periods of accelerations and decelerations; quantified using the amplitude of peak-to-trough in bpm

Fetal scalp blood sampling—A small blood sample taken from the fetal scalp using a capillary tube. The sample is analyzed for the pH level by a blood gas machine.

Intrauterine growth restriction (IUGR)—A decreased rate of fetal growth, most commonly related to inadequate placental perfusion resulting from preexisting or coexisting maternal or placental factors

Late deceleration—A gradual decrease in the FHR, at least 30 seconds to the nadir, which occurs after the

Continued

Assessment of fetal well-being has evolved over the past decades and has become very sophisticated. This chapter will discuss the assessment procedures and how they obtain accurate data about the developing fetus.

I. Ultrasound

Ultrasonography is a safe, noninvasive technique of antepartum fetal assessment using high-frequency sound waves to produce a multidimensional view of the area being scanned. Obstetric ultrasounds may be performed transvaginally or abdominally.
A. Transvaginal ultrasound

A probe covered with a sterile sheath is inserted into the vagina with the patient in a lithotomy position. This method is used to view the pelvic organs and/or an early intrauterine pregnancy. The patient may feel pressure during the ultrasound but generally no pain. First-trimester ultrasounds may be performed to confirm pregnancy, assess gestational age, guide procedures, and determine the source of vaginal bleeding.
B. Abdominal ultrasonography

This assessment requires a full bladder to visualize the uterus in the first 20 weeks of pregnancy. The abdominal method is generally performed during the second and third trimesters. This may be used to evaluate fetal presentation, number of fetuses, anomalies, amniotic fluid volume, cardiac activity, fetal growth, and position of the placenta.

II. Doppler Blood Flow Study

Doppler blood flow studies use noninvasive ultrasound to study the blood flow in the fetus and placenta. The purpose of this ultrasound is to assess placental perfusion and possibly assess a fetus that has **intrauterine growth restriction.** Velocity waveforms are displayed from the umbilical and uterine arteries. These are reported as systolic/diastolic (S/D) ratios that normally decrease as pregnancy progresses due to the declining resistance in the umbilical and uterine arteries. Placental insufficiency is confirmed if the S/D ratio is above the 95th percentile for gestational age or a ratio above 3 or if end-diastolic blood flow is absent or reversed.

DID YOU KNOW?

Intrauterine growth restriction (IUGR) may occur due to placental insufficiency.

III. Amniotic Fluid Volume/Index

Amniotic fluid volume (AFV) measures the vertical depth of the largest pocket of amniotic fluid. Amniotic fluid index (AFI) is the combined total of the deepest amniotic fluid pocket in all four quadrants. A normal AFI is 10 to 25 cm.
A. Hydramnios/polyhydramnios

Excessive amniotic fluid is diagnosed when the vertical depth of the largest pocket of amniotic fluid is greater than 8 cm. Conditions linked to polyhydramnios are fetal hydrops, neural tube anomalies, multiple gestation, and chromosomal anomalies. The AFI measures greater than 25 cm.
B. Oligohydramnios

A reduction in amniotic fluid is diagnosed when the vertical depth of the largest pocket of amniotic fluid is less than 2 cm. Conditions related to oligohydramnios include umbilical cord compression, IUGR, ruptured membranes, and fetal abnormalities. The AFI measures less than 5 cm.

IV. Amniocentesis

In an **amniocentesis,** a needle is inserted transabdominally into the uterine cavity, guided by ultrasound, and amniotic fluid and fetal cells are withdrawn (Fig. 12.1). This procedure is generally performed between 14 and 20 weeks gestation for fetal karyotyping (genetic testing) and assessing the fetus for infection. An amniocentesis may be performed during the third trimester to assess fetal lung maturity. Testing is 99% accurate.
A. Nursing actions
1. Explain the procedure to the client. A full bladder may be necessary if less than 20 weeks gestation.
2. Explain the use of a local anesthetic to minimize discomfort.
3. Provide comfort measures and emotional support during the procedure.

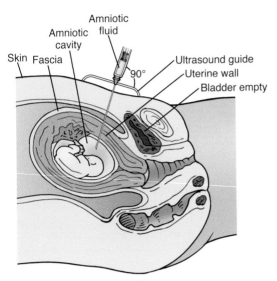

Fig 12.1 Amniocentesis procedure.

4. Prep abdomen with an antiseptic.
5. Assess fetal and maternal well-being pre- and postprocedure.
6. Label specimens that are obtained during procedure.
7. Instruct client to report leaking of fluid, abdominal pain, bleeding, decreased fetal movement, or fever to the care provider.
8. Administer Rh_0D immunoglobulin to Rh-negative women postprocedure as ordered.

> **(!) ALERT** If the client is Rh-negative, then the Rh_0D immunoglobulin is administered after an amniocentesis due to a risk of fetomaternal hemorrhage.

V. Nonstress Test

The **nonstress test (NST)** is a noninvasive antepartum evaluation of fetal well-being (Fig. 12.2). This method of evaluation is widely used since it is inexpensive, easy to perform, and accurate. Fetal movement and fetal heart rate **accelerations** correlate with adequate oxygenation. Normal function of the autonomic nervous system and adequate oxygenation is observed in a fetus through reactivity of the fetal heart rate. The woman is placed in a semi-Fowler's or side-lying position with an ultrasound transducer placed to record the fetal heart rate (FHR). The FHR is recorded for 20 minutes but may be extended to 40 minutes, with the goal of obtaining two FHR accelerations of 15 beats per minute above the baseline, lasting at least 15 seconds each. The NST results are reactive or nonreactive. The preterm fetus (less than 32 weeks) may achieve only two accelerations of 10 bpm above the baseline, lasting at least 10 seconds each to be considered a reactive NST. The NST is reactive if the fetus demonstrates 2 accelerations within a 20-minute tracing.

VI. Vibroacoustic Stimulation

Vibroacoustic stimulation (VAS) is an auditory stimulation method used to elicit an acceleration, increase **fetal heart rate variability,** or change the fetal sleep/wake cycle during an NST or fetal monitoring. After obtaining 5 minutes of baseline, an artificial larynx is placed near the fetal head and the stimulus is applied for 1 to 3 seconds. If no fetal response is observed, the stimulus may be repeated at 1-minute intervals for up to three times.

> **(!) ALERT** Do not use VAS during episodes of **bradycardia** or during a deceleration!

VII. Biophysical Profile (BPP)

The **biophysical profile** is an assessment combining real-time ultrasound with an NST to score five physiological components of the fetus (Table 12.1 and Table 12.2). These components include fetal breathing movement, gross body movement, fetal tone, AFV, and FHR reactivity. An

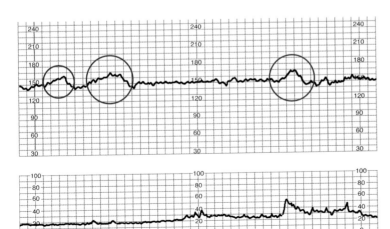

Fig 12.2 Reactive NST.

Table 12.1 Biophysical Profile Scoring

Biophysical Component	Normal Score (2 Points)	Abnormal Score (0 Points)
Fetal breathing movement	Minimum of 1 occurrence of fetal breathing movement in 30 seconds	Absent fetal breathing movement or no occurrences greater than 30 seconds in 30 minutes
Gross body movement	Minimum of 3 body/limb movements in 30 minutes	Less than 3 body/limb movements in 30 minutes
Fetal tone	Minimum of 1 episode of active extension and flexion of fetal limbs/trunk (e.g., opening and closing of hand)	Absent movement; slow extension and return with partial flexion
Reactive FHR	Minimum of 2 FHR accelerations of at least 15 bpm, lasting at least 15 seconds within 30 minutes	Less than 2 accelerations of FHR or accelerations less than 15 bpm within 30 minutes
Qualitative AFV	Minimum of 1 pocket of amniotic fluid that measures at least 2 cm in two perpendicular planes	No amniotic fluid pockets or less than 2 cm in 2 perpendicular planes

Table 12.2 Biophysical Profile Scoring

Score	Interpretation	Treatment
8–10	Reassuring	None (increase frequency of testing with risk factors present)
6	Equivocal	Term—consider delivery Preterm—repeat BPP within 24 hours
4 or less	Nonreassuring	Consider delivery and further evaluation

MAKING THE CONNECTION

Fetal Stress Response

Fetal activity will decrease to preserve energy and oxygen consumption during times of stress, hypoxia, or hypoxemia. As fetal hypoxemia worsens, fetal activity decreases and FHR reactivity will gradually decrease from moderate to minimal with no interventions, to eventually absent. The BPP score will correlate with these findings.

NST is performed with an additional 30 minutes of observation by ultrasound of the other four parameters. Each category is given a score of either 0 or 2. Interventions are based on the overall score. A BPP score of 8 to 10 with adequate AFV indicates normal fetal oxygenation.

VIII. Contraction Stress Test

A **contraction stress test (CST)** or oxytocin challenge test was the first evaluation technique developed to assess the fetus using electronic fetal heart rate monitoring (Table 12.3). The purpose of the test is to detect **late decelerations** with uterine contractions due to chronic uteroplacental insufficiency, which indicates a chronically stressed fetus. However, this test has a high false-positive rate. The CST is positive if the fetus demonstrates late decelerations with at least 50% of the contractions in 10 minutes. The CST is negative if the fetus does not demonstrate any late or significant variables with contractions. Contraindications to the CST include preterm labor,

Table 12.3 Interpreting the Contraction Stress Test

Results	Interpretation	Recommendation
Negative/normal	No late or significant variable decelerations	Routine weekly testing and follow-up
Positive	Late decelerations occur with at least 50% of the contractions, even if fewer than 3 contractions in 10 minutes	Hospital admission, further evaluation, possible delivery
Equivocal–suspicious	Prolonged, variable, or late decelerations occur with less than 50% of the contractions	Repeat testing
Equivocal–hyperstimulatory	Decelerations occur with uterine contractions more frequently than every 2 minutes or lasting longer than 90 seconds	Repeat testing
Equivocal–unsatisfactory	Unable to produce 3 contractions in 10 minutes, or poor FHR tracing	Repeat testing

incompetent cervix, placenta previa, multiple gestations, previous classical uterine incision or extensive uterine surgery, previous uterine rupture, and preterm rupture of membranes. The test may be performed by nipple stimulation or administering exogenous oxytocin.

A. Nursing actions
1. Explain the procedure to the client.
2. Position the patient in semi-Fowler's position.
3. Monitor vital signs before and every 15 minutes during the test.
4. Provide comfort measures and emotional support.
5. Monitor FHR and contractions.
6. If no spontaneous contractions, have patient brush or massage one nipple for 10 minutes. She may apply a warm cloth prior to massaging the nipple.
7. Safely administer oxytocin if nipple stimulation is ineffective. Avoid uterine **tachysystole** (more than five uterine contractions in 10 minutes).

(1) ALERT If the nipple stimulation causes tachysystole (at least 5 contractions within 10 minutes or contractions lasting longer than 90 seconds), have the patient discontinue the stimulation.

IX. Fetal Movement Count (FMC)

A fetal movement count, also called a *fetal kick count,* is considered a cost-effective approach to assessing fetal well-being after 28 weeks gestation. The mother is instructed to count all fetal movements over a specific amount of time and to contact her care provider if a minimum amount of movements are not felt. Teach the woman to lie on her side and count all movements over 1 to 2 hours. If the woman feels a minimum of four movements in 1 hour, the assessment is reassuring. If fetal movement is decreased, the woman should be instructed to eat and rest. Mothers should be taught about factors that may affect fetal activity: exercise, chronic maternal anxiety or stress, smoking, and caffeine use. Nurses should teach women how to record fetal movements and when to report concerns to their care providers.

(1) ALERT If a mother does not feel at least three movements in an hour, she should call her provider for further evaluation.

X. Chorionic Villus Sampling

Chorionic villus sampling is a procedure that removes a tissue specimen from the fetal side of the placenta for genetic studies (karyotyping) and is preferably performed between 10 and 13 weeks gestation. This procedure may be performed using a transabdominal or transcervical method. Chorionic villus sampling is diagnostically as accurate and has similar risks as the amniocentesis.

A. Transcervical
The transcervical procedure is performed by inserting a sterile catheter into the cervix, guided by ultrasound, to aspirate tissue from the fetal side of the placenta.

B. Transabdominal
The transabdominal method is guided by ultrasound and uses a spinal needle with a stylet. A sample of chorionic tissue is obtained once placement is confirmed.

(1) ALERT If the client is Rh-negative, she should receive immunoglobulin after the procedure to prevent isoimmunization. There is always a risk of fetomaternal hemorrhage!

XI. Percutaneous Umbilical Blood Sampling (PUBS)

PUBS is the removal of fetal blood from the umbilical cord, generally during the second trimester of pregnancy. A needle is inserted into the umbilical vein guided by ultrasound and blood is withdrawn to use for diagnostic testing and/or transfusion. The blood may be tested for fetal karyotyping, metabolic disorders, hematological disorders, and infection. Complications are similar to an amniocentesis.

A. Nursing actions
1. Educate the client about the procedure.
2. Position the client laterally to avoid supine hypotension.
3. Assess fetal well-being pre- and postprocedure.
4. Label specimens collected during the procedure.

XII. Fetal Oxygen Saturation Monitoring

Fetal oxygen saturation monitoring, also called *fetal pulse oximetry,* is performed by inserting a small sensor beside the fetal temple or cheek and connecting it to a monitor for continuous readings. The normal range for a healthy fetus 36 weeks gestation or older is between 30% and 70%. To apply the sensor accurately, the mother must have ruptured membranes and the fetus must be in a vertex

---

MAKING THE CONNECTION

Importance in Obtaining Fetal Heart Rate Baseline

Establish a baseline of your fetal heart rate prior to the procedure. This may be difficult to obtain under 24 weeks gestation. If a complication arises postprocedure, you may have difficulty determining a change if you did not evaluate your fetus before the procedure. You may not be able to obtain a tracing with an external fetal monitor; however, you can determine the **baseline fetal heart rate** using a Doppler or ultrasound.

position. This form of monitoring is not widely used and not currently endorsed in clinical practice by the American College of Obstetricians and Gynecologists (ACOG).

XIII. Fetal Scalp Blood Sampling

Fetal scalp blood sampling tests fetal pH, P_{O_2}, and P_{CO_2} levels and is not widely used in the United States. The sample is collected using capillary blood from the fetal scalp, which requires a dilated cervix. There are limitations, which include cervical dilation, rupture of membranes, repetitive testing, difficulty performing procedure, and indecision related to results.

XIV. Electronic Fetal Monitoring

Electronic fetal monitoring (EFM) detects FHR baseline, variability, accelerations, and decelerations for clinicians to evaluate the status of fetal oxygenation. Another major purpose of EFM is for clinicians to observe contraction patterns of pregnant women. EFM may be performed on an intermittent or continuous basis.

A. Monitoring techniques

There are two methods of EFM, which include external and internal monitoring. External monitoring requires the use of a Doppler ultrasound transducer and tocodynamometer, which is applied on the abdomen to record contractions and the FHR. The components used for internal monitoring include a fetal spiral electrode (FSE) and an intrauterine pressure catheter (IUPC). The FSE is inserted into the fetal scalp or presenting part and produces a fetal electrocardiogram. The IUPC is placed into the uterine cavity to monitor uterine contraction frequency, duration, intensity, and resting tone. Internal monitoring is invasive and requires ruptured membranes and a dilated cervix for proper placement. The IUPC and FSE are generally inserted by the practitioner. In some states, the RN may be allowed to insert the IUPC and FSE after competency training.

B. FHR patterns

1. Baseline FHR: The FHR is controlled by the autonomic and central nervous systems. The clinician obtains the FHR baseline by averaging the fetal heart rate between contractions during a 10-minute tracing, excluding periods of marked variability, accelerations, or decelerations. To determine an accurate FHR baseline, the clinician needs at least 2 minutes of baseline data. Also, the mean is rounded to the closest 5 bpm instead of documenting the baseline as a range.

2. Variability: Baseline variability is the fluctuation of the baseline FHR in amplitude and frequency (Table 12.4). The variability is determined by viewing a 10-minute FHR tracing (excluding

accelerations and decelerations) and quantifying the amplitude from peak to trough in bpm.

3. Reassuring FHR
   - Normal FHR baseline: 110 to 160 bpm
   - Baseline FHR variability: moderate
   - No late or variable decelerations (Table 12.5)
   - **Early decelerations** may or may not be present.
   - Accelerations may or may not be present.

4. Nursing management and intrauterine resuscitation

   Intrauterine resuscitation techniques are used for abnormal FHR patterns. The goal is to promote fetal oxygenation, maximize uterine and umbilical blood flow, and support labor progress. The nurse should understand which techniques to implement based on the FHR pattern. For example, a nurse should reposition a patient in an attempt to resolve an umbilical cord compression causing variable decelerations (Box 12.1).

Table 12.4 Degrees of FHR Variability

Degree	Description
Absent	Undetectable amplitude
Minimal	Amplitude range 5 bpm or fewer (visually detectable)
Moderate	Amplitude range 6–25 bpm
Marked	Amplitude range greater than 25 bpm
Sinusoidal	Smooth, sine wavelike undulating pattern, cycling 3–5 minutes at a time and persisting for at least 20 minutes

Table 12.5 Types of FHR Decelerations

Type	Description
Early deceleration	A *gradual* decrease and return of the FHR associated with a uterine contraction. To be gradual, the onset to the nadir (lowest point of the FHR drop), is at least 30 seconds. The lowest point of the deceleration occurs at the peak of the contraction. This deceleration mirrors the contraction.
Late deceleration	A *gradual* decrease and return of the FHR associated with a uterine contraction. The deceleration is delayed and the nadir occurs *after* the peak of the contraction.
Variable deceleration	An *abrupt* decrease in the FHR of at least 15 bpm and lasting at least 15 seconds. To be abrupt, the onset to the nadir is less than 30 seconds.
Prolonged deceleration	A decrease in the FHR from the baseline that is at least 15 bpm, lasting longer than 2 minutes but less than 10 minutes.

Intrauterine Resuscitation Techniques

Maternal reposition
Reduce uterine activity
IV fluid bolus
Correct maternal hypotension
Administer oxygen
Amnioinfusion
Discontinue oxytocin
Discontinue or modify pushing

5. Leopold's maneuvers

Leopold's maneuvers include a four-part assessment method that involves abdominal palpation by the clinician (Fig. 12.3). The assessment determines the fetal part in the fundus, location of the fetal back, fetal presentation (Pawlik's maneuver), and fetal position. By determining the fetal position, the clinician can identify the location to auscultate fetal heart tones, which is the fetal back. The practitioner uses the palmar surface of the hands using gentle but firm pressure.

a) First maneuver: The first maneuver is performed to determine whether the fetal head or buttocks are positioned in the uterine fundus. The practitioner faces the woman's head and places the hands on the top and side of the fundus with focus on the upper region. The head feels firm and round. The buttocks feel soft and less defined.

b) Second maneuver: The second maneuver assesses the location of the fetal back. The clinician continues to face the woman. One hand is placed on the side of the abdomen to stabilize the fetus during palpation. The other hand is used to palpate the fetal spine down the side, which will feel firm and consistent. The small parts will feel irregular or protruding; fetal kicks may possibly be noted.

c) Third maneuver: The third maneuver, also called *Pawlik's maneuver,* identifies the presenting part and is performed with the clinician facing the woman. The middle finger and thumb are used to grasp the part of the fetus situated in the lower uterine segment or pelvic brim. The clinician determines whether the head or buttocks are the presenting part.

d) Fourth maneuver: The fourth maneuver is performed with the clinician facing the woman's feet. Both hands are placed on the sides of the uterus and move in a downward motion toward the symphysis pubis. The fingertips press deeply toward the pelvic inlet to feel for the fetal head (if the fetus is in a cephalic position). If the presenting part does not move, the fetus is engaged. If the presenting part is moveable, engagement has not occurred.

(!) **ALERT** Leopold's maneuvers should be performed without the woman in a supine position. Slightly elevate her head and place a wedge under one hip to avoid compression of the maternal vena cava.

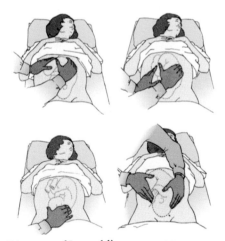

Fig 12.3 Diagram of Leopold's maneuver.

CASE STUDY: Putting It All Together

Mrs. Martin, age 38, is currently 34 weeks gestation and is a gravida 3, para 2. She was diagnosed this pregnancy with gestational diabetes, which is controlled by diet. Mrs. Martin's physician has sent her to the L&D unit for an NST today and repeat NST twice a week until delivery.

Objective Data

Vital signs
Blood pressure: 136/72
Pulse: 85
Respiration: 20
Temperature: 98.2
Level of consciousness: Awake, alert, and oriented times three
Fundal height: 39 cm

Subjective Data

Mrs. Martin stated previously that she has been working long hours, often skipping lunch to get off work in time to get her other kids after school. She isn't sure if she can come twice a week for these tests. She also asks, "My baby hasn't been moving much the last two days, so is that why my doctor wants me to have this test?" Mrs. Martin was monitored for 45 minutes with external monitors. The tracing of the fetal heart rate was 135 bpm baseline, no accelerations, moderate variability, no decelerations. Mrs. Martin's fetal surveillance during her stay in Labor and Delivery concluded that the fetus was not in distress.

Case Study Questions

1. Why was Mrs. Martin scheduled for this test?

2. Was this NST reactive or nonreactive? Give rationale for your answer.

3. What further testing would you anticipate being ordered? Why?

4. Discharge instructions included fetal kick counts. How would you explain this test to Mrs. Martin?

REVIEW QUESTIONS

Be sure to read the Introduction for valuable test-taking tips.

1. The nurse is caring for a client who is scheduled to have an amniocentesis. Which intervention is *most* important for the nurse to perform after the procedure?
   1. Evaluate need for Rh_0D immunoglobulin
   2. Clean site
   3. Administer pain medication
   4. Perform vital signs

2. An NST is performed on a client who is G6T3P1A1L4 38 weeks gestation. After the patient has been on the external monitor for 30 minutes, the nurse sees three fetal heart rate accelerations of 15 bpm lasting 5 seconds in association with fetal movement. The nurse documents this finding as which of the following?
   1. Unsatisfactory
   2. A reactive NST
   3. A nonreactive nonstress test
   4. Equivocal–suspicious

3. A client with diabetes mellitus is at 37 weeks gestation. She has had weekly NSTs for the last 3 weeks, and the results have been reactive. This week, the NST was nonreactive after 40 minutes. The nurse anticipates which of the following will be performed for the client based on these results?
   1. Scheduled for an immediate ultrasound
   2. Scheduled for a biophysical profile
   3. Admitted to the hospital for induction of labor
   4. Scheduled for a follow-up appointment for NST in 2 days

4. The nurse is caring for a client with a suspected breech presentation. When the nurse performs Leopold's maneuvers, which maneuvers determine the fetal presentation? *Select all that apply.*
   1. First
   2. Second
   3. Third (Pawlik's maneuver)
   4. Fourth
   5. All maneuvers

5. The nurse is preparing to teach a client how to perform daily fetal kick counts. Which instruction is *most* important for the nurse to give the client?
   1. Count fetal kicks prior to eating a meal
   2. Lie on back when counting kicks
   3. Call provider if at least three movements are not felt in 1 hour
   4. Count all movements over 1 hour

6. The nurse is caring for a pregnant client who was sent to the hospital for a biophysical profile. She is 37 weeks gestation with her second child, has gestational diabetes, and complains of decreased fetal movement for the last 24 hours. Which action should the nurse take *first*?
   1. Perform vital signs
   2. Call physician
   3. Perform glucose
   4. Place on fetal monitor

7. The nurse is admitting a client, who reports, "My water broke yesterday, and I haven't felt my baby move any today." She is 38 weeks with a history of gestational diabetes. Which assessment data is of *most* concern to the nurse on admission?
   1. Maternal vital signs: T 100.2, HR 104, RR 20, BP 136/82
   2. Pain score 6/10
   3. Minimal variability and variable decelerations
   4. 5 cm/80% effaced/0 station

8. The nurse is caring for a client who had a contraction stress test. Which change in assessment requires immediate notification of the health care provider?
   1. No late decelerations
   2. Late decelerations with at least 50% of the contractions
   3. Accelerations with contractions
   4. No contractions produced

9. The nurse reports a nonreactive NST to the physician. The physician orders vibroacoustic stimulation. Which does the nurse understand the appropriate application for the vibroacoustic stimulation to be? *Select all that apply.*
   1. Clap loudly by the fetal head
   2. Apply a sterile drape to abdomen prior to stimulation
   3. Apply the artificial larynx stimulus by the fetal head
   4. Limit the use of the artificial larynx stimulus to three times
   5. Do not apply the stimulus during episodes of bradycardia or during a deceleration.

10. The nurse is caring for a client being monitored for oligohydramnios. The NST is nonreactive. Which findings correlate with these results?
   1. Less than 2 accelerations in 20 to 40 minutes
   2. Accelerations of at least 15 bpm lasting at least 15 seconds (more than 32 weeks gestation)
   3. Accelerations of at least 10 bpm lasting at least 10 seconds (less than 32 weeks gestation)
   4. Four accelerations in 20 to 40 minutes

11. Which laboratory is important to know when a client is having an amniocentesis?
    1. Blood type
    2. CBC
    3. Rh
    4. PT and PTT

12. A client presents to Labor & Delivery for an ultra-sound at 16 weeks gestation for vaginal bleeding. She asks the nurse if the procedure will harm her baby. Which is appropriate for the nurse to tell the client?
    1. "Since you are already bleeding, we cannot guarantee that the ultrasound will not have any negative effects on your pregnancy."
    2. "Ultrasounds use sound waves to view your baby, not radiation, so the procedure will not harm your baby."
    3. "There are no guarantees when you have a proce-dure performed."
    4. "The doctor wouldn't try to order a test that would hurt your baby."

13. The nurse has admitted a client who is 30 weeks gestation with suspected intrauterine growth restriction. The physician has ordered a Doppler blood flow study. What does the nurse suspect if the results show an S/D ratio above the 95th percentile for the gestational age, a ratio above 3, or end-diastolic blood flow that is absent or reversed?
    1. Decreased blood pressure
    2. Placental insufficiency
    3. Increased amniotic fluid
    4. Decreased fetal movement

14. The nurse is caring for a 45-year-old client who is scheduled to have a chorionic villus sampling. Which information is *most* important for the nurse to obtain from the client before the procedure?
    1. NPO status
    2. Blood type and Rh
    3. Weeks of gestation
    4. Maternal bleeding disorders

15. The nurse is teaching her client about the methods of electronic fetal monitoring during labor. Her client asks which method has the fewest risks to her baby and allows her the most freedom. What is the most appropriate response by the nurse?
    1. "Internal and external monitoring have equal risks. You will have to remain in the bed with both of these methods."
    2. "Internal monitoring is a more invasive method, but we only use internal monitoring if we have difficulty obtaining accurate information with external monitoring."
    3. "External monitoring will allow you the most freedom of movement and does not require any invasive procedures for you or your baby."
    4. "External monitoring is not invasive but you have to remain in the bed."

16. The nurse is preparing to assist with the insertion of an intrauterine pressure catheter and a fetal spiral electrode. What is required for proper placement by the practitioner? *Select all that apply.*
    1. Rupture of membranes
    2. Dilated cervix
    3. Vertex fetus
    4. Moderate variability
    5. Late decelerations

17. The nurse is caring for a client in labor with her third baby. She is 39 weeks gestation, 6 cm dilated, 80% effaced, and 0 station, with minimal variability and recurrent variable decelerations. What action is the *highest* priority for the nurse?
    1. Administer oxygen
    2. Change maternal position
    3. Perform fetal scalp stimulation
    4. Perform vaginal examination

18. The nurse is evaluating a client's response to a contraction stress test. The client performed nipple stimulation and produced 2 contractions in 10 min-utes. The fetus demonstrated no late decelerations. The nurse notifies the practitioner regarding which results of the CST?
    1. They are positive.
    2. They are negative.
    3. They are equivocal–suspicious.
    4. They are equivocal–unsatisfactory.

19. The nurse is caring for a client in labor and notices a gradual decrease in the FHR that occurs after the peak of the contraction and returns to baseline 30 seconds after the contraction ends. The nurse is aware that this is which type of periodic change in the FHR?
    1. Prolonged deceleration
    2. Acceleration
    3. Early deceleration
    4. Late deceleration

20. The nurse assesses uterine contractions using the intrauterine pressure catheter. Which information can be obtained from the IUPC?
    1. FHR, contraction frequency, contraction intensity, acceleration
    2. Contraction intensity, late deceleration, variable deceleration, uterus resting tone
    3. Contraction frequency, contraction duration, contraction intensity, uterus resting tone
    4. Uterus resting tone, fundal height, contraction intensity, contraction frequency

REVIEW QUESTION ANSWERS

1. ANSWER: 1
Rationale

1. During the procedure, there is a risk of maternal and fetal blood mixing. If a woman is Rh-negative, she should be given RhoGAM after the amniocentesis to prevent her Rh-negative antibodies from reacting to Rh-positive fetal cells.
2. After the procedure, the nurse should clean any prepping solution from the client's abdomen. However, this would not be considered the most important intervention.
3. A local anesthetic may be used prior to the amniocentesis to minimize discomfort, but pain medication after the procedure should not be necessary.
4. Maternal vital signs and fetal heart rate should be taken prior to the amniocentesis. After the procedure, the fetal heart rate should be monitored to assess for fetal distress.

TEST-TAKING TIP: Always identify the key word in the stem that sets priority, such as *most important*. If woman is Rh-negative, the Rh_0D immunoglobulin is administered after a procedure. Not administering may result in mixing of the maternal and fetal blood and increasing the risk of fetomaternal hemorrhage.

Cognitive Level: Application
Client Needs: Health Promotion and Maintenance; Disease Prevention
Integrated Process: Nursing Process—Implementation
Content Area: Amniocentesis; Antepartum
Concept: Pregnancy
Reference: Perry, S. E., Hockenberry, M. F., Lowdermilk, D. L., & Wilson, D. (2014). Maternal child nursing care. 5th ed. St. Louis, MO: Elsevier.

2. ANSWER: 2
Rationale

1. An unsatisfactory test cannot be interpreted because of the inadequate FHR tracing data or the absence of fetal movement.
2. A reactive nonstress test indicates a well-oxygenated fetus.
3. A nonreactive NST is described as less than two accelerations or accelerations of less than 15 beats per minute or lasting less than 15 seconds in duration with any fetal movement.
4. This term is used when interpreting a CST.

TEST-TAKING TIP: Use the process of elimination. Answer 3 can be eliminated because it does not contain the name of the test you are performing. From the remaining options, remember that a reactive NST shows that the fetus is reacting to movement. It is described as two or more FHR accelerations of at least 15 bpm, lasting at least 15 seconds from the beginning of the acceleration to the end of the acceleration in a 20-minute period.

Cognitive Level: Application
Client Needs: Health Promotion and Maintenance; Antepartum Care
Integrated Process: Nursing Process—Implementation
Content Area: NST; Antepartum
Concept: Pregnancy
Reference: Perry, S. E., Hockenberry, M. F., Lowdermilk, D. L., & Wilson, D. (2014). Maternal child nursing care. 5th ed. St. Louis, MO: Elsevier.

3. ANSWER: 2
Rationale

1. The abdominal ultrasound is generally performed during the second and third trimesters to evaluate fetal presentation, number of fetuses, anomalies, AFV, cardiac activity, fetal growth, and position of the placenta. Ultrasound is one component of a biophysical profile. The scoring system of the biophysical profile will give the health care professional more information as fetal well-being.
2. A biophysical profile will provide additional information concerning fetal well-being.
3. There is not enough data in the questions to indicate that immediate delivery of the fetus is necessary.
4. Repeating the NST at a later time is not a safe intervention, especially considering that the previous test results were reactive and the one performed today was not reactive and may put the fetus in jeopardy.

TEST-TAKING TIP: Always focus on the issue, which in this stem is a change in test results from reactive to nonreactive. Option 4 can be eliminated because repeating the NST at a later time is not a safe intervention. An ultrasound is part of the biophysical profile; however, it does not include a scoring system to guide further interventions. A BPP is a prenatal ultrasound evaluation of fetal well-being involving a scoring system. It is often done when an NST is nonreactive or for other obstetrical indications.

Cognitive Level: Analysis
Client Needs: Physiological Integrity; Reduction of Risk Potential; Diagnostic Test
Integrated Process: Nursing Process—Planning
Content Area: NST; Antepartum
Concept: Pregnancy
Reference: Durham, R. F., & Chapman, L. (2014). Maternal-newborn nursing: The critical components of nursing care. 2nd ed. Philadelphia: F.A. Davis.

4. ANSWER: 1, 3
Rationale

1. The first maneuver is performed to determine whether the fetal head or buttocks are positioned in the uterine fundus.
2. The second maneuver assesses the location of the fetal back. This maneuver does not take into consideration the presenting part.
3. This maneuver identifies the presenting part and is performed with the clinician facing the woman.
4. This maneuver is assessing engagement of the presenting part. If the presenting part does not move, the fetus is engaged. If the presenting part is moveable, engagement has not occurred. The presenting part could be the fetus's head, buttock, or shoulder.
5. All maneuvers combined determine fetal lie, position, presentation, and the best site to auscultate FHR.

TEST-TAKING TIP: Use the process of elimination. Recalling the purpose and procedure of Leopold's maneuvers will eliminate answers 2 and 4. From the remaining options, it is necessary to know that options 1 and 3 will determine fetal lie.

Cognitive Level: Application
Client Needs: Health Promotion and Maintenance; Antepartum Care

Integrated Process: Nursing Process—Assessment
Content Area: Leopold's Maneuvers; Antepartum
Concept: Pregnancy
Reference: London, M. L., Ladewig, P. A., Davidson, M. R., Ball, J. W., Bindler, R. C., & Cowen, K. J. (2014). Maternal & child nursing care. 4th ed. New Jersey: Pearson.

5. **ANSWER: 3**
Rationale
1. The best time to count fetal kicks is 1 hour after a meal.
2. Lie in a side-lying position.
3. It is very important for the nurse to discuss with the client how to record fetal movements and when to report concerns.
4. Movement varies with each fetus. The client should be instructed that fetal movements should be felt at least 10 times in a 3-hour period.

TEST-TAKING TIP: The question is associating four specific teaching points to the client. The three that involve teaching on how to monitor for fetal movement are incorrect. When to call the provider is always a priority. Review all teaching points regarding fetal kick counts.

Cognitive Level: Application
Client Needs: Health Promotion; Self-Care
Integrated Process: Nursing Process—Education
Content Area: Fetal Kick Counts; Antepartum
Concept: Pregnancy
Reference: London, M. L., Ladewig, P. A., Davidson, M. R., Ball, J. W., Bindler, R. C., & Cowen, K. J. (2014). Maternal & child nursing care. 4th ed. New Jersey: Pearson.

6. **ANSWER: 4**
Rationale
1. If the client was in physical distress, then maternal vital signs would be appropriate for the initial assessment.
2. The nurse must first gather assessment data prior to calling the physician.
3. The client's complaints are of decreased fetal movement, not signs and symptoms of hypo- or hyperglycemia.
4. A significant reduction or sudden alteration in fetal movement is an important clinical sign of fetal well-being. The nurse should immediately place a fetal monitor on the client for assessment data and immediate intervention if necessary.

TEST TAKING TIP: In the stem of the question, always note *who* the question's referring to—the mother or the fetus. In this question, it clearly states the chief complaint is decreased fetal movement, so immediate assessment would be to evaluate fetal heart tones. Answers 1 and 3 would be assessment directed to the mother. You would call the physician when you had assessment data to report.

Cognitive Level: Application
Client Needs: Health Promotion and Maintenance
Integrated Process: Nursing Process—Assessment
Content Area: Decreased Fetal Movement; Antepartum
Concept: Pregnancy
Reference: London, M. L., Ladewig, P. A., Davidson, M. R., Ball, J. W., Bindler, R. C., & Cowen, K. J. (2014). Maternal & child nursing care. 4th ed. New Jersey: Pearson.

7. **ANSWER: 3**
Rationale
1. The client would not be considered febrile until her temperature is 100.4. She does have tachycardia; however, she is in active labor and her pain score is 6/10. Her respiration rate and blood pressure are within normal limits.
2. The client is in active labor, so you would expect her pain score to be high.
3. Variable decelerations mean cord compression and may warrant only turning the patient to her left side. Persistently minimal or absent FHR variability appears to be the most significant intrapartum sign of fetal compromise.
4. This assessment information indicates that the client is in active labor. The client is term (38 weeks gestation), so this would not be the most concerning piece of assessment data.

TEST-TAKING TIP: Answering a test question that asks you to establish a priority (i.e., which is most important, best, initial, and first) requires you to make a decision using clinical judgment. The question in option 4 requires you to use critical thinking to arrive at the correct answer. The key concept in this question is which piece of assessment would be of most concern to the nurse. The key phrase in the question is, "My water broke yesterday, and I haven't felt my baby move any today." To pick the correct option, you would choose the data that directly relates to what is happening.

Cognitive Level: Analysis
Client Needs: Safe and Effective Care Environment; Management of Care
Integrated Process: Nursing Process—Assessment
Content Area: Decreased Fetal Movement; Antepartum
Concept: Pregnancy
Reference: London, M. L., Ladewig, P. A., Davidson, M. R., Ball, J. W., Bindler, R. C., & Cowen, K. J. (2014). Maternal & child nursing care. 4th ed. New Jersey: Pearson.

8. **ANSWER: 2**
Rationale
1. This is the desired result. A negative CST exists when three contractions of good quality last 40 or more seconds in 10 minutes without evidence of late decelerations.
2. This is not a desired result. A positive CST exists when there are repetitive persistent late decelerations with more than 50% of the contractions. The health care provider would need to be contacted with the results of the CST.
3. Accelerations are short-term rises in the heart rate of at least 15 bpm, lasting at least 15 seconds. Accelerations are normal and indicate that the fetus has adequate oxygen supply.
4. This is not a valid CST because no contractions were produced.

TEST-TAKING TIP: Identify the key word in the stem that sets priority, such as *immediate notification*. A CST is performed near the end of pregnancy to determine how well the fetus will cope with the contractions of labor and birth. During uterine contractions, fetal oxygenation is decreased. Late decelerations in FHR occurring during uterine contractions are associated with increased fetal death rate, growth retardation, and neonatal depression. This CST assesses FHR in response to uterine contractions via electronic fetal monitoring and tocodynamometer.

Cognitive Level: Analysis
Client Needs: Safe and Effective Care Environment; Management of Care
Integrated Process: Nursing Process—Intervention

Content Area: Contraction Stress Test; Antepartum
Concept: Pregnancy
Reference: Durham, R. F., & Chapman, L. (2014). Maternal-newborn nursing: The critical components of nursing care. 2nd ed. Philadelphia: F.A. Davis.

9. **ANSWER: 3, 4, 5**
Rationale
1. Clapping loudly will not stimulate the fetus to move.
2. This is not a sterile procedure.
3. Fetal vibroacoustic stimulation is a simple, noninvasive technique where a device is placed on the maternal abdomen over the region of the fetal head and sound is emitted at a predetermined level for several seconds.
4. The fetal vibroacoustic sound stimulus should be activated for 2 to 5 seconds; if no accelerations occur, it is then repeated at 1-minute intervals for up to three times.
5. Application of the fetal vibroacoustic stimulator is contraindicated during episodes of bradycardia or during a deceleration.

TEST-TAKING TIP: When answering a "select all that apply" question, realize this is actually a "true or false" type of question! Therefore, you proceed to answer each option by responding either with a yes or a no, or whether it applies or does not apply to what the question is asking. Go down the list one by one and ask yourself if it is a correct answer; then look at the next choice and do the same thing. Treat each choice as a possible answer separate to the other choices. Don't group or link the choices to one another. They should not be answered as a group.
Cognitive Level: Application
Client Needs: Health Promotion and Maintenance; Reduction of Risk Potential
Integrated Process: Nursing Process—Intervention
Content Area: Vibroacoustic Stimulation; Antepartum
Concept: Pregnancy
Reference: Durham, R. F., & Chapman, L. (2014). Maternal-newborn nursing: The critical components of nursing care. 2nd ed. Philadelphia: F.A. Davis.

10. **ANSWER: 1**
Rationale
1. A nonreactive test is when there are less than two accelerations that occur within a 20-minute period.
2. A reactive NST is when accelerations of at least 15 bpm last at least 15 seconds (greater than 32 weeks gestation).
3. A reactive NST is when accelerations of at least 10 bpm last at least 10 seconds (less than 32 weeks gestation).
4. Four accelerations in 20 to 40 minutes would be considered a reactive or "reassuring" test.

TEST-TAKING TIP: Always focus on the issue, which in this stem is the parameters of a nonreactive test. Options 2, 3, and 4 all indicate a reactive test. Before week 32 of pregnancy, results are considered normal (reactive) if the fetus heartbeat accelerates to a certain level twice or more for at least 10 seconds each within a 20-minute window. At week 32 of pregnancy or later, the fetus's heartbeat should accelerate to a certain level twice or more for at least 15 seconds each within a 20-minute window; the results are considered reactive.
Cognitive Level: Application
Client Needs: Physiological Integrity; Reduction of Risk Potential

Integrated Process: Nursing Process—Assessment
Content Area: NST; Antepartum
Concept: Pregnancy
Reference: Perry, S. E., Hockenberry, M. F., Lowdermilk, D. L., & Wilson, D. (2014). Maternal child nursing care. 5th ed. St. Louis, MO: Elsevier.

11. **ANSWER: 3**
Rationale
1. A blood type is a classification of blood based on the presence or absence of inherited antigenic substances on the surface of red blood cells. Human blood is grouped into four types: A, B, AB, and O. Each letter refers to a kind of antigen, or protein, on the surface of red blood cells.
2. A complete blood count (CBC) is a blood test used to evaluate a client's overall health and detect a wide range of disorders and consists of several components such as red blood cells, white blood cells, hemoglobin, hematocrit, and platelets.
3. The Rh system is the second most significant blood-group system in human-blood transfusion. Rh immunoglobulin after amniocentesis helps to prevent the mother from producing antibodies against fetal blood cells.
4. Partial thromboplastin time (PTT) is a blood test that measures the time it takes a client's blood to clot. A PTT test can be used to check for bleeding problems.

TEST-TAKING TIP: Focus on the subject (amniocentesis). If the stem mentioned that the client was bleeding or had an infection, then the other options would apply. Remember that if a client has an Rh-negative blood type (i.e., A, B, AB, or O negative), she should be given an intramuscular shot called Rh(D) immune globulin (RhoGAM) after amniocentesis. This shot helps protect future pregnancies against problems that can develop if the client is Rh-negative and is pregnant with a fetus who is Rh-positive.
Cognitive Level: Application
Client Needs: Physiological Integrity; Reduction of Risk Potential
Integrated Process: Nursing Process—Assessment
Content Area: Amniocentesis; Antepartum
Concept: Pregnancy
Reference: Perry, S. E., Hockenberry, M. F., Lowdermilk, D. L., & Wilson, D. (2014). Maternal child nursing care. 5th ed. St. Louis, MO: Elsevier.

12. **ANSWER: 2**
Rationale
1. This is not a patient-centered response and is inaccurate for the procedure.
2. This response is patient-centered because it gives the client correct information.
3. This is not a patient-centered response. The role of the nurse is to be a patient advocate and to alleviate anxiety.
4. This is not a patient-centered response. Risks and benefits are discussed for tests/procedures.

TEST-TAKING TIP: Use knowledge of therapeutic communication techniques. First eliminate options that do not support the patient's expression of feelings. Any option that is not patient centered should be eliminated next. Option 4 minimize the patient's concerns because it implies there is nothing to worry about. Focusing on the patient's feelings will direct you to the correct option.

Cognitive Level: Analysis
Client Needs: Health Promotion and Maintenance
Integrated Process: Nursing Process—Assessment
Content Area: Ultrasound; Antepartum
Concept: Pregnancy
Reference: Perry, S. E., Hockenberry, M. F., Lowdermilk, D. L., & Wilson, D. (2014). Maternal child nursing care. *5th ed.* St. Louis, MO: Elsevier.

13. ANSWER: 2
Rationale
1. Doppler blood flow studies do not assess blood pressure.
2. The purpose of this ultrasound is to assess placental perfusion and possibly assess if the fetus has intrauterine growth restriction. Velocity waveforms are displayed from the umbilical and uterine arteries. These are reported as systolic/diastolic (S/D) ratios that normally decrease as pregnancy progresses due to the declining resistance in the umbilical and uterine arteries. Placental insufficiency is confirmed if the S/D ratio is above the 95th percentile for gestational age or a ratio above 3 or if end-diastolic blood flow is absent or reversed.
3. Increased amniotic fluid is measured by ultrasound.
4. Decreased fetal movement is detected by fetal kick counts.
TEST-TAKING TIP: Focus on the subject—Doppler blood flow studies. Recall knowledge of the reason for study and what the results indicate.
Cognitive Level: Application
Client Needs: Physiological Integrity; Reduction of Risk Potential
Integrated Process: Nursing Process—Assessment
Content Area: Doppler blood flow studies; Antepartum
Concept: Pregnancy
Reference: Durham, R. F., & Chapman, L. (2014). Maternal-newborn nursing: The critical components of nursing care. *2nd ed. Philadelphia: F.A. Davis.*

14. ANSWER: 2
Rationale
1. Chorionic villus sampling does not require the client to be NPO.
2. If the client is Rh-negative, she should receive immunoglobulin after the procedure to prevent isoimmunization. There is always a risk of fetomaternal hemorrhage.
3. Weeks of gestation is important because the test is usually performed between 10 and 12 weeks gestation. However, the priority information the nurse should obtain is blood type and Rh.
4. Maternal bleeding disorders would not be a contraindication for having this procedure.
TEST-TAKING TIP: Identify key words in the stem that set a priority: *first, initially, best, safest, most.* Next rank all options in order of importance and eliminate the lower information.
Cognitive Level: Analysis
Client Needs: Safe and Effective Care Environment; Management of Care
Integrated Process: Nursing Process—Assessment
Content Area: Chorionic Villus Sampling; Antepartum
Concept: Pregnancy
Reference: London, M. L., Ladewig, P. A., Davidson, M. R., Ball, J. W., Bindler, R. C., & Cowen, K. J. (2014). Maternal & child nursing care. *4th ed.* New Jersey: Pearson.

15. ANSWER: 3
Rationale
1. False statement. Internal monitoring has more risks associated with the procedure than external monitoring. External monitoring allows freedom of movement, whereas with internal monitoring the client has to stay in bed and is not allowed to get up.
2. Internal monitoring is a more invasive method and is used only if there is difficulty obtaining accurate information with external monitoring. However, the client is not only asking about risk to baby but also freedom of movement.
3. This answer addresses the concern of the client and is an accurate statement.
4. External monitoring is not invasive and allows freedom of movement.
TEST-TAKING TIP: Focus on what is being asked by the client in the stem. Begin by eliminating options 1 and 4 because they are false statements. Option 2 is a true statement but does not address what the client is asking, which is what method has the fewest risks to her baby and allows her more freedom of movement.
Cognitive Level: Application
Client Needs: Health Promotion and Maintenance
Integrated Process: Nursing Process—Education
Content Area: Fetal Monitoring; Antepartum
Concept: Pregnancy
Reference: London, M. L., Ladewig, P. A., Davidson, M. R., Ball, J. W., Bindler, R. C., & Cowen, K. J. (2014). Maternal & child nursing care. *4th ed.* New Jersey: Pearson.

16. ANSWER: 1, 2
Rationale
1. To place internal monitoring (fetal spiral electrode and intrauterine pressure catheter), the amniotic membranes must be ruptured and the cervix must be dilated at least 2 cm.
2. To place internal monitoring (fetal spiral electrode and intrauterine pressure catheter), the amniotic membranes must be ruptured and the cervix must be dilated at least 2 cm.
3. If fetal presenting part is unable to be identified, internal fetal scalp electrodes should not be placed over fontanelles, genitalia, or the face. The presenting part must be down against the cervix and the presenting part must be known to the examiner.
4. Moderate variability is not a criteria for placing internal monitors. Internal monitoring may be used when external monitoring of the FHR and contractions tracings are inadequate or closer surveillance is needed.
5. Internal monitoring may be placed for late decelerations. However, internal monitoring may also be used when external monitoring of the fetal heart rate and contractions tracing is inadequate.
TEST-TAKING TIP: Remember internal RHR monitoring uses an electronic transducer connected directly to the presenting part. A wire electrode is attached through the cervical opening and is connected to the monitor. This type of electrode is sometimes called *spiral* or *scalp electrode.* Internal monitoring provides a more accurate and consistent transmission of the FHR than

external monitoring because factors such as movement do not affect it. Internal monitoring may be used when external monitoring of the FHR is inadequate or when closer surveillance is needed. During labor, uterine contractions are usually monitored along with the FHR. Internal uterine pressure monitoring is sometimes used along with internal FHR monitoring. A catheter is placed through the cervical opening into the uterus beside the fetus and transmits uterine pressure readings to the monitor.

Cognitive Level: *Analysis*
Client Needs: *Physiological Integrity; Reduction of Risk Potential*
Integrated Process: *Nursing Process—Implementation*
Content Area: *Fetal Monitoring; Antepartum*
Concept: *Pregnancy*
Reference: *London, M. L., Ladewig, P. A., Davidson, M. R., Ball, J. W., Bindler, R. C., & Cowen, K. J. (2014). Maternal & child nursing care. 4th ed. New Jersey: Pearson.*

17. ANSWER: 2
Rationale
1. Administration of oxygen would be an intervention for late decelerations.
2. Maternal position change would be an intervention for variable decelerations.
3. Fetal scalp stimulation would be an intervention for fetal bradycardia.
4. A vaginal examination would be an intervention for late decelerations.

TEST-TAKING TIP: For variable decelerations, the usual priority is changing maternal position (side to side, knees to chest). If decelerations are severe, discontinue oxytocin if infusing, administer oxygen at 8 to 10 L/min with tight face mask, assist with vaginal or speculum examination to assess for cord prolapse, assist with amnioinfusion if ordered, assist with fetal oxygen saturation monitoring if ordered, and assist with birth (vaginal assisted or cesarean) if pattern cannot be corrected. Review nursing management for variables and late decelerations.

Cognitive Level: *Analysis*
Client Needs: *Safe and Effective Care Environment; Management of Care*
Integrated Process: *Nursing Process—Implementation*
Content Area: *Fetal Monitoring; Antepartum*
Concept: *Pregnancy*
Reference: *London, M. L., Ladewig, P. A., Davidson, M. R., Ball, J. W., Bindler, R. C., & Cowen, K. J. (2014). Maternal & child nursing care. 4th ed. New Jersey: Pearson.*

18. ANSWER: 4
Rationale
1. Positive CST is considered if late decelerations follow 50% or more of contractions (even if the contraction frequency is fewer than three in 10 minutes).
2. A negative CST is when there are no late or significant variable decelerations.
3. An equivocal–suspicious CST is when there are late decelerations with fewer than 50% of contractions or significant variable decelerations. It requires repeat testing on following day.

4. An equivocal–unsatisfactory CST is when there are fewer than three contractions in 10 minutes or when a tracing is not interpretable.

TEST-TAKING TIP: The contraction stress test is based on the response of the FHR to uterine contractions. It is believed that fetal oxygenation will be transiently worsened by uterine contractions. In the fetus with suboptimal oxygenation, the resulting intermittent worsening in oxygenation will, in turn, lead to the FHR pattern of late decelerations. Uterine contractions also may provoke or accentuate a pattern of variable decelerations caused by fetal umbilical cord compression, which in some cases is associated with oligohydramnios. Review interpretation of CST.

Cognitive Level: *Application*
Client Needs: *Physiological Integrity; Reduction of Risk Potential*
Integrated Process: *Nursing Process—Implementation*
Content Area: *Contraction Stress Test; Antepartum*
Concept: *Pregnancy*
Reference: *Durham, R. F., & Chapman, L. (2014). Maternal-newborn nursing: The critical components of nursing care. 2nd ed. Philadelphia: F.A. Davis.*

19. ANSWER: 4
Rationale
1. Prolonged deceleration is a decrease in FHR of more than 15 bpm measured from the most recently determined baseline rate. The deceleration lasts at least 2 minutes but less than 10 minutes.
2. An acceleration is an abrupt increase in FHR above baseline with onset to peak of the acceleration less than 30 seconds and less than 2 minutes in duration. The duration of the acceleration is defined as the time from the initial change in heart rate from the baseline to the time of return to the FHR to baseline.
3. Early deceleration is a gradual decrease in FHR with onset of deceleration to nadir greater than 30 seconds. The nadir occurs with the peak of a contraction.
4. Late deceleration is a gradual decrease in FHR with onset of deceleration to nadir greater than 30 seconds. Onset of the deceleration occurs after the beginning of the contraction, and the nadir of the contraction occurs after the peak of the contraction.

TEST-TAKING TIP: Episodic patterns are those not associated with uterine contractions. Periodic patterns are those associated with uterine contractions. Early and late decelerations (with some exceptions, such as supine hypotension) are periodic.

Cognitive Level: *Application*
Client Needs: *Physiological Integrity; Reduction of Risk Potential*
Integrated Process: *Nursing Process—Implementation*
Content Area: *Fetal Monitoring; Antepartum*
Concept: *Pregnancy*
Reference: *Durham, R. F., & Chapman, L. (2014). Maternal-newborn nursing: The critical components of nursing care. 2nd ed. Philadelphia: F.A. Davis.*

20. ANSWER: 3
Rationale
1. FHR and acceleration are measured by a fetal spiral electrode. IUPC gives accurate information on contraction frequency and contraction intensity.

2. Late deceleration and variable deceleration are indicated by the placement of a fetal spiral electrode. IUPC gives accurate information on uterus resting tone and contraction intensity.

3. IUPC gives information about contraction frequency, contraction duration, contraction intensity, and uterus resting tone.

4. IUPC gives information about uterus resting tone, contraction intensity, and contraction frequency. However, fundal height is determined by the health care provider using a metric-based measurement tape to measure along the top (longitudinal axis) of the pregnant uterus (or fundus).

TEST-TAKING TIP: When answers have options that contain two or more facts, identify a statement that is incorrect and eliminate that answer. By deleting distractors, you increase your chance of selecting the correct answer.
Cognitive Level: Analysis
Client Needs: Physiological Integrity; Reduction of Risk Potential
Integrated Process: Nursing Process—Implementation
Content Area: Fetal Monitoring; Antepartum
Concept: Pregnancy
Reference: London, M. L., Ladewig, P. A., Davidson, M. R., Ball, J. W., Bindler, R. C., & Cowen, K. J. (2014). Maternal & child nursing care. *4th ed. New Jersey: Pearson.*

Antepartum at Risk

Abruptio placenta—Premature separation of the placenta after 20 weeks of gestation but prior to delivery. The premature rupture results in bleeding, which can be internal or external.

AIDS—Immune disorder that is caused by HIV. Persons with AIDS have impaired immunity and can develop opportunistic infections.

Cerclage—Suturing of the cervix for cervical incompetency. This is used to prevent preterm birth.

Chorioamnionitis—Inflammation of the amnion and chorion from ascending bacteria

Coombs test—Blood test to determine if an Rh-negative mother is developing antibodies to an Rh-positive fetus. The direct Coombs test checks the baby's blood for antibodies on the red blood cells. The indirect Coombs test examines the maternal blood for the number of Rh antibodies.

Eclampsia—New onset of grand mal seizures in women with pre-eclampsia. Eclampsia can occur in the antepartum or postpartum period.

Erythroblastosis fetalis—A hemolytic disease of the newborn resulting in anemia, jaundice, enlargement of the liver and spleen, and generalized edema

HIV—The virus responsible for AIDS. HIV is passed from one person to the other through contact with blood or body fluid.

Hydrops fetalis—Occurs when fetal hemolysis develops in severe cases of Rh isoimmunization. The infant develops severe anemia, cardiac decompensation, cardiomegaly, and hepatosplenomegaly, resulting in fetal hypoxia. Due to a drop in oncotic pressure, fluid leaks out of the intravascular space, resulting in severe edema and placental swelling. Fluid can enter the pericardium and lungs and result in fetal death.

Kernicterus—A form of jaundice occurring in newborns. The basal ganglia and other areas of the brain are infiltrated with bilirubin.

Lecithin/sphingomyelin ratio—The ratio of lecithin to sphingomyelin in the amniotic fluid is used to assess maturity of the fetal lung.

Macrosomia—In the newborn, birth weight above the 90th percentile on the intrauterine growth curve, or 4,000 grams.

Placenta previa—Abnormal implantation of the placenta in the lower uterine wall close to or covering the cervical os

Polycythemia—An excess of red blood cells. In a newborn, it may reflect hemoconcentration due to hypovolemia or prolonged intrauterine hypoxia.

Pre-eclampsia—A multisystem disorder characterized by hypertension in pregnancy, generally a blood pressure (BP) of 140/90 or higher. The patient typically presents with proteinuria and generalized edema.

I. Problems During Pregnancy

Pregnancy is a normal process, but for women with certain conditions, pregnancy can be life-threatening. During the prenatal and antepartum period, it becomes very important to identify these women for risk factors such as age, parity, blood type, socioeconomic status, psychological health, or preexisting chronic illness. Some women have health problems that arise during pregnancy (gestational), and other women have health problems before (pregestational). It is very important for women to receive health care before and during pregnancy to decrease the risk of pregnancy complications.

A. Diabetes mellitus

Diabetes mellitus (DM) is an endocrine disorder of carbohydrate metabolism that results in insufficient insulin production in the beta cells of the islets of Langerhans in the pancreas. Insulin lowers blood glucose levels by enabling glucose to move from the blood into muscle and adipose tissue cells. Diabetes may be categorized into three categories—type 1, type 2 (pregestational), and gestational.

1. Gestational diabetes

   Gestational diabetes is a condition in which the glucose level is elevated and other diabetic symptoms appear during pregnancy in a woman who has not previously been diagnosed with diabetes. All diabetic symptoms disappear following delivery. Gestational diabetes is not caused by an absolute lack of insulin but by insulin resistance, which is attributed to the blocking effects of hormones produced by the placenta.

   a) Metabolic changes occur in normal pregnancy in response to the increase in nutrient needs of the fetus and the mother.

   b) Progressive insulin resistance begins near mid-pregnancy and advances through the third trimester to the level that approximates the insulin resistance seen in individuals with type 2 diabetes mellitus.

   c) The insulin resistance results from placental secretion of progesterone, cortisol, human placental lactogen, prolactin, and growth hormones. These hormones shift the primary energy sources to ketones and free fatty acids.

   d) Because of the insulin resistance during pregnancy, the pancreatic beta cells secrete compensatory insulin to overcome the insulin resistance of pregnancy. As a result, circulating glucose levels are kept within normal limits.

   e) If there is a maternal defect in insulin secretion and in glucose utilization, then **gestational diabetes mellitus (GDM)** will occur as the diabetogenic hormones rise to their peak levels.

2. Influence of pregnancy on diabetes

   a) In the first trimester, insulin needs are decreased because fetal needs are minimal and the woman may consume less food because of nausea and vomiting.

   b) Insulin requirements begin to rise in the second trimester because glucose use and storage by the woman and fetus increase.

   c) Insulin requirements may double or quadruple by the end of pregnancy as a result of placental maturation and human placental lactogen (hPL) production.

   d) Increased energy needs during labor may require increased insulin to balance intravenous (IV) glucose.

   e) Usually an abrupt decrease in insulin requirement occurs after delivery of the placenta and the resulting loss of hPL in maternal circulation.

   f) A decreased renal threshold for glucose leads to a higher incidence of **glycosuria.**

   g) The woman with DM may be at risk for ketoacidosis because of lower serum glucose levels. Ketones are formed by the breakdown of fat and protein, which are used for the woman's and fetus's energy needs.

3. Maternal risk of diabetes

   a) Hydramnios (increase in volume of amniotic fluid) can occur as the result of excessive urination by the fetus because of fetal hyperglycemia. When a woman has hydramnios, she is at a risk for premature rupture of membranes and preterm labor.

   b) Pre-eclampsia/**eclampsia** occurs more often in women with gestational diabetes.

   c) Hyperglycemia, due to insufficient amounts of insulin and causing an increase in serum glucose.

   d) Cesarean delivery due to large for gestational age infant (greater than 90% percentile).

   e) Monilial vaginitis and urinary tract infections (UTIs) because of increased glycosuria, which contributes to a favorable environment for bacterial growth.

ALERT Encourage the patient to use preventive measures to prevent UTIs, such as increasing intake of water and cranberry juice, wearing cotton underwear, wiping perineum from front to back, voiding frequently, and voiding before and immediately after sexual intercourse. The nurse should also instruct the patient on the signs and symptoms of UTI infection, such as urinary frequency, dysuria, cloudy urine, hematuria, lower back pain, and foul-smelling urine.

4. Fetal risk of maternal diabetes

   a) Macrosomia (weight over 4,000 grams): when an infant is considerably larger than normal. All of the nutrients the fetus receives come directly from the mother's blood. If the maternal blood has too much glucose, the fetus's pancreas senses the high glucose levels and

MAKING THE CONNECTION

Diabetes Screening

All women should be assessed for risk factors at the first prenatal visit. Maternal obesity, family history of diabetes, previous gestational diabetes, or infant with a birth weight over 4,000 grams place a woman at risk of gestational diabetes. Overweight and obese women are advised to lose weight with healthy eating prior to conception. In women at risk for diabetes, screening for diabetes should be done earlier than 26 weeks gestation for early identification and intervention.

produces more insulin in an attempt to use this glucose. The fetus converts the extra glucose to fat. Even when the mother has gestational diabetes, the fetus is able to produce all the insulin it needs. The combination of high blood glucose levels from the mother and high insulin levels in the fetus results in large deposits of fat, which cause the fetus to grow excessively large.

b) Shoulder dystocia: resulting from large for gestational age fetus (see Chapter 16).

c) Hypoglycemia: low blood sugar in the newborn immediately after delivery. This problem occurs if the mother's blood sugar levels have been consistently high, causing the fetus to have a high level of insulin. After delivery, the newborn continues to have a high insulin level but no longer has the high level of glucose from its mother, resulting in the newborn's blood glucose level becoming very low.

d) Congenital anomalies: cardiac, skeletal, neurological, genitourinary, and gastrointestinal abnormalities related to maternal hyperglycemia. Hyperglycemia is noted to be a potential teratogen, which may alter molecular signaling pathways and embryogenesis.

e) Respiratory distress syndrome: caused by high levels of fetal insulin, which inhibit some fetal enzymes necessary for surfactant production.

f) **Polycythemia** (excessive number of red blood cells): in the newborn this is mainly due to the diminished ability of glycosylated hemoglobin in the mother's blood to release oxygen.

g) Hyperbilirubinemia: results from the inability of immature liver enzymes to metabolize the increased bilirubin resulting from the polycythemia.

h) Intrauterine growth restriction (IUGR) may occur because of vascular changes in the mother, resulting in decreased efficiency of placental perfusion.

MAKING THE CONNECTION

Prenatal Counseling for Diabetes

Congenital defects observed in fetuses of diabetic mothers is a result of early embryonic insult. Most of the anomalies in the fetuses of diabetic mothers occur sometime during the fourth to seventh week of gestation. Therefore, good prenatal counseling is imperative for women who have diabetes or who are at risk for developing gestational diabetes.

5. Screening for gestational diabetes
   a) Screen for undiagnosed type 2 diabetes at the first prenatal visit in those with risk factors, using standard diagnostic criteria.
      (1) Criteria for testing at first prenatal visit
         • Test should be considered in all women who are overweight (body mass index [BMI] over 25 kg/m^2 or over 23 kg/m^2 in Asian Americans) and have additional risk factors
         • Physical inactivity
         • First-degree relative with diabetes
         • High-risk race/ethnicity (i.e., African American, Latino, Native American, Asian American, Pacific Islander)
         • Women who delivered a baby weighing more than 9 lb or who were diagnosed with GDM
         • Hypertension (140/90 mg/dL or higher or on therapy for hypertension)
         • HDL cholesterol level lower than 35 mg/dL and/or a triglyceride level greater than 2 mg/dL
         • Women with polycystic ovary syndrome
         • Glycosylated hemoglobin A1C (HbA1C) 5.7% or higher
         • History of cardiovascular disease
   b) Women with diabetes in the first trimester should be classified as having type 2 diabetes.
   c) Women who are at low risk should be screened between 24 and 28 weeks, because at this point in gestation the diabetogenic effect of pregnancy is manifest.
   d) GDM can be diagnosed by using either of two strategies recommended by the American Diabetes Association (ADA) and the National Institutes of Health (NIH), as shown in Box 13.1.
6. Glucose monitoring
   a) Self-monitoring of blood glucose is recommended for women with GDM. The goal of monitoring is to detect glucose concentrations elevated enough to increase perinatal mortality (Box 13.2).
7. Antepartum clinical management
   a) Initial treatment begins with nutrition therapy, exercise, and glucose monitoring. Between 70% and 85% of women diagnosed with GDM can control it with lifestyle modification.
   b) The goal of nutrition therapy is to provide adequate nutrition for the mother and fetus, provide sufficient calories for appropriate maternal weight gain, maintain normoglycemia, and avoid ketosis. In general, there is not an increased energy requirement during the

Box 13.1 Criteria for Diagnosing GDM at 24 to 28 Weeks Gestation

One-Step Strategy

- *Perform a 75-gram oral glucose tolerance test (OGTT), with plasma glucose measurement when woman is fasting and at 1 and 2 hours.*
- *The OGTT should be performed in the morning after an overnight fast of at least 8 hours.*
- *The diagnosis of GDM is made when any of the following plasma glucose values are met or exceed:*
  - *Fasting: 92 mg/dL*
  - *1 hour: 180 mg/dL*
  - *2 hour: 153 mg/dL*

Two-Step Strategy

Step 1: Perform a 50-gram glucose tolerance test (GTT) (non-fasting), with plasma glucose measurement at 1 hour. If the plasma glucose level measured at 1 hour after the load is 140 mg/dL or higher, then proceed to a 100-gram OGTT.

Step 2: The 100-gram OGTT should be performed when the patient is fasting. The diagnosis of GDM is made if at least two of the four plasma levels (measured after fasting and 1 hour, 2 hours, and 3 hours after the OGTT) are met or exceeded:

- *Fasting: 105 mg/dL*
- *1 hour: 190 mg/dL*
- *2 hour: 165 mg/dL*
- *3 hour: 145 mg/dL*

Source: National Diabetes Data Group.

Box 13.2 Glycemic Target for Gestational Diabetes

- *Fasting: less than 90 mg/dL*
- *Preprandial: 105 mg/dL or less*
- *1-hour postmeal: 130–140 mg/dL or less*
- *2-hours postmeal: 120 mg/dL or less*

Glycemic Target for Preexisting Type 1 or Type 2 Diabetes During Pregnancy

- *Premeal, bedtime, and overnight glucose: 60–99 mg/dL*
- *Peak postprandial glucose: 100–129 mg/dL*
- *A1C: less than 6%*
- *Note: Recommended as the optimal glycemic goals if this can be achieved without excessive hypoglycemia.*

first trimester of pregnancy. However, most normal-weight women require an additional 300 kcal/day in the second and third trimesters.

(1) In normal-weight women with GDM, the recommended daily caloric intake is 30 kcal/kg/day based on their present pregnant weight. In women with GDM who are overweight (BMI higher than 30 kg/m²), a recommended daily caloric intake is 25 kcal/kg/day based on their present pregnant weight.

(2) Women should be advised to distribute carbohydrates throughout the day and to eat three small- to moderate-sized meals and three snacks per day.

(3) The bedtime snack is very important to prevent nighttime hypoglycemia and should consist of protein and complex carbohydrates.

c) Based on the potential benefits of exercise in women with GDM, the ADA recommends starting or continuing a program of moderate exercise in women without medical or obstetrical contraindications.

d) Insulin therapy is usually ordered when nutritional therapy fails to maintain blood glucose levels at the recommended ranges.

(1) The type and dose of insulin is individualized to meet the woman's needs.

(2) Glyburide (a second-generation sulfonylurea) and metformin (a biguanide) are safe and effective in treating women with gestational diabetes.

ALERT When administering insulin, nurses should use two patient identifiers, administer at the correct time, and monitor the client after administration. Nurses should have documentation signed by two licensed nurses.

e) Fetal assessment during the antepartum period is important in determining fetal well-being, size, and maturation and planning the course and timing of birth.

(1) Maternal serum alpha-fetoprotein is recommended at 16 to 20 weeks gestation because of the increased risk of neural tube defects.

(2) At 18 weeks gestation, an ultrasound is recommended to confirm gestational age and to detect fetal anomalies. Ultrasound is repeated again at the beginning of 28 weeks gestation to monitor for IUGR or macrosomia.

(3) A nonstress test (NST) or biophysical profile may be performed in the third trimester to further evaluate fetal well-being. The NST is usually begun weekly or biweekly at 28 weeks gestation. If the NST is nonreactive, then a biophysical profile may be performed (see Chapter 12 for further discussion).

8. Intrapartum clinical management

a) Timing of birth: most women with diabetes are allowed to carry their fetus to term (40 weeks gestation).

- However, some health care providers may choose to induce labor in a client at term to avoid risks related to decreased perfusion of the placenta.

- Cesarean birth may be indicated if signs of fetal distress exist.
- Prior to induction, fetal lung maturity may be obtained by amniocentesis to evaluate the **lecithin/sphingomyelin ratio** (see Chapter 12 for further discussion).

b) Labor management
- Frequently, maternal insulin requirements decrease dramatically during labor.
- Maternal glucose levels are measured hourly to determine insulin needs.
- The primary goal in controlling maternal glucose levels is to prevent neonatal hypoglycemia.
- Often two IV lines are used, one with 5% dextrose solution and one with a saline solution. The saline solution is then available for piggybacking insulin or if a bolus is needed. During the second stage of labor and the immediate postpartum period, the client may not need additional insulin.

DID YOU KNOW?
Because insulin clings to plastic IV bags and tubing, the tubing should be flushed with insulin before the prescribed amount is added.

9. Postpartum management
There is usually a significant decrease in circulating glucose because hormone levels fall after placental separation and because of the anti-insulin effect. For the first 24 hours postpartum, women with diabetes typically require little insulin and are usually managed with a sliding scale.

B. Anemia
Anemia is defined as hemoglobin/hematocrit of less than 11/33 in the first and third trimesters and hemoglobin/hematocrit of less than 10/32 mg in the second trimester. Anemia is one of the most common complications during pregnancy.
1. Physiological anemia
   a) Occurs because the expansion of plasma volume is quicker than the production of red blood cells.
   b) Iron needs for pregnant women are 1,000 mg per day. Although iron is available in many foods, it is difficult to take in 1,000 mg of iron for most women. Iron supplementation through prenatal vitamins or iron supplements may be advised. Most women do not have sufficient iron stores, due to blood loss during menstruation.
2. Assessment of iron deficiency anemia
   a) The woman experiencing anemia may be pale, fatigued, and lethargic or have headaches. Her lips may appear inflamed.

b) The blood smear will show microcytic red blood cells.
   c) Plasma iron and ferritin will be low, and total iron binding capacity will be high.
3. The treatment for iron deficiency anemia is to encourage intake of iron-rich foods such as green leafy vegetables, red meat, and raisins.
   a) Most prenatal vitamins contain iron. For some women, the amount of iron in the prenatal vitamin may not be sufficient. If iron supplementation is needed, ferrous sulfate 325 mg per day is usually prescribed.
   b) Iron is best absorbed if taken without meals, but many women find it difficult to take iron on an empty stomach.
   c) Vitamin C is often prescribed with iron tablets to increase absorption.
   d) For women who have hemoglobin levels of 8.5 or less who cannot take iron, intravenous iron may be ordered.
4. Women with iron deficiency anemia may be fatigued and should be encouraged to rest.
5. For women planning pregnancy, it is important to eat well and ensure adequate intake of iron and folic acid prior to becoming pregnant. Anemia in pregnancy has been associated with preterm birth.

C. Heart disease
1. Cardiovascular disease in pregnancy warrants early identification and monitoring to decrease incidence of maternal or fetal complications.
2. Women who have cardiovascular disease may be at increased risk during pregnancy due to increased cardiac demands of pregnancy (increased blood volume and increased cardiac output).
3. Congenital cardiac anomaly and valvular disorders are the most commonly seen cardiovascular disease in a pregnant client.
4. Cardiac disease during pregnancy includes congenital and acquired diseases.
5. Women with congenital heart disease are at increased risk for arrhythmia and heart failure, and their infant is at increased risk for IUGR and preterm delivery.
6. Preconception counseling should include full evaluation and plans for cardiac management during the antepartum, intrapartum, and postpartum period.
   a) New York Heart Association's Functional Classification of heart disease is used to guide health care providers in the management of a pregnant or postpartum client (Table 13.1).
   b) Evaluate clients at 3 and 7 months gestation to determine appropriate treatment and to assess functional ability during the antepartum, intrapartum, and postpartum periods.

Table 13.1	New York Heart Association's Classification of Heart Disease	
Class I	Exhibits no symptoms with activity	Client should have a normal pregnancy and delivery.
Class II	Symptoms with ordinary exertion	Client should have a normal pregnancy and delivery.
Class III	Symptoms with minimal exertion	Total bedrest may be indicated during pregnancy.
Class IV	Symptoms at rest	Pregnancy not advised.

7. Risk factors
   - Preterm labor
   - Miscarriage
   - IUGR
8. Nursing management
   a) Antepartum
      (1) Teach signs and symptoms of cardia decomposition: increasing fatigue; difficulty breathing; frequent cough; palpitations; and edema of face, feet, legs, and fingers.
      (2) Assessment for cardiac decomposition: irregular, weak pulse (100 bpm or higher); progressive generalized edema; crackles at base of lungs; orthopnea; rapid respirations (25 breaths/min or more); moist, frequent cough; cyanosis of lips and nails.
      (3) Frequent prenatal visits to assess for proper weight gain to ensure appropriate fetal weight gain and to avoid excessive weight gain of the mother, which could lead to increased workload of the heart.
         (a) Iron supplements may lead to constipation, so the client should be instructed to eat foods high in fiber and to increase fluid intake. However, some clients may be on fluid restriction because of a specific cardiac condition. These clients should be referred to a dietitian.
         (b) A stool softener may be prescribed.
         (c) The client should be instructed to avoid straining during defecation. The straining may cause the client to do the Valsalva maneuver (forced expiration against a closed airway). When expiration is released, blood rushes to the heart and overloads the cardiac system.
      (4) Nutritional education indicating the need for a diet high in iron and low in sodium to prevent anemia and fluid retention.
      (5) Avoid/reduce stress and anxiety.
      (6) Encouragement of sufficient nighttime sleep and daytime rest periods.
         (a) Clients with class I or II cardiac disease need 10 hours of sleep every night and 30 minutes of rest after meals.
         (b) Clients with class III or IV cardiac disease usually need bedrest for most of each day.
      (7) Explanation of fetal surveillance testing (see Chapter 12 for further discussion).
      (8) Educate the client regarding the signs and symptoms of complications and when to call provider. Infections (e.g., respiratory, urinary, and gastrointestinal) complicate heart disease by accelerating the heart rate and by spreading organisms directly to the heart.

DID YOU KNOW?

At 28 and 32 weeks gestation, hemodynamic changes reach their peak. The nurse must have knowledge of the disease process and be able to assess the hemodynamic changes that occur during pregnancy.

   b) Intrapartum
      (1) The nursing assessment is focused on assessing the client and fetus for decreased cardiac output.
         - Decreased and/or irregular pulse
         - Increased respiratory rate
         - Dyspnea
         - Chest pain
         - Abnormal breath sounds, crackles at the base of the lungs
         - Decreased BP
         - Decreased urinary output (less than 30 mL/hr)
         - General edema of hands, face, and feet
         - Abnormal heart sounds, diastolic murmur at the heart's apex
         - Signs of air hunger—anxiety
         - Decreased oxygen saturation—less than 95%. If oxygen is required, administer via a rebreather mask at 10 L/min.
         - Cool, clammy, cyanotic skin
         - Increased capillary refill time—greater than 3 seconds
         - EKG changes
         - Mental changes—disorientation, fatigue, syncope

(2) Nursing care
- Continuous fetal monitoring
- Client's head and shoulders elevated to support cardiac function
- Side-lying position to facilitate uterine perfusion
- Open glottis pushing should be encouraged; closed glottis pushing (Valsalva maneuver) reduces diastolic ventricular filling and obstructs left ventricular outflow.

c) Postpartum
(1) Assess for decompensation because cardiac output increases rapidly as extravascular fluid is shifted into the vascular compartments.
(2) Elevate the head of the bed and have the client in a side-lying position.
(3) Have the client ambulate as tolerated to prevent deep vein thrombosis.
(4) Recommend stool softeners, fiber, and fluid to reduce straining when stooling.

D. Substance abuse problems
1. Substance abuse during pregnancy impacts the health of both the mother and fetus. Approximately 5% of pregnant women (ages 15 to 44) reported substance use in the previous 30 days.
2. The American College of Obstetricians and Gynecologists (ACOG) Clinical Guidelines[1] recommends routine screening of substance abuse through interviews and validated tools with evidence-based interventions for referral and treatment.
   a) Guidelines state that all women should be screened regardless of age, gender, or ethnicity. This should be done early and throughout the pregnancy. Early intervention is essential to reduce fetal exposure to substances and to allow for timely supportive services to assist with substance abuse.
   b) Screening is also essential at various time points, since women may be more likely to reveal their substance abuse when they become comfortable with the provider. Screening every patient as part of routine health assessment helps to lessen the stigma. Warning signs of drug abuse are not receiving prenatal care, late entry to prenatal appointments, and missed appointments.
   c) Many providers will used standardized self-report questionnaires about drug use, and others will ask questions, using a structured

interview. With either method, the staff must be trained to intervene and be nonjudgmental in their approach.
3. Intimate partner violence (IPV) is a well-known phenomenon that may begin or worsen during pregnancy. Since pregnant woman have frequent contact with health care providers, it is important to screen and identify this risk factor, so intervention and referral can take place.
   a) IPV is associated with pregnancy complications, lack of prenatal care, and higher use of alcohol, tobacco, and other drugs.
4. Smoking during pregnancy poses many risks to the mother and fetus. Smoking has been linked to IUGR and premature birth.
5. Drinking alcohol has a known negative effect on the fetus. Prenatal alcohol exposure is linked to fetal alcohol spectrum disorders.
6. Cannabis is one of the most frequently used drugs. The effects of prenatal cannabis exposure are not well documented in the literature. Some researchers report that in utero, cannabis exposure may impair growth, especially head circumference and neurodevelopment.[2]
   a) Cannabis can be detrimental and damaging to the undeveloped brain, especially in adolescence.
   b) To the fetus exposed in utero, there also appears to be damaging effects, which may persist through childhood and impact future growth and development.
   c) Cessation of cannabis use is recommended. If cessation is not possible, reducing its use during pregnancy is suggested. Health care providers have the duty to provide information on the harmful effects of heavy usage to promote healthy growth and development.

E. HIV/AIDS
1. The most common way that **HIV** is transmitted is through sex with an HIV-infected male partner. In 2011, the majority of new HIV infections were in women aged 25 to 44.
2. Risk factors for HIV infections include unprotected sex and sharing needles during drug use. HIV is more easily transmitted from men to women.
3. It is recommended that all pregnant women be tested for HIV at the first prenatal visit in states where opt-out policies are legal. If the results are positive, immediate treatment should begin.

[1] American College of Obstetricians and Gynecologists (ACOG). (2015). ACOG guidelines at a glance: Key points about 4 perinatal infections. Retrieved from http://contemporaryobgyn.modernmedicine.com/contemporary-obgyn/news/acog-guidelines-glance-key-points-about-4-perinatal-infections-0.

[2] Jaques, S. C., Kingsbury, A., Henshcke, P., Chomchai, C., Clews, S., Falconer, J., ... Feller, J. M. (2014). Cannabis, the pregnant woman and her child: Weeding out the myths. *Journal Perinatol, 34*: 249-267. doi:10.1038/jp.2013.180.

4. In women who are high risk, it is suggested that testing be done again in the third trimester of pregnancy. Although women can opt out of the test, carefully discussing their reasons for opting out is indicated.
5. Mother-to-child transmission or perinatal transmission of HIV has decreased in the past 20 years with the advent of antiretroviral therapy.
6. If the results of the testing are unavailable or the patient did not get tested prenatally, rapid testing on admission to labor and delivery is recommended. If the rapid test is reactive, the patient should immediately begin retroviral therapy while confirmatory testing is being processed.[3]
7. Current guidelines recommend antiretroviral therapy, no breastfeeding, and elective cesarean section before the onset of labor to reduce perinatal transmission.
8. A vaginal delivery places the fetus at increased risk of vertical transmission, so it is recommended that all women with viral loads of 1,000 copies/mL be offered a cesarean section at 38 weeks gestation.
9. The provider should limit the use of fetal scalp electrodes or invasive intrauterine pressure monitor since it increases the risk of vertical transmission.
10. After delivery, the infant should be handled with gloves until all fluids have been wiped off and the infant receives the first bath.

DID YOU KNOW?

Women should also be aware that some antiretroviral drugs reduce the effectiveness of birth control pills. Additionally, women should be told that pregnancy may affect how the body processes HIV medications and they may need to change dosages. Pregnant women should be aware of the Antiretroviral Pregnancy Registry and can voluntarily enroll through their health care provider. The registry tracks birth defects related to antiretroviral therapy. Currently, it is believed that the risk of fetal injury from antiretrovirals is low and the benefits outweigh the risk.

11. Women who are HIV positive and contemplating pregnancy should be on a maximally suppressive antiretroviral regimen. If the partner is also infected with HIV (concordant couple), the infected partner should maintain maximum suppression prior to conception. Both partners should be screened and treated for genital tract infections prior to attempting conception.

12. If couples are discordant in HIV status, preconceptional counseling is recommended to explore the most current options and recommendations. Discordant partners must be aware that combination antiretroviral therapy (cART) for the infected partner may not fully protect against sexual transmission of HIV. The administration of periconception antiretroviral pre-exposure prophylaxis for partners who are not infected with HIV may offer an additional tool to reduce the risk of sexual transmission.
13. General principles regarding antepartum care include the following:
    a) All HIV-positive women should have an assessment of HIV disease status and recommendation of initiation of cART or the need for any modification of their current regime.
    b) Current guidelines state that "all women should receive cART, regardless of plasma HIV RNA copy number of CD4 lymphocyte count."[4]
    c) Combined antepartum, intrapartum, and infant antiretroviral (ARV) therapy is recommended because ARV drugs reduce perinatal transmission by several mechanisms, including lowering maternal antepartum viral load and providing infant and postexposure prophylaxis.
    d) All women should be counseled about the benefits and risks of antiretroviral therapy.
    e) The guidelines also state the importance of educating pregnant women on the need to continually take the medications. If needed, social service agencies and support services for pregnant women should be provided to encourage adherence to the medication regimen. If the woman has substance abuse issues, referral to the appropriate treatment center is indicated.
F. Abortions
    1. **Abortion** is the loss of fetus before it is viable.
        a) The general medical consensus is that 20 weeks gestation or a fetus weighing less than 500 grams is considered an abortion. Spontaneous abortion is defined as a loss of a fetus without interference by an instrument or person.
        b) Symptoms include vaginal bleeding, which may be followed by abdominal pain or cramping, pelvic pressure, or low back pain. Pain or cramping with vaginal bleeding is likely to accompany a spontaneous abortion.

[3] American College of Obstetricians and Gynecologists (ACOG). (2014). New guidelines address screening, prevention of HIV in women. Retrieved from http://www.acog.org/Resources-And-Publications/Committee-Opinions/Committee-on-Gynecologic-Practice/Routine-Human-Immunodeficiency-Virus-Screening.

[4] American College of Obstetricians and Gynecologists (ACOG). (2014). New guidelines address screening, prevention of HIV in women. Retrieved from http://www.acog.org/Resources-And-Publications/Committee-Opinions/Committee-on-Gynecologic-Practice/Routine-Human-Immunodeficiency-Virus-Screening.

c) Many women experience bleeding during the first trimester of pregnancy. The bleeding may be light and is referred to as *spotting* or it may be moderate. Any woman experiencing bleeding or spotting during the first trimester should notify her care provider immediately.

d) The nurse should ask the woman to note the amount, color (bright red or brownish red), onset, and duration of bleeding.

e) The woman should also be asked to report accompanying symptoms such as uterine cramping, pelvic pain, abdominal pain, or back pain.

f) Labs are drawn for beta-human chorionic gonadotropin level and progesterone to see if they correlate with gestational age.

g) Spontaneous abortion is further defined by the following categories: inevitable, threatened, complete, incomplete, missed, and recurrent.

 (1) Inevitable abortion occurs when the membrane ruptures and the cervix is open. Fluid is expelled through the vaginal opening and there is spontaneous bleeding. At this point, no interventions would be effective and the fetus must be allowed to pass. Nursing care includes providing the woman and her partner with support. The nurse should monitor for excessive bleeding or infection.

 (2) Threatened abortion is defined by spontaneous bleeding with a closed cervix.

 (3) Complete abortion is when all the products of conception are expelled. After this occurs, active bleeding ends. The pregnancy test will be negative as the hormone levels fall.

 (4) Incomplete abortion is when only some of the products of conception are expelled, placing the mother at risk for infection and excessive bleeding. The products of conception will be very small if this is early in the gestational process.
 - If all the products of conception pass, the diagnosis changes to a complete abortion.
 - In incomplete abortions, bleeding continues because the retained products do not allow the uterus to contract completely.
 - Initial treatment is aimed at stabilizing the cardiothoracic system.
 - Blood is drawn for hemoglobin/ hematocrit and type and cross are obtained.
 - An intravenous line is started and intravenous fluids provided.

 - If the pregnancy is less than 14 weeks and the woman is stable, a dilation and curettage (D&C) is usually performed to remove fetal tissue.
 - Pitocin and/or Methergine may be given to control bleeding (see Chapter 18).
 - If the pregnancy is greater than 14 weeks, a D&C will not be performed because of the danger of excessive bleeding. Instead, prostaglandin and oxytocin may be administered until all products of conception are passed.

 (5) Missed abortion occurs when the fetus dies in utero but products of conception are retained.
 - This generally happens during the first half of pregnancy.
 - Maternal symptoms of pregnancy such as nausea, breast swelling, and urinary frequency disappear.
 - The fetal heartbeat is absent and uterine size usually decreases. The human chorionic gonadotropin (hCG) level will decrease.
 - The patient may present with bleeding and or cramping. Bleeding may be brownish red or dark red in color or may be absent.
 - In most cases the fetus will be expelled. However, since this may be emotionally devastating to the woman, surgical intervention may be employed.
 - A D&C may be performed in the first trimester. If this occurs later, dilation and evacuation or prostaglandin (PGE2 or misoprostol) may be needed to induce uterine contractions to expel the fetus.
 - If the patient experiences fever or abdominal pain, or if there is an odor, cultures should be obtained to determine the presence of infection.
 - If infection is suspected, antimicrobial therapy should be initiated before labor induction.

 (6) Recurrent spontaneous abortion is defined as two or more spontaneous abortions.
 - The primary cause is usually genetic or reproductive. Some reproductive causes are the presence of a bicornuate uterus and incompetent cervix. Other theories believe there is an inadequate luteal phase with insufficient progesterone and immunological factors.
 - The insufficient immunological factors may be due to sharing of human

leukocyte factors of the female ovum and male sperm. Because of this sharing, the female fails to produce immunological factors to protect the fetus.

- Additional factors include sexually transmitted infections and recurrent abortions. Systemic diseases such as lupus and diabetes also place the fetus at risk.

2. Risk factors for spontaneous abortion include congenital malformations, maternal infections, maternal endocrine problems, and problems with the reproductive track. The highest risk factors are advanced maternal age and previous pregnancy loss. Parental age is also considered a risk factor for spontaneous abortion. A higher intake of folic acid with supplements during prepregnancy was associated with a lower risk of spontaneous abortion.

3. For women with suspected spontaneous abortion, usually a pregnancy test and ultrasound are ordered. The pregnancy test may be quantitative to determine if the level of serum β-hCG is rising.

4. Management
   a) All clients with vaginal bleeding during pregnancy should be advised to contact their care provider or go to the emergency department for evaluation.
   b) The client should be instructed to void in a bedpan and save any tissue expelled. Most women experiencing first trimester spontaneous abortions will expel the products of conception within 8 weeks.
   c) The client will be placed on bedrest and encouraged to drink fluids.
   d) Women should contact their provider if bleeding becomes heavy. This is defined as saturation of one pad in 1 hour.
   e) Women are usually discharged home with pain medications in case cramping or pain occurs.
   f) Some providers may order follow-up pregnancy tests or ultrasounds to confirm loss of pregnancy.
   g) If there is an incomplete loss, the woman may be scheduled for a D&C or suction curettage to remove fetal tissue.
   h) Misoprostol, a prostaglandin E1 analogue, may be ordered for complete expulsion and may be given orally or vaginally.
      (1) The recommended initial dose of misoprostol is 800 micrograms vaginally. One repeat dose may be administered as needed, no earlier than 3 hours after the first dose and typically within 7 days if there is no response to the first dose.

   (2) Prescriptions for pain medications should be provided to the patient.
   (3) Women who are Rh(D)-negative and unsensitized should receive Rh(D)-immune globulin within 72 hours of the first misoprostol administration.
   (4) Follow-up to document the complete passage of tissue can be accomplished by ultrasound examination, typically within 7 to 14 days. Serial serum β-hCG measurements may be used instead in settings where ultrasonography is unavailable. Patient-reported symptoms also should be considered when determining whether complete expulsion has occurred.
   (5) If misoprostol fails, the patient may opt for expectant management (for a time determined by the woman and her health care provider) or suction curettage.

5. Surgical treatment of spontaneous abortion
   a) According to the ACOG guidelines, women experiencing infection, hemodynamic instability, or bleeding disorders should have surgical intervention.
      (1) According to the new guidelines, suction curettage is preferable to sharp curettage. Suction curettage may be performed in the office setting without use of local anesthesia.
      (2) Women who are Rh-negative should receive RhoGAM D, 50 micrograms immediately after surgical intervention within 72 hours of a confirmed pregnancy loss to prevent isoimmunization.

6. Patient teaching after a spontaneous abortion
   a) Women should be told to monitor for excessive blood loss (saturating one pad in 1 hour) or feeling weak or dizzy.
   b) Women should be told to monitor vaginal bleeding for foul-smelling odor and to report fever, since these may be signs of infection.
   c) Women should not have sexual intercourse until they have a return visit with the primary care provider. Contraception should be discussed at this visit if the woman wishes to avoid pregnancy.
   d) A spontaneous abortion will be dealt with differently by each woman and her family. It is normal to experience grieving after the loss. Nurses should allow the woman and partner to express their feelings regarding the loss. Many hospitals offer support groups to deal with the loss.

G. Ectopic pregnancy
   Ectopic pregnancy is defined as the implantation of the fertilized ovum outside the uterus. As the ovum begins to grow, it places the mother at significant risk (Fig. 13.1).
   1. An ectopic pregnancy is the cause of 6% of maternal deaths. It is estimated that in 90% of ectopic pregnancies, the ovum is in the fallopian tube; therefore, the term *tubal pregnancy* is often used to refer to this type of pregnancy.
   2. Risk factors for ectopic pregnancy
      - History of sexually transmitted diseases or pelvic inflammatory disease
      - Previous ectopic pregnancy
      - Endometriosis
      - Use of an intrauterine device
      - In vitro fertilization or other method of assisted reproduction
   3. Ectopic pregnancies place the woman at risk for hemorrhage and infertility.
   4. The symptoms of an ectopic pregnancy include abdominal pain, spotting or vaginal bleeding, and missed menstrual period. Symptoms usually occur 6 weeks after the last menstrual period. Many women report a period that is delayed 1 to 2 weeks or is lighter than usual.
   5. Many women go to the emergency department for pain or bleeding and should be evaluated for an ectopic pregnancy. A pregnancy test should be performed.
   6. Management
      a) A client with a suspected ectopic pregnancy should be assessed for acute bleeding, which could indicate a ruptured fallopian tube.
      b) Bleeding can also be internal. Symptoms may include shoulder pain (caused by internal bleeding irritating the diaphragm), vertigo, and hypotension.
      c) A vaginal examination should be done only once, since there may be a palpable mass.

🚫 ALERT Vaginal examination should be done with caution and light pressure, since pressure can cause the rupture of the tube.

      d) If the fallopian tube has ruptured, it should be surgically removed (salpingectomy). Surgical management will be determined by size and location of the pregnancy and the client's desires for future pregnancies.
      e) In uncomplicated ectopic pregnancies, methotrexate may be given to stop cell production and destroy remaining tissue.
         (1) Clients eligible for this management of care must have an unruptured ectopic mass measuring 1.6 inches (4 cm) or less on ultrasound examination, no cardiac activity, and an hCG level less than 1,000 milli-international units. The client must also be willing to comply with follow-up.
         (2) Methotrexate is an antimetabolite that dissolves rapidly dividing cells and is a folate antagonist. It is excreted from the body in urine up to 72 hours after administration and in feces up to 7 days.
            - The woman should be taught to avoid getting urine on the toilet seat and to flush twice with the lid down after urinating.

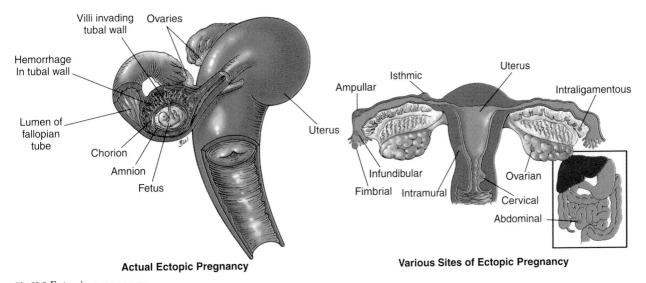

Actual Ectopic Pregnancy

Various Sites of Ectopic Pregnancy

Fig 13.1 Ectopic pregnancy.

- Side effects of the drug include nausea, vomiting, stomatitis, and dizziness.
- The client should avoid eating foods high in folic acid or gaseous food.
- The client should avoid sun exposure.
- The client should be instructed to call her provider if she experiences severe abdominal pain, which may be a sign of tubal rupture.
- The client should not take any medication stronger than acetaminophen because certain pain medications may mask the symptoms of tubal rupture.
    (3) The client is required to follow up with her health care provider to check hCG levels.
    - Weekly quantitative HCG levels will be drawn to make sure hCG levels continue to decrease.
    - Complete resolution of an ectopic pregnancy can take 3 to 6 weeks.

H. Gestational trophoblastic disease

1. **Gestational trophoblastic disease** is the proliferation of trophoblastic cells and includes hydatidiform invasive moles.
2. It is the overgrowth of the trophoblast, the outermost layer of embryonic cells. The placenta forms with grapelike clusters of cells.
    a) This occurs in about 1 in 1,500 pregnancies in the United States.
    b) The complete mole develops from a nuclear egg without genetic material.
    c) It is fertilized and duplicated before the first cell division.
    d) The other type, a hydatidiform mole, develops from a normal ovum that is fertilized by two sperm or a sperm before it has undergone meiosis and contains 46 chromosomes. Partial moles are sometimes recognized after spontaneous abortion.
    e) Signs and Symptoms
        - Vaginal bleeding occurs with almost all molar pregnancies and may be dark brown or bright red.
        - It may begin as early as the first trimester.
        - Absence of fetal heartbeat occurs in complete moles (about 50% of cases) occurring with symptoms of pregnancy. It is extremely rare to have a live birth with a partial molar pregnancy.
        - Uterine enlargement is much larger than gestational age.
        - HCG levels are markedly elevated.
        - Hyperemesis often occurs with molar pregnancies.

- Levels of alpha serum protein are low.
- **Pre-eclampsia** may occur with molar pregnancy.
- Ultrasound is used to diagnose a molar pregnancy. It is usually diagnosed at 6 to 8 weeks when the villi are large enough.

3. Management
    a) Molar pregnancies are believed to increase the risk of uterine cancer.
    b) Treatment begins with suction removal of the molar pregnancy and curettage to ensure the placenta is removed. The early evacuation of the molar pregnancy is better.
    c) Follow-up care should include serial β-hCG levels because this hormone is secreted by molar cells.
    d) hCG levels should be assessed every 1 to 2 weeks until hCG is undetectable on two separate blood levels.
    e) Follow-up should continue and should consist of hCG level measurement every 1 to 2 months for at least 1 year.
    f) The client should be advised to use contraception during this time to prevent pregnancy and increasing hCG levels associated with pregnancy.

I. Hyperemesis gravidarum

1. Hyperemesis gravidarum is defined as nausea and vomiting so severe that the woman's weight is 5% less than pregnancy weight. Although it is relatively rare, affecting approximately less than 2% of pregnant women, it is one of the most frequent causes of hospitalization during the antenatal period.
    a) Severe hyperemesis gravidarum is associated with fetal IUGR and maternal morbidity and mortality.
    b) Many women with hyperemesis gravidarum report symptoms lasting throughout the pregnancy and some symptoms that continue postpartum. Most women report that the symptoms were worse during the first 3 months of pregnancy.
    c) Women with the most severe weight loss— at least 15% less than prepregnancy weight— reported the most severe symptoms. Women who are younger in age, have multiple gestations, or fetal anomalies are at higher risk.
2. Approximately 80% of women experience nausea and/or vomiting in pregnancy. It is believed that nausea and vomiting occur in response to the rising level of hCG.
    a) For most women, this is a short-term problem. For about 30% of women, the nausea and

vomiting can be severe and impact daily activities. In a smaller number, approximately 1% to 5%, the nausea and vomiting is so severe, they require hospitalization.

    (1) Risk factors for developing hyperemesis gravidarum include clinical hyperthyroid disorders, molar pregnancy, multiple gestation, diabetes, gastrointestinal disorders, and previous pregnancy with hyperemesis gravidarum.

    (2) Some studies suggest that prior to planning future pregnancies, the woman should take folic acid and vitamin B supplements and eat smaller, more frequent meals.

3. Women with hyperemesis gravidarum present with weight loss and electrolyte imbalances, often requiring hospitalization.

    a) The patient may be hypotensive due to the loss of fluids. Initially, the patient usually loses hydrochloric acid from vomiting with resulting alkalosis. If the vomiting continues, there is a loss of alkaline fluids. If the patient's potassium level is low, it will interfere with the kidney's ability to concentrate urine and disrupt cardiac functioning. It is important to check for ketonuria.

    b) The woman's electrolytes and fluid balance need to be checked frequently.

    c) Pyridoxine is often used as a first-line treatment and is considered safe in pregnancy. Other medications that may be taken include Zofran, Reglan, or Phenergan.

    d) Vitamin B_6 and B_{12} deficiencies can also develop and can lead to neuropathy.

4. If nausea and vomiting continues for 3 to 4 weeks, women can develop Wernicke's encephalopathy with ataxia and dementia due to thiamine deficiency. If this is not detected and treated, it can become a permanent disability.

    a) It is important to correct the thiamine deficiency before giving dextrose in fluids, since this can lead to Wernicke's encephalopathy. Oral or intravenous thiamine supplementation may be ordered.

5. During hospitalization, the client should receive IV therapy and electrolyte replacement. Initially, she will be kept NPO to allow the bowel to rest. Foods will be reintroduced slowly. A goal of treatment is to keep urinary output greater than 1,000 mL/day.

6. Treatment includes early identification and monitoring. Clients are instructed to eat small, frequent meals and avoid triggers. If the hyperemesis continues, nutritional supplementation may be necessary. The client should:

    • Avoid spicy, odiferous foods.

    • Eat simple, small servings of carbohydrates.

    • Drink clear carbonated liquids.

J. Hypertensive disorders

1. Elevated blood pressure in pregnancy is linked to increased maternal and neonatal mortality worldwide. Hypertension is the most common medical problem in pregnant women.

    a) Women identified as hypertensive during pregnancy are at greater risk throughout their lifetime and should be provided education on reducing risk.

    b) Hypertension during pregnancy places the client at future risk of cardiovascular disease and stroke.

2. The ACOG Task Force on Hypertension in Pregnancy classifies hypertensive disorders during pregnancy, as shown in Table 13.2.

Table 13.2 Classification of Hypertension in Pregnancy	
Chronic hypertension	Hypertension diagnosis prior to becoming pregnant or before the 20th week of pregnancy and persisting beyond the 84th day postpartum.
Pre-eclampsia/eclampsia	Pre-eclampsia (PE) or eclampsiais is a disorder of pregnancy characterized by high blood pressure and a large amount of protein in the urine. The disorder usually occurs in the third trimester and gets worse over time. May result in eclampsia, which is seizure activity.
Pre-eclampsia superimposed on chronic hypertension	Superimposed Pre-eclampsia is a hypertensive disorder that usually develops after the 20th week of pregnancy and is characterized by chronic hypertension and proteinuria (protein in the urine).
Gestational hypertension	Gestational hypertension is defined as hypertension that occurs after 20 weeks in a woman with normal blood pressure that usually returns to normal after pregnancy. Gestational hypertension places women at risk for hypertension later in life.
Transient hypertension	Transient hypertension is high blood pressure near the end of pregnancy. Women with transient hypertension do not have any signs of having Pre-eclampsia. These women will have normal blood pressure again after they have their baby.

3. Pre-eclampsia is identified as hypertension (at least 140/90 mm Hg) and the presence of proteinuria, at least 300 mg in a 24-hour urine specimen.

4. Risk factors include primiparity; previous pre-eclampsia; increased BMI prior to pregnancy; multiple gestations; underlying medical conditions such as diabetes, chronic hypertension, renal disease, and obesity; family history; African American ethnicity; and pregnancies that result from insemination. Age is also reported as a risk factor (younger than 19 years and older than 40 years).

5. Pre-eclampsia involves multiple systems, including immune, cardiac, and renal. It is characterized by placental insufficiency during early pregnancy, vascular dysfunction, and vasospasm. Prompt identification and intervention of the disorder is essential.

6. Fetal risks include IUGR, prematurity, and death.

7. Classification of pre-eclampsia is divided into clinical manifestations of the disease based on end-organ effects.

   a) Hemolysis, elevated liver enzymes and low platelet levels (HELLP) syndrome is a variation of severe pre-eclampsia and is based on laboratory values. Blood pressure may be mildly elevated and proteinuria may be absent (Table 13.3).

8. Management

   a) Clients diagnosed with mild Pre-eclampsia can often be managed at home.

Table 13.3 Assessment Findings of Pre-eclampsia

Mild Pre-eclampsia	Severe Pre-eclampsia	Eclampsia	HELLP Syndrome
Begins after the 20th week of gestation	Begins after the 20th week of gestation	Begins after the 20th week of gestation	Diagnosed by laboratory tests
Elevated blood pressure at 140/90 or greater on two occasions at least 4 hours apart OR Systolic increase of 30 mm Hg or a diastolic increase of 15 mm Hg from prepregnancy baseline	Elevated blood pressure that is 160/100 mm Hg or greater on two occasions at least 4 hours apart	Symptoms of severe pre-eclampsia with onset of seizure activity or coma	H: Hemolysis resulting in anemia and jaundice
Protein greater than or equal to 300 mg/24 hours or protein/creatinine ratio greater than or equal to 0.3 or dipstick reading greater than or equal to 1+	Proteinuria 3 to 4+	Usually preceded by headache, severe epigastric pain, hyperreflexia, and hemoconcentration	E: Elevated liver enzymes such as elevated alanine aminotransferase or elevated aspartate transaminase Epigastric pain Nausea and vomiting
No edema	Extensive peripheral edema		LP: Low platelets (<100,000/mm³), abnormal bleeding and clotting time, bleeding gums, petechiae, and possibly disseminated intravascular coagulation (DIC)
Normal urinary output	Oliguria		
Serum creatinine normal	Elevated serum creatinine greater than 1.2 mg/dL		
Transient headache No visual complaint	Cerebral or visual disturbances (headache and blurred vision)		
Normal reflexes	Hyperreflexia with possible ankle clonus		
Pulmonary and cardiac assessment normal	Pulmonary or cardiac involvement		
Normal hepatic function	Hepatic dysfunction (epigastric and right upper-quadrant pain)		
Normal platelet count	Thrombocytopenia		

b) Prior to discharge, it is very important that the client understand the importance of keeping all prenatal appointments and that she must notify her health care provider if she has:
- Increase in BP (client should be taught to take her BP at home every day).
- Visual changes.
- Epigastric pain.
- Nausea and vomiting.
- Bleeding gums.
- Headaches.
- Increased edema of the hands and face.
- Decreased urinary output.
- Decreased fetal movement.

Weekly or biweekly nonstress may be required. Weight is taken daily at the same time to identify edema. Client should be instructed to call her provider if she gains 3 pounds in 1 day or 4 pounds over the course of 3 days.

c) Severe pre-eclampsia should always be managed in the hospital because of the risk to the mother and fetus.

d) Medications used:
   (1) Magnesium sulfate
   - Magnesium is a central nervous system depressant.
   - Used for seizure prophylaxis.
   - Should be used cautiously with any degree of renal insufficiency because magnesium sulfate is excreted by the kidneys.
   - Side effects include drowsiness, decreased respiration, bradycardia, hypotension, diarrhea, muscle weakness, flushing, sweating, and hypothermia.
   - Administered intravenously by secondary fusion on volumetric infusion pump.
   - Initial loading dose of 4 to 6 grams infused over 15 to 30 minutes followed by a maintenance dose of 2 grams/hour.

   The patient should be assessed frequently to identify toxicity. Therapeutic serum magnesium level of 4 to 7 mEq/L.

   (a) Signs of magnesium toxicity are lethargy, muscle weakness, decreased or absent deep tendon reflexes (DTRs), decreased respirations (less than 12), double vision, and slurred speech.
   (b) The nurse must monitor pulse, BP, and respirations every 15 to 30 minutes (depending on client's condition) while administering magnesium sulfate.
   (c) Continuously monitor fetal heart rate and contraction pattern.
   (d) Monitor neurological status before and throughout therapy. Patellar reflex should be assessed every hour (or hospital protocol). If there is no response, no additional doses should be administered and health care provider should be notified.
   (e) After delivery, the neonate should be monitored closely for hypotension, hyporeflexia, and respiratory depression.
   (f) Monitor intake and output. Output should be at least 30 mL/hour. Restrict fluid intake to a total of no more than 125 mL/hour.
   (g) Assess for presence of headache, visual disturbances, level of consciousness, and epigastric pain at least every hour (indicates worsening).
   (h) Emergency drugs and intubation equipment should be available, side rails up, lights dim, and environment quiet.

(!) ALERT If magnesium toxicity is suspected, the magnesium sulfate infusion should be stopped immediately and calcium gluconate (antidote) should be given intravenously.

   (i) Hypertension medication used in pregnancy includes methyldopa, labetalol, hydralazine, and nifedipine (Table 13.4).

DID YOU KNOW?

For acute-onset, severe hypertension during pregnancy, ACOG Guidelines recommend the patient be given IV labetalol, IV hydralazine, or oral nifedipine if elevations persist. If IV access is not established, a 200-mg dose of labetalol can be given orally and repeated in 30 minutes. If elevations persist for 15 minutes or more, 20 mg of IV labetalol should be administered over 2 minutes. Repeat BP measure in 10 minutes if the threshold is still exceeded, administer 40 mg of IV labetalol over 2 minutes, and repeat BP in 10 minutes. If the threshold is not exceeded, continue to monitor.

K. Rh(D) isoimmunization
1. Isoimmunization is defined as the development of antibodies against the antigens of another individual of the same species.
2. Rh isoimmunization is the development of antibodies against RH antigens found on the surface red blood cell (RBC). The Rh antigen responsible for the most frequent cause for Rh isoimmunization is the Rhesus D antigen.
3. During pregnancy, the Rh-positive RBCs of the fetus gain entry into the Rh-negative circulation of the mother. The reticuloendothelial system

Table 13.4 Medication for Hypertension

Medication	Indication	Nursing Considerations
Hydralazine	Antihypertensive Direct-acting peripheral arteriolar vasodilator	• *Monitor blood pressure and pulse frequently during initial administration because may cause precipitous drops in blood pressure.* • *May cause positive direct Coombs test results.* • *Caution client to avoid sudden changes in position to minimize orthostatic hypotension.* • *If giving multiple doses, wait 20 minutes after first dose to assess client's response.*
Methyldopa	Antihypertensive Stimulates central nervous system's alpha-adrenergic receptors, resulting in decrease in sympathetic outflow to heart, kidneys, and blood vessels	• *Monitor blood pressure and pulse frequently during initial administration because may cause precipitous drops in blood pressure.* • *May cause positive direct Coombs test result.* • *Caution client to avoid sudden changes in position to minimize orthostatic hypotension.*
Labetalol	Antihypertensive Blocks stimulation of beta 1 and beta 2 receptor sites	• *Do not give to clients with a history of bronchial asthma or heart failure.* • *Monitor blood pressure and pulse during administration.* • *Assess for orthostatic hypotension when assisting client out of bed.*
Nifedipine	Antihypertensive Inhibits calcium transport into myocardial and vascular smooth muscles cells, resulting in systemic vasodilation	• *Do not administer to clients with known coronary artery disease.* • *Monitor blood pressure and pulse frequently during initial administration because may cause precipitous drops in blood pressure.* • *May cause positive direct Coombs test result.* • *Caution client to avoid sudden changes in position to minimize orthostatic hypotension.* • *If giving multiple doses, wait 20 minutes after first dose to assess client's response.* • *Do not administer sublingually.* • *Do not administer if client is on magnesium sulfate because of skeletal muscle blockade.*

recognizes these antigens as foreign and develops antibodies in response.

4. During the first pregnancy, these antibodies do not usually harm the fetus. In subsequent pregnancies where the fetus is positive, the number of antibodies can increase and cross the placenta and result in fetal anemia.

5. In order to prevent this from happening, the Rh-negative mother, who gives birth to an Rh-positive fetus, receives Rh immune globulin (a solution of immune globulin that contains Rh antibodies) within 72 hours of giving birth.
   a) Rh immune globulin promotes lysis of the infant's RBCs, before the mother can develop antibodies, which is known as *maternal sensitization.*
   b) In the first pregnancy, the Rh-negative mother who has an Rh-positive baby is usually not problematic. In subsequent pregnancies, there will be an increase in antibodies formed if RhoGAM is not administered, resulting in isoimmunization.

6. If isoimmunization occurs, the antibodies can cross the placenta and attack the fetus's RBCs. This can result in severe hemolytic anemia if the mother's antibodies attack the RBCs. The placenta is usually able to clear the bilirubin.

However, in some cases, there is a buildup, creating jaundice.

7. The infant responds to the hemolysis of RBCs by creating large immature RBCs. This is known as **erythroblastosis fetalis.**
   a) If the hemolysis is really severe, the infant develops **hydrops fetalis.** In this condition, the infant develops severe anemia, cardiac decompensation, cardiomegaly, hepatosplenomegaly, and/or **kernicterus.**
   b) There is severe hypoxia, and due to lower oncotic pressure, fluid leaks out of the intravascular space, resulting in severe edema and placental swelling.

8. Assessment
   a) All women should be tested for blood group, have Rh factor and routine antibody screening, and should be checked for history of previous miscarriage and blood transfusions.
      (1) Maternal blood is drawn for the indirect Coombs test. This test determines if the Rh-negative woman has developed antibodies to the Rh antigen.
      (2) Newborn blood is drawn from the umbilical cord shortly after birth for the direct Coombs test. This test determines if maternal antibodies are attached to fetal RBCs.

9. Medication
   a) Rh$_0$Dimmune globulin (RhoGAM) provides passive immunity by preventing production of anti-Rh$_0$D antibodies in Rh$_0$-negative women who were exposed to Rh$_0$D-positive blood. It also prevents hemolytic disease of newborns in future pregnancies of women who have conceived an Rh$_0$D-positive fetus.
      (1) Abortions, ectopic pregnancy, chorionic villi sampling, fetal-maternal hemorrhage due to amniocentesis, obstetrical manipulation procedures, and trauma when pregnant with Rh$_0$-positive fetus are all risk factors when exposed.
   b) For an unsensitized Rh-negative mother, administer 1 vial (300 mcg) intramuscularly in the deltoid or gluteal muscle (or can be give IV). This should be sufficient to prevent maternal sensitization.
      (1) Given at 25 weeks gestation and 72 hours after birth.
      (2) If a large fetomaternal transfusion is noted, the dosage of RhoGam is determined by Kleihauer-Betke test. This test can detect the amount of fetal blood in maternal circulation.
10. Nursing considerations for administration of RhoGAM:
    • Standard dose 28 weeks prophylaxis or after exposure
    • Within 72 hours after delivery if infant is Rh-positive
    • Verify that client is Rh-negative and has not been sensitized by indirect Coombs test, and verify that direct Coombs test is negative and newborn is Rh-positive
    • Signed consent to receive human plasma, verify dosage and lot number, observe for 20 minutes after administration

L. Preterm labor
   1. Preterm labor is a major cause of infant morbidity and mortality.
      a) Preterm labor is defined as the onset of regular contractions between 20 and 37 weeks of gestation.
      b) There is no definitive cause for why preterm labor occurs, but factors associated with increased risk of preterm labor include previous preterm birth, multiple gestations, history of induced abortions, psychological distress.
      c) Many women experience preterm birth without any risk factors. All women should be taught signs and symptoms of preterm labor and should notify their health care provider if they experience any of these symptoms. Signs and symptoms of preterm labor include:
         • Contractions occurring more than once every 10 minutes and lasting for 1 hour or more.
         • Uterine contractions that may or may not be painful.
         • Pain or pressure in thighs or cervical area.
         • Lower abdominal cramping (may also have diarrhea).
         • Dull low backache (lower lumbar and sacral area).
         • Pelvic pressure that feels like the "baby is coming out."
         • Vaginal discharge that has a change in character or amount (e.g., thicker, thinner, bloody, brown, increased amount, or has odor).
         • Rupture of membranes.
      d) If a woman experiences signs and symptoms of preterm labor, it is important to delay delivery until corticosteroids can be administered to facilitate lung development of the fetus. The client should be transferred to a hospital with a high-level neonatal intensive care unit.
         (1) Recommendation for corticosteroid administration is for clients between 24 and 32 weeks who are at risk for delivery within 7 days.
      e) Women experiencing preterm labor are treated with tocolytics for short-term protection (up to 48 hours) to allow for the administration of corticosteroids for fetal lung maturity (Table 13.5).
M. Preterm premature rupture of membranes (PPROM)
   1. Defined as the rupture of membranes prior to 37 weeks gestation.
   2. The woman may experience a gush of fluid or small amount of leakage from the vagina after rupture of the amniotic sac.
   3. The earlier the rupture of the membranes, the worse the outcome for the fetus, because of the risk of **chorioamnionitis** and preterm delivery.
   4. The time between rupture of the membrane and delivery is known as the *latency period.*
   5. If PPROM occurs before 34 weeks gestation, attempts may be made to prolong latency, as long as there are no signs of active labor, infection, or significant vaginal bleeding and if fetal status is reassuring.
   6. If the latency period can be prolonged, corticosteroids can be administered to the mother to promote fetal lung development. If the infant can be delivered later in the pregnancy, there should be fewer neonatal complications. However, prolonging the latency period increases the risk of infection.

Table 13.5 Medications for Preterm Labor

Medication	Dosage and Route	Adverse Effects	Nursing Considerations
Terbutaline sulfate (beta-adrenergic receptor agonist) Unlabeled use for relaxation of uterine smooth muscles Bronchodilator	0.25 mg subcutaneous injection every 4 hours	Nervousness, restlessness, tremor, headache, insomnia, pulmonary edema, tachycardia, palpitations, nasal congestion, nausea, vomiting, hyperglycemia, hypokalemia	• *Assess lung sounds, respiratory pattern, pulse, and blood pressure prior to administration* • *Monitor fetal heart rate and contractions prior to and after administration* • *Assess for maternal pulmonary edema (increased respiratory rate, dyspnea, rales/crackles, frothy sputum)*
Indomethacin (nonsteroidal anti-inflammatory) Relaxes uterine smooth muscles by inhibiting prostaglandins	Oral loading dose of 50 mg Maintenance oral dose of 25–50 mg every 6 hours for 48 hours because longer administration may constrict ductus arteriosus of the fetus	Nausea, vomiting	• *Only used if gestational age of fetus is less than 32 weeks* • *Do not administer longer than 48 hours* • *Can mask maternal fever*
Nifedipine (calcium channel blocker) Relaxes uterine smooth muscles	Oral loading dose of 10–20 mg every 3 to 6 hours until decrease in contractions Maintenance oral dose of 30–60 mg every 8–12 hours	Hypotension, headache, flushing, nausea	• *Do not administer with magnesium sulfate* • *Assess blood pressure prior to administration*
Magnesium sulfate (central nervous system depressant) Relaxes uterine smooth muscles	Loading dose: intravenous administration of 4–6 grams over 20–30 minutes Maintenance dose: 1–4 grams/hour	Hot flashes, nausea, vomiting, burning at IV insertion site, dry mouth, drowsiness, blurred vision, diplopia, headache, lethargy, hypocalcemia, shortness of breath, transient hypotension	• *Intravenous fluid should be 40 grams in 1,000 mL, secondary setup piggyback to primary infusion by controller pump* • *Obtain maternal and fetal baseline information prior to administration* • *Monitor serum magnesium levels for toxicity (therapeutic range 4–7.5 mEq/L)* • *Have calcium gluconate (antidote) available if toxicity occurs*

7. If PPROM occurs between 34 and 36 weeks, active labor is usually pursued. At 32 to 33 weeks, it will depend on fetal lung maturity and maternal risk of infection.
8. In clients experiencing PPROM, nurses need to closely monitor maternal and fetal status.
9. Nonstress testing and biophysical profile are done to assess fetal well-being.
   a) The mother should be taught to assess for daily fetal movement counts.
   b) A decrease in daily fetal movement counts is a sign of fetal distress and should immediately be reported to the health care provider.
10. A 7-day course of antibiotics will be prescribed. Treatment of patients experiencing PPROM with antimicrobials has shown to increase the latency period and reduce the risk of chorioamnionitis.
11. Maternal infection is another possible complication of PPROM.
    a) Maternal temperature should be monitored frequently and the mother should be taught to keep her genital area clean.
    b) The client should be instructed to not introduce anything into the vagina.
    c) The client should be taught to watch for and report foul-smelling vaginal discharge or odor and maternal or fetal tachycardia.
    d) The client should be told to immediately report increased temperature, foul-smelling vaginal odor or discharge, or increased pulse to her provider.
    e) Tocolytics may be administered until safe transport to a hospital with a neonatal intensive care unit.
12. Chorioamnionitis is a bacterial infection of the amnionic cavity.
    a) It can occur at any gestational age but is more common with PPROM. Chorioamnionitis is also associated with prolonged rupture of the membranes and frequent vaginal examinations during labor.
    b) Treatment of chorioamnionitis includes prompt administration of intravenous antibiotics.
    c) Usually broad-spectrum antibiotics such as penicillin and gentamycin are ordered.
    d) After delivery, the mother should receive coverage for anaerobic organisms with drugs such as metronidazole or clindamycin.

N. Incompetent cervix
1. An incompetent cervix is a painless dilation of the cervix without uterine contractions due to a structural or functional defect of the cervix and usually occurs around 20 weeks gestation. The woman is usually unaware of the dilation and presents with bulging membranes.
2. Risk factors include congenital, acquired, or hormonal factors. Congenital factors include the presence of a bicornuate uterus and in utero exposure to diethylstilbestrol (DES). Acquired factors include multiple gestations, inflammation or infection, cone biopsy, subclinical uterine activity, or second-trimester abortions. The hormone relaxin may be an endocrine cause of cervical incompetence.
3. Based on a woman's obstetric history (previous obstetric losses, previous preterm births, history of multiple gestation, cone biopsies, or other cervical procedures), close observation of cervical length via transvaginal ultrasound may be recommended.
4. On assessment, physical findings that may be noted are pink-stained vaginal discharge or bleeding and/or possible rupture of membranes.
5. Medical management
   a) Suturing of the cervix in the late first or early part of the second trimester. In women with a history of losses, **cerclage** may be done at 12 to 14 weeks gestation.
   b) If there are no complications, the cerclage will be removed at 36 weeks gestation to allow for vaginal delivery (Fig. 13.2).
6. Discharge instructions
   a) Bedrest for the first few days and abstain from sexual intercourse until after the post-op check. After the post-op check, the health care provider will advise the client about activity level and if sexual activity may resume.
   b) Hydration to promote a relaxed uterus (dehydration stimulates uterine contractions).
   c) Education on signs of impending birth, bedrest, serial ultrasounds, progesterone supplementation, and inflammatory drugs if prescribed. If the client experiences a rupture of the membranes, contractions that are 5 minutes apart, perineal pain, or the urge to push, she should immediately go to the hospital.

O. Placenta Previa
1. **Placenta previa** is an abnormal implantation of the placenta in the lower uterine wall close to or covering the cervical os. The abnormal implantation results in bleeding during the third trimester of pregnancy as the cervix begins to dilate and efface (Fig. 13.3).
2. Risk factors include a previous placenta previa, cesarean section, history of induced or spontaneous abortions, and cocaine use.
3. Fetal risk factors include hypoxia and preterm birth.

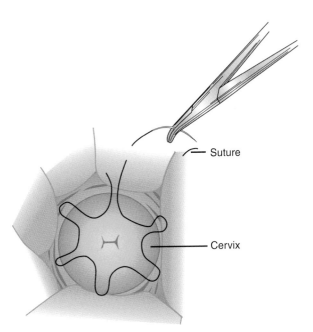

Fig 13.2 Cerclage.

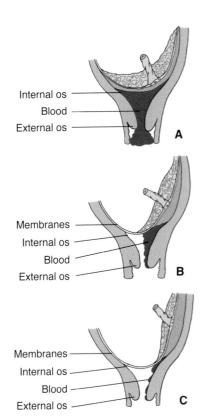

Fig 13.3 Types of placenta previa.

4. The presence of placenta previa is usually determined in the prenatal period during a routine ultrasound.

5. All clients who present with vaginal bleeding in the second trimester should be assessed for placenta previa.

⊘ ALERT Vaginal examination is contraindicated in cases of placenta previa, since the examiner could cause the placenta to separate, which could lead to excessive bleeding.

6. Care should include bedrest; frequent monitoring of fetal heart rate, maternal vital signs, blood loss; and strict intake of fluid and output of urine.

7. Potential complications of placenta previa include risk of abruptio, premature rupture of the membranes, preterm birth, and hemorrhage.

8. Discharge instructions include not putting anything in the vagina, not douching, and not engaging in intercourse because of possible placenta tearing.

9. Placenta accreta, placenta percreta, and placenta increta are placentas that attach to the endometrium in a weakened area. This results in an abnormal adherence to the endometrium.
   a) Confirmed via ultrasound during the antenatal period.
   b) The abnormal adherence to the uterus places the woman at risk of postpartum hemorrhage, especially if an attempt is made to manually extract the placenta after delivery. In cases where placenta accrete is known or suspected, no attempt should be made to pull on the placenta after delivery.

P. Placental abruption
   1. Placental abruption is defined as the placenta's detachment from the uterine wall, causing bleeding and interfering with the exchange of oxygen and nutrients to the fetus.
   2. Hypertension, substance abuse, smoking, intrauterine infection, and recent trauma are risk factors for **abruptio placenta.**
      a) Maternal hypertension and cocaine use are the most significant risk factors for placental abruption.
      b) Clinical signs of abruptio placenta include pain, vaginal bleeding, and uterine pain and tenderness.
         (1) If the placenta separates from the decidua, the blood flows out from the vagina. In some cases it may be concealed behind the placenta and in many cases both types of bleeding occur (Fig. 13.4).
         (2) Pain can be moderate to severe. Localized to one area or over the entire abdomen. The abdomen may be boardlike.

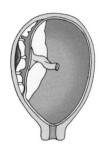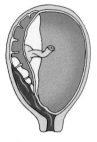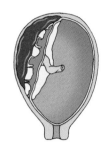

Partial separation (concealed hemorrhage) Partial separation (apparent hemorrhage) Complete separation (concealed hemorrhage)

Fig 13.4 Abruptio placentae.

         (3) If bleeding occurs between the placenta and uterine wall, it may produce a Couvelaire uterus.
   3. Medical management
      a) In cases where the bleeding is moderate to severe, a large-bore (16- to 18-gauge) needle should be in place in case a transfusion is indicated.
      b) Maternal vital signs are monitored frequently to detect excessive bleeding indicated by an increased pulse rate and declining BP.
      c) Serial blood studies of Hgb/Hct and clotting factors are done as well.
      d) A urinary catheter should be inserted for accurate measurement of urine output.
      e) Continuous fetal monitoring is indicated to observe fetal status.
      f) If abruption is mild and occurs between 20 and 34 weeks gestation, conservative treatment may be initiated. The client will be monitored closely for blood loss. The fetus will have nonstress testing and biophysical profiles done frequently to detect any changes.

Q. Perinatal infections
   1. Cytomegalovirus (CMV) is a herpesvirus that is transmitted through sexual contact with an infected person or direct contact with blood, urine, and secretions such as saliva.
      a) The incubation period from exposure to symptom development is 28 to 60 days. Many individuals with cytomegalovirus can be asymptomatic or some may have monolike symptoms.
      b) After exposure, CMV can lie dormant and be reactivated.
      c) Primary or secondary CMV can be transferred to the fetus via transplacental infection, exposure to secretions during delivery, or via breastfeeding.
      d) With primary CMV infection, the biggest risk of transmission is in the third trimester. Approximately one-third of infants exposed to CMV will be affected.

e) The fetus exposed to CMV may be asymptomatic at delivery or present with thrombocytopenia, petechiae, or myocarditis.

f) After secondary infection, the infant may present with congenital hearing loss and neurological sequelae. Many may develop cerebral palsy or intellectual disability.

g) Currently, universal screening for CMV is not recommended because there is no current treatment for transmission.[5] There is some data to suggest that women working with children are at higher risk. Women are encouraged to wash hands carefully after touching a child's body fluids to reduce risk of transmission.

2. Parvovirus B19 is the virus that causes childhood exanthema erythema infectiosum, also known as *fifth disease*. Children with fifth disease may present with reddened cheeks, a lacelike rash on their extremities, joint pain, and sometimes fever.

a) Most children and adults recover completely. Transmission is generally through respiratory secretions and hand-to-mouth contact and generally occurs 5 to 10 days prior to the appearance of the rash. Once the rash appears, the child is no longer contagious.

b) There is likely an increased risk of transmission of the virus to individuals living in the same household. Risk of transmission in childcare or classroom settings is believed to be 20% to 50%.

c) Maternal to fetal transmission is estimated to be 17% to 33%. Most transmission does not cause harmful effects, but infection with the virus is believed to increase the risk for hydrops fetalis, abortion, and stillbirth. Severe infections are more prevalent in infections occurring before 20 weeks gestation.[6]

d) Currently, routine screening for parvovirus B19 is not recommended since there is a low risk of seroconversion and there is no treatment for the virus. In areas of endemic outbreaks, women should have testing, since more careful monitoring of the fetus is recommended.

e) In women who seroconvert when pregnant, it is suggested they have ultrasound testing for fetal anemia. In severe cases, intrauterine transfusions may be recommended. In addition, the infant should be screened for hydrops fetalis.

3. Varicella zoster virus is responsible for the transmission of varicella or chickenpox. Most women should have immunity via varicella immunization or documentation of varicella infection earlier in life.

a) In cases where status is uncertain, varicella immunoglobulin titers can be drawn and sent to the laboratory to determine if immunity exists. Although the rate of vertical transmission from mother to fetus remains low, there are mixed findings regarding the impact on the fetus/newborn.

b) Ultrasound findings that suggest varicella infection in the fetus include hydrops, hyperechogenic foci in the liver and bowel, cardiac malformations, limb deformities, microcephaly, and fetal growth restriction.[7] Infants without anatomical defects on ultrasound appeared to have normal neurodevelopment.

c) If a pregnant woman develops varicella during pregnancy, administration of oral acyclovir may be recommended. If acyclovir is administered within 24 hours of the eruption of the rash, it has been shown to reduce the number of new lesions formed and to reduce the number of lesions and symptoms (ACOG, 2015). Although acyclovir may diminish symptoms in pregnant women, it does not appear to diminish the harmful effects on the fetus.

d) Infants born to mothers infected with varicella 5 days before delivery to 2 days after treatment should be given varicella immune globulin. Infants who develop varicella infection should be treated with intravenous acyclovir (ACOG, 2015).

e) In general, all women should be counseled on the benefits of varicella immunization if there is no documentation of varicella vaccine, infection, or immune titers.

f) It is recommended to give two immunizations. The second should be given 4 to 8 weeks after the initial dose. When receiving the live attenuated varicella virus vaccine, women should be encouraged to receive reproductive counseling and delay pregnancy for 3 months.

g) There is a small risk of contracting a mild form of the disease that could impact the developing fetus. In general, documenting and recommending varicella immunization should be part of preconception care, postpartum care, and after any fetal loss or abortion.

---

[5] American College of Obstetricians and Gynecologists (ACOG). (2015). ACOG guidelines at a glance: Key points about 4 perinatal infections. Retrieved from http://contemporaryobgyn.modernmedicine.com/contemporary-obgyn/news/acog-guidelines-glance-key-points-about-4-perinatal-infections-0.

[6] American College of Obstetricians and Gynecologists (ACOG). (2015). ACOG guidelines at a glance: Key points about 4 perinatal infections. Retrieved from http://contemporaryobgyn.modernmedicine.com/contemporary-obgyn/news/acog-guidelines-glance-key-points-about-4-perinatal-infections-0.

[7] American College of Obstetricians and Gynecologists (ACOG). (2015). ACOG guidelines at a glance: Key points about 4 perinatal infections. Retrieved from http://contemporaryobgyn.modernmedicine.com/contemporary-obgyn/news/acog-guidelines-glance-key-points-about-4-perinatal-infections-0.

4. Group beta streptococcus (GBS) infection is a leading cause of preterm birth and fetal death in the United States.
   a) Infection of the maternal genital tract with GBS is considered a precursor to chorioamnionitis, fetal infection, and neonatal sepsis.
   b) Intrapartum antibiotic treatment is recommended for women who have:
      • Delivered a previous GBS-positive infant.
      • A GBS-positive bacteria in the current pregnancy.
      • An unknown GBS status and delivered before 37 weeks.
      • An intrapartum temperature of 100.4 or greater.
      • Ruptured membranes for 18 hours or longer.
   c) Penicillin is the recommended antibiotic of choice, with ampicillin an acceptable alternative. The infants of mothers with suspected GBS should be evaluated for signs of sepsis. If maternal chorioamnionitis is suspected, the infant should also be evaluated. In some cases, the infant may need treatment with antibiotic therapy.

MAKING THE CONNECTION

GBS Recommendations

In 2002, the Centers for Disease Control and Prevention (CDC) first recommended routine rectal–vaginal screening for GBS at 35 to 37 weeks. In 2010, those guidelines were updated and confirmed the need to screen all women at 35 to 37 weeks gestation and implement antibiotic therapy if cultures are positive. Clinical Guidelines regarding treatment for GBS were also reviewed and updated.

5. According to the CDC, herpes simplex virus (HSV) is estimated to affect one in six persons aged 14 to 49 in the United States.[9]
   a) This virus can cause painful lesions in the genital tract and even on the cervix. Neonatal herpes infection occurs in 1 in 35, 000 births.
   b) If the primary infection occurs in the first trimester, there is an increased risk of abortion.
   c) If the primary infection occurs in the second or third trimester preterm labor, IUGR and neonatal infection are a greater risk. It is estimated that 80% of new infections are caused by HSV-1. If the HSV-1 or HSV-2 lesion is acquired close to the time of birth, there is a risk of 30% to 60% transmission with a vaginal birth.
   d) Women with active or recurrent herpes simplex receive acyclovir at 36 weeks of gestation or later in pregnancy. Acyclovir is believed to decrease viral shedding, reduce recurrences, decrease chances of neonatal infection, and lower the chance for needing a cesarean delivery.
   e) In women with active genital lesions or prodromal symptoms such as pain or itching of the vulva, it is recommended they deliver via cesarean section, since these may be signs of impending outbreak.
   f) Breastfeeding is contraindicated in women with herpes lesions on the breast.[10]

---

[9] Centers for Disease Control and Prevention (CDC). (2015). 2014 Sexually transmitted disease surveillance. Retrieved from http://www.cdc.gov/std/stats14/other.htm#herpes.
[10] American College of Obstetricians and Gynecologists (ACOG). (2012). Management of herpes in pregnancy. ACOG Practice Bulletin No. 82: Management of Herpes in Pregnancy. Obstetrics & Gynecology, 109(6). doi:10.1097/01.AOG.0000263902.31953.3e.

CASE STUDY: Putting It All Together

Subjective Data

Jennifer, a 26-year-old primigravida G1T0P0A0L0, is at her first prenatal visit. She reports that her immunizations are up to date.

Objective Data

Vital Signs	
Blood pressure: 120/68 (initial visit); 140/90 (subsequent visit) Urine trace protein, glucose: negative	BMI: 30 Blood type: Rh negative

_____ **Case Study Questions** _____

1. What blood tests should be done?

CASE STUDY: Putting It All Together (Continued)

_____ **Case Study Questions** _____

2. What kinds of teaching should be done?

At 28 weeks gestation, Jennifer returns for her prenatal visit. Her blood pressure is 140/90 and she has facial swelling. Her urine is 1-plus for protein and negative for glucose. She is diagnosed with pre-eclampsia.

3. Identify risk factors that Jennifer has for pre-eclampsia.

4. What other pregnancy-related complications is she at risk for because of the pre-eclampsia?

Jennifer is started on labetalol orally to treat the hypertension. After 2 days of treatment, her blood pressure decreases to 120/84. She is placed on home blood pressure monitoring.

5. What will her patient teaching involve?

At 36 weeks gestation, Jennifer's blood pressure is again elevated. On admission to the labor and delivery unit, her blood pressure is 160/110. She is advised to lie on her left side and a magnesium sulfate bolus is given. She is to be maintained on 2 g/hr of magnesium sulfate.

6. What kind of nursing assessments and interventions are needed?

Six hours after the magnesium sulfate, Jennifer complains of blurred vision and her blood pressure is 140/90. Her reflexes are 3-plus, her urine output is 80 cc in the past 2 hours, and her respiratory rate is 16.

7. What is the most appropriate nursing intervention?

REVIEW QUESTIONS

1. Which factor places the client at the highest risk of pre-eclampsia?
   1. White race
   2. Multiparity
   3. Obesity
   4. Infertility

2. The nurse is caring for a woman with a history of a previous preterm birth. Based on current knowledge related to cervical incompetency, which should the nurse do?
   1. Prepare the woman for an abdominal ultrasound
   2. Place the patient on her left side to increase perfusion to the fetus
   3. Be prepared to discuss the action and side effects of progesterone
   4. Monitor the patient's blood pressure closely

3. The nurse is caring for a client who is at 24 weeks gestation. Which assessment requires further intervention?
   1. Hemoglobin 11 and hematocrit 33
   2. Blood pressure of 130/80
   3. Patient has slight pedal swelling
   4. Urine dipstick for protein 3+

4. The nurse is assessing a client who has been diagnosed with gestational diabetes. Which should the nurse monitor closely because of her diagnosis?
   1. Edema
   2. Blood pressure, pulse, and respiration
   3. Urine for glucose and ketones
   4. Hemoglobin and hematocrit

5. A nurse has just completed an assessment on a client with mild pre-eclampsia. Which data indicate that her pre-eclampsia is worsening?
   1. Blood pressure of 155/95
   2. Urinary output is greater than 30 mL/hr
   3. Deep tendon reflexes +2
   4. Client complains of blurred vision

6. The nurse is caring for a woman who is suspected of having chorioamnionitis. Which of the following are risk factors for chorioamnionitis? *Select all that apply.*
   1. Changing cat litter
   2. Frequent vaginal examination during labor
   3. Gestational diabetes
   4. Preterm premature rupture of the membranes
   5. pre-eclampsia and eclampsia

7. The nurse is monitoring a woman with signs and symptoms of preterm labor. Which does the nurse include in the teaching plan?
   1. Importance of performing daily fetal movement counts
   2. Need to refrain from putting any objects in the vagina
   3. Need to take a daily stool softener
   4. The need to decrease fluid intake

8. The nurse is providing discharge instructions to a 28-year-old client who received methotrexate for an ectopic pregnancy. Which should the discharge instructions include?
   1. Make sure to take folic acid
   2. Make an appointment to see her provider in 6 weeks
   3. Flush the toilet twice after she urinates for the next 24 hours
   4. Resume all activity in 48 hours

9. A nurse is caring for a client who is 32 weeks gestation who comes to the emergency department for painful bleeding. Which is the *priority* nursing assessment?
   1. Monitor for contractions
   2. Assess pain level
   3. Assess for hemorrhage
   4. Provide emotional support

10. The nurse is caring for a client with a suspected hydatidiform mole. Based on the diagnosis, what does the nurse anticipate? *Select all that apply.*
    1. Dark brown vaginal bleeding
    2. Strong fetal heart tones
    3. Fundal height larger than expected
    4. Elevated blood pressure
    5. Severe abdominal pain

11. The nurse is caring for a 35-year-old client with gestational diabetes. Which teaching should be included? *Select all that apply.*
    1. Telling the client the importance of consuming a bedtime snack
    2. Informing the patient she is at high risk of type 2 diabetes after the pregnancy
    3. Informing the patient that her labor may have to be induced
    4. Teaching the patient to drink plenty of fresh fruit drinks to stay hydrated
    5. Teaching the patient how to test her A1C level every day

12. During an assessment of a client at 32 weeks gestation with a history of congenital ventral septal defect, a nurse notes that the client is experiencing a nonproductive cough on minimal exertion. The nurse knows that this assessment finding may indicate which of the following?
    1. Orthopnea
    2. Pulmonary edema
    3. Anemia
    4. Decreased blood volume

13. A nurse is monitoring a client with type 2 diabetes mellitus. Her blood work reveals a glycosylated hemoglobin (HbA1c) of 10%. The nurse knows this blood work indicates which of the following?
    1. A normal value indicating that the client is managing blood glucose control well
    2. A low value indicating that the client is not managing blood glucose control very well
    3. A high value indicating that the client is not managing blood glucose control very well
    4. The value does not offer information regarding client management of her disease

14. The labor and delivery nurse reviews a client's prenatal records and notes that the client had a positive GBS culture at 27 weeks gestation. Based on current guidelines, what is the recommended plan?
    1. Send a GBS to the laboratory immediately
    2. Prepare to administer penicillin prophylactically
    3. Determine if a follow-up culture was done at 38 weeks gestation
    4. Determine if the patient received antibiotics for the positive strep

15. The nurse is caring for a client in labor who is HIV positive. Which nursing care should be included? *Select all that apply.*
    1. Administering antiretroviral drugs as ordered
    2. Assisting the woman on a labor ball to help with natural descent of the fetus
    3. Handling the newborn with gloves until it receives its first bath
    4. Encouraging the mother to breastfeed soon after delivery
    5. Assigning the patient to a private room to prevent transmission

16. The nurse is caring for a patient who is receiving magnesium sulfate for pre-eclampsia. Which assessments will be of the highest *priority*?
    1. Assessing lung sounds
    2. Assessing blood sugar level
    3. Encouraging fluid intake
    4. Assessing for pitting edema

17. The nurse is caring for a client with severe hyperemesis gravidarum. She is 10 weeks gestation and has a 10% weight loss. The client is being admitted for fluid and electrolyte replacement. The nurse is aware it is important to check which deficiency that puts the client at risk for Wernicke's encephalopathy?
    1. Folic acid
    2. Vitamin D
    3. Thiamine
    4. Glucose

18. The doctor suspects that the client is in preterm labor. Which symptom is consistent with this diagnosis?
    1. Severe pain in the lower quadrant
    2. Severe pain and hard abdomen to palpation
    3. Painless vaginal bleeding
    4. Abdominal cramping and lower back pain

19. A 17-year-old client has been admitted to the hospital for hyperemesis gravidarum. Which factor likely caused her condition?
    1. Having high levels of hCG
    2. Having high blood pressure
    3. Being an adolescent
    4. Being underweight

20. A client who is 30 weeks pregnant comes into the labor and delivery unit complaining of having a gush of fluid come from her vagina. Which complication is this client at risk for?
    1. Infection
    2. Fluid volume deficit
    3. Hypotension
    4. Decreased urinary output

21. A nurse is caring for a client who is G1P0 and 36 weeks gestation who has been diagnosed with severe pre-eclampsia. Her blood pressure is 165/110. The physician has ordered hydralazine. The nurse knows she should do which of the following when administering this medication? *Select all that apply.*
    1. Position the client supine with the head of the bed elevated 30 degrees.
    2. Get baseline blood pressure and pulse and monitor frequently during administration.
    3. Administer medication every 5 minutes until blood pressure is stabilized.
    4. Inform the client that this may cause a positive direct Coombs test result.
    5. Instruct client that she may get a headache and feel flushed after administration.

228 Unit 3 Antepartum

22. Which postpartum client should receive RhoGAM?
    1. A postpartum client who has a negative indirect Coombs test and is A-positive
    2. A postpartum client who is B-negative and has just delivered an infant who is B-positive and has a positive direct Coombs test
    3. A postpartum client who is B-negative and has just delivered an infant who is B-positive and has a negative direct Coombs test
    4. A postpartum client who has just delivered an infant who is A-negative and has a negative direct Coombs test.

23. A nurse is caring for a woman who is on magnesium sulfate for pre-eclampsia. Her assessment reveals absent DTRs, respirations 10 per minute, decreased level of conscious, and urinary output less than 20 mL/hour. What medication would the nurse anticipate the physician to order?
    1. Naloxone
    2. Oxytocin
    3. Labetalol
    4. Calcium gluconate

24. A nurse is caring for a client who has type 1 diabetes that is not well controlled. The nurse understands that the client is a risk for which of the following? *Select all that apply.*
    1. Large for gestational age newborn
    2. Polyhydramnios
    3. Premature rupture of membranes
    4. Hyperemesis gravidarum
    5. Generalized edema

25. The nurse is caring for a client with severe pre-eclampsia. Which is an important intervention for the nurse to perform?
    1. Make sure calcium gluconate is ordered.
    2. Pad the client's bed rails and headboard.
    3. Keep lights on for visualization of client's breathing pattern.
    4. Have tongue blade within easy reach.

1. ANSWER: 3
Rationale
1. Whites are not at high risk for developing pre-eclampsia.
2. Multiparity is not a high risk factor for developing pre-eclampsia.
3. Obesity places the woman at risk of pre-eclampsia.
4. Infertility is not a high risk factor for developing pre-eclampsia.
TEST-TAKING TIP: Obesity; being African American, an adolescent mother, and a mother over the age of 35; and first-time pregnancies are high risk factors for developing pre-eclampsia.
Content Area: Pre-eclampsia; Antepartum at Risk
Integrated Process: Nursing Process—Assessment
Client Need: Physiological Integrity—Reduction of Risk Potential
Cognitive Level: Comprehension
Concept: Pregnancy
Reference: Lowdermilk, D. L., Perry, S. E., Cashion, K., & Alden, K. R. (2016). Maternity & women's health care. 11th ed. St. Louis, MO: Elsevier.

2. ANSWER: 3
Rationale
1. Transvaginal ultrasound would be used to confirm cervical incompetency.
2. Generally there is no issue with fetal perfusion or blood pressure, so these choices are incorrect.
3. The woman with cervical incompetency can be treated with cerclage or progesterone to retain the pregnancy.
4. Generally there is no issue with fetal perfusion or blood pressure, so these choices are incorrect.
TEST-TAKING TIP: Risk factors include congenital, acquired, or hormonal factors. Congenital factors include the presence of a bicornuate uterus and in utero exposure to diethylstilbestrol. Acquired factors include multiple gestations, inflammation or infection, cone biopsy, subclinical uterine activity, or second-trimester abortions. The hormone relaxin may be an endocrine cause of cervical incompetence.
Content Area: Incompetent Cervix; Antepartum at Risk
Integrated Process: Nursing Process—Implementation
Client Need: Safe and Effective Care Environment—Management of Care
Cognitive Level: Application
Concept: Pregnancy
Reference: Lowdermilk, D. L., Perry, S. E., Cashion, K., & Alden, K. R. (2016). Maternity & women's health care. 11th ed. St. Louis, MO: Elsevier.

3. ANSWER: 4
Rationale
1. This assessment is within normal limits and does not warrant further intervention.
2. This assessment is within normal limits and does not warrant further intervention.
3. This assessment is within normal limits and does not warrant further intervention.
4. This assessment is related to the clinical finding of pre-eclampsia.

TEST-TAKING TIP: Pre-eclampsia is identified as hypertension (140/90 mm Hg or higher) and presence of proteinuria, 300 mg or higher in a 24-hour urine specimen.
Content Area: Hypertensive Disorders; Antepartum at Risk
Integrated Process: Nursing Process—Assessment
Client Need: Physiological Integrity
Cognitive Level: Application
Concept: Perfusion
Reference: Murray, S. S., & McKinney, E. S. (2014). Foundations of maternal-newborn and women's health nursing. 6th ed. St. Louis, MO: Elsevier.

4. ANSWER: 3
Rationale
1. Edema is a clinical manifestation of pre-eclampsia.
2. Blood pressure, pulse, and respiration are assessment components that need to be performed at every prenatal visit.
3. Hyperinsulinemia will cause glucose and ketones to be present in the urine.
4. Hemoglobin and hematocrit should be followed closely if the client had a diagnosis of anemia.
TEST-TAKING TIP: Use the process of elimination, focusing on the client's diagnosis. Option 3 is the only assessment specifically related to gestational diabetes.
Content Area: Diabetes; Antepartum at Risk
Integrated Process: Nursing Process—Assessment
Client Need: Physiological Integrity
Cognitive Level: Application
Concept: Metabolism
Reference: Lowdermilk, D. L., Perry, S. E., Cashion, K., & Alden, K. R. (2016). Maternity & women's health care. 11th ed. St. Louis, MO: Elsevier.

5. ANSWER: 4
Rationale
1. Mild pre-eclampsia is defined as BP of 140/90 and severe pre-eclampsia is BP of 160/100.
2. Worsening pre-eclampsia would manifest as oliguria or decreased urinary output.
3. A client with severe pre-eclampsia would have +4 deep tendon reflexes or clonus.
4. Client complaints of headache or blurred vision indicate worsening of pre-eclampsia.
TEST-TAKING TIP: Focus on "worsening." To answer this question, you need to understand the difference in clinical presentation for mild and severe pre-eclampsia. Options 1, 2, and 3 are all assessment findings in a client with mild pre-eclampsia.
Content Area: Hypertension in Pregnancy; Antepartum at Risk
Integrated Process: Nursing Process—Evaluation
Client Need: Physiological Integrity
Cognitive Level: Analysis
Concept: Perfusion
Reference: Ward, S. L., & Hisley, S. M. (2016). Maternal-child nursing care. 2nd ed. Philadelphia: F.A. Davis.

6. ANSWER: 2, 4
Rationale
1. Changing cat litter is a risk factor for developing toxoplasmosis.

2. Frequent vaginal examination during labor is a risk factor for developing ascending infections.

3. Having gestational diabetes is not a risk factor for the development of chorioamnionitis.

4. Women who have preterm premature rupture of the membranes or who have membranes ruptured for more than 24 hours are at increased risk of chorioamnionitis.

5. Pre-eclampsia/eclampsia is not a risk factor for the development of chorioamnionitis.

TEST-TAKING TIP: Chorioamnionitis can occur at any gestational age but is more common with PPROM. It is also associated with prolonged rupture of the membranes and frequent vaginal examination during labor. Treatment of chorioamnionitis includes prompt administration of intravenous antibiotics—usually broad-spectrum antibiotics such as penicillin and gentamycin.

Content Area: Preterm Premature Rupture of Membranes; Antepartum at Risk
Integrated Process: Nursing Process—Assessment
Client Need: Physiological Integrity—Physiological Adaptation: Pathophysiology
Cognitive Level: Application
Concept: Infection
Reference: Durham, R. F., & Chapman, L. (2016). Maternal-child nursing care. 2nd ed. Philadelphia: F.A. Davis.

7. ANSWER: 2
Rationale
1. Education on daily fetal movement counts would be indicated to assess for fetal well-being. Decreased fetal movement is not a sign and symptom of preterm labor.

2. Education should be given concerning abstaining from sexual intercourse and nipple stimulation.

3. Education on the need for a daily stool softener would be correct if the client was constipated.

4. The client should be educated on maintaining hydration with an increase in fluid intake. Dehydration may lead to preterm contractions.

TEST-TAKING TIP: All women should be taught signs and symptoms of preterm labor and to notify their health care provider if they experience any of these symptoms. Signs and symptoms of preterm labor include contractions, pain or pressure in the thighs or cervical area, and rupture of the amniotic sac or a gush of fluids.

Content Area: Preterm Labor; Antepartum at Risk
Integrated Process: Nursing Process—Implementation
Client Need: Physiological Integrity—Physiological Adaptation: Pathophysiology
Cognitive Level: Application
Concept: Pregnancy
Reference: Lowdermilk, D. L., Perry, S. E., Cashion, K., & Alden, K. R. (2016). Maternity & women's health care. 11th ed. St. Louis, MO: Elsevier.

8. ANSWER: 3
Rationale
1. The client should avoid foods high in folic acid.

2. Weekly quantitative hCG levels will be drawn to make sure the level continues to decrease.

3. Methotrexate is excreted in the urine and feces. Special instructions are given to reduce risk to others.

4. There is no activity limitation when taking methotrexate.

TEST-TAKING TIP: The client needs to return within 1 week for follow-up. She needs to avoid gaseous foods and foods high in folic acid. The client will need to be monitored weekly for hCG levels to make sure she is no longer pregnant.

Content Area: Ectopic Pregnancy; Antepartum at Risk
Integrated Process: Nursing Process—Implementation
Client Need: Physiological Integrity—Pharmacological and Parenteral Therapies: Medication Administration
Cognitive Level: Application
Concept: Medication
Reference: Durham, R. F., & Chapman, L. (2016). Maternal-child nursing care. 2nd ed. Philadelphia: F.A. Davis.

9. ANSWER: 3
Rationale
1. Assessing for hemorrhage and shock is a higher priority assessment.

2. Assessing for pain would not be the priority assessment.

3. Clients with bleeding should be assessed for hemorrhage.

4. Providing emotional support would be an intervention, not an assessment.

TEST-TAKING TIP: Remember that the clinical signs of placental abruption include pain, vaginal bleeding, and uterine pain and tenderness. Maternal vital signs should be monitored frequently to detect excessive bleeding.

Content Area: Placental Abruption; Antepartum at Risk
Integrated Process: Nursing Process—Assessment
Client Need: Physiological Integrity—Physiological Adaptation: Medical Emergencies
Cognitive Level: Application
Concept: Perfusion
Reference: Lowdermilk, D. L., Perry, S. E., Cashion, K., & Alden, K. R. (2016). Maternity & women's health care. 11th ed. St. Louis, MO: Elsevier.

10. ANSWER: 1, 2
Rationale
1. Vaginal discharge the color of prune juice is a clinical manifestation of hydatidiform molar pregnancy.

2. Hydatidiform mole is not a viable fetus, so there is no fetal heartbeat.

3. The uterus of a client with a molar pregnancy is significantly larger for the actual weeks gestation because of the accelerated growth of the trophoblastic cells.

4. Elevated blood pressure is not a clinical manifestation of a molar pregnancy.

5. Abdominal pain is not a symptom of a molar pregnancy. The client may present with menstrual-like cramps.

TEST-TAKING TIP: Remember gestational trophoblastic disease is the proliferation of trophoblastic cells and includes hydatidiform or invasive mole, which causes prunelike vaginal discharge, nausea and vomiting (hyperemesis gravidarum), and abdominal cramps.

Content Area: Hydatidiform Mole; Antepartum at Risk
Integrated Process: Nursing Process—Assessment
Client Need: Physiological Integrity—Physiological Adaptation: Pathophysiology
Cognitive Level: Application
Concept: Assessment
Reference: Ward, S. L., & Hisley, S. M. (2016). Maternal-child nursing care. 2nd ed. Philadelphia: F.A. Davis.

11. ANSWER: 1, 2, 3
Rationale
1. A good bedtime snack of complex carbohydrates and protein is recommended to help prevent hypoglycemia and ketosis during the night.
2. Research shows that women with gestational diabetes have a high risk of developing type 2 diabetes later.
3. Induction of labor is a possibility because of poor glycemic control, large fetus (macrosomia), or nonreassuring fetal assessment.
4. Fresh fruit juices are high in sugar. Patients with diabetes should eat fresh fruit in moderation. Fresh fruit has the benefit of fiber and is usually lower in sugars.
5. The nurse should teach the client to test her blood glucose each day with a glucose meter.
TEST-TAKING TIP: Gestational diabetes is a condition in which the glucose level is elevated and other diabetic symptoms appear during pregnancy in a woman who has not previously been diagnosed with diabetes. All diabetic symptoms disappear following delivery. Gestational diabetes is not caused by a lack of insulin but by blocking effects of hormones, produced by the placenta, on the insulin that is produced, a condition referred to as *insulin resistance*.
Content Area: Diabetes; Antepartum at Risk
Integrated Process: Nursing Process
Client Need: Health Promotion and Maintenance—Teaching/Learning
Cognitive Level: Application
Concept: Metabolism
Reference: Ward, S. L., & Hisley, S. M. (2016). Maternal-child nursing care. *2nd ed. Philadelphia: F.A. Davis.*

12. ANSWER: 2
Rationale
1. Breathlessness in the recumbent position would be an assessment finding in orthopnea. It is relieved by sitting or standing.
2. One of the first assessment findings of pulmonary edema is a nonproductive cough.
3. An assessment finding of anemia would be fatigue.
4. Increased blood volume would occur in a patient with congestive heart failure.
TEST-TAKING TIP: The cough occurs in response to fluid filling the alveolar spaces. Pulmonary edema develops as a result of left ventricular failure or acute fluid overload.
Content Area: Heart Disease; Antepartum at Risk
Integrated Process: Nursing Process—Assessment
Client Need: Physiological Integrity—Physiological Adaptation: Pathophysiology
Cognitive Level: Analysis
Concept: Perfusion
Reference: Murray, S. S., & McKinney, E. S. (2014). Foundations of maternal-newborn and women's health nursing. *6th ed. St. Louis, MO: Elsevier.*

13. ANSWER: 3
Rationale
1. This is not a normal level. A HbA1C of 10% is a high level.
2. This is not a low level.

3. The HbA1c should be 6 or less, with elevated levels indicating poor glucose control.
4. Hemoglobin A1c blood test results are an average of blood glucose control over the past 2 to 3 months. This test is used along with daily blood glucose monitoring to make adjustments in diabetes management.
TEST-TAKING TIP: Glycosylated hemoglobin is a measure of glucose control during the past 6 to 8 weeks. It is not influenced by dietary management a day or two before the test is done.
Content Area: Diabetes; Antepartum at Risk
Integrated Process: Nursing Process—Evaluation
Client Need: Physiological Integrity—Physiological Adaptation: Illness Management
Cognitive Level: Analysis
Concept: Metabolism
Reference: Ward, S. L., & Hisley, S. M. (2016). Maternal-child nursing care. *2nd ed. Philadelphia: F.A. Davis.*

14. ANSWER: 2
Rationale
1. Sending another culture for GBS is not necessary or appropriate.
2. The nurse should prepare to administer penicillin.
3. The client should be treated with penicillin.
4. Intrapartum antibiotic treatment is recommended for women who have a GBS-positive bacteria in the current pregnancy.
TEST-TAKING TIP: Current guidelines state that all women who are positive at any point during the pregnancy or positive in a previous pregnancy should receive antibiotics in the current pregnancy.
Content Area: Perinatal Infections; Antepartum at Risk
Integrated Process: Nursing Process—Implementation
Client Need: Physiological Integrity—Physiological Adaptation: Alterations in Body Systems
Cognitive Level: Analysis
Concept: Infection
Reference: Ward, S. L., & Hisley, S. M. (2016). Maternal-child nursing care. *2nd ed. Philadelphia: F.A. Davis.*

15. ANSWER: 1, 3
Rationale
1. Antiretroviral drugs should be administered to reduce risk of vertical transmission to the fetus.
2. The infant should be delivered by cesarean, so placing the patient on a birthing ball is not necessary.
3. Nurses and other personnel should wear protective equipment and gloves to prevent transmission.
4. Breastfeeding is contraindicated since HIV can be transmitted in breast milk.
5. A private room is not necessary.
TEST-TAKING TIP: Current guidelines recommend antiretroviral therapy, no breastfeeding, and elective cesarean section before the onset of labor to reduce perinatal transmission.
Content Area: HIV/AIDS; Antepartum at Risk
Integrated Process: Nursing Process—Implementation
Client Need: Physiological Integrity—Reduction of Risk Potential: Potential for Complications of Diagnostic Tests; Treatments; Procedures

Cognitive Level: Application
Concept: Infection
Reference: *Lowdermilk, D. L., Perry, S. E., Cashion, K., & Alden, K. R. (2016). Maternity & women's health care. 11th ed. St. Louis, MO: Elsevier.*

16. **ANSWER: 1**
Rationale
1. Pulmonary edema can occur in patients receiving magnesium sulfate, so lungs should be assessed frequently.
2. Fluids are at times restricted in patients with pre-eclampsia.
3. Hypertension does not affect glucose levels.
4. Pitting edema should be assessed but is not the highest priority assessment.

TEST-TAKING TIP: Magnesium sulfate causes vasodilation. In pre-eclampsia there is decreased perfusion of the kidneys resulting in an increase of edema and magnesium toxicity and/or pulmonary edema.
Content Area: Pre-eclampsia; Antepartum at Risk
Integrated Process: Nursing Process—Assessment
Client Need: Physiological Integrity—Reduction of Risk Potential: Potential for Complications of Diagnostic Tests; Treatments; Procedures
Cognitive Level: Application
Concept: Oxygenation
Reference: *Durham, R. F., & Chapman, L. (2016). Maternal-child nursing care. 2nd ed. Philadelphia: F.A. Davis.*

17. **ANSWER: 3**
Rationale
1. Folic acid is not a deficiency associated with hyperemesis gravidarum.
2. Vitamin D is not a deficiency associated with hyperemesis gravidarum.
3. Persistent nausea and vomiting can lead to thiamine deficiency.
4. Glucose is not a deficiency associated with hyperemesis gravidarum.

TEST-TAKING TIP: If nausea and vomiting continues for 3 to 4 weeks, women can develop Wernicke's encephalopathy with ataxia and dementia due to thiamine deficiency. If this is not detected and treated, it can become a permanent disability. It is important to correct the thiamine deficiency before giving dextrose in fluids, since this can lead to Wernicke's encephalopathy. Oral or intravenous thiamine supplementation may be ordered.
Content Area: Hyperemesis Gravidarum; Antepartum at Risk
Integrated Process: Nursing Process—Assessment
Client Need: Physiological Integrity—Physiological Adaptation: Pathophysiology
Cognitive Level: Application
Concept: Fluid and Electrolyte Balance
Reference: *Lowdermilk, D. L., Perry, S. E., Cashion, K., & Alden, K. R. (2016). Maternity & women's health care. 11th ed. St. Louis, MO: Elsevier.*

18. **ANSWER: 4**
Rationale
1. This is a symptom of an ectopic pregnancy.
2. This is a symptom of placental abruption.

3. This is a symptom of placenta previa.
4. Abdominal cramping and lower back pain can be a sign of preterm labor.

TEST-TAKING TIP: Many women experience preterm birth without any risk factors. All women should be taught signs and symptoms of preterm labor and to notify their health care provider if they experience any of these symptoms: contractions occurring more than one every 10 minutes and last for 1 hour or more, uterine contractions that may or may not be painful, pain or pressure in the thighs or cervical area, lower abdominal cramping (may also have diarrhea), dull low backache (lower lumbar and sacral area), vaginal discharge that has a change in character or amount (thicker, thinner, bloody, brown, increase in amount, or has odor), or rupture of membranes.
Content Area: Preterm Labor; Antepartum at Risk
Integrated Process: Nursing Process—Assessment
Client Need: Health Promotion and Maintenance—Ante/Intra/Postpartum and Newborn Care
Cognitive Level: Analysis
Concept: Pregnancy
Reference: *Durham, R. F., & Chapman, L. (2016). Maternal-child nursing care. 2nd ed. Philadelphia: F.A. Davis.*

19. **ANSWER: 1**
Rationale
1. High levels of estrogen and hCG have been associated with the development of hyperemesis gravidarum.
2. Having high blood pressure does not make a client at risk for developing hyperemesis gravidarum.
3. Young maternal age is not a risk factor associated with the development of hyperemesis gravidarum.
4. Weight is not a risk factor associated with the development of hyperemesis gravidarum.

TEST-TAKING TIP: Risk factors for developing hyperemesis gravidarum also include clinical hyperthyroid disorders, molar pregnancy, multiple gestation, diabetes, gastrointestinal disorders, and previous pregnancy with hyperemesis gravidarum.
Content Area: Hyperemesis Gravidarum; Antepartum at Risk
Integrated Process: Nursing Process—Assessment
Client Need: Health Promotion and Maintenance—Health Promotion; Disease Prevention
Cognitive Level: Application
Concept: Pregnancy
Reference: *Lowdermilk, D. L., Perry, S. E., Cashion, K., & Alden, K. R. (2016). Maternity & women's health care. 11th ed. St. Louis, MO: Elsevier.*

20. **ANSWER: 1**
Rationale
1. The earlier the rupture of the membranes occurs, the worse the outcome for the fetus, because there is greater risk of chorioamnionitis and preterm delivery.
2. Fluid volume deficit is not a complication of rupture of membranes but would be a complication from vaginal bleeding (hemorrhage).
3. The client will not develop hypotension from rupture of membranes but it would be a complication from vaginal bleeding (hemorrhage).

4. The client will not experience decreased urinary output from rupture of membranes but this would be a complication from vaginal bleeding (hemorrhage).

TEST-TAKING TIP: Rupture of membranes may be a gush of fluid or small amount of leakage from the vagina after rupture of the amniotic sac. Maternal temperature should be monitored frequently and the mother should be taught to keep her genital area clean, not introduce anything into the vagina, watch for and report foul-smelling vaginal discharge or odor, and report increased temperature or increased pulse immediately to her provider.

Content Area: Preterm Premature Rupture of Membranes; Antepartum at Risk
Integrated Process: Nursing Process—Assessment
Client Need: Physiological Integrity—Physiological Adaptation: Alterations in Body Systems
Cognitive Level: Application
Concept: Pregnancy
Reference: Ward, S. L., & Hisley, S. M. (2016). Maternal-child nursing care. 2nd ed. Philadelphia: F.A. Davis.

21. **ANSWER: 2, 4, 5**
Rationale
1. The client must be maintained in a lateral position for adequate maternal and fetal perfusion.
2. A precipitous drop can lead to shock and placental abruption.
3. Medication must be administered for at least 20 minutes in order to assess the effects of the initial dose.
4. Medication may cause positive direct Coombs test results.
5. Maternal side effects include headache, flushing, palpitations, and tachycardia.

TEST-TAKING TIP: Hydralazine is an antihypertensive direct-acting peripheral arteriolar vasodilator. It is very important for the nurse to understand the maternal and fetal effects and nursing actions involved when administrating this medication.

Content Area: Pre-eclampsia; Antepartum at Risk
Integrated Process: Nursing Process—Implementation
Client Need: Physiological Integrity—Pharmacological and Parenteral Therapies: Medication Administration
Cognitive Level: Application
Concept: Medication
Reference: Ward, S. L., & Hisley, S. M. (2016). Maternal-child nursing care. 2nd ed. Philadelphia: F.A. Davis.

22. **ANSWER: 3**
Rationale
1. RhoGAM should be given to an Rh-negative woman who has had an Rh-positive newborn and a negative indirect Coombs test.
2. A positive direct Coombs test indicates that Rh sensitization has occurred so the woman is not a candidate for RhoGAM.
3. A negative Coombs indicates the Rh sensitization has not occurred so the woman is a candidate for RhoGAM.
4. The question does not indicate if the woman is negative or positive. However, the newborn is negative and there is

not the possibility of antibody production from the woman.

TEST-TAKING TIP: A blood test can determine if an Rh-negative mother is developing antibodies to an Rh-positive fetus. The direct Coombs test looks at the baby's blood for antibodies on the red blood cells. An indirect Coombs test examines maternal blood for the number of Rh antibodies.

Content Area: Rh(D) Isoimmunization; Antepartum at Risk
Integrated Process: Nursing Process—Assessment
Client Need: Physiological Integrity—Pharmacological and Parenteral Therapies: Medication Administration
Cognitive Level: Application
Concept: Medication
Reference: Lowdermilk, D. L., Perry, S. E., Cashion, K., & Alden, K. R. (2016). Maternity & women's health care. 11th ed. St. Louis, MO: Elsevier.

23. **ANSWER: 4**
Rationale
1. Naloxone is an opiate antagonist administered to reverse respiratory depression.
2. Oxytocin is a hormone that stimulates uterine contraction and milk letdown.
3. Labetalol is a beta-blocking medication causing vasodilation to decrease muscle tone and peripheral resistance in high blood pressure.
4. Calcium gluconate should be administered for magnesium toxicity.

TEST-TAKING TIP: If magnesium toxicity is suspected, the magnesium sulfate infusion should be stopped immediately and calcium gluconate (antidote) should be given intravenously. Signs of magnesium toxicity are lethargy, muscle weakness, decreased or absent DTRs, decreased respirations less than 12, double vision, and slurred speech.

Content Area: Pre-eclampsia; Antepartum at Risk
Integrated Process: Nursing Process—Implementation
Client Need: Physiological Integrity—Physiological Adaptation: Medical Emergencies
Cognitive Level: Application
Concept: Medication
Reference: Lowdermilk, D. L., Perry, S. E., Cashion, K., & Alden, K. R. (2016). Maternity & women's health care. 11th ed. St. Louis, MO: Elsevier.

24. **ANSWER: 1, 2, 3**
Rationale
1. Poor glycemic control increases the rate of fetal growth.
2. Increased glucose concentration in amniotic fluid results from fetal hyperglycemia.
3. Polyhydramnios and urinary tract infection may result in premature rupture of membranes.
4. This client is not at risk for developing hyperemesis gravidarum.
5. Generalized edema is a clinical manifestation of pre-eclampsia.

TEST-TAKING TIP: Maternal obesity, family history of diabetes, previous gestational diabetes, or infant with birth weight over 4,000 grams place a woman at risk of gestational diabetes.

Content Area: Diabetes; Antepartum at Risk
Integrated Process: Nursing Process—Assessment
Client Need: Physiological Integrity—Physiological
Adaptation: Pathophysiology
Cognitive Level: Application
Concept: Medication
Reference: Lowdermilk, D. L., Perry, S. E., Cashion, K., & Alden, K. R.
(2016). Maternity & women's health care. 11th ed. St. Louis, MO: Elsevier.

25. **ANSWER: 2**
Rationale
1. Calcium gluconate is the antidote for a client on
magnesium sulfate. The stem does not indicate that this
medication is being administered or ordered.
2. Severe pre-eclampsia can lead to eclampsia (seizures).
3. Light should remain dim and nurse should decrease
stimulation as much as possible.

4. Using a tongue blade is not a standard protocol when
someone is having a seizure.
TEST-TAKING TIP: If a client has a seizure, emergency
management should consist of keeping the airway
patent (turn head to one side and place pillow under
one shoulder or back), calling for assistance, protecting
with padded side rail up, and observing and recording
seizure activity.
Content Area: Pre-eclampsia; Antepartum at Risk
Integrated Process: Nursing Process—Implementation
Client Need: Physiological Integrity—Physiological
Adaptation: Medical Emergencies
Cognitive Level: Analysis
Concept: Critical Thinking
Reference: Lowdermilk, D. L., Perry, S. E., Cashion, K., & Alden, K. R.
(2016). Maternity & women's health care. 11th ed. St. Louis, MO: Elsevier.

Intrapartum

Process of Labor and Birth

I. Onset of Labor

The onset of labor is multifactorial and involves a decrease in progesterone and an increase in estrogen and prostaglandins, overdistention of the uterus, an increased intrauterine pressure, and aging of placenta. Fetal hormones are also thought to contribute to labor onset.

A. Signs of impending labor
   1. **Lightening:** fetal head descending into the pelvis
      • Woman able to breathe easier due to the rib cage expanding more easily.
      • Pressure on bladder causes urinary frequency.
      • May occur during the first stage of labor in multiparous women.
   2. Irregular contractions—Braxton Hicks (false labor)
      • These may cause women experiencing preterm labor to delay seeking care.
   3. Pain in the lower back or sacroiliac joint from relaxation of pelvic joints

   4. Increase in vaginal discharge of cervical mucus
      • Bloody show—brownish red mucus
   5. Weight loss of 0.5 to 1.5 kg
   6. Surge of energy
B. Assessment for rupture of membranes
   1. May be assessed by vaginal examination or obvious leaking of fluid from the vagina. Confirmed with:
      • Nitrazine paper: changes from yellow to dark blue due to alkaline nature of amniotic fluid (pH 7 to 7.5).
      • Ferning: amniotic fluid dried on slide and observed under microscope, reveals fernlike pattern. More conclusive than nitrazine.
      • Sterile speculum examination may be done in cases of preterm labor.
      • Immunoassay tests may also be used: detects small amounts of proteins that are present in amniotic fluid.
        a) Normal amniotic fluid is clear with white flecks (vernix) and is not foul-smelling.

b) Green color suggests **meconium** staining—
assess for fetal distress.
  • Normal for fetus in breech presentation
c) Cloudy or foul-smelling fluid may suggest
infection.
d) Bloody drainage heavier than bloody show
may suggest placenta previa or placental
abruption. Assess for fetal distress.

2. Rupture of fetal membranes
  a) **Spontaneous rupture of membranes:**
  Membranes rupture without intervention.
  b) **Artificial rupture of membranes (AROM)**
  or amniotomy: Performed with amnihook to
  stimulate labor.

🛇 **ALERT** The priority assessment before and after the
rupture of fetal membranes is evaluation of the fetal
heart rate. This can be accomplished with continuous
fetal monitoring or intermittent auscultation.

  c) Chart the time of the rupture of membrane,
  response of fetus, and characteristics of fluid.
  d) Assess maternal temperature every 2 hours to
  assess for the possibility of infection of the
  membranes (chorioamnionitis).

C. Vaginal examinations
  1. Leopold's maneuvers prior to examination to
  determine fetal presentation and **position**
  a) Perform sterile vaginal examination as indicated. With sterile glove and water-soluble
  lubricant, insert index and middle fingers into
  the woman's vagina to determine:
  Cervical **dilation:** opening of the cervix measured in centimeters (0, or closed, to 10 cm,

or full dilation) and estimated based
on the measurement of the examiner's
fingers.
Effacement: shortening and thinning of
the cervix, measured from 0% to 100%.
An uneffaced (0%) cervix is approximately
2 to 3 cm long, while fully effaced (100%) it
is thin on palpation (Fig. 14.1).
Station: amount of descent of the presenting
part (PP) in centimeters above or below
the ischial spines, the narrowest part of the
maternal pelvis.
  • Negative stations (–3, –2, –1) represent
  approximate centimeters *above* the ischial
  spines.
  • The PP at zero station is **engagement.**
  • Positive stations (+1, +2, +3) represent
  approximate centimeters below the
  ischial spines. For example, if the examiner assessed that the fetus's presenting
  part was 2 cm below the ischial spines,
  this would be documented as +2 station
  (Fig. 14.2).
  • Floating: fetal head is too high or
  may be ballotable, meaning it moves
  away, then comes back toward examiner's
  hand.
  b. Fetal presenting part (Table 14.1)
  c. Position
  • Sutures on fetal head can be palpated
  to determine fetal position, which is the
  relation of the fetal head to the maternal
  pelvis.

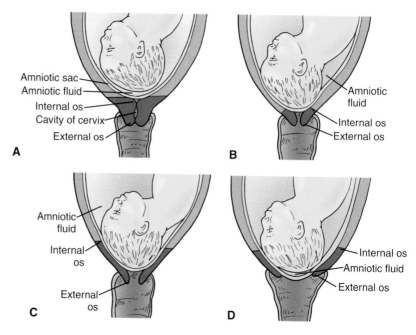

Fig 14.1 Cervical effacement and dilation.

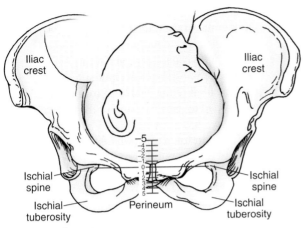

Fig 14.2 Fetal station.

MAKING THE CONNECTION

Vaginal Examinations and Active Bleeding

Vaginal examinations should not be performed with active vaginal bleeding because the placenta might be implanted near or over the cervical os (placenta previa) or prematurely separating from the uterine wall (abruptio placenta), or the fetal blood vessels might be overlying the cervical os (vasa previa).

II. Factors Affecting Labor

Factors affecting labor are powers, passage, passenger, presentation, and psyche (5Ps).

A. Powers
1. First stage of labor (beginning of labor until full cervical dilation). Contractions are the force that helps fetal descent and dilation.
2. Second stage of labor (full dilation until birth of the baby). Propulsive efforts of pushing are added. Urge to bear down is very strong now and the woman my report rectal pressure.

DID YOU KNOW?

The pressure on the posterior vagina causes release of the hormone oxytocin, which causes an increased urge to bear down, known as the Ferguson reflex.

B. Passage
1. Maternal pelvis and soft tissues (cervix, vagina, pelvic floor)
2. Maternal pelvis
   a) False pelvis: top of pelvis, not significant in childbirth
   b) True pelvis: bottom of pelvis, important during birth; different dimensions in each level:
      - Inlet: upper border of the true pelvis
      - Midpelvis: curved passage, coccyx is the posterior section, which is movable at end of pregnancy
      - Outlet: lower border of the pelvis
   c) The hormone relaxin helps relax the ligaments in the pelvis.
3. Four types of pelvis. Most women have mixed features of two or more pelvises.
   - Gynecoid: round, wide pubic arch; most common and best for delivery.
   - Anthropoid: long and narrow, anterior/posterior (AP) diameter greater than transverse diameter, narrow pubic arch, larger outlet.
   - Android: heart or triangular shaped, narrow pubic arch, with a narrow distance between the spines. May have longer labor.
   - Platypelloid: flat and wide, transverse diameter greater than AP diameter, wide pubic arch; this type is uncommon and the woman may have longer and more difficult labor.

C. Passenger
1. Fetal head is rigid but presence of membranous sutures and fontanels allow for overlapping or molding of skull bones during delivery.
2. Shoulders are usually able to conform to the birth canal but may develop into shoulder dystocia.

Table 14.1 Fetal Presentations

Presentation	Variant	Presenting Part
Cephalic: head down, feels hard and round on palpation or vaginal examination. Most common presentation.	Vertex: head flexed on the chest	Occiput
	Face: head and neck in hyperextension	Mentum (chin)
	Brow: midway between flexion and hyperextension	Frontal bone
Breech: buttocks or feet down, feels softer, less regular on palpation or vaginal examination. Approximately 3% to 4% of pregnancies.	Complete breech: both hips and knees flexed	Sacrum
	Frank breech: hips flexed, knees extended	Sacrum
	Footling Single: one hip flexed, one extended with that foot presenting Double: both hips and knees extended with both feet presenting	Foot/feet
Shoulder: transverse lie or the head to tailbone axis is at a 90-degree angle to the woman. Occurs in less than 1% of pregnancies.		Scapula

DID YOU KNOW?

Shoulder dystocia is a condition that occurs during vaginal delivery after delivery of the fetal head, where the anterior shoulder cannot pass under the symphysis pubis. This is an obstetrical emergency that requires manipulation in order to facilitate delivery and is associated with fetal and maternal morbidity. More detail about shoulder dystocia can be found in Chapter 16.

D. Fetal presentation

Factors that facilitate vaginal delivery include vertex presentation, which allows the smallest diameter of the fetal head to present to the pelvis and vaginal opening.

1. Fetal **attitude:** optimal is with fetal flexion: back rounded, legs and arms flexed onto the body, and head flexed onto the chest. Extension of the fetus is the opposite of flexion.
2. Fetal **lie:** the relationship of the long axis (spine) of the fetus to the long axis of the mother.
   a) Longitudinal: long axes are parallel; fetus is vertical in the uterus.
      • Cephalic and breech presentation
   b) Transverse: long axes are perpendicular; fetus is horizontal in the uterus.
      • Shoulder presentation

E. Fetal position (in cephalic presentation)

1. The preferred position is occiput anterior, where the back of the fetal head (or occiput) is positioned toward the front of the maternal pelvis.
2. Occiput posterior (OP) is where the back of the fetal head (or occiput) is positioned toward the back of the maternal pelvis.
3. Occiput transverse (OT) is where the back of the fetal head (or occiput) is positioned toward the side of the maternal pelvis.

Both OP and OT make delivery difficult (Fig. 14.3).

F. Psyche

1. Anxiety, fear, fatigue, inability to deal with pain, and lack of a support person can all negatively affect the progress of labor. Catecholamines secreted can inhibit uterine activity and cause longer and more dysfunctional labor.
2. Previous birth experience and cultural issues can also affect the woman's labor experience.

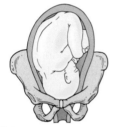
Right occiput anterior (ROA)

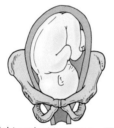
Right occiput transverse (ROT)

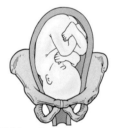
Right occiput posterior (ROP)

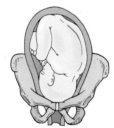
Left occiput anterior (LOA)

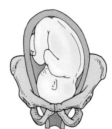
Left occiput transverse (LOT)

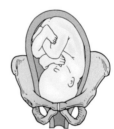
Left occiput posterior (LOP)

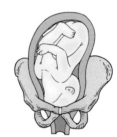
Right mentum anterior (RMA)

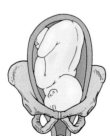
Right mentum posterior (RMP)

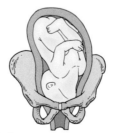
Left mentum anterior (LMA)

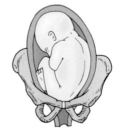
Left sacrum anterior (LSA)

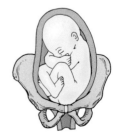
Left sacrum posterior (LSP)

Fig 14.3 Fetal presentations and positions.

III. True Labor Versus False Labor

See Table 14.2.

IV. Mechanism of Labor

There are seven cardinal movements of labor, which are positional changes that allow the fetus to fit through the mother's pelvis.
A. Descent
  - Fetus progresses through the pelvic inlet
  - Occurs concurrently with other mechanisms
  - Measured by station
B. Engagement
  - Biparietal diameter of the fetal head passes the pelvic inlet
  - Occurs before labor in primiparous woman
C. Flexion
  - Flexion of the fetal chin to the chest to bring a smaller diameter to the outlet
D. Internal rotation
  - Allows the largest (AP) diameter of fetal head to align with largest diameter of maternal pelvis
  - Sagittal suture is transverse or oblique
E. Extension
  - Allows the fetal head to line up with the pelvic outlet
  - Occiput passes under the symphysis pubis
  - Head is delivered in extension
F. External rotation
  - After the head is born, it aligns with the fetal shoulders
G. Expulsion
  - The fetal shoulders and body are delivered

V. Stages of Labor

The **stages of labor** are as follows.
A. First stage of labor
  1. Latent phase: 0 to 3 cm
    a) Labor support
      - Assess maternal medical and obstetric history, vital signs.
      - Collect laboratory specimens: blood type and Rh, complete blood count, urinalysis, and other laboratory results as dictated by clinical status.
      - Evaluate fetal heart rate and contraction pattern.
      - Establish therapeutic relationship between nurse and patient.
      - Determine family's birth plan.
      - Support person is important to physical and psychological well-being.
        - Partner, family, nurse, doula, friend
        - Can provide encouragement, distraction, and nonpharmacological pain relief and can assist with personal hygiene
      - Allow woman to ambulate if not contraindicated.
  2. Active phase: 4 to 7 cm
    a) Position changes
      - Avoid supine position; change positions for maternal comfort.
      - Vertical maternal positions improve fetal descent.
    b) Comfort measures
      - Make labor room comfortable, cool cloth on head, perineal care, keep bladder empty.
      - Perform mouth care, give ice chips and oral hydration with clear fluids per policy
    c) Assess for preferred method of pain relief: pharmacological and nonpharmacological.
    d) Asses fetal heart rate in labor.
      - Intermittent auscultation (IA): determines rate, accelerations, and decelerations
      - Continuous electronic fetal heart rate monitoring (EFM): determines baseline rate, variability, accelerations, and decelerations
      - Continuous internal fetal monitoring (Table 14.3)
        - Invasive placement of fetal scalp electrode for continuous EFM
        - Determines baseline rate, variability, accelerations, decelerations

Table 14.2 **True vs. False Labor**	
True Labor	**False Labor**
Contractions increase in intensity despite change in activity	Contractions decrease in intensity when walking or changing position
Contractions become stronger, last longer, and are more regular	Contractions are irregular
Cervix becomes softer, with an increase in dilation and effacement	No appreciable cervical change in dilation and effacement

Table 14.3 **Continuous External Fetal Monitoring**		
	First Stage (Active Phase)	**Second Stage**
Low-risk women	Every 30 minutes	Every 15 minutes Every 5 minutes
High-risk women: continuous EFM recommended	Every 15 minutes	At least every 5 minutes

3. Transition phase: 8 to 10 cm
   a) Client may have a loss of control and need increased nursing support with instruction and reinforcement.
   b) May have urge to push before full dilation and need to change method of breathing to panting.
   c) Assess for signs of hyperventilation; dizziness or circumoral or extremity numbness. Encourage woman to slow down rate of breathing.
B. Second stage of labor
   This stage is from full dilation until the baby's birth.
   1. Pushing is more effective when the woman has a strong urge to push. Squatting is optimal for pushing. Use a birthing ball, toilet, or squatting bar on bed.
   2. Encourage open glottis pushing.

DID YOU KNOW?

Do not encourage prolonged pushing with the woman holding her breath. Sustained pushing with the glottis closed can initiate the Valsalva maneuver, which decreases fetal blood flow. Allowing women to push spontaneously is more beneficial to the fetus and can lessen maternal fatigue.

3. Episiotomy
   a) **Episiotomy** is when an incision of the perineum is made at the time the fetal head is crowning, just before birth
      - Median (midline): easier repair and may be less painful but associated with more third- or fourth-degree **lacerations** as the episiotomy extends toward the rectum
      - Mediolateral: more painful and difficult to repair, may have more blood loss
   b) Episiotomy may be used for shoulder dystocia, for operative vaginal birth (forceps or vacuum extractor), and for less traumatic delivery of the fetal head, particularly with the preterm infant. However, rates of performance of routine episiotomies have steadily declined.
   c) There is less chance of blood loss, infection, and perineal pain with an intact perineum.
4. Lacerations of the perineum
   a) First degree: extends through skin and vaginal mucous membrane
   b) Second degree: extends through the fascia and muscle
   c) Third degree: extends through to involve the anal sphincter
   d) Fourth degree: extends through the rectal mucosa

C. Third stage of labor
   This involves the delivery of the placenta and is the shortest portion of labor.
   1. Observe for sudden gush of blood, lengthening of umbilical cord, and change in shape of the uterus to globular shape.
   2. Woman may feel fullness in the vagina.
   3. Active management of the third stage of labor to prevent postpartum hemorrhage includes:
      - Administering oxytocin after delivery of the anterior shoulder.
      - Clamping cord within 2 to 3 minutes of birth.
      - Delivering the placenta with controlled cord traction while supporting the uterus.
      - Performing vigorous fundal massage after delivery of the placenta for at least 15 seconds.[1]
   4. At this time, the initial infant assessment is performed.
D. Fourth stage
   This stage is after the delivery of the placenta for 1 to 2 hours after birth.
   1. Care of mother
      a) Assess the amount of lochia to evaluate for possible postpartum hemorrhage. Weighing of all obstetric items to quantify that blood loss is superior to visual estimation.
      b) Assess for firmly contracted uterine fundus. If it is not firm, massage gently until it firms. Record fundal height in relation to the umbilicus.
         - If bleeding occurs with a firmly contracted uterus, consider laceration of the genital tract.

MAKING THE CONNECTION

Estimating Blood Loss During Delivery

Lack of accurate estimation of blood loss following delivery is very common. Overestimation can lead to unnecessary treatments, while underestimation can lead to a delay in evaluation and treatment of women who are hemorrhaging. Subjective visual estimation has been shown to be inaccurate and should be replaced with the more accurate method of quantification of blood loss. This can be accomplished by measuring blood loss with calibrated drapes and canisters and weighing blood-saturated obstetric items.[2]

[1] Association of Women's Health, Obstetric and Neonatal Nurses. (2014). *Perinatal nursing.* 4th ed. K. R. Simpson, & P. A. Creehan (Eds.). Philadelphia: Lippincott Williams & Wilkins.
[2] Association of Women's Health, Obstetric and Neonatal Nurses (AWHONN). (2014). Quantification of blood loss: AWHONN practice brief number 1. Retrieved from http://www.pphproject.org/downloads/awhonn_qbl.pdf.

- Oxytocin administered as per order of physician or nurse midwife.

c) Vital signs should be assessed every 15 minutes for the first hour.

d) Assess bladder for distention. Assist woman to void or catheterize her if needed.

DID YOU KNOW?

Fundal examination of the postpartum woman may reveal the uterine fundus to be above the umbilicus and to the right if the bladder is full. Emptying of the bladder will assist in keeping the uterus contracted.

e) Observe perineum to assess episiotomy, laceration, edema, ecchymosis, or rectal hemorrhoids.
- Perineal care is administered for patient comfort.
- Ice packs are applied to the perineum to treat or prevent edema.
  - Assess cultural norms, as some women prefer not to be exposed to anything cold.

f) Apply warm blanket, as shivering is common. Not related to fever or infection.

g) Allow for bonding with infant and initiation of breastfeeding. Skin-to-skin contact with infant may occur immediately after birth.

h) Assess the need for pain medication. Allow client to eat or drink unless clinical status does not allow.

2. Care of the infant
a) Clear the airway and clean and dry the newborn.
- Drying stimulates the infant crying and expansion of lungs.
- If infant is stable, skin-to-skin contact is adequate; otherwise, place the infant under a radiant warmer. The infant's head should be covered with a hat.
- Assess for any obvious congenital abnormalities.
- Facilitate early breastfeeding in stable infants.
- Assess infant's weight and length.
- Administer eye prophylaxis and vitamin K.
- Staff working in the delivery room should be trained in neonatal resuscitation.

b) **Apgar scores** are assigned at 1 and 5 minutes after birth (Table 14.4).

c) Apply identification bands to mother, primary support person, and newborn. These identification bands should include the mother's name and preprinted numbers. The primary nurse should ensure that all information is correct.

See Box 14.1 for items to note when determining gravida and para of a woman.

Table 14.4 **Apgar Scores**

Parameter	0 points	1 point	2 points
Heart rate	Absent	Below 100 beats/minute	100 beats/minute or higher
Respiratory effort	No spontaneous respirations	Slow, irregular respirations or weak cry	Vigorous cry
Muscle tone	Limp or absent	Minimal flexion of extremities, sluggish movement	Active movement
Reflex response	No response to suction	Minimal response to suction (grimace, pull away)	Active motion (sneeze, cough,
Color	Pallor or cyanosis	Body pink, extremities blue	Completely pink

Box 14.1 **Obstetric History Using Gravida and Para**

G (Gravida): the total number of pregnancies, including a present one. The length of gestation, the outcome (live birth or not), or the number of fetuses (single, twin, etc.) does not affect this number.
P (Para): the number of deliveries; subdivided into TPAL:
  T (Term): a pregnancy (single or multiple fetuses) that is delivered at 37 to 42 weeks, including stillborn
  P (Premature): a pregnancy (single or multiple fetuses) that ends at 20 to 37 weeks, including stillborn
  A (Abortion): a pregnancy (single or multiple fetuses) that ends before 20 weeks gestation (not viable). This can be an elective termination of pregnancy or spontaneous (miscarriage)
  L: the number of live children

CASE STUDY: Putting It All Together

Subjective Data

A 35-year-old gravida 1 para 0 female who is 38 weeks pregnant presents to the labor and delivery unit stating that she has had uterine contractions every 6 minutes but they are still irregular. She has had leakage of dark bloody mucus since yesterday. She has no known allergies and her current medications consist of prenatal vitamins (one tab daily) and ferrous sulfate (one tab daily).

Vital Signs

Height: 5'9" (175.3 cm)
Current weight: 190 lb (86.2 kg)
Prepregnancy weight: 155 lb (70.3 kg)
Temperature: 99°F (37.2°C)
Blood pressure: 98/65
Heart rate: 82 bpm, regular
Respiratory rate: 18 breaths per minute
Pulse oximetry: 99% on room air

Laboratory Results

Blood type and Rh: O negative
Antibody screen: Negative
Rubella: Nonimmune
Hepatitis (HbsAg): Negative
HIV (3rd trimester): Negative
WBC: 16,000 per mm³

Objective Data

Nursing Assessment

Leopold's maneuvers demonstrate a soft defined round object in the fundus. Sterile vaginal examination reveals the cervix to be 4 cm dilated, 70% effaced, −1 station

Health Care Provider's Orders

Continuous external fetal monitoring
Blood type and Rh
CBC
V/S every 2 hours
Intake and output
Insert IV of Lactated Ringer's solution at 100 mL/hr
Diet: NPO

Case Study Questions

1. What *subjective* assessment findings indicate that the client is experiencing a change in clinical status?

2. What *objective* assessment findings indicate that the client is experiencing a change in clinical status?

3. What interventions should the nurse plan and/or implement to meet this client's needs?

REVIEW QUESTIONS

Be sure to read the Introduction for valuable test-taking tips.

1. Which of the following are signs of impending labor? *Select all that apply.*
   1. Weight gain
   2. Surge of energy
   3. Increase in urinary frequency
   4. Dyspnea
   5. Pain in lower back
   6. Increase in bloody show

2. The onset of labor is multifactorial. These reasons include which of the following? *Select all that apply.*
   1. Increase in progesterone
   2. Increase in estrogen
   3. Increase in human chorionic gonadotropin
   4. Aging of placenta
   5. Fetal hormones
   6. Decrease in prostaglandins

3. A 29-year-old gravida 1, para 0 woman who is 35 weeks pregnant is admitted to the labor and delivery unit. She states that there is fluid leaking from her vagina but she is not sure if it is urine. What should the nurse do to make the determination?
   1. A nitrazine test is the most conclusive test.
   2. Nitrazine paper changes from yellow to dark blue due to the acidic nature of amniotic fluid.
   3. Ferning is more conclusive than nitrazine paper testing.
   4. Note if there is fluid leaking from the perineal area.

4. A woman's pelvis is described as long and narrow with an anteroposterior diameter greater than the transverse diameter. This is known as which type of pelvis?
   1. Platypelloid
   2. Android
   3. Anthropoid
   4. Gynecoid

5. Which female pelvis is most suitable for vaginal delivery?
   1. Gynecoid
   2. Android
   3. Platypelloid
   4. Anthropoid

6. An infant was born 1 minute ago and the Apgar score is being assigned. The infant has blue extremities, minimal flexion, a weak cry, a heart rate of 110 beats per minute, and coughs and pulls away when suctioned. How many points should be assigned? Record your answer using a whole number:

   _____.

7. A 35-year-old gravida 1, para 0 is admitted to the labor and delivery unit. She reports intense rectal pressure. Which stage of labor is probable?
   1. First stage, latent
   2. Second stage
   3. Third stage
   4. Fourth stage

8. The nurse has just performed a sterile vaginal examination on her patient and reports the examination as 4 cm, 50%, –1. What does this represent?
   1. Effacement, station, and dilation
   2. Dilation, station, and fetal lie
   3. Dilation, effacement, and status of membranes
   4. Dilation, effacement, and station

9. A primigravida has just been examined. The examination revealed engagement of the fetal head. The nurse is aware that this means which of the following?
   1. The biparietal diameter of the fetal head is at the level of the ischial spines.
   2. The biparietal diameter of the fetal head is at –2 station.
   3. The fetal head is well flexed.
   4. The fetal head is unable to pass under the pubic arch.

10. The nurse midwife caring for a multiparous client who is 5 cm dilated requests intermittent auscultation (IA) of the fetal heart rate. The woman's history reveals no risk factors. How often should IA be performed in this patient?
    1. Every 15 minutes
    2. Every 5 minutes
    3. Every 20 minutes
    4. Every 30 minutes

11. On admission to the labor unit, a primigravid woman at 38 weeks gestation states, "I need to urinate more now but at least I can breathe easier." The nurse is aware that this is likely due to which physiological process?
    1. Onset of labor
    2. Effacement
    3. Lightening
    4. Rupture of membranes

12. A 40-year-old G2, P1 woman is admitted to the labor and delivery unit with contractions 6 minutes apart. She is 36 weeks pregnant, has a history of placenta previa, and is currently experiencing moderate vaginal bleeding. What should the nurse be prepared to do?
    1. Perform a vaginal examination to determine cervical dilation
    2. Assist the health care provider to perform artificial rupture of the membranes
    3. Initiate external fetal monitoring
    4. Encourage patient to ambulate to intensify labor

13. A 28-year-old woman without risk factors has now reached the second stage of labor. What is the optimal position for her at this point?
    1. Supine
    2. Lateral recumbent
    3. Lithotomy
    4. Squatting

14. A nurse performs a vaginal examination on her patient in early labor and determines that the head is ballotable. What is this defined as?
    1. Floating
    2. Zero station
    3. +1 station
    4. –2 station

15. A sterile vaginal examination completed on a patient revealed the presenting part to be the mentum. What is this presentation known as?
    1. Face presentation
    2. Breech presentation
    3. Vertex presentation
    4. Shoulder presentation

16. A fetus is positioned in a longitudinal lie with its head in the fundus with both hips and knees flexed. Which presentation is this known as?
    1. Frank breech
    2. Complete breech
    3. Vertex
    4. Transverse

17. A fetus is positioned in the occiput anterior position. The nurse determines that the fetus is positioned in which way?
    1. The fetal shoulder is closest to the vaginal opening.
    2. The fetal head is closest to the vaginal opening and the occiput is directed toward the maternal symphysis.
    3. The fetal head is closest to the uterine fundus and is directed toward the maternal symphysis.
    4. The fetal head is closest to the vaginal opening and is directed toward the maternal sacrum.

18. A woman who is 39 weeks pregnant presents to the labor and delivery unit stating that she thinks she is in labor. Her contractions are irregular at 7 to 10 minutes apart. Which sign is definitive for true labor?
    1. Pain decreases when walking.
    2. Cervical dilation is occurring.
    3. The fetal membranes rupture.
    4. The fetal head is at –1 station.

19. Arrange the seven cardinal movements of labor, in order.
    1. Descent
    2. Expulsion
    3. Extension
    4. External rotation
    5. Engagement
    6. Flexion
    7. Internal rotation

20. A fetus is in the occiput anterior position. During the cardinal movement of *extension*, which events are occurring? *Select all that apply.*
    1. The fetal head lines up with the pelvic outlet.
    2. The occiput passes under the symphysis pubis.
    3. The fetal head is engaged.
    4. The head is delivered.
    5. The fetus is progressing through the pelvic inlet.

21. Which of the following is a function of a doula during labor?
    1. Administration of oral pain medications
    2. Assess fetal heart rate
    3. Perform vaginal examination with the mother's permission
    4. Provide nonpharmacological pain relief

22. A patient who is 8 cm dilated develops circumoral numbness and dizziness. What is the nurse's *priority* intervention?
    1. Call the health care provider immediately.
    2. Increase intravenous fluid, as these are signs of hypovolemia.
    3. Have the patient slow down her breathing.
    4. Have her start pushing, as these are signs of the beginning of the second stage.

23. A patient admitted to the labor unit asks the nurse to discuss the episiotomy procedure with her. Which is true regarding episiotomy?
    1. An episiotomy is required for all vaginal births.
    2. A midline episiotomy is associated with more third- and fourth-degree lacerations.
    3. A mediolateral episiotomy is easier to repair than a medial episiotomy.
    4. A midline episiotomy is associated with more blood loss.

24. A patient sustained a third-degree perineal laceration during a vaginal delivery. Which is this associated with?
    1. Extension through skin and vaginal mucous membrane
    2. Extension through the fascia and muscle
    3. Extension through involving the anal sphincter
    4. Extension through the rectal mucosa

25. A G1, P0 patient delivered an infant after a prolonged second stage of labor. During the fourth stage of labor, the uterine fundus is examined and found to be boggy with an increase in lochia. Which is the *first priority* intervention for the nurse to perform?
    1. Call the health care provider.
    2. Administer oxytocin to help contract the uterus.
    3. Massage the uterus firmly.
    4. Weigh all pads to determine the amount of blood loss.

REVIEW QUESTION ANSWERS

1. ANSWER: 2, 3, 5, 6
Rationale
1. Weight gain does not occur but weight loss of 0.5 to 1.5 kg may occur.
2. A surge of energy is very common preceding labor.
3. Increase in urinary frequency occurs due to pressure on the urinary bladder (lightening).
4. Dyspnea is lessened and not increased due to the baby descending into the birth canal and creating less pressure on the rib cage (lightening).
5. Pain in the lower back occurs due to relaxation of pelvic joints.
6. Increase in bloody show can occur prior to labor and increases with dilation and effacement.

TEST-TAKING TIP: Review signs of impending labor if you answered this question incorrectly.
Content Area: Process of Labor and Birth
Integrated Processes: Nursing Process—Assessment
Client Need: Health Promotion and Maintenance
Cognitive Level: Comprehension
Concept: Pregnancy
Reference: Murray, S. S., & McKinney, E. S. (2014). Foundations of maternal-newborn and women's health nursing. 6th ed. St. Louis, MO: Elsevier/Saunders.

2. ANSWER: 2, 4, 5
Rationale
1. Hormonal changes that occur prior to labor are an increase in estrogen and prostaglandins with a decrease in progesterone.
2. Hormonal changes that occur prior to labor are an increase in estrogen and prostaglandins with a decrease in progesterone.
3. Human chorionic gonadotropin is not elevated at the end of pregnancy.
4. The placenta ages as pregnancy progresses.
5. The fetal hypothalamic-pituitary-adrenal axis has an effect on the beginning of labor.
6. Hormonal changes that occur prior to labor are an increase in estrogen and prostaglandins with a decrease in progesterone.

TEST-TAKING TIP: Review onset of labor if you answered this question incorrectly.
Content Area: Process of Labor and Birth
Integrated Processes: Nursing Process—Assessment
Client Need: Health Promotion and Maintenance
Cognitive Level: Application
Concept: Pregnancy
Reference: Lowdermilk, D. L., Perry, S. E., Cashion, K., & Alden, K. R. (2016). Maternity & women's health care. 11th ed. St. Louis, MO: Elsevier.

3. ANSWER: 3
Rationale
1. Factors that may cause false-positive results with nitrazine are the presence of blood, mucus, or semen, so ferning is a more conclusive test than nitrazine.
2. Recall that amniotic fluid is alkaline in nature with a pH of 7 to 7.5. It turns nitrazine paper blue.
3. Due to the possibility of false-positive tests with nitrazine, ferning is a more conclusive test.
4. The fluid leaking may be urine due to the pressure of the fetal head on the bladder. Urine is acidic in nature with a pH of 6.

TEST-TAKING TIP: Review assessment of rupture of membranes if you answered this question incorrectly. Review the alkalinity of amniotic fluid and different tests that are used to determine its presence.
Content Area: Process of Labor and Birth
Integrated Processes: Nursing Process—Assessment
Client Need: Health Promotion and Maintenance
Cognitive Level: Application
Concept: Pregnancy
Reference: Lowdermilk, D. L., Perry, S. E., Cashion, K., & Alden, K. R. (2016). Maternity & women's health care. 11th ed. St. Louis, MO: Elsevier.

4. ANSWER: 3
Rationale
1. A platypelloid pelvis is flat and wide with a transverse diameter greater than the anteroposterior (AP) diameter and a wide pubic arch.
2. An android pelvis is heart or triangular shaped with a narrow pubic arch.
3. An anthropoid pelvis is long and narrow with an AP diameter greater than the transverse diameter, a narrow pubic arch, and a larger outlet.
4. A gynecoid pelvis is round, wide, and most suitable for delivery.

TEST-TAKING TIP: Review the four types of pelvises in the "Passenger" section if you answered this question incorrectly. Recall the parameters that can be assessed with each pelvis.
Content Area: Process of Labor and Birth
Integrated Processes: Nursing Process—Assessment
Client Need: Health Promotion and Maintenance
Cognitive Level: Knowledge
Concept: Pregnancy
Reference: Lowdermilk, D. L., Perry, S. E., Cashion, K., & Alden, K. R. (2016). Maternity & women's health care. 11th ed. St. Louis, MO: Elsevier.

5. ANSWER: 1
Rationale
1. A gynecoid pelvis is round, wide, and most suitable for delivery.
2. An android pelvis is heart or triangular shaped with a narrow pubic arch, which may lead to a longer labor.
3. A platypelloid pelvis is flat and wide with a transverse diameter greater than the AP diameter and a wide pubic arch. It is uncommon and associated with a longer and more difficult labor.
4. An anthropoid pelvis is long and narrow with an AP diameter greater than the transverse diameter, a narrow pubic arch, and a larger outlet. There is a poorer prognosis for delivery.

TEST-TAKING TIP: Review the four types of pelvises under the "Passenger" section if you answered this question incorrectly. Recall the parameters that can be assessed with each pelvis.
Content Area: Process of Labor and Birth
Integrated Processes: Nursing Process—Assessment
Client Need: Health Promotion and Maintenance

Cognitive Level: Knowledge
Concept: Pregnancy
Reference: Lowdermilk, D. L., Perry, S. E., Cashion, K., & Alden, K. R.
(2016). Maternity & women's health care. 11th ed. St. Louis, MO: Elsevier.

6. ANSWER: 7 POINTS

Rationale

One point for color, 1 point for muscle tone, 1 point for respiratory effort, 2 points for heart rate, and 2 points for reflex response = 7.

Parameter	0 Points	1 Point	2 Points
Heart rate	Absent	Below 100 beats/minute	100 beats/minute or higher
Respiratory effort	No spontaneous respirations	Slow, irregular respirations or weak cry	Vigorous cry
Muscle tone	Limp or absent	Minimal flexion of extremities, sluggish movement	Active movement
Reflex response	No response to suction	Minimal response to suction (grimace)	Active motion (sneeze, cough, pull away)
Color	Pallor or cyanosis	Body pink, extremities blue	Completely pink

TEST-TAKING TIP: Review the assignment of Apgar scores if you answered this question incorrectly. Recall the points that can be assessed with each parameter.
Content Area: Process of Labor and Birth
Integrated Processes: Nursing Process—Assessment
Client Need: Health Promotion and Maintenance
Cognitive Level: Analysis
Concept: Pregnancy
Reference: Lowdermilk, D. L., Perry, S. E., Cashion, K., & Alden, K. R.
(2016). Maternity & women's health care. 11th ed. St. Louis, MO: Elsevier.

7. ANSWER: 2

Rationale

1. In the first stage, latent phase rectal pressure is not usually felt, because the fetal head has not yet reached the pelvic floor.
2. In the second stage, the urge to push is much more intense.
3. The third stage of labor is the delivery of the placenta, and the fetus can no longer cause an urge to push.
4. The fourth stage is the period after delivery when homeostasis is being established.

TEST-TAKING TIP: Review the four stages of labor if you answered this question incorrectly. Recall what occurs during each stage.
Content Area: Process of Labor and Birth
Integrated Processes: Nursing Process—Assessment
Client Need: Health Promotion and Maintenance

Cognitive Level: Analysis
Concept: Pregnancy
Reference: Lowdermilk, D. L., Perry, S. E., Cashion, K., & Alden, K. R.
(2016). Maternity & women's health care. 11th ed. St. Louis, MO: Elsevier.

8. ANSWER: 4

Rationale

1. The order of these is incorrect.
2. Dilation is recorded as 0–10 cm, effacement as 0%–100%, and fetal lie as longitudinal or transverse.
3. Dilation is recorded as 0–10 cm, effacement as 0%–100%, and membranes as intact or ruptured.
4. Dilation is recorded as 0–10 cm, effacement as 0%–100%, and station as –3, –2, –1, 0, +1, +2, or +3, so this answer is correct.

TEST-TAKING TIP: Review vaginal examinations if you answered this question incorrectly. Recall that assessments made during the vaginal examination include dilation, effacement, station, presentation, position, and status of membranes, but be aware of the meaning of the labels: cm, %, and – or +. Effacement is recorded as 0%–100%; station as –3, –2, –1, 0, +1, +2, or +3; and dilation as 0–10 cm.
Content Area: Process of Labor and Birth
Integrated Processes: Nursing Process—Assessment
Client Need: Health Promotion and Maintenance
Cognitive Level: Comprehension
Concept: Pregnancy
Reference: Durham, R. F., & Chapman, L. (2014). Maternal-newborn
nursing: The critical components of nursing care. 2nd ed. Philadelphia:
F.A. Davis.

9. ANSWER: 1

Rationale

1. Engagement of the fetal head occurs when the largest diameter (usually biparietal) reaches the level of the ischial spines, so this is correct.
2. Flexion of the fetal head does not determine the station.
3. A –2 station is 2 cm above the ischial spines.
4. The pubic arch is below the ischial spines; the inability to pass under it does not refer to engagement.

TEST-TAKING TIP: Review vaginal examinations and engagement if you answered this question incorrectly. Recall that assessments made during the vaginal examination include dilation, effacement, station, presentation, position, and status of membranes.
Content Area: Process of Labor and Birth
Integrated Processes: Nursing Process—Assessment
Client Need: Health Promotion and Maintenance
Cognitive Level: Comprehension
Concept: Pregnancy
Reference: Durham, R. F., & Chapman, L. (2014). Maternal-newborn
nursing: The critical components of nursing care. 2nd ed. Philadelphia:
F.A. Davis.

10. ANSWER: 4

Rationale

1. An assessment time of 15 minutes is too frequent.
2. An assessment time of 5 minutes is too frequent.
3. An assessment time of 20 minutes is too frequent.
4. An assessment time of 30 minutes is the recommended time frame for a woman without risk factors in the active phase of the first stage of labor.

TEST-TAKING TIP: Review fetal assessment in labor if you answered this question incorrectly.
Content Area: Process of Labor and Birth
Integrated Processes: Nursing Process—Assessment
Client Need: Health Promotion and Maintenance
Cognitive Level: Comprehension
Concept: Pregnancy
Reference: Association of Women's Health, Obstetric and Neonatal Nurses. (2014). Perinatal nursing. 4th ed. K. R. Simpson, & P. A. Creehan (Eds.). Philadelphia: Lippincott Williams & Wilkins.

11. **ANSWER: 3**
Rationale
1. Lightening may precede the onset of labor by 2 weeks in a primigravida.
2. Effacement is thinning and shortening of the cervix and does not affect pressure on the bladder.
3. Lightening occurs when the fetal head descends into the maternal pelvis, causing decreased pressure on the rib cage and increased pressure on the bladder. This creates increased ease of breathing and urinary frequency.
4. Lightening may not be related to rupture of membranes.
TEST-TAKING TIP: Review the signs of impending labor if you answered this question incorrectly.
Content Area: Process of Labor and Birth
Integrated Processes: Nursing Process—Assessment
Client Need: Health Promotion and Maintenance
Cognitive Level: Comprehension
Concept: Pregnancy
Reference: Durham, R. F., & Chapman, L. (2014). Maternal-newborn nursing: The critical components of nursing care. 2nd ed. Philadelphia: F.A. Davis.

12. **ANSWER: 3**
Rationale
1. A vaginal examination is contraindicated in this patient, who has vaginal bleeding. In this case it is associated with placenta previa.
2. AROM would be contraindicated, as it is too invasive and could cause further bleeding. The patient is also 36 weeks pregnant, so if the fetus is not in distress and bleeding could be curtailed, it would be wise to maintain the pregnancy as long as the clinical picture is stable.
3. External fetal monitoring is appropriate, as it is noninvasive and necessary to ascertain fetal status in this high-risk pregnancy.
4. The patient should be placed on bedrest in the lateral position to improve placental blood flow. Ambulation is contraindicated.
TEST-TAKING TIP: Review the vaginal examination and contraindications if you answered this question incorrectly.
Content Area: Process of Labor and Birth
Integrated Processes: Nursing Process—Intervention
Client Need: Physiological Integrity—Reduction of Risk Potential
Cognitive Level: Analysis
Concept: Pregnancy
Reference: Lowdermilk, D. L., Perry, S. E., Cashion, K., & Alden, K. R. (2016). Maternity & women's health care. 11th ed. St. Louis, MO: Elsevier.

13. **ANSWER: 4**
Rationale
1. Supine positioning eliminates the effects of gravity and can lead to maternal supine hypotension due to pressure of the fetus, uterus, and amniotic fluid on the great vessels.
2. Lateral recumbent position eliminates the effects of gravity but can help prevent maternal supine hypotension.
3. Lithotomy has the same effects of a supine position except discomfort may occur when the mother's legs are in stirrups.
4. Squatting uses the effects of gravity and can help to open the maternal pelvis. It may also be a comfortable position for a woman in labor.
TEST-TAKING TIP: Review maternal positioning in labor if you answered this question incorrectly.
Content Area: Process of Labor and Birth
Integrated Processes: Nursing Process—Intervention
Client Need: Physiological Integrity—Reduction of Risk Potential
Cognitive Level: Analysis
Concept: Pregnancy
Reference: Lowdermilk, D. L., Perry, S. E., Cashion, K., & Alden, K. R. (2016). Maternity & women's health care. 11th ed. St. Louis, MO: Elsevier.

14. **ANSWER: 1**
Rationale
1. When the presenting part is not descending into the maternal pelvis and is too high, it is known as *floating* or *ballotable*. It moves away, then comes back toward the examiner's hand during the vaginal examination.
2. Zero station is engaged and the fetal head is down in the pelvis at the level of the ischial spines.
3. A +1 station is 1 cm below the level of the ischial spines, which is lower than floating.
4. A –2 station is 2 cm above the level of the ischial spines but still not high enough to be floating.
TEST-TAKING TIP: Review vaginal examination in labor if you answered this question incorrectly.
Content Area: Process of Labor and Birth
Integrated Processes: Nursing Process—Assessment
Client Need: Health Promotion and Maintenance
Cognitive Level: Comprehension
Concept: Pregnancy
Reference: Lowdermilk, D. L., Perry, S. E., Cashion, K., & Alden, K. R. (2016). Maternity & women's health care. 11th ed. St. Louis, MO: Elsevier.

15. **ANSWER: 1**
Rationale
1. The mentum or chin is the presenting part in a face presentation.
2. The sacrum is the presenting part in a breech presentation.
3. The occiput is the presenting part in a vertex presentation.
4. The acromion process of the scapula is the presenting part in a shoulder presentation.
TEST-TAKING TIP: Review fetal presentations of face, vertex, and transverse/shoulder if you answered this question incorrectly.
Content Area: Process of Labor and Birth
Integrated Processes: Nursing Process—Assessment

Client Need: Health Promotion and Maintenance
Cognitive Level: Comprehension
Concept: Pregnancy
Reference: Durham, R. F., & Chapman, L. (2014). Maternal-newborn nursing: The critical components of nursing care. 2nd ed. Philadelphia: F.A. Davis.

16. ANSWER: 2

Rationale

1. In a frank breech, the fetus is positioned in a longitudinal lie with its head in the fundus with hips flexed and knees extended.
2. In a complete breech, the fetus is positioned with a longitudinal lie with its head in the fundus with both hips and knees flexed.
3. In a vertex presentation, the fetus is positioned in a longitudinal lie with the head down.
4. In a transverse presentation, the fetus is in a transverse lie.

TEST-TAKING TIP: Review fetal presentations of vertex, breech, and transverse if you answered this question incorrectly.

Content Area: Process of Labor and Birth
Integrated Processes: Nursing Process—Assessment
Client Need: Health Promotion and Maintenance
Cognitive Level: Comprehension
Concept: Pregnancy
Reference: Durham, R. F., & Chapman, L. (2014). Maternal-newborn nursing: The critical components of nursing care. 2nd ed. Philadelphia: F.A. Davis.

17. ANSWER: 2

Rationale

1. This defines the fetal shoulder presentation, not the occiput anterior position.
2. In the occiput anterior position, the fetus must be in cephalic presentation with the occiput facing the anterior portion of the maternal pelvis (position).
3. This describes a breech presentation, as the head is up in the fundus.
4. This describes an occiput posterior position, as the fetus is in cephalic presentation with the occiput facing the posterior portion of the maternal pelvis (position).

TEST-TAKING TIP: If you answered this question incorrectly, review fetal positions of occiput anterior and posterior and presentations of cephalic and breech. Differentiate between fetal presentation and position.

Content Area: Process of Labor and Birth
Integrated Processes: Nursing Process—Assessment
Client Need: Health Promotion and Maintenance
Cognitive Level: Comprehension
Concept: Pregnancy
Reference: Durham, R. F., & Chapman, L. (2014). Maternal-newborn nursing: The critical components of nursing care. 2nd ed. Philadelphia: F.A. Davis.

18. ANSWER: 2

Rationale

1. Pain decreases with walking in false labor.
2. Cervical dilation is an absolute sign that true labor has started.

3. The fetal membranes may rupture during pregnancy or as late as birth, so this does not define true labor.
4. The station of the fetus does not define a stage of labor.

TEST-TAKING TIP: Review the differences between true and false labor if you answered this question incorrectly.

Content Area: Process of Labor and Birth
Integrated Processes: Nursing Process—Assessment
Client Need: Health Promotion and Maintenance
Cognitive Level: Comprehension
Concept: Pregnancy
Reference: Durham, R. F., & Chapman, L. (2014). Maternal-newborn nursing: The critical components of nursing care. 2nd ed. Philadelphia: F.A. Davis.

19. ANSWER: 5, 1, 6, 7, 3, 4, 2

Rationale

The order of the seven cardinal movements are engagement, descent, flexion, internal rotation, extension, external rotation, and expulsion (engagement occurs at the same time as descent and flexion).

TEST-TAKING TIP: Review the seven cardinal movements of labor if you answered this question incorrectly.

Content Area: Process of Labor and Birth
Integrated Processes: Nursing Process—Assessment
Client Need: Health Promotion and Maintenance
Cognitive Level: Knowledge
Concept: Pregnancy
Reference: Durham, R. F., & Chapman, L. (2014). Maternal-newborn nursing: The critical components of nursing care. 2nd ed. Philadelphia: F.A. Davis.

20. ANSWER: 1, 2, 4

Rationale

1. During extension, the fetal head lines up with the pelvic outlet, passes under the symphysis pubis, and is delivered.
2. During extension the fetal head lines up with the pelvic outlet, passes under the symphysis pubis, and is delivered.
3. Engagement occurs earlier than extension.
4. During extension the fetal head lines up with the pelvic outlet, passes under the symphysis pubis, and is delivered.
5. The fetus passes through the pelvic inlet during descent.

TEST-TAKING TIP: Review the seven cardinal movements of labor if you answered this question incorrectly.

Content Area: Process of Labor and Birth
Integrated Processes: Nursing Process—Assessment
Client Need: Health Promotion and Maintenance
Cognitive Level: Knowledge
Concept: Pregnancy
Reference: Durham, R. F., & Chapman, L. (2014). Maternal-newborn nursing: The critical components of nursing care. 2nd ed. Philadelphia: F.A. Davis.

21. ANSWER: 4

Rationale

1. Doulas are not licensed and are not permitted to give medications to the woman in labor.
2. Doulas are not licensed, trained, or permitted to assess the fetal heart rate.
3. Doulas are not licensed, trained, or permitted to perform vaginal examinations even if they have permission from the mother.

4. One of the functions of doulas is to provide nonpharmacological pain relief to women in labor.

TEST-TAKING TIP: Review labor support if you answered this question incorrectly. Remember that a doula is a layperson who is in attendance only for physical comfort and emotional support. They are not permitted to make clinical decisions or have responsibility for direct communication with the care provider.

Content Area: Process of Labor and Birth
Integrated Processes: Nursing Process—Intervention
Client Need: Health Promotion and Maintenance
Cognitive Level: Analysis
Concept: Pregnancy
Reference: *Durham, R. F., & Chapman, L. (2014).* Maternal-newborn nursing: The critical components of nursing care. *2nd ed. Philadelphia: F.A. Davis.*

22. **ANSWER: 3**
Rationale
1. There is no need to call the health care provider, as this is a common occurrence in labor, which can be treated with a simple intervention.
2. These symptoms are not related to hypovolemia.
3. This is a common occurrence in labor related to hyperventilation, so having the patient slow down her breathing would increase $PaCO_2$ toward normal and ameliorate symptoms.
4. The patient is not fully dilated and is therefore not in the second stage of labor. The patient should not be encouraged to push at this time.

TEST-TAKING TIP: Review care of the woman in the active/transition stage of labor if you answered this question incorrectly. Recall that hyperventilation can cause circumoral or extremity numbness or dizziness due to hypocapnia (decrease in arterial $PaCO_2$).

Content Area: Process of Labor and Birth
Integrated Processes: Nursing Process—Intervention
Client Need: Physiological Integrity
Cognitive Level: Analysis
Concept: Pregnancy
Reference: *Durham, R. F., & Chapman, L. (2014).* Maternal-newborn nursing: The critical components of nursing care. *2nd ed. Philadelphia: F.A. Davis.*

23. **ANSWER: 2**
Rationale
1. An episiotomy is not needed for all vaginal births, and research has not supported the benefit of performing them.
2. A midline episiotomy is associated with more third- and fourth-degree lacerations due to the extension from the episiotomy down toward the rectum.
3. A midline, not a mediolateral, episiotomy is easier to repair.
4. A mediolateral, not a midline, episiotomy is associated with more blood loss.

TEST-TAKING TIP: Review episiotomy in labor if you answered this question incorrectly. Review the two different types of episiotomies and reasons for performing them along with advantages and disadvantages of each.

Content Area: Process of Labor and Birth
Integrated Processes: Nursing Process—Assessment
Client Need: Physiological Integrity—Physiological Adaptation
Cognitive Level: Analysis
Concept: Pregnancy
Reference: *Lowdermilk, D. L., Perry, S. E., Cashion, K., & Alden, K. R. (2016).* Maternity & women's health care. *11th ed. St. Louis, MO: Elsevier.*

24. **ANSWER: 3**
Rationale
1. Extension through the skin and vaginal mucous membrane describes a first-degree laceration.
2. Extension through the fascia and muscle describes a second-degree laceration.
3. Extension involving the anal sphincter describes a third-degree laceration.
4. Extension through the rectal mucosa describes a fourth-degree laceration.

TEST-TAKING TIP: Review episiotomy in labor if you answered this question incorrectly. Review the two different types of episiotomies and reasons for performing them along with advantages and disadvantages of each.

Content Area: Process of Labor and Birth
Integrated Processes: Nursing Process—Assessment
Client Need: Physiological Integrity—Physiological Adaptation
Cognitive Level: Analysis
Concept: Pregnancy
Reference: *Lowdermilk, D. L., Perry, S. E., Cashion, K., & Alden, K. R. (2016).* Maternity & women's health care. *11th ed. St. Louis, MO: Elsevier.*

25. **ANSWER: 3**
Rationale
1. Although the health care provider may need to be called, it is not the first priority. The nurse needs to make sure the uterus becomes and remains contracted to prevent hemorrhage.
2. The nurse needs to make sure the uterus becomes and remains contracted to prevent hemorrhage and should assess if uterine atony can first be corrected with massage. Oxytocin may need to be administered, which can occur shortly after massage.
3. The first priority of the nurse is to be sure the uterus becomes and remains contracted to prevent hemorrhage.
4. Although all pads should be weighed to determine the amount of blood loss, it is not the first priority. The nurse needs to make sure the uterus becomes and remains contracted to prevent hemorrhage. Weighing can occur when the patient is more stable.

TEST-TAKING TIP: Review care of the patient in the fourth stage of labor if you answered this question incorrectly.

Content Area: Process of Labor and Birth
Integrated Processes: Nursing Process—Intervention
Client Need: Physiological Integrity—Physiological Adaptation
Cognitive Level: Analysis
Concept: Pregnancy
Reference: *Lowdermilk, D. L., Perry, S. E., Cashion, K., & Alden, K. R. (2016).* Maternity & women's health care. *11th ed. St. Louis, MO: Elsevier.*

Nursing Care During Labor and Birth

I. Maternal Assessment During Labor

The labor process is a time of great physiological stress for mother and fetus as well as psychological stress for mother and support person. Nurses need to be encouraging, supportive, and cognizant of these issues when caring for a woman in labor. This chapter will discuss nursing management focus throughout labor and birth, with the goal of ensuring the best possible outcome for all involved.

A. Prenatal data

This should be reviewed for parity status, estimated date of birth, history of current pregnancy, status, past obstetric history, past health history, past family history, prenatal education, and list of medications. Laboratory studies collected upon admission usually include a urinalysis to check for the presence of protein, glucose, and ketones. A complete blood count (CBC) should be done to look for the following:

- Hemoglobin and hematocrit: assess for anemia or as baseline laboratory value
- White blood cell count: may be elevated to levels as high as 20,000 to 30,000/mm^3 without an infection
- Platelet count: may decrease in pre-eclampsia

- Blood type and Rh factor: RhoGAM will need to be administered to Rh-negative mother (if baby is Rh-positive)
- Hepatitis B: to determine need for treatment of baby
- HIV: to determine need for treatment of mother and baby
- Blood glucose level: indicated if the mother is diabetic

B. Physical examination

This should include a general assessment, uterine activity, status of membranes, cervical dilation and degree of effacement, fetal status, and pain level.

1. Perform **Leopold's maneuvers** to assess presentation of the fetus. This is done by palpating the maternal abdomen (see Chapter 12 for further discussion).
2. Cervical assessment may be performed to determine cervical **dilation, effacement,** and **station,** fetal position and presentation, and **rupture of membranes (ROM).**
   a) Cervical assessment is a sterile procedure.
   b) Dilation is confirmed by assessment of the cervical os and is measured in centimeters (see Chapter 14 for further discussion):
      - 0 cm (cervical os is closed) to 10 cm (fully dilated, which denotes the first stage of labor)

- 0–3 cm: the latent phase of labor
- 4–7 cm: the active phase of labor
- 8–10 cm: the transition phase of labor

c) Effacement is confirmed by assessment of the thinning of the cervix and shortening of the endocervical canal.

d) Station is the decent of the fetus's head in relation to the ischial spines of the maternal pelvis.
- Zero station is when the biparietal diameter of the fetal head is at the level of spines. This is also known as *engagement*.
- Negative numbers are above the spines and positive numbers are below the spines. For example, if the examiner assessed that the fetus's presenting part was 2 cm below the spines, this would be documented as +2 station.
- *Presentation* refers to the fetal part that enters the pelvis first.

e) Rupture of fetal membranes should be assessed during the initial cervical assessment.
- The color of amniotic fluid is clear with white particles.
- Fetal membranes may rupture spontaneously or artificially by the health care provider.
- To verify ROM, litmus paper may be used. Alkaline pH of the amniotic fluid will turn the paper from yellow to blue. This indicates that the membranes have ruptured.
- Another method to verify ROM is ferning. When amniotic fluid is viewed through a microscope, it gives the appearance of ferning.
- AmniSure is a rapid immunoassay test used for detecting ruptured fetal membranes. It uses monoclonal antibodies to assess a protein called *placental alpha microglobulin-1 protein*. This protein is found in increased amounts in amniotic fluid. The test is said to be accurate even in the presence of urine and semen and does not require a speculum examination.

C. Electronic fetal monitoring
1. External fetal monitoring is noninvasive and can be applied by the nurse.
   a) An ultrasound transducer is placed over the point where the FHR can be best heard.
   - If the fetus is in a cephalic presentation, the FHR will be heard below the umbilicus.
   - If the fetus is in a breech presentation, the FHR will be heard above the umbilicus.
   b) A tocodynamometer or tocotransducer placed on the uterine fundus (top of uterus) provides a reading of uterine activity (UA).
   - Increment is the building of the contraction.
   - Acme is the peak of the contraction.

Fetal Monitoring

The fetal monitor provides the practitioner with a visual interpretation of the fetal heart rate (FHR) and the maternal contraction pattern. Two monitors are placed on the maternal abdomen—an ultrasound transducer to assess the FHR and a tocotransducer to assess uterine contractions. Both are displayed on a monitor strip. The top part of the strip displays the FHR. The bottom section displays a pattern of the frequency and duration of uterine contractions. There is a pressure-sensitive portion on the side of the tocotransducer in contact with the abdomen. As the contraction increases, force on the pressure-sensitive portion of the transducer causes a pattern to display on the monitor. An important consideration is the ability to assess the FHR in relation to the uterine contractions.

- Decrement is the descent or relaxation of the contraction.
- Frequency is the time from the beginning of one contraction to the beginning of the next contraction. The frequency of the contraction is measured in minutes.
- Duration is the time from the beginning of a contraction to the end of the same contraction. The duration is measured in seconds.

2. Internal fetal monitoring (Fig. 15.1) is invasive and requires cervical dilation and rupture of membranes.
   a) A fetal spiral electrode is placed onto the presenting part to measure FHR.
   b) Intrauterine pressure catheter (IUPC) sits in the uterine cavity and records UA in mm Hg. This

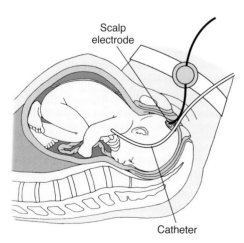

Scalp electrode

Catheter

Fig 15.1 Internal fetal monitor.

gives an objective measurement of intensity, duration, and frequency of uterine contractions.
3. The normal baseline FHR range is 110 to 160 beats per minute (bpm) (Fig. 15.2).
4. Normal FHR baseline and uterine contractions:
   a) Less than 110 = fetal bradycardia
      - Causes: hypoxemia may be the cause or the result of bradycardia. Assess for complete heart block in the fetus (rare). Sudden profound bradycardia may follow placental abruption, umbilical cord prolapse, rupture of the uterus, or rupture of vasa previa.
5. Fetal tachycardia
   a) Greater than 160 = fetal tachycardia. Assess for:
      - Maternal fever, infection, hyperthyroidism.
      - Fetal hypoxemia, anemia, arrhythmia, heart failure.
      - Parasympatholytic and beta-sympathetic drugs.

DID YOU KNOW?
Maternal fever causes accelerated fetal metabolism, which increases the FHR.

6. Baseline FHR **variability** is a baseline fluctuation of FHR in amplitude and frequency.
   a) Determined in a 10-minute window, excluding accelerations, decelerations, or periods of marked variability.
   b) Represented by a wavy, irregular line on the monitor.
      - Absent variability: amplitude range undetectable
      - Minimal: less than 5 bpm
      - Moderate: 6 to 25 bpm; considered normal
      - Marked: higher than 25 bpm
   c) Absence of variability is suggestive of fetal compromise.
   d) Causes of decreased variability include fetal metabolic acidosis, opioids, tranquilizers,

magnesium sulfate, betamethasone, fetal sleep cycles, anencephaly, congenital neurological abnormality, or prematurity.

ALERT Moderate variability is associated with a well-oxygenated fetus. Absent or minimal FHR variability is a significant intrapartum sign of fetal compromise, especially when associated with variable or **late decelerations.**

DID YOU KNOW?
When documenting variability, the nurse should use the terms *absent, minimal, moderate,* or *marked.*

7. Accelerations are a visually apparent increase in FHR of 15 bpm above baseline and lasting for at least 15 seconds but less than 2 minutes.
   a) Accelerations are considered evidence of fetal well-being.
8. Decelerations are a visually apparent decrease in FHR (Table 15.1).
   a) Episodic decelerations: not associated with uterine contractions
   b) Periodic decelerations: associated with uterine contractions
   c) Recurrent decelerations: those that occur in 50% or more of uterine contractions in any 20-minute window
   d) Early decelerations: decrease in the fetal heart rate where the nadir (lowest point) occurs at the same time as the peak of the contraction
   e) Variable decelerations: visually apparent, abrupt decrease in fetal heart rate from the baseline
   f) Late decelerations: decrease in the fetal heart rate where the nadir (lowest point) occurs after the contraction is over

ALERT To decrease anxiety and the perception of pain, the nurse should always explain assessment findings to the client and her birth partner.

   g) The National Institute of Child Health and Human Development describes terminology and nomenclature for FHR tracings and uterine contractions in a three-tier FHR interpretation system.
      (1) Category I
         - Baseline FHR of 110 to 160 with moderate variability
         - No variable or late decelerations
         - **Early decelerations** present or absent
         - Accelerations present or absent
      (2) Category II
         - FHR tracing that is considered indeterminate and includes a wide variety of possible tracings that do not fit in either Category I or Category III

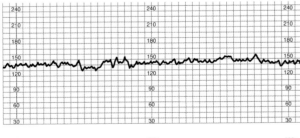
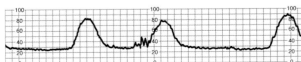

Fig 15.2 Normal FHR baseline and uterine contractions.

Table 15.1 Classification of Fetal Heart Rate Decelerations

Classification of Decelerations	Appearance on Monitor Strip	Cause	Nursing Intervention
Early	Gradual decrease and return to baseline of the FHR	Vagal stimulation: head compression, pushing	• Considered benign and no nursing intervention necessary
Late	Gradual decrease and return to baseline of the FHR. Nadir (lowest point) of contraction occurs after the peak of the contraction.	Uteroplacental insufficiency or decreased oxygen being transferred to the fetus	• Position client on side • Increase IVF rate to correct hypotension • Discontinue oxytocin if infusing • Administer oxygen at 8 to 10 L/min via nonrebreather face mask • Notify obstetric provider
Variable	Wide, deep, abrupt decrease from baseline Resembles U, V, or W shape. May occur at any time of the contraction cycle (episodic) or may be associated with uterine contractions (periodic)	Umbilical cord compression	• Recurrent: change maternal position (side to side or knee chest) • Assess baseline variability • Discontinue oxytocin if infusing • Administer oxygen at 8 to 10 L/min via nonrebreather face mask
Prolonged	Decrease of FHR at least 15 bpm for greater than 2 minutes but less than 10 minutes	Uteroplacental insufficiency or decreased transfer of oxygen to fetus	• Assist client to position to improve FHR (side to side, knee chest) • Discontinue oxytocin if infusing • Administer oxygen at 8 to 10 L/min via face mask • Increase IVF • Anticipate cesarean birth if FHR pattern does not resolve

• The classification of Category II tracings includes the following: bradycardia with variability, tachycardia, minimal variability, no variability with no recurrent decelerations, marked variability, absence of induced accelerations even after fetal stimulation, recurrent variable decelerations with minimal or moderate baseline variability, prolonged decelerations lasting more than two minutes but less than ten minutes, recurrent late decelerations with moderate variability, variable decelerations with other characteristics such as slow return to baseline, overshooting the baseline, or "shoulders."

(3) Category III
  • Absent baseline variability with any of the following:
    • Recurrent late decelerations
    • Recurrent **variable decelerations,** bradycardia
    • Sinusoidal pattern—uniform fluctuations in FHR without variability

DID YOU KNOW?
The findings from the first assessment upon admission form a baseline against which the nurse can compare all future assessment findings throughout labor.

II. Management of Discomfort During Labor and Birth

A. Nonpharmacological
  1. Maternal position
     a) Upright (including squatting) or ambulatory, as tolerated by maternal and fetal condition
     b) Use of birthing ball in sitting position or having arms and chest draped over the ball
     c) Turn client side to side if on bedrest

  (!) ALERT The nurse must make sure that the client avoids the supine position, as this may result in maternal hypotension. This is caused by compression of the maternal vena cava from the gravid uterus with subsequent decreased venous return to the heart. Signs and symptoms may include severe hypotension, tachycardia, dizziness, pallor, nausea, and diaphoresis. The first priority of the nurse should be to immediately turn the client to her left side.

  2. Breathing techniques
     a) Breathing techniques are usually taught in prenatal classes.
     b) Encourage slow, deep breathing at the start of the contraction to increase oxygen to the client and fetus.
     c) As labor progresses, breathing may increase but should be no more than two times the normal

rate. Client may use pant-blow breaths, which are three to four pants followed by exhaling.

d) Assess for hyperventilation with signs of dizziness, tingling, and circumoral numbness.

DID YOU KNOW?

Hyperventilation is a state of respiratory alkalosis. To reverse the effects, the nurse can instruct the clients to slow her breathing.

3. Massage and touch
   a) Hold hand or stroke, with attention to cultural preferences
   b) Hand or foot massage
4. Counterpressure
   a) Counterpressure is implemented with the use of a tennis ball or fist over the client's sacrum for pain relief.
   b) This may help pain associated with the occiput posterior position.
5. Effleurage
   a) **Effleurage** is a light stroking of the abdomen, used as distraction.
6. Music
   a) Music chosen prior to labor by the client/ support person that promotes relaxation
   b) May decrease anxiety associated with perception of pain
7. Relaxation
   a) Use the senses to promote relaxation by focusing on a pleasing object; make room lighting dim and have pleasing sounds.
8. Guided imagery
   a) Focus client's attention on pleasant scene or favorite activity. This involves all the senses, the imagination, and the whole body.
9. Hydrotherapy
   a) Immersion in warm water, which promotes relaxation and comfort
   b) More opportunity to move around
   c) Appropriate for uncomplicated, low-risk pregnancies
   d) Maternal and fetal evaluation, including assessing for maternal temperature and fetal tachycardia for signs of hyperthermia
   e) May also use warm shower
10. Hypnotherapy
    a) Attainment of deeply relaxed mental and physical state
    b) Should practice throughout pregnancy and may need to use tapes or videos
11. Aromatherapy
    a) Use of essential oils that are inhaled or applied to the skin
    b) Highly concentrated; need to assess if they are contraindicated in pregnancy

c) Cochrane reviews demonstrated that there is insufficient evidence from randomized controlled trials about the benefits of aromatherapy on pain management in labor.

12. Application of heat and cold
    a) Use heat packs, warm blankets, heating pads, warm shower, ice packs, or cold cloths to decrease pain or tension.
    b) Assess cultural preferences that do not allow the use of cold.
    c) Caution applying heat or cold; do not apply directly to skin or over anesthetized areas.
13. Biofeedback
    a) Use monitoring equipment to detect physio-logical responses (e.g., skin temperature, muscle tension) in order to increase relaxation techniques.
14. Transcutaneous electrical nerve stimulation
    a) Low-voltage electrical stimuli delivered to skin through a stimulator to two sets of electrodes placed on the client's back
    b) May not decrease pain but poses no safety concerns
15. Intradermal injections of sterile water
    a) Four injections of 0.05 to 0.1 mL of sterile water over the client's sacrum
    b) Use of counterirritation to offset pain along the same dermatome
16. Acupressure
    a) Pressure on certain points of the body using fingers, hands, or fists
    b) Layperson can be trained to do this
17. Acupuncture
    a) Ancient Chinese therapy targeting specific parts of the body are stimulated, usually with the use of needles, to restore the flow of qi (energy)
    b) Need trained acupuncturist, which might be difficult on a labor unit
    c) Might provide pain relief
B. Pharmacological
   1. **Analgesic** medications
      a) An *agonist* is a molecule that binds to one or more cell receptors to trigger a physiological reaction.
      b) An *antagonist* is a molecule that binds to one or more cell receptors without eliciting a physiological reaction. Blocks binding by agonists.
      c) *Agonist–antagonists* initiate mixed reactions.
   2. Opioid agonist analgesics
      a) Morphine sulfate's primary effect is heavy sedation. It is not sensitive to labor pain.
         • Relatively long-acting, shorter half-life, and more rapid plasma clearance than Demerol

- No published randomized controlled clinical trials addressing the effect of morphine on labor
- Used as part of regional analgesia
- Duramorph—preservative-free morphine that is administered by the intrathecal or **epidural** route
  - Provides pain relief for extended times with loss of motor, sensory, or sympathetic function.
  - Pruritus is a common side effect that can be treated with nalbuphine or low-dose naloxone infusion. Diphenhydramine is not effective.

(!) ALERT Opioids should be administered with caution, and many of these medications must be administered by a person trained in giving anesthetic agents.

  b) Sublimaze (Fentanyl)
  - Potent opioid agonist for moderate to severe pain
  - Greater analgesic potency than morphine
  - Action: binds to opiate receptors in the central nervous system (CNS), altering the response to and perception of pain; produces CNS depression
  - Side effects: bradycardia, hypotension, confusion, drowsiness, dizziness, rash, nausea and vomiting, urinary retention
  - Rapidly crosses placenta
  - Short-term diminished FHR variability
  - Can be given intravenously or as neuraxial anesthesia (spinal or epidural)
  - Nursing considerations: assess for respiratory depression. Have naloxone readily available as antidote.
  c) Sufentanil citrate (Sufenta)
  - For epidural administration: as an analgesic combined with low-dose bupivacaine during labor and vaginal delivery
  - Also used in general anesthesia where patient must be intubated and ventilated
  - Assess for respiratory depression and muscle stiffness
  d) Remifentanil (Ultiva)
  - Ultra-short-acting fentanyl analog.
  - Potent respiratory depressant; may also cause hypotension, hypertension, bradycardia, tachycardia, or skeletal muscle rigidity (including chest wall).
  - Given by intravenous route by trained personnel and primarily used for general

anesthesia. Contraindicated for spinal or epidural use.
  - Client needs continuous vital sign and oxygen monitoring.
  - Intubation equipment and narcotic antagonist needs to be readily available.
  - Caution in morbidly obese patients.
3. Opioid agonist–antagonist analgesics
  a) Butorphanol
  - High-potency labor analgesic.
  - Actions: alters pain perception and produces generalized CNS depression.
  - Side effects: somnolence, sedation, respiratory depression that can be reversed by naloxone.
  - Higher doses do not provide additional pain relief but do increase side effects.
  - May produce impaired sucking in neonate.

(!) ALERT Butorphanol is contraindicated in clients who are opioid dependent since antagonist effects may precipitate withdrawal symptoms.

  b) Nalbuphine
  - Potent analgesic equivalent to morphine on a milligram-to-milligram basis
  - Chemically, it is related to the opioid agonist oxymorphone
  - Produces sedation, nausea, vomiting, respiratory depression treatable with naloxone
  - May produce impaired sucking in neonates
4. Opioid antagonist
  a) Naloxone
  - Opioid antagonist
  - Reverses opioid-induced respiratory depression but will cause pain to return suddenly
  - Shorter duration of action than most opioids, so caution for return of opioid depression
  - Can be given to the mother or the newborn
  - Caution in opioid-dependent client to avoid withdrawal symptoms
5. Regional blocks
  a) Local perineal infiltration
  - Indication: used before birth for episiotomy or after birth for repair of lacerations
  - Local injection of anesthetic such as 1% lidocaine
  - Nursing assessment: observe perineum for bruising, discoloration, hematoma, or signs of infection

b) Pudendal nerve block
- Indication: administered late in second stage for episiotomy, forceps, or vacuum extraction. Administered during third stage for repair of episiotomy or lacerations.
- Relieves pain in lower vagina, vulva, and perineum.
- Does not relieve pain from uterine contractions.
- Nursing assessment: Monitor for signs of infection and urinary retention.

6. Regional anesthesia (neuraxial anesthesia)
   a) Regional analgesia alleviates pain during labor and vaginal delivery. The block extends to the T10 dermatome or umbilicus.
   b) Regional anesthesia for cesarean delivery requires more concentrated medication and extends to the T4 dermatome or nipple line.
   c) Regional anesthesia is the preferred method for surgical procedures in obstetrics due to high morbidity and mortality associated with general anesthesia.
   d) Have the patient void prior to the procedure and encourage voiding as least every 2 hours. May need insertion of indwelling urinary catheter.
   e) Informed consent is needed for anesthesia.

7. Spinal block (subarachnoid)
   a) Injection of local anesthetic alone or in combination with opioid agonist medication into the subarachnoid space
   b) Preferred method of anesthesia for cesarean section due to the rapid onset of anesthesia, short duration of action
   c) Assess for any coagulopathy

   d) Technically easier to perform than an epidural
   e) Performed in sitting or side-lying position (Fig. 15.3)
   f) Effect lasts 1 to 3 hours
   g) Caution: marked hypotension due to loss of sympathetic tone and pooling of venous blood, ineffective breathing, impaired placental perfusion
   - Place wedge under right hip or turn patient to left lateral position
   - Assess maternal vital signs every 5 to 10 minutes
   - Assess FHR for bradycardia, decelerations, decreased variability
   - Have emergency resuscitation equipment nearby, including the medications phenylephrine and ephedrine for treatment of hypotension

---

MAKING THE CONNECTION

Spinal Headache

A postdural puncture headache or spinal headache occurs when cerebrospinal fluid leaks from a dural puncture. This usually occurs from an inadvertent dural puncture with an epidural needle, which is a larger gauge than a spinal needle. Other symptoms include tinnitus, blurred vision, and photophobia. The pain is intensified with an upright position and is relieved or reduced when supine. Treatment includes a blood patch where the patient's blood (15 to 20 mL) is withdrawn from a vein and injected into the epidural space by the anesthesia provider. This forms a clot that seals the puncture in the dura and relieves that pain.

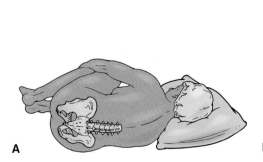

A

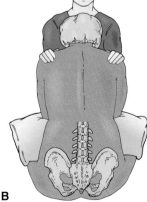

B

Fig 15.3 Positions for spinal and epidural blocks.

- Monitor site leakage of spinal fluid, development of hematoma, or postdural headache

8. Lumbar epidural block
   a) Administration of local anesthetics with or without opioids and/or epinephrine into the space above the dura. A catheter is usually inserted so that more medication can be injected as the block starts to wear off.
   b) Has a slower onset than a spinal and more volume needs to be injected.
   c) High spinal block: significant side effects can occur with inadvertent injection into subarachnoid space or systemic circulation. Test dose of lidocaine may be administered first.

9. Combined spinal epidural
   a) Combines rapid onset with spinal anesthesia with the ability to inject medication through the epidural catheter

   b) Small amount of medication is injected into subarachnoid space; then epidural is administered as usual
   c) Affords pain relief without loss of motor function
   d) Contraindications to regional anesthesia: severe maternal hemorrhage, maternal hypotension, coagulopathy, injection site infection, and allergy to medication

10. General anesthesia
    a) For emergencies such as the need for expeditious delivery of the neonate
    b) When spinal or epidural is contraindicated
    c) Higher risk of aspiration. Anesthesia provider may order clear antacid (Bicitra, H2 receptor blocker; famotidine, ranitidine) to decrease gastric acid
    d) Difficult intubation with morbidly obese patients

CASE STUDY: Putting It All Together

Subjective Data

A 30-year-old gravida 1, para 0 presents to the labor and delivery unit complaining of "abdominal tightening" and "leakage of urine" without burning or urgency. She is 34 weeks pregnant with a singleton pregnancy and has been receiving prenatal care since early in the first trimester. She has a history of hypothyroidism. She has no known allergies and her current medications are prenatal vitamins (one tablet daily) and levothyroxine (150 mcg daily).

Vital Signs

Height: 5'5" (165 cm)
Current weight: 185 lb (83.9 kg)
Prepregnancy weight: 148 lb (67 kg)
Temperature: 99°F (37.2°C)
Blood pressure: 130/88
Heart rate: 100 bpm, regular
Respiratory rate: 24 breaths per minute
Pulse oximetry: 98% on room air

Laboratory Results

Blood type and Rh: A negative
Antibody screen: Negative
Rubella: Immune
Hepatitis (HbsAg): Negative
HIV (3rd trimester): Negative
WBC: 12,000 per mm^3

Objective Data

Nursing Assessment

Leopold's maneuvers demonstrate the fetus to be in cephalic presentation. Sterile vaginal examination reveals the cervix to be 2 cm dilated, 50% effaced, 0 station.

Health Care Provider's Orders

- Continuous external fetal monitoring
- Blood type and Rh
- CBC in a.m.
- TSH, T_3, T_4
- Betamethasone 12 mg IM every 12 hours, x2 doses
- V/S every 2 hours
- Intake and output
- Insert IV of Lactated Ringer's solution at 100 mL/hr
- Diet: NPO

CASE STUDY: Putting It All Together (Continued)

_____ **Case Study Questions** _____

1. What *subjective* assessment findings indicate that the client is experiencing a change in clinical status?

2. What *objective* assessment findings indicate that the client is experiencing a change in clinical status?

3. After analyzing the data that has been collected, what primary nursing diagnosis should the nurse assign to this client?

4. What interventions should the nurse plan and/or implement to meet this client's needs?

5. What client outcomes should the nurse use to evaluate the effectiveness of the nursing interventions?

REVIEW QUESTIONS

Be sure to read the Introduction for valuable test-taking tips.

1. The nurse is monitoring her patient during labor and is aware that the only way to determine the objective measurement of uterine contractions is through the use of which modality?
   1. Tocodynamometer
   2. Fetal spiral electrode
   3. IUPC
   4. Palpation

2. Which is an opioid medication administered by the intrathecal or epidural route that can provide prolonged pain relief but does not interfere with movement or sensation?
   1. Meperidine
   2. Preservative-free morphine (Duramorph)
   3. Fentanyl
   4. Remifentanil

3. The nurse is about to perform Leopold's maneuvers on her patient, who was admitted in early labor. Which statement by the patient demonstrates understanding of the procedure?
   1. "This will be done to determine the stage of my labor."
   2. "You will be able to determine the baby's age."
   3. "This is an invasive procedure."
   4. "You will be able to tell if my baby is in breech presentation."

4. A patient admitted to the labor and delivery unit is reported to have a fetus that is in the breech position. Which of the following is a nursing priority?
   1. Maternal temperature of 101°F (38.3°C)
   2. FHR of 150 bpm without accelerations
   3. Rupture of the fetal membranes
   4. Maternal blood pressure of 100/60

5. Members of the labor and delivery unit are reviewing principles of electronic fetal monitoring. Which facts are regarded as accurate? *Select all that apply.*
   1. The normal FHR is 110 to 160 bpm.
   2. An FHR of 130 is considered fetal tachycardia.
   3. An acceleration of the FHR from the baseline of 120 bpm to 135 bpm for 20 seconds is considered abnormal.
   4. Accelerations in the FHR are considered a sign of fetal well-being.
   5. A deceleration of the FHR may be benign, depending on when it occurs in relation to uterine contractions.

6. A 40-year-old primiparous woman who is 38 weeks pregnant has been on the labor unit for an hour when she starts to complain of feeling dizzy, light-headed, and nauseous. Her blood pressure is 90/60. What should be the *first* response of the nurse?
   1. Give the patient a bolus of intravenous fluid.
   2. Turn the patient to her left side.
   3. Call the obstetrician or nurse midwife.
   4. Give the patient an antiemetic medication for the nausea.

7. What are late FHR decelerations caused by?
   1. Altered cerebral blood flow
   2. Umbilical cord compression
   3. Uteroplacental insufficiency
   4. Meconium fluid

8. The nurse who will care for a patient in labor receives a report and is told that the patient's status is as follows: 4 cm, 50%, and +1 station. What should be the nurse's interpretation of this information?
   1. The cervix is effaced 4 cm, is dilated to 50%, and is 1 cm below the ischial spines.
   2. The cervix is dilated 4 cm, is effaced to 50%, and is 1 cm above the ischial spines.
   3. The cervix is dilated 4 cm, is effaced to 50%, and is 1 cm below the ischial spines.
   4. The cervix is effaced 4 cm, is dilated to 50%, and is 1 cm above the ischial spines.

9. Which is fetal tachycardia likely caused by?
   1. Compression of the umbilical cord
   2. Maternal infection
   3. Compression of the fetal head
   4. Maternal hypertension

10. A patient in active labor starts to complain of circumoral numbness and tingling in her fingertips. What should the nurse do?
    1. Increase intravenous fluids.
    2. Give the woman pain medication.
    3. Obtain an arterial blood gas.
    4. Encourage the woman to slow down her breathing.

11. The woman's partner is lightly stroking her abdomen as an alternative to medication for pain relief in labor. What is this known as?
    1. Counterpressure
    2. Effleurage
    3. Guided imagery
    4. Biofeedback

12. Which is an expected characteristic of amniotic fluid?
    1. Deep yellow color
    2. Clear, with small white particles
    3. Nitrazine test: acidic result
    4. Absence of ferning

13. A 35-year-old patient is admitted to the delivery room having contractions 6 minutes apart. Upon palpation of the abdomen, the nurse feels a hard round object in the uterine fundus and a soft object in the pelvis. What should be anticipated?
    1. Cesarean section
    2. Imminent delivery
    3. Normal progressive labor and delivery
    4. FHR to be heard below the umbilicus

14. Five minutes after delivery of the infant, the umbilical cord is protruding more from the woman's vaginal introitus and there is a sudden gush of blood with a contracted uterus. What does this signal to the nurse?
    1. Laceration of the genital tract
    2. The second stage of labor
    3. Separation of the placenta
    4. Postpartum hemorrhage

15. A patient who is 38 weeks pregnant presents to the labor and delivery unit. Upon vaginal examination, it is determined the fetus is engaged. What is the correct interpretation by the nurse?
    1. The cervix is completely effaced.
    2. The lie is longitudinal.
    3. The fetal head is flexed.
    4. The biparietal diameter of the fetal head is at the level of the ischial spines.

16. The patient who has received a dose of preservative-free morphine (Duramorph) is beginning to experience pruritus. Which medication is used to treat this?
    1. Low-dose naloxone infusion
    2. Diphenhydramine
    3. Dilaudid
    4. Sublimaze

17. A patient in labor is undergoing an epidural block and is given intravenous fluid. What is the purpose of this?
    1. To treat hypotension that results from hemorrhage
    2. To increase urine output
    3. To treat insensible fluid losses
    4. To treat hypotension that results from sympathetic blockade

18. A patient who is about to undergo a cesarean section for breech presentation without fetal distress asks her nurse what kind of anesthesia would be best for her. The nurse explains that which of the following is the preferred method of anesthesia in this nonemergent case?
    1. Spinal block
    2. Epidural block
    3. General anesthesia
    4. Intravenous sedation

19. The nurse is caring for a patient who is in labor and being externally monitored. What should the nurse do after noting early decelerations of the FHR?
    1. Anticipate a cesarean birth
    2. Turn the patient onto the left side
    3. Continue to monitor the patient
    4. Notify the physician or nurse midwife immediately

20. A patient who was admitted to the delivery room undergoes an ultrasound, which reveals that the sacrum is the presenting part; the lie is longitudinal, with both the hips and knees in flexion. Which describes this fetal presentation?
    1. Cephalic
    2. Complete breech
    3. Frank breech
    4. Footling breech

REVIEW QUESTION ANSWERS

1. ANSWER: 3
Rationale
1. A tocodynamometer is the device used to externally monitor the mother for uterine contractions, which does not give an objective measure of pressure. Reasons for this include maternal obesity, placement of monitor, or maternal movement.
2. A fetal spiral electrode is the device to measure the fetal heart rate.
3. The IUPC is an internal device that can objectively measure uterine contractions and is measured in mm Hg.
4. Palpation is the external assessment of uterine contractions and is a subjective measurement.
TEST-TAKING TIP: Review principles of continuous external fetal monitoring in labor if you were unable to answer the question correctly.
Content Area: Internal Monitoring; Nursing Care During Labor and Birth
Integrated Processes: Nursing Process—Assessment
Client Need: Physiological Integrity—Reduction of Risk Potential
Cognitive Level: Comprehension
Concept: Pregnancy
Reference: Lowdermilk, D. L., Perry, S. E., Cashion, K., & Alden, K. R. (2016). Maternity & women's health care. 11th ed. St. Louis, MO: Elsevier.

2. ANSWER: 2
Rationale
1. Meperidine is not administered via the intrathecal or epidural route and does not provide prolonged pain relief without readministration.
2. Duramorph can be administered (by trained personnel) for pain relief after cesarean section via the intrathecal or epidural route. Patients are able to ambulate and maintain normal sensation.
3. Fentanyl is a short-acting opioid narcotic.
4. Remifentanil is a short-acting opioid narcotic, which is a potent respiratory depressant. It is contraindicated for spinal or epidural use.
TEST-TAKING TIP: Review narcotic medications used in labor if you were unable to answer the question correctly. Recall that although trained anesthesia personnel administer many of these medications, the nurse caring for the client must be aware of the medications' effects.
Content Area: Pain Management; Nursing Care During Labor and Birth
Integrated Processes: Nursing Process—Planning
Client Need: Physiological Integrity—Pharmacological and Parenteral Therapies
Cognitive Level: Comprehension
Concept: Pregnancy
Reference: Anderson, D. (2011). A review of systemic opioids commonly used for labor pain relief. Journal of Midwifery and Women's Health, 56(3): 222-239.

3. ANSWER: 4
Rationale
1. The stage of labor can be determined by vaginal examination, not Leopold's maneuvers.

2. Gestational age can be determined by using the date of the last menstrual period or by ultrasound measurements, not Leopold's maneuvers.
3. Leopold's maneuvers are not invasive; they are a form of external palpation.
4. Leopold's maneuvers are performed by the nurse or other trained health care provider. They are a form of abdominal palpation that helps determine the fetal presentation, position, lie, engagement, and flexion of extension of the fetal head.
TEST-TAKING TIP: Review the process of the four maneuvers involved with Leopold's maneuvers. Recall that it is an examination done to determine presentation and position of the fetus.
Content Area: Leopold's Maneuvers; Nursing Care During Labor and Delivery
Integrated Processes: Nursing Process—Assessment
Client Need: Health Promotion and Maintenance
Cognitive Level: Analysis
Concept: Pregnancy
Reference: Lowdermilk, D. L., Perry, S. E., Cashion, K., & Alden, K. R. (2016). Maternity & women's health care. 11th ed. St. Louis, MO: Elsevier.

4. ANSWER: 3
Rationale
1. Maternal temperature needs to be assessed for possible infection but is not the priority here.
2. FHR of 150 bpm falls within the expected range of 110 to 160 bpm.
3. Rupture of fetal membranes is not a nursing action. ROM may initiate labor, and this patient may need to be scheduled for a cesarean section due to breech presentation.
4. A blood pressure of 100/60 should be monitored but is not the priority and may be within the patient's normal range.
TEST-TAKING TIP: Review steps needed after rupture of membranes. Focus on the priority, remembering that signs that point to a problem may not always mean the fetus is in distress but an untoward change in FHR would.
Content Area: Rupture of Membranes; Nursing Care During Labor and Delivery
Integrated Processes: Nursing Process—Analysis
Client Need: Health Promotion and Maintenance
Cognitive Level: Application
Concept: Pregnancy
Reference: Lowdermilk, D. L., Perry, S. E., Cashion, K., & Alden, K. R. (2016). Maternity & women's health care. 11th ed. St. Louis, MO: Elsevier.

5. ANSWER: 1, 4, 5
Rationale
1. The normal fetal heart rate is 110 to 160 bpm.
2. Fetal tachycardia is defined as a rate greater than 160 bpm, so 130 is normal.
3. An acceleration of the FHR from the baseline of 120 bpm to 135 bpm for 20 seconds is considered an acceleration and is normal.
4. FHR accelerations are indicative of fetal well-being, but their absence is not considered pathological.
5. A late deceleration is always abnormal. A variable deceleration needs further investigation for frequency of

occurrence and heart rate variability but may be benign. An early deceleration is usually a result of descent and pressure on the fetal head and is considered benign. Assessment of descent may be assessed by vaginal examination but no other treatment is generally needed.

TEST-TAKING TIP: Review principles of FHR monitoring if you were unable to answer the question correctly.
Content Area: Electronic Fetal Monitoring; Nursing Care During Labor and Delivery
Integrated Processes: Nursing Process—Analysis
Client Need: Physiological Integrity—Reduction of Risk Potential
Cognitive Level: Knowledge
Concept: Pregnancy
Reference: Lowdermilk, D. L., Perry, S. E., Cashion, K., & Alden, K. R. (2016). Maternity & women's health care. 11th ed. St. Louis, MO: Elsevier; Macones, G. A., Hankins, D. V., Spong, C. Y., Hauth, J., & Moore, T. (2008). The 2008 National Institute of Child Health and Human Development workshop report on electronic fetal monitoring: Update on definitions, interpretation, and research guidelines. Journal of Obstetric, Gynecologic and Neonatal Nursing, 37(5): 510-515.

6. **ANSWER: 2**
Rationale
1. A bolus of IV fluid is likely not necessary and is not the priority intervention.
2. Dizziness, light-headedness, and nausea associated with a drop of blood pressure in a pregnant woman are usually caused by maternal supine hypotension, which is easily treated by turning the patient onto her left side. This is the priority intervention.
3. Treatment with an antiemetic is usually not needed.
4. Calling the health care provider is not the first priority.

TEST-TAKING TIP: Review maternal supine hypotension if you were unable to answer the question correctly. Recollect that there is a simple treatment to do before calling the health care provider and you must prioritize actions.
Content Area: Maternal Supine Hypotension; Nursing Care During Labor and Delivery
Integrated Processes: Nursing Process—Implementation
Client Need: Physiological Integrity—Physiological Adaptation
Cognitive Level: Application
Concept: Pregnancy
Reference: Lowdermilk, D. L., Perry, S. E., Cashion, K., & Alden, K. R. (2016). Maternity & women's health care. 11th ed. St. Louis, MO: Elsevier.

7. **ANSWER: 3**
Rationale
1. Altered cerebral blood flow from head compression produces early decelerations.
2. Umbilical cord compression produces variable decelerations.
3. Late FHR patterns are caused by uteroplacental insufficiency.
4. Meconium fluid may be caused by fetal distress, which may or may not produce changes in the FHR.

TEST-TAKING TIP: Review principles of FHR monitoring if you were unable to answer the question correctly.
Content Area: Late Decelerations; Nursing Care During Labor and Delivery

Integrated Processes: Nursing Process—Analysis
Client Need: Physiological Integrity—Reduction of Risk Potential
Cognitive Level: Knowledge
Concept: Pregnancy
Reference: Lowdermilk, D. L., Perry, S. E., Cashion, K., & Alden, K. R. (2016). Maternity & women's health care. 11th ed. St. Louis, MO: Elsevier.

8. **ANSWER: 3**
Rationale
1. Parameters for effacement and dilation are interchanged.
2. The station of +1 refers to a position below the spines.
3. This defines the parameter given for dilation, effacement, and station.
4. Parameters for effacement and dilation are interchanged and the station is −1.

TEST-TAKING TIP: The vaginal examination monitors cervical dilation measured in centimeters (cm), effacement measured by percentage (%), and station measured by plus (+) or minus (−), which represents how many centimeters above or below the ischial spines the presenting part is located. Review elements of labor progression defining dilation, effacement, and station if you were unable to answer the question correctly. Eliminate the incorrect answers because they contain incorrect measurements.
Content Area: Maternal Assessment; Nursing Care During Labor and Delivery
Integrated Processes: Nursing Process—Assessment
Client Need: Health Promotion and Maintenance
Cognitive Level: Comprehension
Concept: Pregnancy
Reference: Lowdermilk, D. L., Perry, S. E., Cashion, K., & Alden, K. R. (2016). Maternity & women's health care. 11th ed. St. Louis, MO: Elsevier.

9. **ANSWER: 2**
Rationale
1. Compression of the umbilical cord causes variable decelerations.
2. Fetal tachycardia may have many causes, including maternal or fetal infection, fetal anemia, maternal hyperthyroidism, fetal cardiac arrhythmias, beta sympathetic or parasympatholytic drugs, cocaine, methamphetamines, or caffeine.
3. Compression of the fetal head causes early decelerations.
4. Maternal hypertension is not a direct cause of fetal tachycardia.

TEST-TAKING TIP: Review principles of FHR monitoring if you were unable to answer the question correctly. Recall that tachycardia in the fetus can be caused by the same processes that can cause it to happen in the mother.
Content Area: Fetal Tachycardia; Nursing Care During Labor and Delivery
Integrated Processes: Nursing Process—Analysis
Client Need: Physiological Integrity—Reduction of Risk Potential
Cognitive Level: Knowledge
Concept: Pregnancy
Reference: Lowdermilk, D. L., Perry, S. E., Cashion, K., & Alden, K. R. (2016). Maternity & women's health care. 11th ed. St. Louis, MO: Elsevier.

10. ANSWER: 4
Rationale
1. Administering IV fluids would not treat this problem caused by hyperventilation and hypocarbia (low $PaCO_2$).
2. If pain is an issue, then the woman should be treated with medication, depending on maternal preference, provider order, and stage of labor.
3. An arterial blood gas would only be indicated with severe respiratory distress.
4. Hyperventilation resulting in circumoral and fingertip numbness is common in a laboring woman, especially as labor becomes more active and breathing increases in rate and depth. Encouraging her to slow down her breathing is the priority and a simple first action.
TEST-TAKING TIP: Recall that hyperventilation is common in labor and simple measures can combat the untoward effects.
Content Area: Nursing Management; Nursing Care During Labor and Delivery
Integrated Processes: Nursing Process—Implementation
Client Need: Health Promotion and Maintenance
Cognitive Level: Application
Concept: Pregnancy
Reference: Lowdermilk, D. L., Perry, S. E., Cashion, K., & Alden, K. R. (2016). Maternity & women's health care. 11th ed. St. Louis, MO: Elsevier.

11. ANSWER: 2
Rationale
1. Counterpressure is accomplished with the use of firm pressure over the woman's sacrum with a fist or tennis ball.
2. Effleurage is accomplished by lightly stroking the maternal abdomen.
3. Guided imagery is accomplished by focusing attention on a pleasant scene or favorite activity. It involves all the senses, the imagination, and the whole body.
4. Biofeedback uses monitoring equipment to detect physiological signs in order to increase relaxation.
TEST-TAKING TIP: Review nonpharmacological methods of pain relief in labor if you were unable to answer the question correctly.
Content Area: Nonpharmacological Pain Management; Nursing Care During Labor and Delivery
Integrated Processes: Nursing Process—Assessment
Client Need: Physiological Integrity—Basic Care and Comfort
Cognitive Level: Comprehension
Concept: Pregnancy
Reference: Lowdermilk, D. L., Perry, S. E., Cashion, K., & Alden, K. R. (2016). Maternity & women's health care. 11th ed. St. Louis, MO: Elsevier.

12. ANSWER: 2
Rationale
1. A deep yellow color results from meconium-stained fluid.
2. Amniotic fluid is normally clear with white particles consisting of fetal vernix and skin.
3. Amniotic fluid is alkaline when tested with nitrazine.
4. Amniotic fluid would have positive ferning on microscopic examination.
TEST-TAKING TIP: Review characteristics of amniotic fluid if you were unable to answer the question correctly.
Content Area: Rupture of Membrane; Nursing Care During Labor and Birth
Integrated Processes: Nursing Process—Assessment
Client Need: Health Promotion and Maintenance
Cognitive Level: Knowledge
Concept: Pregnancy
Reference: Lowdermilk, D. L., Perry, S. E., Cashion, K., & Alden, K. R. (2016). Maternity & women's health care. 11th ed. St. Louis, MO: Elsevier.

13. ANSWER: 1
Rationale
1. Leopold's maneuvers that reveal a hard round object in the fundus suggest that the fetus is in breech presentation and would likely be delivered by cesarean section.
2. There is no need to anticipate an imminent delivery since the patient does not appear to be in active labor. Further assessment of labor progress is needed.
3. Labor would be high risk if it were allowed to progress.
4. The FHR would be heard above the umbilicus in a breech presentation.
TEST-TAKING TIP: Review fetal presentations and Leopold's maneuvers if you were unable to answer the question correctly.
Content Area: Leopold's Maneuvers; Nursing Care During Labor and Birth
Integrated Processes: Nursing Process—Assessment
Client Need: Health Promotion and Maintenance
Cognitive Level: Application
Concept: Pregnancy
Reference: Lowdermilk, D. L., Perry, S. E., Cashion, K., & Alden, K. R. (2016). Maternity & women's health care. 11th ed. St. Louis, MO: Elsevier.

14. ANSWER: 3
Rationale
1. Continuous oozing or loss of blood usually accompanies laceration of the genital tract.
2. The second stage of labor is full dilation to the birth of the infant, during which time the woman is pushing with uterine contractions.
3. Signs of the third stage of labor, which is the separation of the placenta, are changes in shape of the uterus, sudden gush of blood, and lengthening of the umbilical cord from the vagina.
4. Postpartum hemorrhage would occur after delivery of the placenta.
TEST-TAKING TIP: Review the stages of labor, focusing on the signs of the third stage. Note that the "sudden" gush of blood associated with cord lengthening differentiates this from other causes of bleeding.
Content Area: Stages of Labor; Nursing Care During Labor and Birth
Integrated Processes: Nursing Process—Analysis
Client Need: Physiological Integrity—Physiological Adaptation
Cognitive Level: Application
Concept: Pregnancy
Reference: Lowdermilk, D. L., Perry, S. E., Cashion, K., & Alden, K. R. (2016). Maternity & women's health care. 11th ed. St. Louis, MO: Elsevier.

15. ANSWER: 4
Rationale
1. Cervical effacement or thinning of the cervix does not determine engagement.
2. Fetal lie or the axis of the fetus does not determine engagement.
3. Flexion of the fetal head does not determine engagement.
4. The fetus is said to be at zero station or engaged when the biparietal diameter (widest part of the fetal skull) is at the level of the ischial spines of the maternal pelvis.

TEST-TAKING TIP: Review the signs associated with engagement of the fetal head if you were unable to answer the question correctly. Recall that process has to do with fetal descent through the birth canal.
Content Area: Station of Presenting Part; Nursing Care During Labor and Birth
Integrated Processes: Nursing Process—Assessment
Client Need: Health Promotion and Maintenance
Cognitive Level: Comprehension
Concept: Pregnancy
Reference: Lowdermilk, D. L., Perry, S. E., Cashion, K., & Alden, K. R. (2016). Maternity & women's health care. 11th ed. St. Louis, MO: Elsevier.

16. ANSWER: 1
Rationale
1. One of the most common side effects from Duramorph is pruritus, which can be treated with low-dose naloxone infusion or nalbuphine.
2. Pruritus is not effectively treated with diphenhydramine.
3. Dilaudid is an opioid medication, which is not a treatment for pruritus.
4. Sublimaze is an opioid medication, which is not a treatment for pruritus.

TEST-TAKING TIP: Review treatment of side effects of preservative-free morphine. Review the term *pruritus*.
Content Area: Pharmacological Pain Management; Nursing Care During Labor and Birth
Integrated Processes: Nursing Process—Implementation
Client Need: Physiological Integrity—Pharmacological and Parenteral Therapies
Cognitive Level: Application
Concept: Pregnancy
Reference: Anderson, D. (2011). A review of systemic opioids commonly used for labor pain relief. Journal of Midwifery and Women's Health, 56(3): 222-239.

17. ANSWER: 4
Rationale
1. Hemorrhage is not the cause of hypotension in this case.
2. Increasing urine output will not treat the hypotension.
3. Insensible fluid losses would not cause this degree of hypotension.
4. Sympathetic blockade occurs after administration of an epidural anesthesia, which results in hypotension. For this reason, intravenous fluids are administered concurrently with the block.

TEST-TAKING TIP: Review effects and untoward effects of epidural blocks in patients in labor if you were unable to answer the question correctly.
Content Area: Epidural; Nursing Care During Labor and Birth
Integrated Processes: Nursing Process—Planning
Client Need: Physiological Integrity—Pharmacological and Parenteral Therapies
Cognitive Level: Comprehension
Concept: Pregnancy
Reference: Lowdermilk, D. L., Perry, S. E., Cashion, K., & Alden, K. R. (2016). Maternity & women's health care. 11th ed. St. Louis, MO: Elsevier.

18. ANSWER: 1
Rationale
1. Spinal block would be the preferred method of anesthesia for a cesarean section due to the technical ease compared to an epidural.
2. Epidural anesthesia is more difficult to perform than a spinal block.
3. General anesthesia is reserved for an acute emergency due to the associated high morbidity and mortality.
4. Intravenous sedation would not be effective for this abdominal surgery and would cross the placenta.

TEST-TAKING TIP: Review types of anesthesia appropriate for a cesarean section. Realize that this is not an emergency delivery.
Content Area: Spinal Block; Nursing Care During Labor and Birth
Integrated Processes: Teaching/Learning
Client Need: Physiological Integrity—Pharmacological and Parenteral Therapies
Cognitive Level: Application
Concept: Pregnancy
Reference: Witcher, P. M., & McLendon, K. (2013). Anesthesia emergencies in the obstetric setting. In N. A. Troiano, C. J. Harvey, & B. F. Chez (Eds.), High-risk and critical care obstetrics (pp. 175-188). Philadelphia: Lippincott Williams & Wilkins.

19. ANSWER: 3
Rationale
1. There is no need to anticipate a cesarean section, as this is a normal occurrence.
2. Turning the patient onto the left side is the treatment for maternal hypotension.
3. Early decelerations are related to compression of the fetal head and do not require any intervention except continued monitoring, which may include vaginal examination to assess fetal descent.
4. There is no need to immediately notify the health care provider; cervical status and fetal descent should be assessed first.

TEST-TAKING TIP: Review principles of continuous external fetal monitoring in labor if you were unable to answer the question correctly.
Content Area: Decelerations; Nursing Care During Labor and Birth
Integrated Processes: Nursing Process—Implementation
Client Need: Physiological Integrity—Reduction of Risk Potential

Cognitive Level: Application
Concept: Pregnancy
Reference: Lowdermilk, D. L., Perry, S. E., Cashion, K., & Alden, K. R.
(2016). Maternity & women's health care. *11th ed. St. Louis, MO: Elsevier.*

20. **ANSWER: 2**
Rationale
1. In a cephalic presentation, the head is the presenting part.
2. The report suggests that the fetus is in breech position because the sacrum is the presenting part and the lie is longitudinal. With complete breech, the hips and knees are flexed.
3. In frank breech, the hips are flexed with knees extended.
4. In footling breech, one or both hips are extended with a foot or feet as the presenting part.

TEST-TAKING TIP: Review lie and presentation of the fetus, specifically the variations of breech presentation. Recall that the presenting part is the one closest to the vaginal opening.
Content Area: Fetal Presentation; Nursing Care During Labor and Birth
Integrated Processes: Nursing Process—Assessment
Client Need: Physiological Integrity; Physiological Adaptation
Cognitive Level: Application
Concept: Pregnancy
Reference: Lowdermilk, D. L., Perry, S. E., Cashion, K., & Alden, K. R.
(2016). Maternity & women's health care. *11th ed. St. Louis, MO: Elsevier.*

Chapter 16

Labor and Birth at Risk

KEY TERMS

Acynclitic—A fetus who is trying to enter the pelvis diagonally

Amniotic fluid embolism—Collection of fetal cells, vernix, and lanugo that enter maternal circulation

Amniotomy—When a provider ruptures the membranes intentionally

Arrest disorders—Disruptions that cease the progress of labor

Augmentation—Augmentation of a spontaneous labor that has slowed or stopped

Bishop score—A scale that helps determine cervical favorability based on vaginal exam

Cephalopelvic disproportion (CPD)—When the fetal head shape, position, or size is incompatible with that of the maternal pelvis

Cervical ripening—Softening and effacement of the cervix

Cesarean section—Delivery of a fetus from a uterine incision

Dystocia—Abnormal labor that results from abnormalities of the power, passageway, passenger, or psyche factors of labor

Elective—Delivery of an infant, by cesarean section or induction, without medical indication

External version—Correction of a fetal malpresentation by external manipulation

Favorability—Degree to which a cervix is ripened

Hypertonic uterine dysfunction—Strong, frequent, uncoordinated contractions that inhibit normal labor progression; prodromal labor

Hypotonic uterine dysfunction—Contractions that are too weak and infrequent to effectively dilate the cervix

Induction—Purposeful stimulation of uterine contractions before spontaneous labor

Intrauterine fetal demise—When a fetus passes away prior to birth

McRoberts maneuver—Sharp flexion of the maternal thighs onto her abdomen

Oligohydramnios—Amniotic fluid levels that are low for gestational age

Operative vaginal delivery—Vaginal delivery that is assisted by the use of forceps or a vacuum

Placenta accreta—Implantation of the placenta beyond the usual boundary

Placental abruption—Separation of the placenta from the uterine wall before delivery

Placental succenturiata—When the fetal vessels run between the placenta and an accessory lobe

Placenta previa—Partial or total blockage of the cervix by the placenta

Precipitous labor—Completion of the labor and delivery process within 3 hours

Protraction disorders—Disruptions that prolong the process of labor

Shoulder dystocia—Obstetrical emergency where the fetus's anterior shoulder is wedged behind the symphysis pubis

Suprapubic pressure—Downward pressure on the symphysis pubis to relieve a shoulder dystocia

Trial of labor—A planned and timed period in which a woman with cephalopelvic disproportion (CPD) risk factors attempts labor

Trial of labor after cesarean—Trial of labor after a previous cesarean section

Umbilical cord prolapse—Umbilical cord that slips under the fetal presenting part

Uterine rupture—Tear in the uterine wall

Vaginal birth after cesarean—Vaginal delivery after a previous cesarean section

Vasa previa—When the fetal vessels are positioned under the fetal presenting part, blocking the cervix

Velamentous cord insertion—Insertion of the umbilical cord somewhere other than the central portion of the placenta

Labor and birth that are at risk can be linked to a dysfunction of or an imbalance between the power, passageway, passenger, and psyche factors necessary for a successful labor and spontaneous vaginal delivery. **Dystocia** is the abnormal labor that results from the dysfunction of or imbalance of these factors and is the most common reason for primary **cesarean sections.** Maternal and neonatal outcomes are positively correlated with nursing competency during labor and birth at risk. This chapter will review the complications that are associated with the labor and birth process and will highlight the nurse's role in preserving maternal and neonatal health through timely and accurate recognition of each complication and the initiation of pertinent actions.

I. Dystocia

Abnormal labor patterns that occur during the active phase of labor can be classified into two categories: **protraction disorders,** characterized by a labor that is prolonged, and **arrest disorders,** characterized by labor that has ceased. Conditions that increase the likelihood that a woman will experience a dystocia can be related to the following factors: maternal, fetal, power, and psyche. A dystocia can also be precipitated by a combination of conditions that cause abnormal labor patterns.

A. Contributing factors
1. Passageway-related factors: maternal build, position, and health status
   - Short stature or overweight (BMI greater than 30)
   - Android (narrow), platypelloid (flat), or anthropoid (oval) pelvis shape
   - Uterine abnormalities (ex: bicornuate uterus)
   - Maternal dehydration or electrolyte imbalance
   - Maternal position
2. Passenger-related factors: fetal presentation and size
   - Occiput-posterior presentation
   - Face or brow presentation
   - Shoulder or compound presentation
   - Macrosomia (estimated fetal weight greater than 4,500 g)
3. Power-related factors
   - Ineffective contraction patterns or strength
   - Tachysystole (hyperstimulation that results in five or more uterine contractions in a 10-minute window that lasts for 30 minutes) related to oxytocin use
   - Early administration of analgesia or anesthesia
4. Psyche-related factors
   - Maternal exhaustion or fear

B. Dysfunctional labor patterns
Dysfunctional labor patterns are abnormal patterns of uterine contractions that prevent normal cervical dilation or descent of the fetus. Dysfunctional labor is often the result of **hypertonic uterine dysfunction** or **hypotonic uterine dysfunction.**

1. Hypertonic uterine dysfunction
   This is characterized by contractions that are strong and frequent but uncoordinated. Subsequently, the contractions are ineffective at dilating and effacing the cervix. In the early phase of labor, hypertonic uterine dysfunction may be referred to as *prodromal labor.* The primary concerns regarding hypertonic uterine dysfunction are the high risk for maternal exhaustion and fetal intolerance to labor due to the decreased resting intervals between the frequently occurring contractions.
   a) Risk factors: Nulliparous women are more likely to experience hypertonic dysfunction early in their labor.
   b) Assessment findings
      - Strong contractions at frequent intervals that are ineffective at causing cervical dilation and effacement
      - Incomplete uterine relaxation between contractions
      - Indeterminate (Category II) or abnormal (Category III) fetal heart rate (FHR) patterns due to frequent contractions and inadequate relaxation
   c) Independent nursing actions: The primary goals during hypertonic labor is to promote maternal and uterine rest. The nurse can accomplish this by:
      - Assisting with warm shower or bath.
      - Reducing environmental stimuli.
      - Clustering care to provide prolonged rest periods.
      - Continually assessing and interpreting the fetus and uterine contractions.
      - Evaluating labor progress with a sterile vaginal examination (SVE).
      - Keeping the patient and support persons informed regarding progress.
   d) Collaborative care: The best care is provided when the nurse works in collaboration with the patient's primary care provider (PCP). The nurse may need to complete PCP orders for:
      - IV or PO hydration
      - IV pain medication
      - Hydration, accompanied by the administration of pain medicine, can relax both the woman and the uterus, preventing maternal exhaustion and allowing better blood flow to the uterus. Improved perfusion of the uterus and prolonged relaxation often result in the appearance of normal contraction patterns, as a healthy uterus is better able to coordinate its movements.

ALERT Laboring women are typically not allowed to have any food or drink during labor. This is because all laboring women are potential surgical candidates, and emergent cesarean sections are often performed under general anesthesia, necessitating that the stomach be empty to reduce the risk of an aspiration pneumonia. Since dystocias are a primary cause of first-time cesarean sections, the decision to use PO hydration should be weighed heavily against assessment findings and made in collaboration with the patient's PCP.

2. Hypotonic uterine dysfunction

   Hypotonic uterine dysfunction is characterized by uterine contractions that are not strong enough to cause cervical change. Hypotonic labor occurs in active labor after the woman has progressed normally through the latent phase of labor. Maternal risks include exhaustion and infection from the prolonged labor. The fetus is at risk for intolerance to labor due to withstanding contractions for a prolonged period of time.

   a) Risk factors: Multiparous women are more at risk for hypotonic labor. In addition, intense fear during labor causes catecholamine release, which inhibits uterine contractility.

   b) Assessment findings
      - Contractions that are farther apart in frequency and have decreased duration and decreased strength of contractions
      - No cervical change or cervical change that is slower than expected for the patient's parity
      - Signs of increased fear and anxiety in the patient

   c) Independent nursing actions
      - Assess and interpret maternal and fetal status
      - Assess progress via SVE
      - Provide the patient and support persons with information as it is received
      - Provide emotional support to decrease the likelihood that fear will affect the labor progress
      - The nurse can attempt to stimulate a normal labor pattern by:
      - Assisting with ambulation.
      - Assisting with frequent position changes.
      - Helping with ambulation and assisting with frequent position changes. Provide mechanical manipulation of the maternal pelvis and fetal presenting part via gravity and rotation. These interventions are commonly used and effective in stimulating labor because of their ability to encourage descent and create a more optimal cephalopelvic alignment.

   d) Collaborative care: Effective treatment of hypotonic labor often requires PCP dependent actions. The nurse may further assist with stimulation of normal contraction patterns by:
      - Initiating oxytocin per augmentation protocol.
      - Assisting with amniotomy.
      - Administering IV or PO hydration.
      - Assisting with regular perineal care. Although assessment of progress is important, if the PCP decides to perform an amniotomy to stimulate labor, sterile vaginal exams should be limited to reduce the risk of intrauterine infection. Impeccable sterile technique is required when examinations do occur.

3. Precipitous labor and birth: **Precipitous labor** is defined as the completion of the labor and birthing process in less than 3 hours.

   a) Risk factors: Grand multiparous (five or more births) women and women who have had previous precipitous labors are most at risk for this type of labor. When assessing risk factors for any complication, the fact that the patient has experienced the complication previously is always the biggest risk factor for future occurrences.

   b) Assessment findings
      - Contractions that are strong to palpation, occur every 2 minutes or less, and are greater than 60 seconds in duration
      - Possible category II or III FHR tracing
      - Rapid cervical dilation
      - Increased maternal pain and anxiety

   c) Independent nursing actions
      - Assess cervical change frequently per sterile technique
      - Provide emotional support to the patient and support persons to reduce anxiety
      - Prepare for the possibility that the birth will not be attended by the PCP

MAKING THE CONNECTION

Postpartum Hemorrhage

Overdistention of the uterine muscle is often associated with hypotonic labor, as the stretched muscle fibers cannot contract effectively, which is why multigravida are more at risk. The majority of postpartum bleeding is also caused by uterine atony or hypotonicity, meaning that the same conditions that cause hypotonic labor are also risk factors for postpartum bleeding. The nurse can accurately recognize those patients at higher risk for postpartum bleeding by identifying those conditions in their history or events of hospitalization that contribute to decreased uterine tone.

- Continue frequent (every 15 minutes) assessment and interpretation of the FHR tracing
- Prepare for the possibility of postpartum uterine atony or lacerations that increase the mother's risk of postpartum hemorrhage
- Prepare for the possibility of an infant who shows signs of central nervous system depression and respiratory distress
- It is not uncommon for infants who were born via cesarean section prior to the start of labor to need additional help transitioning to extrauterine life. This is because they miss the chest cavity compression that accompanies descent through the birth canal. This compression initiates expulsion of amniotic fluid from the fetal lungs, making spontaneous respirations easier. Infants who are born via precipitous labor often exhibit the same difficulty transitioning due to the short amount of time they had to receive the benefit of being compressed by the birth canal.

4. Fetal dystocias and pelvic dystocias
Fetal dystocias are abnormal labors that occur because of a large fetus, fetal malpresentation (Table 16.1), multifetal pregnancies, or other fetus-based anomalies. Pelvic dystocias are related to the narrowing of the pelvic inlet, outlet, or the midpelvis, preventing fetal descent. The most desirable fetal presentation is vertex. This means the smallest diameter of the fetus's head is presenting first. This position also indicates the fetus's ability to flex forward. This ability to flex is what allows the fetus to maneuver through the birth canal. The ability of the fetus to engage in the maternal pelvis signals that the pelvis is likely adequate.

a) Assessment findings related to fetal dystocias
- FHR heard above the maternal umbilicus (a sign that the infant is not in a cephalic position)
- Palpation of fetal body parts other than the head during SVE
- Lack of fetal descent or engagement

b) Assessment findings related to pelvic dystocias
- Delayed or lack of fetal descent

c) Interventions for fetal dystocia
- At times, a PCP can turn a breech infant into the cephalic position by doing an **external version.** An ultrasound must be done to assess umbilical cord placement before the procedure begins. The patient must also receive a dose of terbutaline to relax the uterus. Ultrasound gel is used on the maternal abdomen to make maneuvering easier. This procedure is not as simple as it seems, and risk factors include cord compression, placental abruption, and fetal distress. This is why the patient is prepped for cesarean section prior to the start of the procedure, just in case. Many providers perform the procedure in the operating room as an extra precaution.

Table 16.1 Fetal Malpresentations

Name of Malpresentation	Description	Implications
Occiput posterior	The fetal occiput is against the maternal sacrum. In this position, the infant descends with the wider diameter of the head as the presenting part. If the fetus does not rotate before delivery, the baby will be born "sunny-side up" or looking at the ceiling instead of the floor as in occiput anterior presentations.	Prolonged labor and a difficult second stage Increased lower back pain compared to normal labor
Face presentation	The fetal head is extended backward instead of flexed. The fetus's face and not occiput is the presenting part. The infant will descend down the birth canal like an olympic skeleton luger.	Prolonged labor and second stage Potential delivery by cesarean Extensive facial bruising
Brow presentation	Described in some texts as military position. The fetal head is neither flexed nor extended but descends down the birth canal as if standing at attention. The widest diameter of the infant's head is presenting first.	Prolonged labor and second stage
Shoulder presentation	The fetal lie is so that the fetal spine is perpendicular to the maternal spine and the fetus's shoulder is presenting at the cervix.	Increased risk for cord prolapse Necessitates cesarean delivery Suspicion that an infant has a shoulder presentation should arise if the nurse can feel no presenting part during a sterile vaginal exam.

Table 16.1 Fetal Malpresentations (Continued)

Name of Malpresentation	Description	Implications
Compound presentation	One or more fetal extremities are lying adjacent to the presenting part. For example, a fetus may present with his hand lying next to his presenting occiput.	Cesarean section may be indicated depending upon the nature of the compound presentation.
Breech presentation	Frank breech: the fetus's hips are completely flexed upward so that the fetal buttocks are the only presenting part and the fetal feet are near its head. Complete breech: the presenting part is the fetal buttocks. The fetal extremities are in a crossed-legged position. Footling breech: Can be double or single. One or both of the fetus's legs present before the buttocks.	Breech position usually requires cesarean delivery to prevent head entrapment. Increased risk of cord prolapse. Some physicians skilled in breech delivery may allow the mother to deliver vaginally if she has a proven pelvis, meaning she has a previous vaginal delivery with no complications that can be linked to CPD.

5. Cephalopelvic disproportion

Cephalopelvic disproportion (CPD) is a combination of maternal and fetal factors that can cause dysfunctional labor when the fetus size, shape, or position is incompatible with that of the maternal pelvis. CPD can occur even when a mother has the preferred gynecoid pelvis shape. For example, a fetus who is in the occiput posterior position travels down the birth canal with a wider diameter of the head presenting first. This mismatch in shape can cause an abnormal labor pattern even though nothing is inherently wrong with the mother's pelvis or the fetus's head. This is similar in effect to what happens when a fetus is **acynclitic.** An acynclitic fetus can cause abnormal labor as it tries to descend through the maternal pelvis diagonally. Early decelerations that occur before the fetal head is engaged in the maternal pelvis can be an early sign of CPD. Early decelerations are caused by head compression, usually against the soft tissue of the birth canal. If the fetus has not yet reached the birth canal, the fetal head may be getting compressed in the pelvic inlet, which is a sign of CPD.

6. Trial of labor

CPD is often difficult to diagnose prior to the start of labor. A **trial of labor** is the planned and often timed (4 to 6 hours) monitoring of a woman's labor when there are known risk factors for CPD. During this time, the nurse is monitoring the woman closely for adequate uterine contractions, fetal well-being, and progression of labor as evidenced by cervical dilation and descent of the fetus. Providing support and keeping the patient and her support persons informed remain priorities.

II. Induction of Labor

Induction refers to the purposeful stimulation of uterine contractions prior to the start of spontaneous labor. Induction of labor can be **elective** (done in absence of a medical indication) or as a means to preserve maternal or fetal health. Induction is not without risk and is associated with increased levels of intervention, continuous fetal monitoring, activity restriction, increased use of analgesia and anesthesia, and prolonged labor and delivery admissions. Furthermore, ultrasounds, even if done early in pregnancy, can underestimate gestational age by as much as 2 weeks. The accuracy of ultrasounds decreases with each passing trimester. Strict rules are in place regarding confirmation of gestational age to be at least 39 weeks for elective inductions and elective cesarean sections. These guidelines are in place to prevent neonatal morbidity associated with unintended preterm delivery.

A. Indications for induction

1. Post-term pregnancy
2. Pregnancy-induced hypertension
3. Pre-eclampsia/eclampsia
4. Maternal medical indications (e.g., diabetes, cardiac disease, pulmonary disease)
5. Premature rupture of membranes (PROM)
6. Chorioamnionitis
7. Fetal stress (e.g., **oligohydramnios,** isoimmunization, intrauterine growth restriction)
8. Fetal demise
9. History of precipitous labor or geographic isolation
10. Psychosocial indications

B. Contraindications to induction

1. Contraindications to vaginal birth
2. Presence of a vertical or transfundal uterine scar
3. Placenta previa or vasa previa
4. Fetal malpresentation
5. Umbilical cord prolapse
6. Active genital herpes
7. Known pelvic abnormalities

C. Risks associated with induction

1. Indeterminant (Category II) or abnormal (Category III) FHR tracings
   a) The extent of fetal stress is positively correlated with the dose of induction medication and can be mitigated by reducing or discontinuing administration in response to the FHR tracing.

2. Water intoxication can occur when high doses of Pitocin (40 mu/min) are given in conjunction with hypotonic IV fluids.

D. Induction methods

There are several labor induction methods available. The decision as to which method is most appropriate depends on the patient's parity, membrane status, cervical status, and whether or not she has a history of cesarean section birth.

1. Oxytocin (Pitocin) induction

Pitocin is the synthetic version of endogenous oxytocin that is produced by the hypothalamus and released by the pituitary gland to spontaneously initiate labor. The hormone is released in response to vaginal and cervical stretching. Pitocin has a half-life of 10 minutes, and the uterus responds to its presence in the bloodstream in as little as 3 to 5 minutes.

a) Assessment prior to initiation
  - The nurse should review the patient's prenatal records for confirmation of gestational age if induction is elective.
  - The nurse should also review the patient's medical records for any contraindications to induction.
  - If preliminary assessments are negative, consent may be obtained for the induction.

b) Administration of oxytocin
  - Patient teaching should precede administration.
  - The infusion is started low (0.5 to 1 mu/min) and increased by 1 to 2 mu/min every 15 to 30 minutes until adequate uterine contractions are achieved. Adequate uterine contractions can be defined as contractions that:
    - Are approximately every 3 minutes in frequency.
    - Last for 40 to 60 seconds.
    - Are 25 to 75 mm Hg in intensity or moderate to strong to palpation.
  - Contractions that are adequate promote cervical dilation of 0.5 cm/hour for primiparous women and 1 cm/hour for multiparous women during the active phase of labor. The reason labor and birth get shorter with each pregnancy is that the cervix becomes more efficient at dilating and effacing at the same time, whereas in primiparous women, the actions happen independently.
  - A uterine resting tone of 20 mm Hg should last for at least 1 minute between contractions.
  - Pitocin must always be administered via infusion pump.
  - Pitocin should be connected to the mainline tubing port that is closest to the IV insertion site. This ensures that Pitocin will stop infusing quickly if the medication needs to be discontinued.
  - Titration is based on maternal and fetal response.

c) Assessment during oxytocin induction
  - Continuous fetal monitoring is typical during Pitocin infusion.
  - The FHR tracing should be assessed, interpreted, and documented every 30 minutes for low-risk patients and every 15 minutes for patients with risk factors.
  - During the second stage of labor, monitoring frequency should increase to every 5 minutes.
  - Uterine contraction assessment and documentation should include frequency, duration, and strength of contractions. In the presence of tachysystole, the nurse should discontinue Pitocin or reduce the infusion rate by half.
  - Fetal documentation should include baseline heart rate, degree of variability, and the presence or absence of accelerations or decelerations. In the event of Category II (indeterminate) or Category III (abnormal FHR tracing) the nurse should:
    - Reposition the patient to a lateral position.
    - Administer an IV fluid bolus of 500 to 1,000 mL of Lactated Ringer's (LR).
    - Administer O_2 per nonrebreather at 10 to 12 L/min.
    - Discontinue oxytocin.
    - Notify the PCP.
    - Discuss the use of terbutaline with the PCP if there is no response to interventions.
  - Monitor vital signs per unit protocol (usually at least every 2 hours).
  - Assess pain management success every 30 minutes.
  - Assess color of amniotic fluid and amount of bloody show.
  - Assess for output that matches input. Signs of fluid overload include:
    - Decreased urine output.
    - Edema.
    - Signs of pulmonary edema (e.g., crackles, difficulty breathing).
    - Increased blood pressure (BP).

d) Safety during oxytocin administration: Nearly half of perinatal legal settlements involve the use of Pitocin. Following administration protocols and recognizing maternal and fetal distress early can reduce maternal and fetal injury related to Pitocin induction.

2. Cervical ripening

   Prior to labor, the cervix is closed and uneffaced. **Cervical ripening** refers to the softening and opening of the cervix in preparation for labor. The **favorability** of the cervix or the degree of ripening that has occurred is the single best predictor of induction success; therefore, the cervix is assessed using the **Bishop score** (Table 16.2). A score of 6 or above is considered favorable. Women with Bishop scores below 6 may be candidates for cervical ripening.

   a) Mechanical cervical ripening: Mechanical cervical ripening agents are inserted inside the cervix (remember its cylindrical shape) and provide manual dilation of the cervix through expansion. Although cervical ripening is intended to be followed with Pitocin administration, it is not uncommon for cervical ripening agents to stimulate the labor process.

      (1) Laminaria, Lamicil, Dilapan
         (a) These agents ripen the cervix by expanding with the absorption of cervical fluids. The expansion provides manual dilation and stimulates prostaglandin release.
      (2) Balloon catheters
         (a) An uninflated balloon catheter is inserted into the cervical canal, where it is then filled with fluid to provide manual dilation and stimulate prostaglandin release.
      (3) Indications for mechanical cervical ripening
         (a) Unripened cervix or little to no effacement
         (b) Previous uterine surgery prevents the use of pharmacological ripening agents
      (4) Risks of mechanical cervical ripening: There is a higher risk of infection and PROM in patients who use mechanical cervical ripening.
      (5) Mechanical dilators are typically in place for 6 to 12 hours before removal by the

PCP. The balloon catheter may dislodge from the cervix on its own, when the patient is approximately 3 centimeters. Nursing responsibilities are similar to those discussed under Pitocin administration:
- Provide education and support.
- Inform the patient that cramping is normal after insertion.
- Assess maternal and fetal status per unit protocol, with maternal temperature being of particular importance.
- Assess for rupture of membranes (ROM) and vaginal bleeding.

   b) Pharmacological cervical ripening: Pharmacological cervical ripening agents are hormonal preparations placed in or near the cervix to soften and thin the cervix (Table 16.3). The indications for pharmacological cervical ripening are the same as those for induction in general. These ripening agents have the potential to produce tachysystole similar to the use of Pitocin. The nursing actions discussed for tachysystole and fetal distress discussed with the use of Pitocin apply here as well. Nursing responsibilities are the same as those indicated for mechanical ripening agents.

3. Stripping the membranes

   Stripping the membranes refers to the separation of the chorionic membrane (the outer membrane of the amniotic sac) from the lower uterine segment and cervical wall. Although there is lack of support for this method of ripening and it is unclear how it works, it is believed to stimulate the release of prostaglandins and endogenous oxytocin. The procedure is most successful in first-time mothers with an unripe cervix. The procedure is done in the PCP's office and the PCP takes responsibility for patient education; however, the nurse should be aware that:
- FHR should be assessed before and after the procedure.
- Spotting and cramping following the procedure are normal.
- Infection and unplanned ROM can result.
- Excessive bleeding may be a sign of undiagnosed placental problems.

4. Amniotomy

   Amniotomy refers to the artificial rupture of membranes by the PCP during a sterile vaginal exam, usually to augment labor. This is most often done with an AmniHook, but finger cots are available for this use as well. The procedure should be avoided in early labor to decrease the risk of cesarean section due to abnormal FHR.

   a) Contraindications include a fetal presenting part that is not engaged (higher than 0 station)

Table 16.2 Bishop Score

	0	1	2	3
Centimeter dilation	0	1–2	3–4	5–6
Percent effaced	0%–30%	40%–50%	60%–70%	80%
Fetal station	−3	−2	−1/0	+1/+2
Cervix consistency	Firm	Medium	Soft	
Cervix position	Posterior	Midposition	Anterior	

Table 16.3 Pharmacologic Cervical Ripening Agents

Medication	Dose	Considerations	Contraindications	MOA	Adverse Effects
Prepidil PGE$_1$ (Dinoprostone Gel)	0.5 mg every 6 hours x3 doses, if indicated. Administration is completed by CNM or MD and assisted by speculum. Gel is inserted into cervical canal but not passed the internal os.	Patient should lie in recumbent position for 30 minutes following insertion. Continuous fetal monitoring necessary for 30 minutes to 2 hours following placement. Oxytocin use is delayed for 6–12 hours following placement.	Previous uterine incision	The onset of uterine contractions occurs within 1 hour and the dose peaks in 4 hours. Tachysystole may be present within 1 hour.	Nausea, vomiting, diarrhea, fever, and tachysystole, which may or may not be accompanied by abnormal FHR pattern. Meconium staining of fluid secondary to fetal distress
Cervidil (Dinoprostone Insert)	10 mg controlled release insert to be removed via attached string after 12 hours is the posterior fornix. Nurses may place if facility allows.	Patient should be lateral or recumbent for 2 hours following placement. Continuous fetal monitoring necessary for duration of use. Oxytocin use can begin 30–60 minutes after removal.	Previous uterine incision.	The onset of contractions occurs within 5–7 hours. Tachysystole may be present within 1 hour. Remove insert for Category II and III tracings. Remove insert if tachysystole noted, even if fetal tracing is normal.	Headache, nausea, vomiting, diarrhea, fever, hypotension, and tachysystole, which may or may not be accompanied by abnormal FHR pattern. Meconium staining of fluid secondary to fetal distress.
Misoprostol PGE$_1$ (Cytotec)	25 mg tablet inserted into the posterior fornix.	Continuous fetal monitoring necessary. Oxytocin use can begin 4 hours after last dose.	Previous uterine incision.	Peaks within 1–2 hours. Onset is variable. Tachysystole most common with Misoprostol.	Nausea, vomiting, diarrhea, fever, and tachysystole, which may or may not be accompanied by abnormal FHR pattern. Meconium staining of fluid secondary to fetal distress. Adverse effects are dose dependent with effects more likely for doses, such as 50 mcg every 6 hours. Reducing the dose and increasing the dosage intervals can mitigate the adverse effects.

and the presence of HIV or active genital herpes infections in the mother.

b) Risks include umbilical cord prolapse, severe variable decelerations, and bleeding from undiagnosed placental abnormalities. The risk for infection increases the longer the woman is ruptured before birth of the infant.

c) Nursing actions include:
- Assessment of FHR before and after the procedure to rule out cord prolapse
- Assessment of maternal temperature
- Assessment of fluid's color, amount, and odor
- Documentation of rupture time
- Assessment of uterine contractions

5. Labor augmentation
Labor **augmentation** refers to the stimulation of uterine contractions after the spontaneous onset of labor in an effort to manage dystocia. Lower doses of oxytocin are needed for augmentation due to a decrease in cervical resistance compared to those women who have not labored at all. The indications, contraindications, risks, and nursing responsibilities are the same as those presented for oxytocin as an induction method.

III. Operative Vaginal Delivery

An **operative vaginal delivery** refers to the use of forceps or a vacuum to shorten the second stage of labor. These procedures can only be performed by PCPs with the hospital privileges to do so. Only one assistive method is recommended per delivery and failed attempts should be followed by cesarean section.

A. Vacuum-assisted delivery
A vacuum-assisted delivery is the delivery of the fetus's head using a suction cup and gentle traction.
1. Compared to forceps use, vacuum deliveries are associated with:
   • Earlier application.
   • Decreased need for additional anesthesia.
   • Decreased maternal soft tissue damage.
   • Fewer fetal injuries.
2. Criteria and guidelines for use
   • The cervix must be completely dilated and the fetal head engaged.
   • Three failed attempts to use the vacuum should be followed by cesarean section. A failed attempt is identified by a "pop off," where the vacuum pops off the fetal head in response to too much pressure being exerted on the fetal head.
   • Only three attempts can be made in 15 minutes.
   • The fetus should be at least 36 weeks gestation.
   • Pressure should be released between contractions.
3. Indications for use
   • Shorten the second stage of labor to avoid prolonged pushing, maternal exhaustion, or fetal compromise
   • A prolonged second stage of labor is defined by no progress after 3 hours of pushing with regional anesthesia for a nulliparous woman (2 hours without anesthesia) and 2 hours of pushing for a multiparous woman (1 hour without anesthesia).
4. Maternal risks
   • Vaginal and perineal lacerations
   • Episiotomy extension
   • Hemorrhage caused by uterine atony or uterine rupture

• Bladder infection
• Perineal wound infection
5. Risks to the neonate
   • Cephalohematoma
   • Intracranial or retinal hemorrhage
   • Scalp lacerations or bruising
6. Nursing actions
   • Document and keep the PCP informed regarding the number of "pop-offs" and the total time period the vacuum has been in use.
   • Emptying the mother's bladder prior to vacuum extraction decreases the likelihood of bladder trauma.
   • Modern vacuum devices (e.g., KIWI) are completely physician controlled and no longer require the nurse to establish vacuum pressure using a pump.

B. Forceps-assisted delivery
A forceps-assisted delivery involves the use of forceps to deliver the fetal head. Two types of forceps can be applied. Outlet forceps are used when the fetal head is on the pelvic floor. Low forceps are used when the fetal head is +2 station or lower but has not reached the pelvic floor.
1. The cervix must be completely dilated and the fetal head must be engaged, just as in vacuum-assisted delivery. The fetus should also be at least 36 weeks gestation.
2. Indications for forceps delivery include the same indications as for vacuum delivery, in addition to:
   • Inability to push due to high regional anesthesia block.
   • Cardiac or pulmonary disease that inhibits the mother from pushing.
3. Maternal risks are the same as those listed for vacuum-assisted delivery in addition to perineal hematoma.
4. Risks to the neonate:
   • Cephalohematoma
   • Craniofacial and brachial plexus nerve damage
   • Facial lacerations or bruising
   • Skull fractures
   • Intracranial hemorrhage

MAKING THE CONNECTION

Neonatal Jaundice
Since neonatal jaundice is caused by an excess of unconjugated bilirubin, a by-product of red blood cell breakdown, infants with a cephalohematoma are at increased risk for developing jaundice. The additional bilirubin produced during the healing of the cephalohematoma adds an extra workload to the immature liver.

5. Nursing actions
   - Additional anesthesia may be required for the use of forceps
   - Emptying the woman's bladder will decrease bladder trauma
   - Document the type of forceps, number of applications, and time the instruments were in use

IV. Obstetric Complications and Emergencies

This section will review the unique causative factors and nursing implications associated with the most common obstetrical complications and emergencies. Positive maternal-fetal outcomes following the situations described below are highly reliant on the obstetric nurse's ability to recognize their presence and intervene effectively. Although each obstetric complication and emergency is distinct, many of the conditions associated with the antepartum period threaten maternal and fetal health in the intrapartum period. Specifically, pre-eclampsia, diabetes, post-term pregnancies, and preterm pregnancies are major factors in several obstetric complications and emergencies. Noting the connection between antepartum and intrapartum health promotes critical thinking and improves the nurse's ability to identify at-risk patients before complications occur.

A. Fetus-related labor and birth complications
   A **shoulder dystocia** is when the infant's head delivers vaginally, but the anterior (top) shoulder is wedged behind the symphysis pubis, preventing expulsion. The condition is unpredictable and unpreventable.
   1. Causative factors
      a) A shoulder dystocia is the result of a mismatch in size, shape, or position between the passageway (mother's pelvis) and passenger (fetus) or CPD.
      b) Gestational onset diabetes mellitus (GODM) is associated with fetal macrosomia and infants that are large for gestational age (LGA). This could potentially create a passenger that is too large for the passageway.
      c) Not all LGA infants are the result of GODM, but GODM is a common cause of fetal macrosomia and shoulder dystocias.
      d) The risk for shoulder dystocia applies to gestational diabetic mothers only. Women who have diabetes prior to pregnancy are more likely to have small for gestational age infants due to the long-term effect of diabetes on circulation. The less the infant is perfused through the placenta, the less nutrition it receives that it needs for growth.
      e) Android (narrow), platypelloid (flat), or anthropoid (oval) pelvis shape
      f) Excessive weight gain
      g) History of shoulder dystocia

2. Implications
   a) The delay in expulsion results in the fetal neck being compressed by the maternal pelvis, which can cause anoxia, asphyxia, increased intracranial pressure, and brain damage.
   b) After approximately 5 minutes of delay, the infant may experience hypoxemia and acidosis. Once the interval approaches 6 minutes and beyond, brain and organ damage becomes permanent.
   c) Brachial plexus nerve damage and clavicular fracture can lead to decreased mobility on the affected side. Although clavicle fractures usually heal well, brachial plexus nerve damage can be permanent and affect facial movements as well.
   d) The patient can suffer lacerations, infection, bladder injury, and postpartum hemorrhage.
   e) The worse outcome, of course, is neonatal death.
3. Warning sign
   Turtle sign, defined as retraction of the fetal head into the perineum after the head is delivered (like a turtle snapping its head back into the shell), is the first sign of a possible shoulder dystocia.
4. Nursing actions
   Since a shoulder dystocia is the result of a mismatch in size, shape, or position between the passageway and passenger, the initial steps to remedy the dystocia involve the manipulation of these two factors.
   a) **McRoberts maneuver** is the sharp flexion of the maternal thighs onto her abdomen. It is performed by using the bottom of the patient's feet to move her knees toward her ears. McRoberts maneuver works to enlarge the angle at the pelvic inlet by straightening the sacrum, allowing more room for the fetus's shoulders to pass under the symphysis pubis.
   b) **Suprapubic pressure** is when downward pressure is applied to the symphysis pubis in attempts to manually dislodge the anterior shoulder (Fig. 16.1).
   c) Fundal pressure during a shoulder dystocia will exacerbate the problem by further pressing the anterior shoulder against the symphysis pubis.
5. Collaborative care
   a) Downward traction on the fetal head by the PCP performed simultaneously with McRoberts maneuver and suprapubic pressure are normally sufficient to relieve the dystocia.
   b) The PCP may also cut a midline episiotomy. An episiotomy increases the diameter of the birth canal, creating more room to pull the infant downward and allow the anterior shoulder to pass under the symphysis pubis.

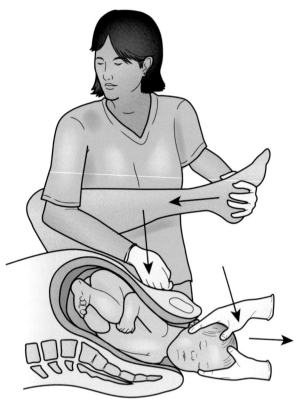

Fig 16.1 McRoberts maneuver and suprapubic pressure.

c) Intentional fracturing of the fetus's clavicle allows the PCP to collapse the anterior shoulder so that it may pass under the symphysis pubis.

d) The Woods corkscrew involves rotating the shoulder 180 degrees (half a turn) at a time until the shoulder is released.

e) Delivery of the posterior arm first may be possible if the PCP can sweep the fetus's arm across its chest to facilitate delivery of the extremity.

f) The Zavanelli maneuver calls for the replacement of the fetus's head back into the pelvis and subsequent cesarean delivery. This should be reserved for the most extreme of cases after all other attempts to deliver the infant have failed.

g) Do not forget to call for assistance. No obstetrical emergency should be handled by a single nurse and PCP.

h) Other important care providers to notify are:
   (1) Anesthesia: An anesthesiologist or certified nurse anesthetist will need to be readily available in case a cesarean section is necessary.
   (2) Newborn care team: Who makes up the newborn care team will vary from facility to facility. Shoulder dystocia deliveries should be attended by a group of health care providers who are designated to care

for the infant only after delivery. Someone on the team should be certified to perform at least intermediate resuscitative newborn care, including intubation.

6. Additional considerations
   a) Being aware of and following the hospital's protocol during any obstetric emergency is extremely important to both the patient's and the health care team's safety.
   b) The time that the infant's shoulder was trapped under the symphysis pubis should be documented. It is the nurse's responsibility to note in the delivery record the time that the shoulder dystocia began and when the shoulder was able to be dislodged.
   c) Follow-up and potential assessment findings or complications may include facial petechiae, Erb's palsy from pressure on the infant's brachial nerve plexus, and corneal hemorrhage. Decreased or no spontaneous movement in one arm should be followed by an x-ray. A broken clavicle can be occult and accidental.

B. Umbilical cord–related labor and birth complications
   1. Umbilical cord prolapse
   An **umbilical cord prolapse** is when the umbilical cord slips under the fetal presenting part. Cord prolapses can be occult and may be discovered prior to rupture of the membranes before the cord is swept into the vagina. However, this complication usually occurs at or soon after ROM. Since the amniotic fluid provides suspension for the fetus, the effect of gravity on the infant is greater when amniotic fluid is lost. The danger in this is that the presenting part of the fetus can descend onto the prolapsed cord and significantly reduce or eliminate blood flow to itself. This is an absolute obstetrical emergency and requires a cesarean section birth as soon as the prolapse is found, unless birth is imminent.
   a) Risk factors: nonmodifiable
      (1) Breech position: Since the fetus's buttocks are not as large as the fetus's head, there is more room for the umbilical cord to slip around and in front of the presenting part when the infant is in a breech position.
      (2) Polyhydramnios: An abundance of fluid means that amniotic fluid will escape the uterine cavity with greater force when rupture of membranes occurs, making it more likely that the umbilical cord will be swept down below the infant.
      (3) High station at time of spontaneous rupture of membranes: The more space that is between the infant's presenting part and the ischial spines of the pelvis, the

more opportunity there is for the umbilical cord to be positioned before the presenting part. On the other hand, if the infant is engaged in the pelvis, there is virtually no opportunity for the cord to slip in front of the presenting part. The higher the infant's station or the higher the infant's presenting part is in the uterine cavity, the greater the risk of cord prolapse.

(4) Preterm gestation: Preterm infants are in a relatively large amount of amniotic fluid compared to their term counterparts, leaving more room for the umbilical cord to be positioned before the fetus and creating a greater degree of suspension. In addition, the preterm infant's small size inhibits the fetus's capability to be engaged in the maternal pelvis. Since engagement serves as protection against umbilical cord prolapse, preterm infants are at higher risk.

(5) High parity

b) Risk factors: modifiable

(1) Ambulation after rupture of membranes and prior to engagement: Fundal pressure during a shoulder dystocia will exacerbate the problem by further pressing the anterior shoulder against the symphysis pubis.

(2) Performing an amniotomy prior to fetal engagement: This complication is affected by fetal station. Therefore, performing an amniotomy or artificial rupture of membranes when the fetus is not engaged in the maternal pelvis increases the risk of cord prolapse.

c) Nursing actions

Since several risk factors for umbilical cord prolapse are unmodifiable, the health care team must be prepared to act in the event of this emergency. The nurse has the critical responsibility of recognizing signs of an umbilical cord prolapse and intervening so that umbilical blood flow can be reestablished or maintained until the infant can be safely delivered by cesarean section.

(1) Placing the patient in Trendelenburg position

(2) Applying counterpressure to the presenting part to relieve cord compression

(3) What the nurse does first in the event of an umbilical cord prolapse is dependent upon whether she sees it first or finds it during a sterile vaginal exam. A nurse who sees an umbilical cord prolapsed outside the birth canal should place the patient in Trendelenburg position. This causes gravity to shift the fetus upward into the uterine cavity, away from the prolapsed cord, allowing pressure to be relieved. After this intervention is completed, the nurse may move on to applying counterpressure on the fetal presenting part. A nurse who finds a prolapsed umbilical cord during a sterile vaginal exam should use the exam fingers to apply counterpressure to the infant's presenting part, relieving pressure on the umbilical cord. This counterpressure cannot be released until the infant is completely delivered from the uterine cavity by cesarean section. Assessment of fetal status should not be discontinued during this time. The nurse can estimate a pulse rate from the umbilical cord as a way to judge infant status and keep the delivery team updated and informed. Do not forget the root cause of the problem. There is usually an ideal solution to a problem, but the nurse's job is to choose the best solution from what is available. When Trendelenburg is not an option, having the patient positioned on her hands and knees with her head lowered can also allow gravity to move the infant upward in the uterus and relieve any pressure on the cord (Fig. 16.2).

d) Fetal monitoring assessment findings

Since variable decelerations are caused by cord compression, it is not usual to see deep variables above uterine contractions after a cord has prolapsed. When contractions push the infant's presenting part down on the cord, there is cord compression that is then relieved when the contraction is over. Remember variables are named for their timing, and variables

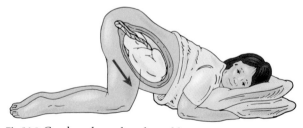

Fig 16.2 Cord prolapse hands and knees position.

are called so because their timing can vary. Just because they are happening with every contraction does not mean they are early decelerations. Variables are identified by their V, W, or U shape, and their abrupt descent and abrupt return to baseline. Cord prolapses are often accompanied by prolonged decelerations (greater than 2 minutes long) or terminal bradycardia as gravity forces the presenting part to exert constant pressure on the cord.

e) Collaborative care

Although the nurse's actions are critical, the nurse should not forget that the best outcome for the fetus depends on collaboration. Using the patient's call light to signal for help while interventions are in progress is critical to timely delivery of the infant.

2. Vasa previa and velamentous cord insertion

Vasa previa is the traversing of unprotected fetal vessels through the amniotic membranes over the cervix. Vasa previas are usually precipitated by **velamentous cord insertion,** where the umbilical cord is inserted into the amniotic membranes instead of the placenta or when the fetal vessels run between placental accessory lobes **(placenta succenturiata).** Fundal pressure during a shoulder dystocia will exacerbate the problem by further pressing the anterior shoulder against the symphysis pubis (Fig. 16.3).

a) Implications
  - Undiagnosed vasa previa is associated with perinatal mortality rates as high as 60%.
  - The fetus is compromised by asphyxia if the vessels are compressed or the neonate can die of exsanguination if the vessels are severed.
  - Diagnosis of vasa previa is commonly made at ROM, when amniotic fluid is noted to be blood tinged or when ROM is proceeded by fetal distress or death.

b) Risk factors
  - Placenta previa
  - Low-lying placenta (marginal previa)
  - Presence of placental accessory lobes
  - Multiple gestation
  - Pregnancies resulting from in vitro fertilization

c) Collaborative care
  (1) Diagnosis of vasa previa should be followed by scheduled cesarean section at 35 weeks prior to the ROM. This practice improves neonatal survival to 95%.
  (2) The nurse may be responsible for the administration of betamethasone (Celestone) to aid in fetal lung maturity in preparation for the early delivery. In

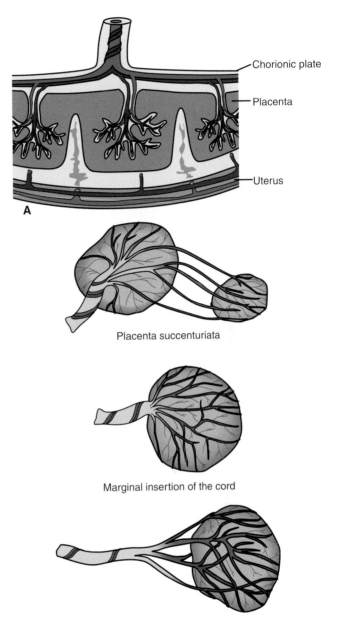

A

Placenta succenturiata

Marginal insertion of the cord

B Velamentous insertion of the cord

Fig 16.3a and 16.3b Vasa previa degrees.

fetal development, the lungs are the last organ system to mature. This usually happens around 34 weeks. No fetus at 34 weeks gestation or later needs to receive Celestone, even though they still may be preterm.

(3) The nurse may also be the first provider to recognize the abnormal bleeding upon examination. Prompt notification of the PCP is required so that the fetus may be delivered by emergent cesarean section if found to have a vasa previa.

C. Placenta-related labor and birth complications

1. **Placental abruption** is defined as the premature separation of the placenta from the uterine wall prior to the infant's birth (Table 16.4). Placental abruptions are almost always an absolute obstetric emergency, as the placenta is the infant's source of oxygen and emergent cesarean section must follow diagnosis. Hemorrhage into the decidua basalis causes hematoma formation and subsequent destruction of the adjacent placental tissue. The management of placental abruptions is based on maternal-fetal status.

   a) Risk factors: The exact cause of premature placental separation is unknown but risk factors can be identified, a number of them associated with vasoconstriction:
      • Pre-eclampsia (vasoconstriction)
      • Cocaine use (intense vasoconstriction)
      • Injury/trauma
      • History of abruption (increases risk by 15%)
      • Preterm premature rupture of membranes
      • Thrombophilia
      • Uterine abnormalities (e.g., fibroids)

   b) Maternal implications
      • Disseminated intravascular coagulation
      • Postpartum hemorrhage and hemorrhagic shock
      • Hypoxic organ damage to liver and kidneys

   c) Fetal and newborn implications
      • Intrauterine growth restriction
      • Preterm birth
      • Hypoxic injury (neurological) or hemorrhagic fetal death
      • Neonatal death (15%)

   d) Assessment findings
      (1) Fetal distress
         The extent of fetal compromise is related to the percentage of the placenta that has detached. Signs of fetal distress may include:
         • Absent to minimal variability.
         • Late decelerations.
         • Tachycardia.
         • Prolonged decelerations.
         • Terminal bradycardia.
         • Undetectable heartbeat.
      (2) Maternal rigid boardlike abdomen.
      (3) If an abruption occurs during the process of labor, the nurse may note that the patient's resting tone between contractions is beginning to rise above the standard 20 mm Hg. After noticing this change, the nurse's first action should be to rezero or reset the resting tone on the fetal monitor, as the display can be affected by movement and maternal position. A uterine resting tone that continues to be elevated after troubleshooting warrants further assessment.
      (4) Dark red vaginal bleeding associated with the involvement of the placental venous sinuses.
      (5) Severe abdominal pain or tenderness.
      (6) Signs and symptoms of hypovolemia.

   e) Nursing actions
      • Monitor for signs of hypovolemic shock.
      • Measure bleeding and assess the uterus for tenderness, rigidity, and distention.
      • Maintain IV access with large-bore needle.
      • Continue assessing fetal status via fetal monitor and by noting trends in ultrasound and Doppler studies. Necessary interventions may include O_2 at 10 to 12 L/min per nonrebreather.
      • Monitor trends in CBC and coagulation studies.
      • Administer RhoGAM if mother is Rh-negative.

   f) Collaborative care
      The presence of a placental abruption can be confirmed with ultrasound if there is equipment, personnel are readily available, and there is time

Table 16.4	Classification of Placental Abruption
Mild: Grade 1	One-sixth of placenta separates.
	Absent uterine tenderness and irritability. Mild lower abdominal and back pain.
	Dark vaginal bleeding. Less than 500 mL estimated blood loss (EBL).
	Fibrinogen 450 mg/dL (normal)
	Normal maternal vitals and FHR pattern
Moderate: Grade 2	One-sixth to one-half of placenta separates.
	Abdominal pain and uterine tenderness present. Increased uterine tone.
	Dark vaginal bleeding. EBL 1,000–1,500 mL. 15%–30% of blood volume lost.
	Fibrinogen 150–300 mg/dL (low). Early signs of DIC.
	Maternal blood pressure normal but accompanied by tachycardia, narrowed pulse pressure, orthostatic hypotension, and tachypnea. Fetus shows signs of compromise.
Severe: Grade 3	Greater than 50% separation
	Constant tearing and knifelike pain. Abdomen rigid to touch.
	Dark vaginal bleeding. EBL greater than 1,500 mL. Greater than 30% of blood volume lost.
	Fibrinogen less than 150 mg/dL. Presence of DIC.
	Low blood pressure, pronounced tachycardia, severe orthostatic hypotension, and an increase in tachypnea. Fetus death is possible.

Vaginal Bleeding and Placental Abruption

Just as in the fourth stage of labor when the uterus maintains an intense constant contraction to control postpartum bleeding, the uterus will do the same in a placental abruption. This intense constant contraction is what causes the rigid and boardlike abdomen. Bleeding is commonly associated with a placental abruption but it is not as reliable as the rigid abdomen as a telltale sign. The presence or absence of vaginal bleeding depends on where the placental abruption has occurred. If the placenta has separated at one of its edges, that makes it possible for blood to leak through the birth canal. If the separation occurs centrally, then the blood is contained by the parts of the placenta that are still attached, meaning that bleeding would not be visible on the outside.

or need to do so. Deteriorating maternal or fetal condition warrants emergent cesarean section. Frequent updates to the PCP are necessary.

ALERT Pregnant women can lose 25% to 30% of their blood volume before signs of hypovolemic shock are visible. Moreover, since the bleeding associated with an abruption can be internal, it is important not to mask signs of blood loss if an abruption is suspected. Terbutaline, which is used to relax the uterus, should not be given to a patient with a suspected abruption. A side effect of terbutaline is maternal tachycardia, making it difficult for care providers to differentiate between the effects of the medication and maternal compensation for a falling blood pressure.

2. Placenta previa

Placenta previa is the implantation of the placenta in the lower uterine segment, near or over the cervix. Placenta previa is diagnosed parentally by ultrasound and is a chronic condition that can be effectively managed. Often the third trimester is the most common time for complications related to placenta previa as the cervix begins to dilate and the arteries that attach the placenta to the lower uterine segment are severed from the stretching of the cervix. Dangerous bleeding can occur with a placenta previa, and it is often critical that care providers be able to differentiate between placenta previas and placental abruptions, which is why the condition is discussed here.

a) Degrees of placenta previa

(1) Marginal (low-lying): A marginal placenta previa is also referred to as a low-lying placenta. The placenta attaches to the uterine wall close to or on the margin of the cervical opening but does not cover the cervix to any extent. This is the only previa type that can attempt a vaginal delivery.

(2) Partial: A partial previa covers just a portion of the cervical opening.

(3) Complete: A complete placenta previa totally covers the cervical opening.

b) Risk factors: Placenta previa risk factors are usually related to one of three conditions: (1) endometrial scarring, (2) impeded endometrial vascularization, and (3) increased placental mass.

(1) Endometrial scarring can be caused by:
- History of placenta previa.
- Previous uterine surgery.
- History of abortion.
- Multiparity.

(2) Endometrial vascularization can be impeded by:
- Uterine abnormalities (e.g., fibroids).
- Maternal age greater than 35.
- Cigarette smoking.
- Diabetes or hypertension.

(3) Increased placental mass can result from:
- Large placenta.
- Multiple gestation.

c) Maternal implications
- Hemorrhagic shock
- Anemia
- Rh sensitization in Rh-negative women

d) Fetal and newborn implications
- Fetal hypoxia due to a lack of placental perfusion. The degree of hypoxia is directly related to the amount of blood loss.
- Fetal death secondary to maternal hemorrhage
- Fetal anemia
- Neonatal morbidity and mortality associated with premature birth

e) Assessment findings
- Pain only if laboring, so abdomen typically soft upon assessment
- Bright red vaginal bleeding
- The first episode of bleeding is rarely life threatening.

f) Nursing actions
- Assessment of maternal hemodynamic stability
- Assessment of fetal well-being
- Evaluation and documentation of bleeding amount and color
- Assessment of uterine activity
- Maintenance of large-bore IV
- Verification of blood product availability

- Assist patient with coping with bedrest and assist to bathroom as condition allows
- Administer betamethasone (Celestone) for lung maturity
- Administer RhoGAM to Rh-negative women
- Monitor trends in CBC and coagulation studies

🛑 ALERT No sterile vaginal exams for women who have been diagnosed with or suspected of having a placenta previa. A digital examination could stretch the cervix, increasing bleeding and decreasing perfusion to both the mother and the fetus. Furthermore, uterine perfusion is greatest in the third trimester. Failure to resolve maternal bleeding related to placenta previa can result in exsanguination in 10 minutes.

g) Collaborative care
   (1) Cesarean sections are indicated in almost all incidences of placenta previa
   (2) The PCP should be notified if:
     - Bleeding returns or increases.
     - BP less than 90/60 mm Hg and/or pulse greater than 120 beats per minute (bpm).
     - Respiratory rate less than 14 breaths per minute (bpm) or greater than 26 bpm.
     - Temperature greater than 100.4°F.
     - Urine output less than 30 mL/hour.
     - O_2 saturation less than 95%.
     - Decreased level of consciousness.
     - Onset of uterine contractions.
     - Indeterminate or abnormal FHR findings.

DID YOU KNOW?

On early ultrasound, it often appears like many women have a placenta previa. This is due to the small uterine cavity. As the uterus stretches and enlarges, the placenta will migrate to an appropriate place in the upper portion of the uterine cavity. A visual example of this can be reproduced with a balloon and a sticker. Place a small sticker on the side wall of a standard party balloon just past the tail that is used for inflation, then blow the balloon up. As the balloon enlarges, the sticker should move away from the tail of the balloon much like the placenta will as the uterus grows during the course of pregnancy.

3. Placenta accreta
   Placenta accreta is when the placenta invades the uterine wall of trophoblasts. Although the condition can be diagnosed by ultrasound in the antenatal period, it is often not confirmed until the placenta is retained (unable to be delivered) in the fourth stage of labor.
   a) Degrees of placenta accreta
     - Placenta accreta: invasion of the trophoblast beyond the normal boundary (80% of cases)
     - Placenta increta: invasion of the trophoblast into the myometrium (15% of cases)
     - Placenta percreta: invasion of the trophoblast through the uterine musculature with the potential to adhere to other pelvic organs (5% of cases)
   b) Maternal implications
     - Approximately 90% of women lose greater than 3,000 mL of blood as a result of placenta accreta.
     - Prompt surgical intervention is required to reduce morbidity and mortality related to blood loss.
     - A hysterectomy may be needed to stop maternal blood loss.

D. Uterine rupture
   Uterine rupture is the tearing of the uterine muscle, either partial or complete.
   1. Partial uterine rupture: also referred to as *uterine dehiscence.* The uterine muscle is torn but the visceral peritoneum remains intact. The visceral peritoneum is the protective layer of connective tissue that covers the outside of the uterus.
   2. Complete uterine rupture: every layer of the uterine wall is separated, including the visceral peritoneum.
   3. The extent of maternal-fetal compromise is related to the extent of the injury. Fetal mortality related to this complication is estimated at 50% to 70%. Five percent of mothers with uterine rupture will not survive the complication.
   4. Risk factors
     - **Trial of labor after cesarean** (attempt of **vaginal birth after cesarean**)
     - Previous vertical uterine scar (includes classical cesarean section scars and T-shaped scars)
     - Multifetal gestation
     - Tachysystole
   5. Other considerations
     a) Notice that the risk factors are based on uterine incisions. It is possible for a mother to have a skin incision that is horizontal or low transverse and a uterine scar that is vertical or classical. It is insufficient to assess the skin as an indication of what type of surgery the client has had before.
   6. Trial of labor after cesarean (TOLAC) and vaginal birth after cesarean (VBAC)
      When certain criteria are met, VBAC risks are less than repeat cesarean risks.
     a) VBAC criteria
       - Only one (two according to some literature) previous low-transverse (horizontal) cesarean section.
       - Clinically adequate pelvis
       - Readily available physician, anesthesia personnel, and operating room staff if emergent cesarean birth is needed

Simulating the Effects of Contractions

The effect of labor contractions on a uterine incision can be reproduced by holding two loose leaf sheets of paper adjacent to each other and gripping them with your forefinger and thumb at both the top and the bottom of the sheets. When you produce "contractions" by pressing downward with your top forefinger and thumb, you should notice that at times the sheets move away from each other, creating a diamond-like hole. That is what it is like to labor with a classical cesarean section. If you place the adjacent sheets horizontally in one palm and push downward on the sheets with the other, the result is nothing really. This is why there is a dramatically decreased risk of uterine rupture in women who have had one previous low-transverse cesarean section.

b) Contraindications to a VBAC
- Previous classical (vertical) cesarean section, T-shaped incision, or other uterus surgeries
- History of uterine rupture
- Inadequate pelvis
- Any preexisting conditions that prohibit vaginal delivery
- Planned birth in a facility that is not equipped for emergent cesarean delivery

c) Important considerations
 (1) The risks to the mother and neonate are reduced when labor is allowed to occur spontaneously. Use of oxytocin for induction of labor in a mother who has decided to have a TOLAC is allowed; however, the use of prostaglandins is contraindicated. While oxytocin can be tightly controlled and titrated per infusion pump, the absorption of prostaglandins like misoprostol cannot be controlled due to the route of administration (vaginally or orally). Use of prostaglandins can cause tachysystole, which can precipitate a uterine rupture.
 (2) When assessing a woman's candidacy for a TOLAC, the nurse should assess the type of uterine incision presence as well as the indication for her last cesarean section. Late decelerations, for example, are situation dependent and have no bearing on future births. However, some delivery complications, like pelvic dystocias, are likely to repeat. The presence of unmodifiable barriers to vaginal delivery increases the risks to mother and baby during labor and may be grounds for a repeat cesarean section, even if the uterine incision is transverse.

7. Implications of uterine rupture
 The maternal implications are associated with hypovolemia secondary to internal hemorrhage. The fetus will display signs of compromise respective to the secondary conditions associated with uterine rupture: placental insufficiency, placental abruption, cord compression, asphyxia, and hypovolemia. Maternal and fetal survival is dependent upon nurse recognition of assessment findings.
 a) Maternal-related implications
 - Signs of hypovolemia (e.g., hypotension, tachycardia, tachypnea, pallor)
 - Severe pain with contractions or reports of burning or stabbing sensations
 - Vaginal bleeding
 b) Fetus-related implications
 - Terminal bradycardia
 - Absent variability
 - Late decelerations
 - Absent fetal heart tones
8. Collaborative care
 The presence of a uterine rupture requires an emergent cesarean section with the possibility of hysterectomy if hemorrhage cannot be controlled. At first recognition of the associated assessment findings, the provider and other assistive personnel should be notified. The nurse can attempt to stabilize the patient's O_2 and IV fluids. A blood transfusion may be necessary during the perioperative period.

E. Amniotic fluid embolism
 An **amniotic fluid embolism** (or anaphylactic syndrome) is a rare condition caused by a collection of fetal cells, lanugo, and vernix that enters the maternal vasculature and begins a cascade of events similar to anaphylactic shock. The end result is maternal cardiorespiratory collapse. This complication can occur during the course of pregnancy, labor, birth, or within the 24 hours following delivery. Maternal death usually occurs within 1 hour of symptom appearance.
 1. Amniotic fluid embolism (AFE) is associated with a two-step process, as shown in Box 16.1.
 2. How the embolism enters the maternal circulation is poorly understood, but it has been hypothesized that it occurs:
 - At the cervix after the ROM.
 - At the placental separation site.
 - At a site of uterine trauma.
 3. Proposed risk factors have been ineffective at predicting the occurrence of AFE.
 4. Assessment findings include:
 - Dyspnea.
 - Seizure.
 - Hypotension.
 - Cyanosis.
 - Cardiopulmonary decompensation.

Box 16.1 Amniotic Fluid Embolism Cascade

First Stage

Fetal cells and tissue enter the maternal circulation › maternal immune mediators are released › pulmonary vasospasm and pulmonary hypotension › increased right ventricular pressure › hypoxia › cardiac and pulmonary capillary damage › left heart failure and acute respiratory distress

Second Stage

Development of DIC and subsequent maternal hemorrhage

- Uterine atony leading to hemorrhage and disseminated intravascular coagulation (DIC).
- Cardiac and respiratory arrest.

5. Collaborative care

Maternal prognosis is often unchanged, even with intervention. Support is aimed at preserving cardiopulmonary function. Massive blood and platelet transfusions may be necessary. Important labs include CBC, clotting factors, and arterial blood gases. A full code is often needed immediately following recognition of symptoms.

F. Fetal demise

Intrauterine fetal demise is defined by fetal death that occurs in utero. A specific cause cannot usually be identified but the occurrence has been linked to:

- Maternal disease processes (e.g., diabetes, cardiac disease, hypertensive disorders, and autoimmune disease).
- Placental abruption.
- Labor occurring before the 24th week of pregnancy.
- Malnutrition.
- Maternal trauma.
- Post-term pregnancy (greater than 42 weeks gestation).
- Accidental umbilical cord compression or compromise.
- Fetal conditions that are incompatible with life, often genetic.

Initial assessment findings may include maternal reports of decreased or no fetal movement. The absence of fetal heart tones is confirmed with ultrasound, and induction is initiated within 24 to 48 hours to avoid maternal complications such as disseminated intravascular coagulation (DIC), sepsis, and infection of the intrauterine cavity (endometritis). The nurse's actions during this time will vary based on patient response and readiness to face the pregnancy loss. All actions should be geared toward keeping the family informed, providing emotional support, and assisting the family with feelings of grief at their own pace. It is imperative that the nurse understand that mothers and fathers grieve differently and not to forget to provide emotional support to the father as well. If ready and receptive, helping partners understand each other's reactions to the death of the fetus can help decrease disruptions in the parents' relationship.

V. Cesarean Section Delivery

Cesarean section is the delivery of a fetus through a uterine incision. Cesarean sections can be classified by their timing and the type of incision used.

A. Scheduled cesarean births

Scheduled cesarean births occur prior to the start of spontaneous labor. A scheduled cesarean birth may be indicated if the woman has had a cesarean section before and if the mother or the fetus has a health condition that could be worsened by vaginal delivery. Cesarean sections may also be scheduled electively.

B. Unscheduled cesarean sections

Unscheduled cesarean sections may be:

- Emergent: denotes need for instantaneous delivery of the infant (e.g., cord prolapse).
- Urgent: denotes prompt delivery of the infant (e.g., active labor with breech presentation with normal fetal heart tones).
- Nonurgent: an unscheduled need for a cesarean without urgency (e.g., dystocia).

C. Uterine incisions may be classical (vertical) or low-transverse (horizontal).

D. Preoperative nursing care

Since this chapter focuses on labor and birth at risk, the nursing care described here is related to unscheduled cesarean sections. Keep in mind that in an emergent cesarean section, some preoperative duties may be foregone.

1. Notify all pertinent providers of the pending birth (e.g., anesthesia, scrub nurse, and the neonatal department).
2. Provide education to the patient and family as time allows. There may not be any time in absolute obstetric emergencies to perform quality teaching. The nurse should give detailed information in the immediate postpartum period and answer remaining questions to help reduce anxiety related to the birth experience.
3. Review admission interview and prenatal records, noting any risk factors that need to be communicated to anesthesia or other pertinent care providers.
4. Verify that consent for the procedure is on the patient's chart.
5. Review CBC results and verify completion of a type and screen.
   a) Damage to the spinal cord can result in maternal platelets being too low to repair the area where the epidural/spinal needle was inserted due to hematoma formation. No client with platelet counts less than 100,000 cmm is a candidate for spinal or epidural anesthesia.

6. Notify anesthesia of the patient's last PO intake.
7. Continue maternal and fetal assessment, intervening as necessary based on findings.
8. Initiate 1,000 mL bolus of LR in preparation for spinal anesthesia in nonemergent cesarean sections.
9. Insert a Foley catheter.
10. Use trimmers to remove hair from the pubic region that may interfere with the incision site.
11. Remove internal fetal monitor parts.
12. Remove any jewelry, hair clips, or clothing items that contain metal.
13. Administer narrow-spectrum antibiotics (e.g., cephazolin, clindamycin, and gentamicin can substitute in case of an allergy).

E. Intraoperative care and anesthesia

Although spinal anesthesia is the primary choice for scheduled cesarean sections, due to their quick onset and total loss of sensation, this type of anesthesia takes time to complete and often requires positioning that is not conducive to certain emergencies, like umbilical cord prolapses. If a patient has labored before her emergency occurred and has an epidural, additional medicine can be given through the epidural catheter to mimic the increased loss of sensation associated with spinal anesthesia. In obstetric emergencies where there is no time to place a spinal, the patient's position cannot be changed, or there is no epidural in place, general anesthesia is the best option. Cesarean sections performed under general anesthesia are done quickly to limit the amount of anesthesia the fetus receives. General anesthesia compromises the infant's respirations in the same way it does the mother's. You may notice that surgeons will gown and glove after the spinal is placed, but when general is used, the surgeons are dressed for surgery before the anesthesia is administered because of the aforementioned time limitation. Regardless of type of anesthesia chosen:

1. Anesthesia will take over the responsibility of monitoring maternal vital signs during the intraoperative period.
2. Anesthesia will also monitor urine output for amount and the presence of blood, give an estimated blood loss, and administer oxytocin once the placenta had been manually removed.
3. The nurse should:
   - Conduct a time-out with the physician.
   - Assist with positioning for spinal anesthesia if there is time.
   - Position the patient in a left tilt on the operating table to avoid vena cava compression and subsequent reduced cardiac output. Compression of the vena cava by the gravid uterus can compromise oxygen delivery to the fetus and cause the woman to feel faint and nauseated.
   - Assess fetal heart tones.
   - Complete the abdominal preparation.

- Apply a grounding pad to the patient's thigh. To avoid risk of electrocution to the patient, the grounding pad should not be applied to an area that is wet from the abdominal prep. If the grounding pad is applied before abdominal preparation, the nurse should be sure not to accidentally wet the grounding pad during the process.
- Secure the patient to operating table.
- Initiate venous thromboembolism prophylaxis.
- Ensure that the neonatal team has the needed care supplies.
- Act as the circulator by retrieving supplies needed by the operating team and helping the scrub nurse manage the instrument, sponge, and needle counts.
- If appropriate, facilitate the presence of the patient's support person during delivery.
- Complete necessary documentation.
- Apply identification bands to the infant and parents. The nurse may facilitate bonding time if the mother's and infant's conditions allow.

F. Postoperative care

During the postoperative period, the nurse will resume care of the patient from anesthesia. Nursing actions during this period include:

- Assessing vital signs per unit protocol.
- Monitoring for signs of complications.
- Assessing urine for amount and the presence of blood.
- Performing fundal massage and peri pad assessments.
- Applying Ted anti-embolism stockings and sequential compression devices if not used during surgery and not contraindicated.
- Assessing pain and initiating pharmacological and nonpharmacological pain relief methods.
- Monitoring the patient's recovery from anesthesia, providing support as necessary (e.g., O_2 for low oxygen saturation following general anesthesia).
- Auscultating lung and bowel sounds, assessing for signs of pulmonary edema and paralytic ileus.
- Assisting with temperature maintenance by using warm linens and fluids if available.
- Assessing abdominal bandage for signs of drainage.
- Advancing diet per orders received from physician.
- Assisting with newborn care when appropriate.
- Assisting with peri care. Women who deliver by cesarean section have the same vaginal lochia as those who deliver vaginally.

G. Associated maternal complications

These include hemorrhage, deep venous thrombosis, pulmonary embolism, atelectasis, paralytic ileus, bladder trauma, infection, and need for hysterectomy.

H. Associated fetal and neonatal complications

include asphyxia from poor placental perfusion (related to regional anesthesia-related hypotension or supine maternal positioning), scalpel lacerations, and respiratory complications.

CASE STUDY: Putting It All Together

Subjective Data

Ms. Jones is a 24-year-old G1 T1 P0 A0 L1 who has been admitted to labor and delivery at 33 weeks plus 6 days gestation for prolonged monitoring. The patient had no complications with her previous pregnancy and delivered a full-term female infant weighing 6 pounds, 1 ounce. The patient has been diagnosed with polyhydramnios this pregnancy and was sent to the labor and delivery unit for observation after a nonstress test at the clinic displayed uterine contractions every 3 to 4 minutes that were mild to moderate to palpation. The patient denied any pain at this time. An ultrasound was done in the clinic, and the fetus was determined to be in a single footling breech position. Her sterile vaginal exam prior to admission was 2 to 3 cm dilated/ 30% effaced/−3 station.

Objective Data

Nursing Assessment

Vital Signs

BP: 117/56 mm Hg

Pulse: 76

Respirations: 20

Temperature: 97.7°F

Pain score: 3/10. Denies the need for pain medicine at this time.

Uterus: Mild to moderate contraction every 3 to 4 minutes

Fetus: FHR in 140s, moderate variability, no accelerations, no decelerations

No abnormal physical assessment findings are noted.

Health Care Provider's Orders

LR 125 mL/hr via 18G IV

Clear liquids

Bedrest with bathroom privileges

Continuous fetal monitoring

While the nurse is at the nurse's station, the patient rings the call light and states that her water has broken. The nurse looks up at the fetal monitor screen and sees that the fetus is now having changes in the FHR. The baseline is still 140s with moderate variability, but with every contraction the FHR drops abruptly to the 50s and rapidly returns to baseline when the contraction is over.

Case Study Questions

1. What subjective data in the case study should alert the nurse of a change in status?

2. What objective or assessment data also support a change in status?

3. What should be the nurse's primary concern for this patient at the end of this case study?

4. What independent and collaborative actions should the nurse anticipate?

REVIEW QUESTIONS

Be sure to read the Introduction for valuable test-taking tips.

1. The labor and delivery nurse is caring for a 27-year-old primigravida with the following vaginal exam: 2 to 3 cm dilated/70% effaced/–2 station. For the last 2 hours the FHR tracing has displayed a Category I tracing and uterine contractions that are every 2 minutes. The contractions are strong to palpation and the patient is now 3/70%/–2. Which is the nurse's next *best* action?
   1. Encourage the patient to ambulate
   2. Request orders to initiate oxytocin
   3. Assist the patient to a warm bath
   4. Document the findings

2. Which is the best explanation for the use of hydration and relaxation in the treatment of hypertonic labor?
   1. Hydration promotes uterine relaxation by diluting endogenous oxytocin.
   2. Hydration improves uterine coordination by increasing perfusion.
   3. Hydration encourages contraction regulation by stimulating catecholamine release.
   4. Hydration stimulates the production of prostaglandins to relax the uterus.

3. The nurse is caring for a 34-year-old gravida 4, para 3 experiencing a prolonged labor. The physician performed an amniotomy 3 hours ago to stimulate the progression of labor. The patient's most recent vaginal exam was 8/80%/0. Which assessment finding should the nurse should be most concerned about?
   1. Pain score of 7/10
   2. FHR baseline of 165
   3. Mild variable decelerations
   4. Increased bloody mucous discharge

4. Which explains why infants who are delivered via cesarean section before the start of labor have more difficulty transitioning to extrauterine life?
   1. The use of warm IV fluids precipitates hyperthermia.
   2. Regional anesthesia causes respiratory depression.
   3. The maternal left tilt position reduces placental blood flow.
   4. Residual amniotic fluid in the lungs makes spontaneous respirations difficult.

5. The nurse is caring for a patient during induction of labor. The oxytocin is currently infusing at 6 mU/min. The fetal heart tracing displays a 130 baseline, moderate variability, and no accelerations or decelerations. Uterine contractions have been every 2 minutes for the last 30 minutes. What is the nurse's next *best* action?
   1. Reduce the oxytocin infusion to 3 mU/min
   2. Delay the next scheduled oxytocin increase
   3. Maintain infusion at 6 mU/min
   4. Discontinue the oxytocin infusion

6. Which is the cervical exam that most indicates the use of misoprostol?
   1. 1 cm dilated, 20% effaced, –3 station, firm and posterior
   2. 3–4 cm dilated, 50% effaced, –2 station, firm and midposition
   3. 5 cm dilated, 80% effaced, 0 station, soft and midposition
   4. 6 cm dilated, 100% effaced, +1 station, soft and anterior

7. Which criteria should be verified prior to vacuum or forceps use? *Select all that apply.*
   1. The woman's bladder is empty.
   2. The fetus must be at least 34 weeks gestation.
   3. There is a Category I tracing.
   4. The cervix must be completely dilated.
   5. The fetal head must be 0 station.

8. Cephalohematoma occurring from an operative vaginal delivery increased a newborn's risk of developing which of the following complications?
   1. Bulging fontanels
   2. Developmental delays
   3. Jaundice
   4. Macrocephaly

9. The nurse is caring for a gravida 5, para 4 who has been 5 centimeters dilated for 2 hours. The uterine contractions are every 5 minutes and mild to palpation. Which is the *most* appropriate nursing action?
   1. Administer ordered IV pain medicine
   2. Assist the patient with frequent position changes
   3. Prepare patient for epidural anesthesia
   4. Prepare patient for a cesarean section delivery

10. Why is precipitous labor most often seen in multiparous women?
    1. The cervix weakens after each delivery.
    2. The cervix can dilate and efface simultaneously.
    3. The multigravida uterus is better able to coordinate muscle movements.
    4. It is more difficult for multiparous women to know when labor begins.

11. While attending the delivery of a patient with GODM, the nurse notices the retraction of the fetal head onto the perineum. What is the nurse's next *best* action?
    1. Apply fundal pressure
    2. Assist the woman to left lateral position
    3. Flex the mother to left lateral position
    4. Assist the woman to hands-and-knees position

12. The patient with which vaginal exam is most at risk for an umbilical cord prolapse?
    1. 1–2 cm dilated, 70% effaced, –1 station
    2. 5 cm dilated, 60% effaced, –3 station
    3. 7–8 cm dilated, 80% effaced, –2 station
    4. 9 cm dilated, 100% effaced, 0 station

13. A gravida 3, para 2 is attempting a vaginal birth without the use of pain medicine or anesthesia. Following spontaneous rupture of membranes, the patient's cervical exam was 5 cm dilated, 60% effaced, –2 station. Which therapeutic intervention is appropriate for this patient?
    1. Ambulation with assistance
    2. Squatting with support from partner
    3. Sitting on birthing ball
    4. Resting on hands and knees

14. A woman presents to labor and delivery at 37 weeks plus 6 days gestation with complaints of constant abdominal pain and dark red bleeding that started 30 minutes ago. Upon examination, the woman's abdomen is consistently rigid and tender. Fetal heart tones are noted to be in the 70s. Which are these findings are associated with?
    1. Placental abruption
    2. Placental accreta
    3. Placenta previa
    4. Placenta succenturiata

15. A gravida 2, para 1 is in active labor at 39 weeks gestation. Her cervical exam is 6 cm dilated, 60% effaced, and 0 station. An amniotomy is performed by the physician. The fluid is noted to be bloody and the fetal heart tones have decelerated to the 50s. What is the nurse's next best action?
    1. Notify the operating team of emergent cesarean delivery
    2. Assist the patient to left lateral position
    3. Apply O_2 at 10–12 L/min per nonrebreather
    4. Administer an IV fluid bolus

16. During an oxytocin induction, which assessment finding is most concerning to the labor and delivery nurse?
    1. A uterine resting tone of 17 mm Hg
    2. A uterine resting tone of 30 mm Hg
    3. Contractions that are every 3 minutes and last 60 seconds
    4. Contractions that are every 5 minutes and last 60 seconds

17. A 24-year-old G4 T1 A2 L1 presents to obstetric triage with complaints of contractions every 3 minutes, accompanied by bright red vaginal bleeding. The woman is 29 weeks gestation with a twin pregnancy. She has had three urinary tract infections during this pregnancy and is currently taking Microbid daily as prophylaxis. Her last baby was born via cesarean section for breech malpresentation. She denies any other significant medical history. What risk factors for placenta previa does this patient have? *Select all that apply.*
    1. Maternal age of 24
    2. Twin gestation
    3. Gestational age of 29 weeks
    4. Previous delivery by cesarean section
    5. History of abortion

18. When caring for a woman with a complete placenta previa, which finding should the nurse report to the physician?
    1. BP of 95/60
    2. Temperature of 100.1°F
    3. Urine output of 40 mL/hour
    4. O_2 saturation less that 95%

19. Which woman is the best candidate for a trial of labor after cesarean (TOLAC)?
    1. A 34-year-old gravida 2, para 1 with one previous classical cesarean section for prematurity
    2. A 21-year-old gravida 2, para 1 with one previous low-transverse cesarean section for CPD
    3. A 31-year-old gravida 4, para 2 with one previous low-transverse cesarean section for late decelerations
    4. A 27-year-old gravida 3, para 2 with one previous T-shaped incision for macrosomia

20. A woman has chosen a trial of labor after cesarean. Which findings indicate the *best* understanding of the nurse's teaching by the patient?
    1. "It is safer for me to be induced at 39 weeks so that my labor can be controlled and monitored carefully."
    2. "I will need to arrive to the hospital the night before my induction so that my cervix can be ripened with prostaglandins."
    3. "If I do not got into labor on my own, I will have to have a cesarean section since Pitocin is contraindicated for me."
    4. "A balloon catheter may be used to manually ripen my cervix, if necessary."

21. Laboring women are often NPO to decrease the risk of which complication?
    1. Aspiration
    2. Diarrhea
    3. Vomiting
    4. Paralytic ileus

22. Why are elective deliveries not performed unless the fetus is confirmed to be 39 weeks gestation or greater?
    1. The lower uterine segment is not developed until 39 weeks gestation.
    2. The mother's oxytocin receptors are immature until 39 weeks gestation.
    3. Delivery before 39 weeks may result in neonatal morbidity related to prematurity.
    4. Delivery before 39 weeks is associated with increased risk for precipitous delivery.

23. The nurse is caring for a 25-week patient who was diagnosed with preterm premature rupture of membranes 8 days ago. After completing a change of shift assessment, which finding should the nurse be most concerned about?
    1. Minimal variability on the FHR tracing
    2. Abdominal tenderness when adjusting external monitors
    3. A gush of amniotic fluid when changing positions
    4. Patient requests to go to the bathroom often

24. Which may the nurse do to preserve fetal well-being during oxytocin induction?
    1. Give O_2 per nonrebreather for absent accelerations
    2. Administer an IV fluid bolus for moderate variability
    3. Turn the patient to a lateral position for late decelerations
    4. Discontinue Pitocin administration for early decelerations

25. Which of the following prohibits a woman from receiving epidural or spinal anesthesia?
    1. HIV positive status
    2. Presence of scoliosis
    3. Presence of lower back tattoos
    4. Thrombocytopenia

REVIEW QUESTIONS ANSWERS

1. ANSWER: 3
Rationale

1. Ambulation is appropriate for hypotonic not hypertonic labor. This patient should be encouraged to rest.
2. Oxytocin is also appropriate for hypotonic labor and is not indicated here, as the patient is having strong contractions every 2 minutes. Oxytocin would exacerbate the situation.
3. Assisting the patient to a warm bath promotes relaxation. Relaxation along with hydration are the primary goals to treat hypertonic labor.
4. Document the findings is an inappropriate best action. The client is in hypertonic labor and is progressing slowly for a primiparous woman. This requires intervention to improve maternal and fetal health outcomes.

TEST-TAKING TIP: There are a few things required to answer this question. The tester needs to be familiar with the normal curve of labor for a primiparous woman, characteristics of hypertonic labor, and interventions for hypertonic labor. This multistep thinking process is often required during testing. If you are missing information needed to answer the question, revisit the question for clues. For example, hypertonic labor is more common in primiparous women in the latent phase of labor, which can be assumed from the patient's cervical examination. The patient in the stem possesses these two characteristics. Also primiparous women should dilate 0.5 cm in 1 hour, and it has taken this patient 2 hours. This indicates that there is an issue, which rules out document the findings as an answer. Nursing interventions should combat dystocias using opposites. Women in hypertonic labor require relaxation and women in hypotonic labor require stimulation, which is why ambulation and oxytocin are incorrect.

Content Area: *Labor and Birth at Risk—Dystocias*
Integrated Process: *Nursing Process—Intervention*
Client Need: *Physiological Integrity*
Cognitive Level: *Application*
Concept: *Pregnancy*
Reference: *Durham, R. F., & Chapman, L. (2014).* Maternal-newborn nursing: The critical components of nursing care. *2nd ed. Philadelphia: F.A. Davis.*

2. ANSWER: 2
Rationale

1. Hydration does not dilute endogenous oxytocin.
2. Hydration increases the oxygen being delivered to the uterus. The muscle requires stimulation, which is why ambulation and oxytocin are incorrect.
3. Catecholamine release can inhibit contractions but the hormone is released in response to fear, not hydration.
4. Prostaglandins would further stimulate contractions.

TEST-TAKING TIP: Each of the answer choices contains words and phrases that are recognizable from the section on dystocias. This is typical for testing options. To eliminate some of the answers, identify the problem that needs to be solved in the stem. The nurse is treating an overstimulated uterus, so prostaglandins would not be helpful. The remaining three all work to decrease uterine stimulation, but only one is plausible. After reviewing the rationales, it is easier to see that although a decrease in oxytocin or an increase in catecholamines is desirable, hydration can do neither of those things. Since this question is specifically about the use of hydration, neither of those can be correct.

Content Area: *Labor and Birth at Risk—Dystocias*
Integrated Process: *Nursing Process—Analysis*
Client Need: *Physiological Integrity*
Cognitive Level: *Analysis*
Concept: *Pregnancy*
Reference: *Durham, R. F., & Chapman, L. (2014).* Maternal-newborn nursing: The critical components of nursing care. *2nd ed. Philadelphia: F.A. Davis.*

3. ANSWER: 2
Rationale

1. The patient is in the transition phase of labor and an increase in pain can be expected.
2. The FHR is higher than the normal range of 110 to 160. Fetal tachycardia is an indication of maternal fever. This would be the most concerning assessment finding since the patient has been ruptured.
3. Mild variable decelerations after rupture of membranes are common since the suspension effect of the amniotic fluid is decreased.
4. Increased bloody show is a normal finding during the progression of labor.

TEST-TAKING TIP: Even without knowing that mild variables were common after rupture of membranes and fetal tachycardia was a sign of maternal fever, of the answer choices given, the FHR was the only thing that was abnormal for the patient's status, meaning it was really the only thing that really should concern the nurse.

Content Area: *Labor and Birth at Risk—Amniotomy*
Integrated Process: *Nursing Process—Assessment*
Client Need: *Physiological Integrity*
Cognitive Level: *Analysis*
Concept: *Pregnancy*
Reference: *Perry, S. E., Hockenberry, M. F., Lowdermilk, D. L., & Wilson, D. (2014).* Maternal child nursing care. *5th ed. St. Louis, MO: Elsevier*

4. ANSWER: 4
Rationale

1. The use of prewarmed fluids improves umbilical pH and Apgar scores.
2. General not regional anesthesia can result in neonatal depression. Regional has the least effects on the infant, and when they do occur are usually due to secondary causes, such as unmanaged hypotension from spinal placement.
3. The left tilt position displaces the uterus and improves maternal cardiac output to the fetus.
4. Infants delivered by cesarean section miss the chest cavity compression that happens in a vaginal delivery, making transition more difficult.

TEST-TAKING TIP: The fetal lungs are not used for respiration in utero, even though practice breaths may be visible on ultrasound. The space is filled with fluid, and approximately 30 mL of amniotic fluid are squeezed from the lungs during labor and delivery. Displacement of the fluid makes it easier for the alveoli to stay open during neonatal respirations, decreasing the work of breathing. If a significant amount of fluid remains at delivery, the wet alveoli collapse and stick together after each inspiration. This increases the work of breathing for the baby because with every breath, he must reinflate the alveoli. Sometimes this work is so great that the infant cannot maintain the work of breathing without assistance. Nasal flaring, grunting, and retractions are signs of respiratory distress in an infant. The grunting is especially significant, as it results from the neonate trying to force the alveoli open by increasing thoracic pressure.

Content Area: Cesarean Section—Newborn Implications
Integrated Process: Nursing Process—Assessment
Client Need: Physiological Integrity
Cognitive Level: Analysis
Concept: Pregnancy
Reference: Durham, R. F., & Chapman, L. (2014). Maternal-newborn nursing: The critical components of nursing care. 2nd ed. Philadelphia: F.A. Davis.

5. **ANSWER: 1**
Rationale
1. Contractions that are every 2 minutes (five or more contractions in a 10-minute window) for 30 minutes are the definition of tachysystole. In the presence of tachysystole, even with normal fetal heart tones, the nurse should decrease the infusion rate by half.
2. This is inappropriate since the patient is having tachysystole, so reduction of the current rate is required.
3. Maintaining contractions this close together compromises fetal blood flow and increases the risk of uterine rupture and placental abruption.
4. Discontinuing the oxytocin is not indicated since the fetal heart tones are reassuring.

TEST-TAKING TIP: The risks of using induction medications are often viewed in regard to the fetus, but there are risks to the mother as well. Just as with prostaglandin insert use, tachysystole alone indicates a need for intervention. Contractions that are every 2 minutes apart are dangerous, even if there are currently no signs of compromise. Removal of the prostaglandin insert or a reduction in the oxytocin infusion rate is indicated in the presence of tachysystole.

Content Area: Labor and Birth at Risk—Oxytocin Induction
Integrated Process: Nursing Process—Analysis
Client Need: Physiological Integrity
Cognitive Level: Application
Concept: Pregnancy
References: Durham, R. F., & Chapman, L. (2014). Maternal-newborn nursing: The critical components of nursing care. 2nd ed. Philadelphia: F.A. Davis.

6. **ANSWER: 1**
Rationale
1. The cervical exam in this option has the lowest Bishop score at 1. It is the least dilated and effaced. The fetus is still high in the abdomen and the cervix is firm in consistency and facing the maternal back.
2. Cervical exam equals a Bishop score of 5.
3. Cervical exam equals a Bishop sore of 9.
4. Cervical exam equals a Bishop score of 9.

TEST-TAKING TIP: The Bishop score chart is not something that providers memorize. Since rationales are provided, it may be a good idea to calculate Bishop scores to compare for practice; however, the calculations are not needed to answer this question correctly. Misoprostol is for cervical ripening, so the question is really just asking the tester to identify which cervix is farthest from desirable. Answer choice 1 would be correct because it has the least desirable qualities of the exams presented.

Content Area: Labor and Birth at Risk—Cervical Ripening
Integrated Process: Nursing Process—Assessment
Client Need: Health Promotion and Maintenance
Cognitive Level: Application
Concept: Pregnancy
Reference: Durham, R. F., & Chapman, L. (2014). Maternal-newborn nursing: The critical components of nursing care. 2nd ed. Philadelphia: F.A. Davis.

7. **ANSWER: 1, 4, 5**
Rationale
1. Emptying the woman's bladder before operative delivery reduces bladder injury from instrument use.
2. The fetus must be at least 36 weeks gestation.
3. The presence of a Category I tracing is not criteria for use. Operative vaginal deliveries are often done because the fetus is showing signs of distress and maternal pushing efforts are not expected to get the fetus delivered before further complication results.
4. The cervix must be completely dilated to avoid cervical lacerations and subsequent maternal hemorrhage.
5. The fetus must be engaged, which means the largest part of the fetal head is at the ischial spines. This is also the definition of 0 station. Applying instruments before this point would be dangerous, as providers could not rule out CPD before this point.

TEST-TAKING TIP: Select-all-that-apply questions are usually difficult for students. In these types of questions, each choice is usually related to the topic in the stem; it is just that the information in some of the choices is incorrect. Since answer 2 has a gestational age stipulation, the student can assume that there is a gestational age stipulation associated with operative vaginal delivery and now needs to decide whether the one presented is correct or not. The same goes for answer 3. There are certain tracing categories associated with vacuum and forceps use and maternal indications for operative vaginal delivery as well, but does it make sense to speed up the delivery of an infant that is showing no signs of distress?

Content Area: Labor and Birth at Risk—Operative Vaginal Delivery
Integrated Process: Nursing Process—Assessment
Client Need: Health Promotion and Maintenance
Cognitive Level: Application
Concept: Pregnancy
Reference: Durham, R. F., & Chapman, L. (2014). Maternal-newborn nursing: The critical components of nursing care. 2nd ed. Philadelphia: F.A. Davis.

8. **ANSWER: 3**
Rationale
1. Bulging fontanels are usually caused by increased intracranial pressure from overproduction of cerebral spinal fluid, not a cephalohematoma. Furthermore, cephalohematomas are contained injuries that cannot cause widespread changes in the infant's head findings.
2. Cephalohematomas are not associated with developmental delays.
3. A cephalohematoma is the collection of blood under the fetal periosteum. As the newborn breaks down this injury that is made of red blood cells, additional bilirubin will be released. The immature liver cannot conjugate the bilirubin fast enough, so it remains fat soluble. Since it cannot be

excreted, it sinks into the skin and other fatty tissues, the most dangerous being the cerebrum.
4. Cephalohematomas are not associated with macrocephaly.

TEST-TAKING TIP: This question is simply about making connections to anticipate risks. The cephalohematoma is a collection of RBCs, and jaundice is the only condition listed that is associated with red blood cells. In order to rule out some of the other answers, the tester could consider the timing of the injury. Answer 4 can be ruled out immediately because an infant would not suddenly have macrocephaly during the second stage of labor; macrocephaly is a preexisting condition. Anatomy may help as well; cephalohematomas cannot cross suture lines because the injury is under the fetal periosteum, and since an infant's skull bones are not fused, there is no way for the injury to be on both sides of a suture line. This also means that the injury could not affect the fontanels, which are spaces between unfused bone.

Content Area: Labor and Birth at Risk—Operative Vaginal Delivery
Integrated Process: Nursing Process—Analysis
Client Need: Health Promotion and Maintenance
Cognitive Level: Analysis
Concept: Pregnancy
Reference: *Durham, R. F., & Chapman, L. (2014). Maternal-newborn nursing: The critical components of nursing care. 2nd ed. Philadelphia: F.A. Davis.*

9. ANSWER: 2
Rationale
1. This patient has the characteristics of hypotonic labor, so giving IV pain medicine would exacerbate the issue.
2. The manipulation of the fetus's position that occurs with frequent position changes can help correct any misalignment that is impeding the process of labor. Fetal engagement can stimulate labor by stimulating the release of prostaglandins as a response to cervical stretching.
3. Epidural anesthesia would also prolong the presence of hypotonic labor. This is why many standing orders require that the woman be in active labor with progressive cervical change to reduce the likelihood that the epidural will prolong labor.
4. There is not enough information to make a decision regarding cesarean delivery.

TEST-TAKING TIP: If one of the answers could be correct if more information was provided, then it is probably not the correct answer. If you have to read into the question to make an answer choice correct, that is a good sign that there is a better option. With this in mind, answer 4 could be eliminated. Since the patient is showing signs of hypotonic labor, neither answer 1 nor 3 would be useful.

Content Area: Labor and Birth at Risk—Operative Vaginal Delivery
Integrated Process: Nursing Process—Interventions
Client Need: Health Promotion and Maintenance
Cognitive Level: Application
Concept: Pregnancy
Reference: *Durham, R. F., & Chapman, L. (2014). Maternal-newborn nursing: The critical components of nursing care. 2nd ed. Philadelphia: F.A. Davis.*

10. ANSWER: 2
Rationale
1. The cervix regains firmness and thickness by the end of the first postpartum week.
2. Labor is quicker in multiparous women because the cervix dilates and effaces simultaneously.
3. Multigravida is also a risk factor for hypotonic labor due to the stretching that occurs with each pregnancy. Therefore, the ability to better coordinate contractions is not a factor.
4. Since they are experienced, multiparous women are often better at recognizing the signs of labor.

TEST-TAKING TIP: Answering test questions accurately requires information from more than one area of nursing. This question also required some knowledge of labor progression and postpartum. When studying weak areas, also study what other topics affect those areas.

Content Area: Labor and Birth at Risk—Dystocias
Integrated Process: Nursing Process—Analysis
Client Need: Physiological Integrity
Cognitive Level: Application
Concept: Pregnancy
Reference: *Durham, R. F., & Chapman, L. (2014). Maternal-newborn nursing: The critical components of nursing care. 2nd ed. Philadelphia: F.A. Davis.*

11. ANSWER: 3
Rationale
1. The retraction of the fetal head onto the perineum is the definition of turtle sign, which is associated with shoulder dystocia delivery. Fundal pressure would exacerbate a shoulder dystocia.
2. Assisting the woman to a lateral position is not recommended, as it has no effect on the placement of the anterior shoulder.
3. McRobert's maneuver involves flexing the mother's thighs onto her abdomen. This position flattens the sacrum and widens the pelvis to facilitate passage of the anterior shoulder under the symphysis pubis.
4. Hands-and-knees position does not benefit a shoulder dystocia.

TEST-TAKING TIP: When studying, it is important to know the correct terms as well as their definitions. Since sometimes certain words are easy to recognize in relation to specific topics, testers are challenged to interpret a situation without the use of key words. Remember, exams are designed to test understanding, not ability to memorize.

Content Area: Labor and Birth at Risk—Fetus-Related Complications
Integrated Process: Nursing Process—Interventions
Client Need: Health Promotion and Maintenance
Cognitive Level: Application
Concept: Pregnancy
Reference: *Durham, R. F., & Chapman, L. (2014). Maternal-newborn nursing: The critical components of nursing care. 2nd ed. Philadelphia: F.A. Davis.*

12. ANSWER: 2
Rationale
1. The most important indicator of umbilical cord prolapse risk is fetal station, with the highest stations being at the greatest risk. This fetus's station is –1.

2. This fetus has the highest station of the presented vaginal exams, making this patient most at risk.
3. The fetus has a higher station but is not as at risk as the fetus in answer 2.
4. The fetus in this option is engaged in the maternal pelvis; this is a protective factor.

TEST-TAKING TIP: When the stem of a question asks for the most or best option, that is an indication that all or nearly all the options are appropriate in some way. Now the tester should be looking for the degree of difference or impact between the answer choices. This question suggests that more than one of the options is at risk, so by knowing that umbilical cord prolapse is associated with high station, the tester just needs to identify which station is the highest.

Content Area: Labor and Birth at Risk—Umbilical Cord–Related Complications
Integrated Process: Nursing Process—Analysis
Client Need: Physiological Integrity
Cognitive Level: Analysis
Concept: Pregnancy
Reference: Durham, R. F., & Chapman, L. (2014). Maternal-newborn nursing: The critical components of nursing care. 2nd ed. Philadelphia: F.A. Davis.

13. ANSWER: 4
Rationale
1. This woman is ruptured with a –2 station. Ambulation increases her risk for cord prolapse due to the pull of gravity.
2. Squatting also increases the downward gravitational pull.
3. Sitting on the birthing ball has the same effect as ambulating and squatting.
4. Resting on hands and knees is appropriate, as it moves the weight of the fetus away from the cervix.

TEST-TAKING TIP: If the nature of a question is unclear, try to find the common link between the answer choices presented. In this question, the answer choices are all positions. Knowing this may stimulate analysis about the ability of each position to affect what is happening in the stem. If that does not help, try and group the answer choices into categories based on similarities. In this case, choices 1 through 3 are upright positions, hinting at the probability that the choice that is different is correct. Figuring out that three of the answers have the same effect may also help establish a connection between the answer choices and the nature of the stem.

Content Area: Labor and Birth at Risk—Umbilical Cord–Related Complications
Integrated Process: Nursing Process—Analysis
Client Need: Health Promotion and Maintenance
Cognitive Level: Application
Concept: Pregnancy
Reference: Durham, R. F., & Chapman, L. (2014). Maternal-newborn nursing: The critical components of nursing care. 2nd ed. Philadelphia: F.A. Davis.

14. ANSWER: 1
Rationale
1. A placenta abruption is noted by a consistently rigid abdomen as the uterus contracts around the separated placenta. This is considered a telltale sign since bleeding may or may not be seen vaginally with an abruption.

2. A placenta accreta can cause bleeding but not until after delivery when it is time for the placenta to separate.
3. Placenta previa bleeding is bright red and the mother's abdomen will only be rigid if she is contracting. The soft uterine resting tone will return when the contraction is over.
4. Placenta succenturiata is defined by a placenta that has accessory lobes and is associated with vasa previa.

TEST-TAKING TIP: Test takers are often challenged to differentiate between incidences of placental abruption and placenta previa since they are both significant bleeding disorders of pregnancy. Knowing the difference between the two in terms of type of bleeding, presence or absence of pain, and assessment findings is essential to this differentiation. Placenta previa bleeding is arterial, so is likely bright red, while placental abruption bleeding is dark red due to venous involvement. Women experiencing placental abruption will always hurt. The separation of the placenta causes intense and constant contraction of the uterus, while women with placenta previa will have this pain only if they are experiencing the contractions of labor. The constant contraction of the uterus during a placental abruption will cause a rigid, boardlike abdomen upon assessment, while the previa will remain soft unless the mother is contracting. The fetus will always display signs of distress when an abruption is present, while the degree of fetal compromise in a previa is directly related to amount of blood loss and maternal ability to compensate for that loss.

Content Area: Labor and Birth at Risk—Placenta-Related Complications
Integrated Process: Nursing Process—Assessment
Client Need: Physiological Integrity
Cognitive Level: Analysis
Concept: Pregnancy
Reference: Durham, R. F., & Chapman, L. (2014). Maternal-newborn nursing: The critical components of nursing care. 2nd ed. Philadelphia: F.A. Davis.

15. ANSWER: 1
Rationale
1. This is the most correct answer. The assessment findings indicate the presence of a vasa previa. If not diagnosed prenatally, vasa previas are often diagnosed at rupture of membranes. Amniotic fluid is blood tinged and ROM may be proceeded by fetal distress or death. Due to how quickly the fetus can exsanguinate, the priority is to deliver the baby as quickly as possible via cesarean section.
2. Since there is a tear in the umbilical cord, improving maternal cardiac return is not a priority when a team is available to deliver the infant by cesarean section.
3. O_2 will not be effectively delivered since the infant is losing its blood volume through a tear in the cord.
4. A bolus will be of little use with a compromised umbilical cord.

TEST-TAKING TIP: Answer test questions as if you were in utopia, if the utopian answer exists. Do not question the question by asking things like, "What if the nurse was alone in a hospital in the woods with no operating team?" Just focus on what is present in the question. This fetus's best outcome relies on rapid delivery, so that is the best answer.

Content Area: Labor and Birth at Risk—Umbilical Cord–Related Complications

Integrated Process: Nursing Process—Assessment
Client Need: Physiological Integrity
Cognitive Level: Analysis
Concept: Pregnancy
Reference: *Durham, R. F., & Chapman, L. (2014).* Maternal-newborn nursing: The critical components of nursing care. *2nd ed. Philadelphia: F.A. Davis.*

16. **ANSWER: 2**
Rationale
1. A uterine resting tone of 20 mm Hg or below is normal and desired.
2. A uterine resting tone of 30 mm Hg is high and suggests that the uterus remains somewhat contracted between uterine activity. This is often the first indication of a placental abruption.
3. Contractions that occur approximately every 3 minutes that last for 40 to 60 seconds are the goal of oxytocin use.
4. Contractions that are every 5 minutes and last 60 seconds are not concerning. It could be a sign of hypotonic labor but more information about their strength and the patient's progression is needed to determine that.
TEST-TAKING TIP: If the question requires the identification of a concern and there is only one abnormal option, then that is the best answer even if the reason is unclear.
Content Area: Labor and Birth at Risk—Placenta-Related Complications
Integrated Process: Nursing Process—Assessment
Client Need: Physiological Integrity
Cognitive Level: Application
Concept: Pregnancy
Reference: *Durham, R. F., & Chapman, L. (2014).* Maternal-newborn nursing: The critical components of nursing care. *2nd ed. Philadelphia: F.A. Davis.*

17. **ANSWER: 2, 4, 5**
Rationale
1. Placenta previa is associated with maternal age greater than 35 due to uterine vascularization compromise.
2. Multiple gestation is a risk factor for placenta previa due to increased placental mass.
3. Preterm gestation is not a risk factor for placenta previa.
4. Previous uterine surgery is a risk factor for placenta previa due to uterine scarring.
5. History of abortion is also a risk factor due to uterine scarring.
TEST-TAKING TIP: Risk for labor and birth complications is higher in the obstetric extremes of age. So young mothers (age 16 or younger) and older mothers (age 35 or older) are commonly at risk for complications.
Content Area: Labor and Birth at Risk—Placenta-Related Complications
Integrated Process: Nursing Process—Analysis
Client Need: Physiological Integrity
Cognitive Level: Analysis
Concept: Pregnancy
Reference: *Durham, R. F., & Chapman, L. (2014).* Maternal-newborn nursing: The critical components of nursing care. *2nd ed. Philadelphia: F.A. Davis.*

18. **ANSWER: 4**
Rationale
1. BP less than 90/60 should be reported.
2. Temperatures higher than 100.4°F should be reported.
3. Urine output less than 30 mL/hour should be reported.
4. O_2 saturations during pregnancy should be maintained at 95% or above. An O_2 saturation less than 95% in a woman with placenta previa is suggestive that too much blood has been lost. Exsanguination can occur within 10 minutes if previa bleeding is not controlled.
TEST-TAKING TIP: Due to the extra fluid volume that mothers acquire in the second trimester, a pregnant woman can lose 25% to 30% of her blood volume before signs of hypovolemic shock appear. Therefore, a small change in maternal hemodynamic stability should be taken seriously.
Content Area: Labor and Birth at Risk—Placenta-Related Complications
Integrated Process: Nursing Process—Assessment
Client Need: Physiological Integrity
Cognitive Level: Application
Concept: Pregnancy
Reference: *Durham, R. F., & Chapman, L. (2014).* Maternal-newborn nursing: The critical components of nursing care. *2nd ed. Philadelphia: F.A. Davis.*

19. **ANSWER: 3**
Rationale
1. The woman in this answer choice is not a candidate because of her classical incision.
2. The woman in this answer choice has the right type of incision, but a previous incidence of CPD suggests that her pelvis may be inadequate for a vaginal delivery.
3. The woman who had the low-transverse cesarean section for late decelerations is the best candidate. She has the incision least associated with a uterine rupture, and the reason for her first cesarean is situational and not related to her ability to have a vaginal delivery.
4. The woman in this answer choice is not a candidate because of her vertical incision.
TEST-TAKING TIP: When analyzing risk factors for uterine rupture, vertical (classical) incisions can be ruled out right away. Of the two remaining women, decide which previous indication for a cesarean section is not likely to repeat.
Content Area: Labor and Birth at Risk—Trial of Labor After Cesarean
Integrated Process: Nursing Process—Analysis
Client Need: Health Promotion and Maintenance
Cognitive Level: Analysis
Concept: Pregnancy
Reference: *Durham, R. F., & Chapman, L. (2014).* Maternal-newborn nursing: The critical components of nursing care. *2nd ed. Philadelphia: F.A. Davis.*

20. **ANSWER: 4**
Rationale
1. It is always safer for women attempting a TOLAC to labor without pharmacological assistance. Induction increases the risk of tachysystole and subsequent abruption.
2. Pharmacological cervical ripening agents are contraindicated in women with a previous uterine scar of any type.

3. Pitocin should be used with caution but is not contraindicated during a TOLAC.
4. If cervical ripening is necessary, balloon catheters are an alternative for women who cannot receive prostaglandins.
TEST-TAKING TIP: There are two answer choices present about cervical ripening. Two answer choices about similar things warrant further evaluation. This question requires the tester to determine which one of those two options about cervical ripening is incorrect when concerning a patient requesting TOLAC.
Content Area: Labor and Birth at Risk—Trial of Labor After Cesarean
Integrated Process: Teaching/Learning
Client Need: Health Promotion and Maintenance
Cognitive Level: Application
Concept: Pregnancy
Reference: Durham, R. F., & Chapman, L. (2014). Maternal-newborn nursing: The critical components of nursing care. 2nd ed. Philadelphia: F.A. Davis.

21. **ANSWER: 1**
Rationale
1. All laboring women are potential surgical candidates. In emergencies, cesarean sections are performed under general anesthesia, increasing the risk for aspiration.
2. Diarrhea is unpleasant but is not a complication.
3. Vomiting is common during labor due to decreased gastric motility and vagal nerve stimulation. Avoiding solid foods may help curtail nausea during labor but it is also not a complication.
4. Paralytic ileus is associated with the postoperative period and is not helped by NPO status prior to surgery.
TEST-TAKING TIP: Laboring women is a broad category of patients. Trying to find the things that all laboring women have in common (e.g., pain) will help you identify the correct answer.
Content Area: Labor and Birth at Risk—Cesarean Section Risks
Integrated Process: Nursing Process—Analysis
Client Need: Health Promotion and Maintenance
Cognitive Level: Application
Concept: Pregnancy
Reference: Durham, R. F., & Chapman, L. (2014). Maternal-newborn nursing: The critical components of nursing care. 2nd ed. Philadelphia: F.A. Davis.

22. **ANSWER: 3**
Rationale
1. The lower uterine segment is developed long before 39 weeks, making low-transverse cesarean delivery possible even if the infant is preterm.
2. Oxytocin receptors are numerous by this point as well.
3. Since ultrasounds can underestimate gestational age by up to 2 weeks, waiting until 39 weeks to perform elective inductions reduces the incidence of unintentional preterm delivery.
4. There is no association between precipitous delivery and previous birth before 39 weeks.
TEST-TAKING TIP: If you are not sure whether some answer choices are actually related to the stem or not, try and determine the degree of seriousness associated with each answer. For example, even if the tester thinks that Pitocin

receptors may not be developed until 39 weeks, morbidity related to prematurity would trump the possibility of a failed induction as a concern.
Content Area: Labor and Birth at Risk—Elective Induction
Integrated Process: Nursing Process—Analysis
Client Need: Health Promotion and Maintenance
Cognitive Level: Application
Concept: Pregnancy
Reference: Durham, R. F., & Chapman, L. (2014). Maternal-newborn nursing: The critical components of nursing care. 2nd ed. Philadelphia: F.A. Davis.

23. **ANSWER: 2**
Rationale
1. Minimal variability at this gestational age is common due to neurological immaturity.
2. Abdominal tenderness is one of the first signs of chorioamnionitis. Chorioamnionitis is a serious condition, and findings should be reported to the PCP immediately, with expectations that induction orders will follow. Chorioamnionitis can be the cause of maternal and fetal death if left untreated.
3. Amniotic fluid continues to be reproduced, swallowed, and eliminated by the fetus. It is normal to have a gush of fluid when intra-abdominal pressure increases during position changes.
4. This patient is in the trimester when frequent trips to the bathroom are at their highest.
TEST-TAKING TIP: Infection is always a priority concern when rupture of membranes is not followed by a timely delivery.
Content Area: Labor and Birth at Risk—Amniotomy
Integrated Process: Nursing Process—Assessment
Client Need: Physiological Integrity
Cognitive Level: Application
Concept: Pregnancy
Reference: Durham, R. F., & Chapman, L. (2014). Maternal-newborn nursing: The critical components of nursing care. 2nd ed. Philadelphia: F.A. Davis.

24. **ANSWER: 3**
Rationale
1. There is no intervention needed for absent accelerations.
2. No intervention is needed for moderate variability since it is desirable.
3. Turning the patient to a lateral position relieves vena cava compression, subsequently improving maternal cardiac output and oxygen delivery to the fetus.
4. Early decelerations need no intervention.
TEST-TAKING TIP: Each of the interventions in the answer choices is valid when preserving fetal well-being. The tester must connect the intervention to the change in FHR that it is most appropriate for.
Content Area: Labor and Birth at Risk—Oxytocin Induction
Integrated Process: Nursing Process—Interventions
Client Need: Health Promotion and Maintenance
Cognitive Level: Application
Concept: Pregnancy
Reference: Durham, R. F., & Chapman, L. (2014). Maternal-newborn nursing: The critical components of nursing care. 2nd ed. Philadelphia: F.A. Davis.

25. ANSWER: 4

Rationale

1. HIV-positive women can receive epidural and spinal anesthesia.
2. Scoliosis makes placement of regional anesthesia difficult but is not a contraindication.
3. Lower back tattoos are not an issue unless newly done. Even then the area can usually be avoided.
4. Thrombocytopenia, or low platelets, is a contraindication to epidural or spinal placement.

TEST-TAKING TIP: No woman with a platelet count less than 100,000 cmm can receive regional anesthesia for birth. The inability to clot can encourage hematoma formation that can compress the spinal nerves and cause permanent damage or disability.

Content Area: Labor and Birth at Risk—Anesthesia
Integrated Process: Nursing Process—Assessment
Client Need: Health Promotion and Maintenance
Cognitive Level: Application
Concept: Pregnancy
Reference: Durham, R. F., & Chapman, L. (2014). Maternal-newborn nursing: The critical components of nursing care. 2nd ed. Philadelphia: F.A. Davis.

Postpartum

Nursing Care of the Postpartum Woman

I. Postpartum Care

The **postpartum** period or **puerperium** is the interval between the birth of the newborn and the return of the reproductive organs to their prepregnant state, which is usually 6 weeks. To provide care during this period, the nurse must synthesize knowledge of the maternal anatomy and physiology and the woman's response to the birth of the newborn. This section focuses on the physiological changes of the postpartum period and

the nursing interventions and education that should be implemented.

A. Uterus
   1. Involution of the uterus
      a) The return of the uterus to a prepregnant state after birth is called **involution** (Fig. 17.1). The involution process begins immediately after expulsion of the placenta with contraction of the uterine smooth muscle.

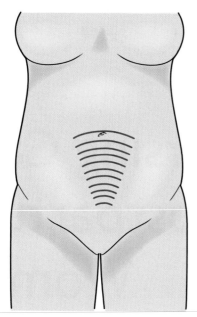

Fig 17.1 Involution of the uterus.

b) After delivery of the placenta, the uterus is in the midline position, approximately 2 cm below the level of the umbilicus.

c) Within 12 hours, the **fundus** portion of the uterus rises to approximately 1 cm above the umbilicus.

d) By 24 hours after birth, the uterus is about the same size as it was at 20 weeks gestation or approximately at the level of the umbilicus.

e) The fundus descends 1 to 2 cm every 24 hours.

f) By the sixth postpartum day, the fundus is normally located halfway between the umbilicus and the symphysis pubis.

g) The uterus should not be palpable abdominally after 2 weeks and should have returned to its prepregnant location by 6 weeks after childbirth.

h) After delivery of the placenta, the decrease in estrogen and progesterone causes a decrease in the pregnancy-induced hypertrophied cells. The additional cells laid down during pregnancy remain and account for the slight increase in uterine size after pregnancy.

2. Contractions

a) Postpartum hemostasis is achieved primarily by compression of intramyometrial blood vessels as the uterine muscle contracts rather than by platelet aggregation and clot formation.

b) The hormone oxytocin, released from the pituitary gland, strengthens and coordinates uterine contractions, promoting hemostasis by compressing the blood vessels. A firm and contracted uterus prevents excessive bleeding and hemorrhage.

c) During the first 1 to 2 hours postpartum, uterine contractions may decrease in intensity and become uncoordinated. Because it is vital that the uterus remain firm and well contracted, exogenous oxytocin (Pitocin) is usually administered intravenously or intramuscularly immediately after expulsion of the placenta.

d) Breastfeeding immediately after birth and in the early postpartum period increases the release of oxytocin, which decreases blood loss and reduces the risk for postpartum hemorrhage.

3. Afterpains

a) **Afterpains** are intermittent contractions, occurring after the delivery of the placenta. These contractions resemble menstrual cramping and help prevent excessive bleeding by compressing the blood vessels in the uterus.

(1) A primipara uterine tone is usually good, so the uterus typically remains firm and the woman generally experiences only mild cramping.

(2) A multipara usually experiences more uterine relaxation due to the repeated overstretching of muscle fibers of previous pregnancy. This loss of muscle tone leads to more vigorous contractions and relaxation of the uterus.

(3) Also at risk for more intense afterpains are women whose uterus has been overstretched from a macrosomic infant, multiple gestation, and polyhydramnios.

(4) Afterpains typically resolve in 3 to 7 days.

4. Placental site

a) Immediately after the placenta and membranes are delivered, vascular compression and thrombosis decrease the placental site. The growth of the endometrium causes sloughing of necrotic tissue and prevents scar formation. This healing process is called *exfoliation* and enables the endometrium to resume its usual cycle of changes, allowing implantation and placental growth in future pregnancies.

MAKING THE CONNECTION

Afterpains During Breastfeeding

Breastfeeding and exogenous oxytocin usually intensify afterpains because both stimulate uterine contractions. Because of the intensity of the pain, some women may choose to stop breastfeeding. It is very important for the nurse to educate and encourage the mother so that she will be successful with breastfeeding. The nurse should advise her to request pain medication 30 minutes prior to breastfeeding to minimize afterbirth pains.

b) Endometrial regeneration is completed by postpartum day 16, except at the placental site, which is not complete until 6 weeks after birth (Table 17.1).
5. Nursing assessment of the uterus
   a) Assess the fundus of the uterus after the third stage of labor for location and tone. To perform this assessment, the nurse should lower the head and foot of the bed so that the patient is in a supine position.

ALERT The nurse must use proper assessment techniques when massaging the uterus. The uterus should always be palpated while supporting the lower uterine segment. Failure to do so may result in uterine inversion and hemorrhage.

   (1) Uterine assessment should be performed:
   - Every 15 minutes for the first hour.
   - Every 30 minutes for the second hour.
   - Every 4 hours for the next 22 hours.
   - Every shift (8 hours) after the first 24 hours.
   - More regularly if the assessment findings are not within normal limits.
   (2) Prior to the assessment of the uterus, it is important for the nurse to:
   - Explain the procedure.
   - Instruct the client to empty her bladder before the procedure.

Table 17.1 Causes That Impede Uterine Involution

Causes	Underlying Pathology
Overdistention of uterus	Overstretching of uterine muscles, as in multiple pregnancies, macrosomic newborns, and hydramnios, can cause uterine atony and excessive bleeding after the cesarean or vaginal delivery.
Grand multiparity	Repeated overstretching of the uterus during pregnancy can lead to diminished tone and muscle relaxation.
Prolonged labor	Muscles become relaxed because of the prolonged time of contraction during labor and may result in decreased response to postpartal administration of Pitocin.
Retained placenta or membranes	A small quantity of tissue affects the ability of the uterus to remain firmly contracted.
Difficult labor and delivery	The uterus may be manipulated excessively, which can lead to muscle relaxation.
Uterine infection	Inflammation interferes with the uterine muscles' ability to contract effectively.
Full bladder	The uterus is pushed up and usually to the right, and the excessive pressure on the uterus interferes with effective contraction.

- Provide privacy.
- Lower the head and foot of the bed so that the client is in a supine position.
   (3) Proper nursing assessment of the uterus should include:
   - Wearing clean gloves.
   - Supporting the lower uterine segment by placing one hand just above the symphysis pubis.
   - Locating the fundus with the other hand using gentle pressure (Fig. 17.2).
   - Determining the tone of the uterus to be either firm (contracted) or soft (boggy).

ALERT A boggy uterus indicates that it is not contracting, which places the woman at risk for excessive blood loss or hemorrhage. The nurse should immediately massage the fundus with the palm of the hand in a circular motion until the uterus is firm and then reevaluate in 30 minutes. If the uterus does not respond to massage, the nurse should give oxytocin according to standing orders and notify the physician or nurse midwife.

   (4) Use a finger to measure the distance between the fundus and umbilicus. Each finger breadth (width) equals 1 cm.
   (5) Determine the position of the uterus (Table 17.2).

ALERT The uterus should be at the midline position. If it has shifted to one side, this may indicate a distended bladder. This can interfere with the ability of the uterus to contract properly and can place the woman at risk for **uterine atony** and an increase for excessive bleeding or hemorrhage. The nurse should immediately assist the woman to the bathroom to void and assist her back to bed. Reassessment of the uterus should be done after the woman is supine in bed.

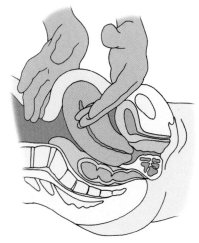

Fig 17.2 Assessment of the postpartum uterus.

Table 17.2 Location, Tone, and Position of Fundus

Day	Location
Immediately after delivery of placenta	Uterine fundus is located at the umbilicus and is firm and at midline.
1 to 2 hours after delivery of placenta	Uterine fundus is midway between umbilicus and symphysis pubis and is firm and at midline.
12 hours after the delivery of placenta	Uterine fundus is located 1 cm above the umbilicus and is firm and at midline.
24 hours after the delivery of placenta	Uterine fundus is located 1 cm below the umbilicus and is firm and at midline.
10 days after delivery of placenta	Uterine fundus descends 1 cm per day and by day 10 the fundus is into the pelvis area and is not palpable.

6. **Lochia** (rubra) is postbirth uterine discharge that is initially bright red and may contain small clots. Lochia rubra progresses to lochia serosa and then to lochia alba. Lochia discharge is like a menstrual discharge and has a musty, stale odor. After birth, the amount of uterine discharge will be like a heavy menstrual period. After that time, the lochia flow will steadily decrease.

7. Nursing assessment of lochia
   a) Lochia should be assessed each time the uterus is assessed. Apply clean gloves, lower the perineal pad, and observe lochia flow as the fundus is palpated.

b) The peri-pad should be inspected and the amount of lochia should be determined, as well as whether clots are found on the pad (Table 17.3).

🛑 **ALERT** Always assess for blood under the woman's buttocks. Although the amount on the perineal pad may be normal for the postpartum day, blood may flow between the buttocks onto the linens beneath the woman. This assessment is essential because excessive bleeding may go undetected.

c) The lochia is assessed as scant, light, moderate, or heavy:
   - Scant is less than 1 inch on the pad.
   - Light is less than 4 inches on the pad.
   - Moderate is less than 6 inches on the pad.
   - Heavy is when the pad is saturated within 1 hour (Fig. 17.3).

🛑 **ALERT** A heavy saturated pad is a sign of excessive bleeding and/or hemorrhage. The nurse should immediately assess the position, tone, and location of the uterus. If the uterus is boggy, the nurse should massage the uterine fundus until firm. If the uterine fundus is firm and heavy bleeding is noted, this may indicate the presence of a genitourinary tract laceration or hematoma (see further discussion in Chapter 18). If the uterus is displaced to the side, the nurse should instruct the patient to void and then reevaluate the uterine fundus. If the fundus is firm, the nurse should apply a clean pad and reevaluate in 15 minutes. If continued bleeding is noted, the nurse should notify the physician or midwife.

(1) Assess for clots on the pad.
   - It is common for the lochia to contain small clots, which occur when the

Table 17.3 Normal Lochia Discharge

Lochia	Time Frame	Appearance	Components	Deviations From Normal
Lochia rubra	1–3 days	Bright red at beginning, then darker red, bloody consistency, clots smaller than a nickel, fleshy odor, moderate to scant amount, increased flow on standing or breastfeeding	Blood with small amounts of mucus, pieces of decidua, epithelial cells, leukocytes, lanugo, or vernix caseosa	Large clots, heavy amount, saturated pads within 15 minutes (sign of hemorrhage), foul odor (sign of infection), placental fragments
Lochia serosa	4–10 days	Pink or brownish, serosanguineous consistency, fleshy odor, scant amount, increased flow during physical activity	Serum, cervical mucus, erythrocytes, leukocytes, pieces of disintegrating decidua, and bacteria	Continuation of rubra stage after 4 days, heavy amount, saturation of pad within 15 minutes (possible hemorrhage), foul odor (sign of infection)
Lochia alba	11–21 days, may persist longer in lactating women	Scant amount, fleshy odor, yellow to white	Leukocytes, decidual cells, epithelial cells, cervical mucus, and bacteria	Bright red bleeding (sign of late postpartum hemorrhage), foul odor (sign of infection)

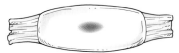

Scant: Blood only on tissue when wiped or 1-inch (2.5-cm) stain on peripad

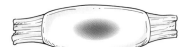

Light: Less than 4-inch (10-cm) stain on peripad

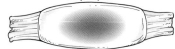

Moderate: Less than 6-inch (15-cm) stain on peripad

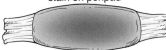

Heavy: Peripad saturated within 1 hour

Fig 17.3 Comparison of scant, light, moderate, and heavy lochia on pad.

lochia has been pooling in the lower uterine segment.

- Small clots (less than the size of a nickel) should be documented in the patient's chart.
- Large clots can interfere with uterine contractions. These clots should be weighed and the findings reported to the physician or midwife. To determine blood loss, weigh the clot in grams. Ten grams equal 10 milliliters of blood loss.
- Clots should be examined for the presence of retained placental tissue, which can inhibit the uterus from contracting efficiently and lead to excessive bleeding and/or hemorrhage.

8. Patient education and discharge teaching concerning the involution of the uterus and risk factors are a very important component of postpartum nursing care. This education must be individualized to the learning capability and readiness of the mother.

a) Involution

(1) Educate the woman on how to monitor and assess her uterus for firmness and about the natural process of involution. For heavy bleeding or a boggy uterus, instruct the patient on how to properly perform fundal massage and to notify the nurse while in the hospital and the physician or midwife after discharge.

(2) Instruct the woman to void frequently to aid in the effectiveness of uterine involution.

(3) Recommend the use of ibuprofen for afterbirth pains.
- Inform the woman that breastfeeding aids in the involution process.
- Instruct the woman to apply a heating pad or lie prone to relieve afterpain. A warm blanket and relaxation techniques help to interfere with the transmission of pain sensations.
- While the client is in the hospital, instruct her to request pain medication 30 minutes prior to breastfeeding to help minimize afterpains from breastfeeding.

b) Lochia

(1) Provide information on the stages of lochia and the variations due to lying or sitting for prolonged periods of time and from excessive exercise.

(2) Instruct the woman to notify the nurse, physician, or nurse midwife of any abnormal variations, such as sudden increase in the amount of lochia, bright red bleeding after rubra stage, or foul odor.

(3) Educate the woman that foul-smelling lochia, increased temperature of 100.4°F or higher, or pelvic or abdominal tenderness indicate a possible infection.

(4) Wash hands before and after performing perineal care.

(5) Teach that perineal hygiene includes frequent voiding and cleansing the perineum from front to back.

(6) Instruct the woman on how to properly use a warm water peri-bottle wash while lochia is present.

MAKING THE CONNECTION

Postpartum Perineal Care

Perineal care after each elimination prevents infection and helps to promote comfort. The client should be instructed to wash her hands before and after changing peri-pads or performing peri-care. Many agencies provide "peri-bottles" that a woman can use to squirt warm tap water over her perineum following elimination. The woman should fill the peri-bottle with warm tap water to approximately 100.4°F (38°C). The woman should be instructed to sit on the toilet seat and position the nozzle of the peri-bottle between her legs. She should then squirt the warm water on her perineum from front to back. To cleanse and dry her perineum, the woman should use moist antiseptic wipes or toilet paper in a blotting (patting) motion, starting in the front of her perineum and proceeding toward the back to prevent contamination from the anal area.

B. Cervix
  1. After delivery of the placenta, the cervix will appear soft, edematous, and dilated and will have little tone. Multiple small lacerations may be seen.
  2. By the end of the first week, the cervix will appear firmer and thicker.
  3. The external os is contracted, only about 1 cm in diameter.
  4. The internal os is close as in the prepregnancy.
  5. The cervix is healed by the fourth to sixth week after delivery.
  6. The external os will remain slightly open and assume a typical transverse slitlike rather than a round shape.
C. Vagina
  1. After a vaginal delivery, the vagina is swollen and has poor tone.
    a) Estrogen increases blood flow to the folds of the vagina so that the elastic connective tissue is better able to expand and stretch during the second stage of labor.
    b) The vagina regains its tone and returns to its original size by the fourth to sixth week of the postpartum period.
    c) The patient can help to improve tone and contractibility of the vaginal orifice by performing Kegel exercises (perineal tightening).
D. Perineum
  1. The perineum is the anatomic area between the urethra, the anus, and the vaginal opening. During the early postpartum period, the soft tissue in and around the perineum may appear edematous, with some bruising. Some women may require a surgical cut called an **episiotomy** when they deliver a baby or the skin may tear (laceration) and require suturing (see Chapter 14 for further discussion).

MAKING THE CONNECTION

Kegel Exercises

Kegel exercises help to tone pelvic muscles. These muscles are weakened by the birth process and should be exercised right after birth. To do Kegel exercise correctly, the woman should gently tighten and then relax the muscles of the perineum (pelvic floor muscles). This can be accomplished while lying down, sitting, or standing. Kegel exercise involves contracting muscles around the vagina (as though stopping the flow of urine), holding tightly for 5 to 10 seconds, and then relaxing for 10 seconds. The woman should work up to 30 contractions relaxation cycles each day. It is important that the nurse encourage and inform the woman that Kegel exercises are difficult at first but will become easier with practice.

Initial healing of the episiotomy or laceration occurs in 2 to 3 weeks after birth.
  2. Nursing assessment
    a) Immediately postdelivery, the perineum should be assessed with the fundus and lochia for redness, edema, ecchymosis, discharge, and approximation of edges of episiotomy or laceration.
      • The nurse should provide privacy and explain the procedure prior to assessing the perineum.
      • Assist the woman to the side-lying position.
      • Lower the peri-pad and separate the buttocks to visualize the perineum. While doing this, assess the rectal area for the presence of hemorrhoids.

DID YOU KNOW?
The nurse should educate the woman concerning the importance of self-evaluation of the perineal area after she is discharged home. Instruct the woman to use a handheld mirror to inspect her perineum for redness, edema, bruising, approximation, and drainage. If the client routinely inspects her perineum, she will be more aware of the changes that could indicate an infection.

  3. Prevention and management
    a) Instruct the client to always wash her hands well before and after cleaning the vaginal area.
    b) In the first 24 hours after delivery, place ice on the perineum to reduce swelling and pain. Ice may be continued at home as needed.
    c) Instruct the woman that when sitting, position squarely on the bed or in the chair, tightening the perineum, buttocks, and thigh muscles. Sitting only on one hip may pull the stitches.
    d) After urination or bowel movements, instruct the woman to cleanse her perineum by squirting warm water from the front to the back toward the rectum. Pat dry with a clean tissue, again from front to back.
    e) Apply clean sanitary pad from the front to back.
    f) For perineal discomfort, instruct the woman that she can place witch hazel pads/compresses between the pad and the stitches (Box 17.1).
    g) Sitz baths may be ordered for three to four times a day for 20 minutes and can be continued at home as needed for comfort.
      (1) A sitz bath is a warm water (102°F to 105°F) bath taken in the sitting position to relieve pain, reduce infection, and promote healing for a woman who has received an episiotomy or experienced a perineal tear during the birthing process (Fig. 17.4).

Box 17.1 **Patient Education and Discharge Teaching**

Instruct the woman how to assess the uterus and the natural process of involution.

Instruct the woman how to massage her uterus if boggy and instruct her to notify the nurse while in the hospital and the physician or midwife after discharge. Excessive lochia (saturating more than one pad in an hour) may indicate hemorrhage.

Provide information about afterpains and comfort measures such as emptying the bladder frequently. A full bladder displaces the uterus, so it cannot contract as well as it should. A warm blanket to the abdomen and relaxation techniques help to interfere with the transmission and sensation of pain.

Provide information on the stages of lochia and the variations due to lying or sitting for prolonged periods of time and from excessive exercise.

Instruct the woman to notify the nurse, physician, or midwife of any abnormal variations such as sudden increase in the amount of lochia, bright red bleeding after rubra stage, or foul odor.

Teach that foul-smelling lochia, temperature of 100.4°F (38°C) or higher, or pelvic or abdominal tenderness indicate a possible infection.

Instruct woman to change peri-pad often, apply peri-pad from front to back, wash hands before and after changing pads.

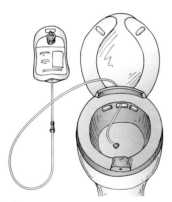

Fig 17.4 Sitz bath.

    h) A topical agent such as Dermoplast Spray may be used for the relief of perineal discomfort. The nurse should instruct the woman to:
- Clean the affected areas first, then simply spray on the area while holding the can 6 to 12 inches away.
- Advise the woman to apply the topical agent after a sitz bath or perineal care.

E. Cardiovascular system
1. After delivery, dramatic changes occur to the circulating blood volume, resulting from the elimination of placental circulation and an increase in venous return. The increase is responsible for profound diuresis in early postpartum and a fall in hematocrit.

Early postpartum time is the greatest risk for heart failure in patients with cardiac disease or limited cardiac reserve.
2. Hematocrit drops because of blood loss during actual delivery. It then usually rises by the third to seventh postpartum day unless substantial blood loss has occurred.
   a) The average blood loss from a vaginal delivery is approximately 300 to 500 mL (10% of blood volume).
   b) The average blood loss from a cesarean is 500 mL to 1,000 mL (15% to 30% of blood volume).
     (1) The diuresis evident between the second and fifth days postpartum plus the blood loss at birth act to reduce the added blood volume the woman accumulated during pregnancy. This reduction occurs so rapidly that by the first or second week postpartum, the blood volume has returned to its normal prepregnancy level.
     (2) The rule of thumb for blood loss is a 2-point drop in hematocrit means blood loss of 500 mL.
3. Cardiac output, which increased during pregnancy, may increase even higher for up to 60 minutes following delivery and can remain elevated for at least 48 hours (this applies for both vaginal and cesarean births).
   a) Cardiac output will rapidly decrease in the first 2 weeks postpartum.
   b) The return of cardiac output to the prepregnancy level takes about 24 weeks.
4. Vital signs during the postpartum period is a critical indication of how the woman's body is adjusting to her prepregnancy state. Vital signs can alert the nurse to high-risk situations such as infection and hemorrhage.
   a) Blood pressure, respiration, and pulse should be taken every 15 minutes during the first hour after vaginal childbirth, then every 30 minutes during the second hour, once during the third hour, and then every 8 hours until discharge.
   b) Temperature should be taken after birth and then in 1 hour. Temperature assessment should then follow the same time frame as the blood pressure, pulse, and respiration. For a cesarean birth, vital signs should be assessed every 30 minutes for 4 hours, then every hour for 3 hours, and then every 8 hours.
   c) Blood pressure should remain consistent with pregnancy baselines. **Orthostatic hypotension** or the feeling of faintness or dizziness immediately after standing can develop in the first 48 hours as a result of splanchnic engorgement that sometimes occurs after birth.

MAKING THE CONNECTION

Orthostatic Hypotension

Orthostatic hypotension is a sudden drop in blood pressure when standing up from a sitting position or when standing up from a lying position. Gravity causes blood to pool in the lower extremities whenever standing. The body compensates for this by increasing the heart rate and constricting blood vessels, thereby ensuring enough blood return to the brain. In individuals with orthostatic hypotension, this compensating mechanism fails and blood pressure falls, leading to symptoms of dizziness, light-headedness, blurred vision, and fainting. During the first few hours after birth, women may have some orthostatic hypotension. This will cause her to have a lower blood pressure reading in a sitting position. Orthostatic hypotension can develop in the first 48 hours as a result of splanchnic engorgement due to the pooling of blood within the blood vessels of the stomach cavity following the birth. The nurse can ensure an accurate blood pressure reading by taking the woman's blood pressure in the same arm and in the same position each time. The best position is to have the client lie on her back with her arm at her side. Because of the increased risk for orthostatic hypotension, the nurse should assist the client the first few times she attempts to get out of bed.

d) Pulse ranging from 50 to 70 beats per minute (bpm) is common during the first 6 to 10 days.
   (1) Tachycardia is related to increased blood loss, temperature elevation, or difficult, prolonged labor and birth.
e) Respiration rate is decreased because of a decrease in intra-abdominal pressure and should remain within the normal range of 12 to 20 respirations per minute.
   (1) Elevated respirations may occur because of pain, fear, exertion, or excessive blood loss.

DID YOU KNOW?

Some women experience shaking chills immediately after childbirth. This physiological response results from pressure changes in the abdomen after the sudden release of pressure on the pelvic nerves and temperature readjustments after the **diaphoresis** of labor. These shaking chills can be uncomfortable. The nurse should reassure the client that this is a normal response and self-limiting. The nurse can provide comfort measures by covering the woman with a warmed blanket.

5. White blood cell (WBC) count increases during labor, resulting in a marked leukocytosis (up to 20,000 to 30,000/μL) in the first 24 hours postpartum. WBC count returns to normal within 1 week.

DID YOU KNOW?

Increased WBCs up to 30,000/mm³ does not necessarily mean infection; however, this increase may also mask the signs of an infection. An increase greater than 30% in 6 hours indicates pathology.

6. Coagulation factors and fibrinogen are increased (hypercoagulability) during pregnancy and remain elevated in the immediate postpartum period. This hypercoagulability aids in reducing the risk of hemorrhage during delivery and the postpartum period.
   a) Damaged vessels, immobility, and hypercoagulability puts the postpartum woman at an increased risk for thromboembolism, especially after cesarean birth.
   b) It is very important for the nurse to assess and educate the client about the risk for deep vein thrombosis in the lower extremities.
      (1) Examine for the presence of warm, red, painful, and/or edematous areas.
      (2) Assess for adequate circulation by checking the pedal pulses and noting temperature and color in both lower extremities.
      (3) Pedal edema is normally present for several days after delivery as fluids in the body shift. However, lasting edema should be reported for further assessment.
      (4) The client should be encouraged to ambulate as soon as possible after delivery. Early ambulation will help to improve circulation and prevent the development of thrombi.
      (5) Instruct to avoid crossing the legs for long periods of time and to keep the legs elevated while sitting.
      (6) Educate and encourage the woman to wear sequential compression devices after delivery if ordered by the physician/midwife.
7. Varicosities may occur because the venous return relies on valves to maintain unidirectional blood flow returning to the heart. Venous blood return is more passive, relying on valves to prevent retrograde flow. Pregnancy creates changes in a woman's vein valve leaflets and inhibits the normal venous flow.
   a) Varicosities can occur in the anus (hemorrhoids), vulva, labia, and legs.
   b) Total regression of varicosities is usually noted after childbirth.
F. Endocrine system
   1. Estrogen and progesterone levels drop rapidly after the delivery of the placenta and reach their lowest levels at 1 week. Decreased estrogen levels are associated with the diuresis of excess extracellular fluid added during pregnancy.

2. Menstruation usually resumes at 7 to 9 weeks for nonlactating women, with 70% experiencing a menstrual period by 12 weeks; the first cycle is usually anovulatory.
   a) The return of ovulation and menstruation are prolonged in lactating women and affected by the length of time the woman breastfeeds and whether formula supplements are used. This time may vary from 2 to 18 months.
G. Urinary system
   1. Urinary output increases the first 12 to 24 hours due to postpartum diuresis. The kidneys must eliminate an estimated 2,000 to 3,000 mL of extracellular fluid. This causes rapid filling of the bladder.
      a) Within 12 hours after delivery, the woman will experience profuse diaphoresis because of the decrease in estrogen. This diaphoresis will usually occur at night and will last for about 2 to 3 days.
      b) Increased bladder capacity and decreased bladder tone can lead to decreased sensation and increased risk of urinary retention and infection.
   2. Nursing assessment
      a) Assess the status of the woman's bladder on admission. The postpartum woman can show signs of bladder distention as soon as 1 to 2 hours after birth.
      b) Review the labor/birth history to detect any risk factors (see Chapter 16).
      c) Ask the woman if she has a normal sensation to void or is experiencing any discomfort or difficulty when voiding.
      d) Signs of urinary retention may include:
         • Difficulty initiating a void.
         • Feeling of bladder fullness after voiding.
         • Dribbling of urine postmicturition.
         • Frequent voiding with small void amounts.
         • Poor flow rate with straining to void.

MAKING THE CONNECTION

Postpartum Bladder Changes
The bladder is a hormone-responsive organ, and its functions are directly related to the fluctuation of hormones during pregnancy and in the postpartum period. Immediately after delivery of the newborn, the bladder becomes hypotonic and can remain so for several days. This reduced tone is a result of physiological hormonal changes such as elevated progesterone levels during normal pregnancy. Because of physiological hormonal changes and possible trauma to the bladder, pelvic floor muscles, and nerves during delivery, the bladder becomes susceptible to retention.

• Urinating more than 2 times a night that is not related to baby feeding.
   e) Check and document the frequency and volume passed with each void.
      (1) For vaginal deliveries, the first void should be no later than 4 to 6 hours after birth; if cesarean birth, it should be no later than 4 to 6 hours after indwelling catheter is removed.
      (2) The postpartum woman may be asymptomatic, especially if she has had an epidural. In some cases, she may have overflow incontinence due to bladder overdistention.
   3. Prevention and management
      a) Encourage voiding every 2 to 3 hours in the immediate postpartum
      b) Supportive measures:
         • Assist patient to bathroom and offer privacy
         • Run water from faucet while patient is trying to void
         • Offer a warm shower
         • Have woman immerse hands in water
         • Encourage ambulation
         • Provide hot tea or fluids of woman's choice
         • Medicate for perineal pain

ALERT Urinary retention can lead to urinary tract infections (UTIs). The nurse should assess the postpartum client for signs of UTI, including tenderness over the costovertebral angle, fever, urinary frequency and/or urgency, and difficult or painful urination. The bladder can become distended and displace the uterus upward and to the side. This prevents the uterine muscles from contracting properly and can lead to a postpartum hemorrhage. Therefore, health care providers must carefully monitor bladder distention, the firmness of the fundus, and bleeding during the postpartum period.

H. Gastrointestinal system
   1. After delivery, the client has decreased gastrointestinal muscle tone and motility due to the effects of progesterone, decreased physical activity, and dehydration from fluid loss during labor. This puts the client at a high risk for constipation.
   2. Women are generally hungry and thirsty after delivery. Food and fluid intake is restricted during labor.
      a) The diaphoresis that occurs during the postpartum period may also lead to increased thirst.
      b) Bowel tone is sluggish as a result of elevated progesterone levels. Some women may be hesitant to have a bowel movement due to pain in the perineal area caused by episiotomy, lacerations, or hemorrhoids.

3. Nursing assessment
   a) Assess bowel sounds each shift
   b) Assess for constipation
      - Question client daily about bowel movements, bloating, abdominal discomfort, and nausea.
      - Observe for signs of distension
   c) Assess for **hemorrhoids,** which can become aggravated by the constipation that commonly follows delivery. They may become swollen and tender, sometimes itch, and may bleed.
4. Prevention and management
   - Encourage early and frequent ambulation
   - Encourage increased fluids and fiber
   - Educate woman to avoid straining
   - Normal bowel patterns should return in 1 to 2 weeks
   a) Health care providers may prescribe stool softeners and/or laxatives to treat constipation and provide perineal comfort during defecation. Docusate is used for the prevention of constipation by promoting the incorporation of water into the stool, resulting in softening and easier passage of stool.
      (1) The nurse should assess for abdominal distention and presence of bowel sounds.
      (2) Administer stool softener with full glass of water or juice; however, softener may be administered on an empty stomach for more rapid results.
   b) To relieve the pain and discomfort of hemorrhoids, educate the woman to:
      - Practice good hygiene, because fecal matter or mucus drainage irritates the skin and hemorrhoid area.
      - Apply an ice pack for 20 to 30 minutes, several times a day as needed for swelling and comfort.
      - Take sitz baths in warm or iced water. Lie down for 15 minutes after a sitz bath.
      - Use witch hazel pads, which can relieve itching, discomfort, irritation, and burning caused by hemorrhoids.
      - Use stool softeners to ease constipation.
      - Drink 8 to 10 glasses of water.
      - Eat unpeeled fruit and vegetables and whole grains to avoid constipation.
      - Avoid using dry toilet paper; instead use hypoallergenic baby wipes or flushable wet wipes.
      - Ask the physician or midwife for a prescription for hemorrhoid medication if these measures do not increase the client's comfort.

I. Breasts
1. After delivery, there is a significant decrease in estrogen and progesterone levels, resulting in the rise of the effects of prolactin.
   a) During pregnancy, **prolactin** also rises; however, lactation is inhibited because of the high levels of estrogen and progesterone.
   b) Before milk production begins, the breasts secrete colostrum, a thin, yellowish fluid that helps maintain the blood glucose level in the breastfeeding infant.
   c) Nipple stimulation by the infant causes the release of the hormone oxytocin from the posterior pituitary gland, which triggers the release of the hormone prolactin from the anterior pituitary.
   d) Prolactin initiates milk production, and the breasts become full (engorged), warm, and tender between postpartum days 3 and 4.
2. Nursing assessment
   a) The first 2 days after delivery, the breasts should be soft and nontender. Changes after the first 2 days depend on whether the client is breastfeeding.
   b) Assessment of the client's breasts whether breastfeeding or not should be performed with each shift assessment.
   c) Inspect the breasts for:
      - Size, symmetry, and shape.
      - Dimpling or thickening.
      - Problems such as flat or retracted nipples.
      - Signs of nipple trauma such as redness, blisters, or fissures.
   d) Gently palpate each breast for firmness and tenderness.
      - Firmness or tenderness indicates increased vascular and lymphatic circulation that may precede milk production.
      - Nodules or "lumpy" breasts also indicate the lobes are beginning to produce milk.
3. Prevention and management
   a) While performing the breast assessment, the nurse should also provide information about breast care.
   b) Care of the breast when breastfeeding
      (1) Wash breasts each day with warm water in the shower or bath. Avoid using soaps, which can cause dry, cracked, and irritated skin. Soaps remove the natural oils produced by the Montgomery glands, which clean and moisturize the nipples and areola.
      (2) Wear a nursing bra or a regular bra that provides support. Cotton fabric is best because it allows the skin to breathe.
      (3) Instruct on proper infant latch and to breastfeed at least every 2 to 3 hours (see Chapter 20).

(4) Proper latch helps to prevent the development of painful breast problems, such as sore nipples, **engorgement,** plugged ducts, and mastitis.

(5) If the client is using breast pads to control leaking breasts, instruct her to change often to prevent sore nipples, thrush, or mastitis.

(6) Instruct the client that she can moisturize her nipples and areola after breastfeeding by rubbing some of her breast milk on them and letting them air-dry. Instruct the client on how to properly remove the newborn from the breast so that trauma to the breast will not occur—that is, the client should place a finger in the corner of the newborn's mouth to break the suction between the infant's mouth and the breast.

(7) If sore nipples develop, instruct the woman to talk to physician/midwife or lactation consultant about using purified lanolin to help soothe the breasts. Do not use any lotions, creams, or sprays without first discussing it with the health care provider, as many products can harm the infant, clog milk ducts, or irritate the skin.

(8) If engorgement develops, instruct the client that frozen cabbage leaves can be placed onto hard, swollen breasts to reduce inflammation and relieve pain. It is theorized that frozen cabbage leaves help decrease tissue congestion by dilating capillaries, which improves the blood flow in and out of the area, allowing the body to reabsorb the fluid trapped in the breasts. Cabbage may also have a type of drawing or wicking action that helps move trapped fluid.

(9) Instruct the woman to continue to perform monthly self-breast examinations even while nursing. Breasts may feel lumpy when full of milk, but the lumps should go away with breastfeeding, pumping, or massaging the breasts. If a lump is noticed and does not diminish on its own within a few days, the woman should contact her physician or midwife.

c) Women who choose not to breastfeed will also experience milk production; however, lactation can be suppressed.

(1) To suppress lactation, instruct the woman to wear a well-fitted bra at all times (even while sleeping) until her breasts become soft.

(2) Avoid any type of nipple stimulation or heat to the breasts, such as warm or hot showers in which the water is allowed to run continuously over the breasts. Breasts that are stimulated or emptied will continue to make milk and will be painful.

(3) Apply ice pack, gel pack, or package of frozen vegetables wrapped in a cloth to the breasts for 15 to 20 minutes every 1 to 2 hours while awake to ease breast discomfort. It generally takes 5 to 7 days for the breasts to stop producing milk.

J. Musculoskeletal system

1. The pelvic ligaments and joints relax during pregnancy. This relaxation is a direct result of the increase in the hormone **relaxin.** After delivery, relaxin levels decrease and return to their prepregnant state. The joints of the feet remain changed, and many women notice a permanent increase in shoe size.

2. During pregnancy, the growing uterus stretches the muscles in the abdomen, causing the muscles that meet in the middle of the abdomen to separate. This separation is called *diastasis recti* or *diastasis recti abdominis.*

   a) This develops in late pregnancy but is usually noticeable after delivery.

   b) Muscle separation often lessens in the months that follow. However, some degree of separation might remain for up to a year after childbirth and beyond (Fig. 17.5).

K. Integumentary system

1. Melanocyte-stimulating hormone (MSH) is responsible for the hyperpigmentation that occurs during pregnancy.

   a) Skin changes caused by increased MSH revert back to the prepregnant state or are permanently altered.

   • Mask of pregnancy (chloasma) usually disappears, and stretch marks (striae gravidarum) and linea nigra fade but generally do not go away.

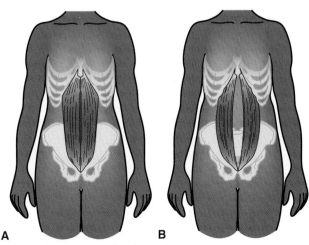

A   **B**

Fig 17.5 Diastasis recti abdominis.

- Hair loss may occur during the postpartum period but usually resolves without the need for intervention.
L. Immune system
  1. There are few changes in the immune system during the postpartum period.
  2. Rh-negative clients should receive Rh immune globulin within 72 hours of delivery to prevent maternal antibody production in response to the Rh-positive antigen received from infants during pregnancy or birth (see Chapter 16).
  3. The rubella vaccine should also be administered to postpartum clients who tested nonimmune or had a rubella titer less than 1:10 prior to delivery.
     - Inform the client that the vaccination is given to prevent fetal anomalies in subsequent pregnancies.
     - The rubella vaccine is a live virus and is contraindicated during pregnancy.
     - The vaccine is administered as a single-dose subcutaneous injection.
     - Inform the client that she may have burning or stinging at the injection site.
     - The vaccine is contraindicated if the client has a sensitivity to neomycin, is immunosuppressed, or has received blood transfusions within the last 3 months.
     - Instruct the client to avoid becoming pregnant for the 4 weeks following the administration of the vaccine.[1]
M. Nursing care for the woman experiencing a cesarean birth
  1. The nursing care for women who undergo a cesarean birth is the same as for women who give birth vaginally. However, nursing care should also include assessments and interventions similar to a patient who has undergone abdominal surgery.
     a) Assist the mother to turn, cough, and take deep breaths. This assists in preventing the pooling of secretions in the lungs.
        - Instruct the woman to hug a pillow snugly against her incision to splint it and reduce the pain and pressure over the incision when she coughs and takes deep breaths.
        - Encourage the client to use an incentive spirometer to help expand the lungs to prevent pneumonia.
        - Encourage the client to flex her knees and to move her feet frequently while in bed to help improve peripheral circulation and to prevent thrombi.
        - Sequential compression devices will probably be ordered to prevent the pooling of blood in the lower extremities.
     b) Constipation is common after any abdominal surgery and is also a side effect of pain medications. Encourage the client to take a stool softener, eat high-fiber foods, and increase activity and ambulation (as ordered by the physician and midwife) each postpartum day.
     c) Instruct the client to rest as much as she can and avoid lifting anything heavier than her newborn.
     d) Reassure the client that mothers who have had a cesarean birth are just as successful at breastfeeding as women who have given birth vaginally.
        - Prescribed pain medications are safe to take while breastfeeding and should be taken as directed to remain comfortable.
        - To increase her comfort during breastfeeding, advise the client to use a pillow to position her baby away from the incision.
     e) Instruct the client to notify her physician or midwife if her incision opens or if it becomes sore and red, has greenish-yellow drainage, or bleeds.

II. Psychological Postpartum Adaptations

A major psychological task for the parents is the process of bonding and attachment with their newborn. Nurses are in an exceptional position to observe and offer support and reassurance. Encouragement and education can help to change negative bonding behaviors and reinforce the positive maternal–infant adaptations. Bonding and attachment are the basis for a strong and healthy family relationship.

A. Restorative period

There are three phases a mother will go through after delivery, from the time of delivery to 4 to 6 weeks postpartum:
  1. Taking-in phase: This lasts approximately 1 to 2 days. During this phase, the mother is focused primarily on her own needs, especially sleeping and eating. She will often be passive and dependent.
     a) This behavior is often a reaction to the concentrated physical energy expended during labor and delivery.
     b) During this time, the mother may have limited interactions, such as using her fingertip to touch her infant or holding her infant in the **en face** position (being face-to-face, approximately 8 inches apart and on the same plane).

1 Centers for Disease Control and Prevention. (2013). Prevention of measles, rubella, congenital rubella syndrome and mumps, 2013: Summary recommendations of the advisory committee on immunization (ACIIP). Retrieved from http://www.cdc.gov/mmWr/preview/mmwrhtml/rr6204a1.htm.

c) During this period, the mother will talk about her delivery experience, which enables her to integrate the birth of her infant with reality.

2. Taking-hold phase: This lasts for about 10 days and is when the woman is striving for independence and autonomy.

   a) The woman's focus of concern is about her bodily functions, such as her bladder, bowels, taking care of her infant, and, if breastfeeding, the amount and quality of her breast milk. This phase may be associated with a great deal of anxiety and mood swings because of trying to accomplish tasks.

3. Letting-go phase: This is the last phase. The woman is trying to realize and accept the physical separation of the infant from her body and to adjust her life and that of the family's to dependency of her infant.

   a) The woman may experience **postpartum blues** caused by hormonal changes that occur during the postpartum period (see Chapter 18). Common manifestations may be irritability, tears, loss of appetite, and difficulty sleeping.

   b) The woman may feel guilty about her emotional displays because she cannot identify why she is crying.

   c) Provide privacy for a crying mother. Let her know there is nothing wrong with her behavior. Crying may even be therapeutic.

B. Nursing assessment

1. The nurse should observe maternal–infant behavior, which should be documented in the mother's and infant's chart. Inappropriate behavior should be viewed on an individual basis and reported to the appropriate health care member.

   a) Positive bonding/attachment signs:
   - Touching
   - Holding
   - Kissing
   - Cuddling
   - Talking and singing
   - Choosing the en face position
   - Expressing pride in the infant and attributing characteristics to family members
   - Attempting to evoke a smile or vocal response from her baby

   b) Negative bonding/attachment signs:
   - Refusing to look at the infant
   - Refusing to touch or hold the infant
   - Refusing to name the infant
   - Finding the infant unattractive or ugly
   - Refusing to respond or responding negatively to infant cues such as crying or smiling

C. Nursing prevention and management

1. Plan nursing activities so that the woman can rest as much as possible; failure to allow the woman to receive adequate rest may lead to irritability, fatigue, and general interference with the normal restorative process.

2. Provide guidance, instruction, and demonstration to woman on self- and infant care. The nurse should allow the client to care for her newborn and reinforce all positive actions.

3. Recognize and interpret the mother's behavior on an individual basis. Not all women act or react the same. The nurse should understand there may be underlying factors influencing the mother's behavior that may not be apparent, such anesthesia, pain, a traumatic birthing experience, cultural beliefs, or current social situation.

CASE STUDY: Putting It All Together

Mrs. Smith, age 30, just delivered 1.5 hours ago and is now a gravida 5, para 5. She was in labor for 30 hours when she delivered a male infant weighing 9 lb, 9 oz. Mrs. Smith was induced with oxytocin at 40 weeks gestation. She had originally wanted to have her baby without any pain medication; however, after 20 hours of labor she asked and received an epidural. During birth, Mrs. Smith sustained a second-degree laceration, which was repaired. Breastfeeding was initiated after delivery. Mrs. Smith states that she is very tired and can't wait to just rest. She has no known allergies and this pregnancy was without complications. Your nursing assessment indicates the following:

Vital Signs
BP: 128/65
Pulse: 75 bpm
Respirations: 15
Temperature: 98.6°F
Level of conscious: Awake, alert, and oriented x3
Uterus: Fundus firm, midline, at umbilicus
Lochia: Moderate rubra with dime-sized clots
Pain scale: 6 out of 10. Patient states, "My bottom hurts and I am cramping so bad!"
Intravenous infusions: Patient has received a total of 2,500 mL of Lactated Ringer's (LR). She is currently receiving her second bag of LR (1,000 mL) with 20 units of Pitocin (exogenous oxytocin).
Urinary output: Has not voided since 4 hours prior to delivery
Extremities postepidural: able to move all extremities
Patient: "I am really tired. I have been up for two nights."

Case Study Questions

1. What findings would warrant further assessment?

2. What intervention should the nurse institute?

REVIEW QUESTIONS

Be sure to read the Introduction for valuable test-taking tips.

1. A postpartum patient comes to the clinic for her 6-week postpartum checkup. When assessing the patient's cervix, how should the nurse expect the cervix to appear?
   1. Noticeable small lacerations
   2. Approximately 3 cm dilated
   3. Symmetrically round external os
   4. Firm and thick

2. A nurse is preparing to perform a fundal assessment on a postpartum client who delivered 12 hours ago. What should the nurse do *first*?
   1. Lower the head of the bed
   2. Locate the level of the fundus
   3. Assist the woman to the bathroom to empty her bladder
   4. Massage the fundus

3. The nurse is assessing her patient, who is 1 day postpartum. The nurse notes that the fundus is firm and at midline, the lochia is moderate in amount, and the presence of rubra with two dime-sized clots is on her peri-pad. What should the nurse determine from these assessment findings?
   1. They are normal.
   2. They indicate the presence of infection.
   3. The physician should be notified of the abnormal findings.
   4. The patient should be instructed to increase her fluid intake.

4. The physician has ordered the rubella vaccine to be given to a postpartum woman who is being discharged. Which should be included when providing education about the vaccine to the woman?
   1. Breastfeeding is contraindicated.
   2. The woman should avoid becoming pregnant after receiving the vaccine.
   3. The vaccine can safely be given to women with egg allergies.
   4. The woman must be separated from her infant for 24 hours after receiving the vaccine.

5. A woman who is 4 days postdelivery calls the nurse's station and states that she is feeling faint and dizzy. Which is an appropriate nursing action?
   1. Notify the physician.
   2. Elevate the woman's legs.
   3. Administer oxygen to increase oxygen concentration.
   4. Instruct the woman to request help when getting up.

6. The nurse is preparing to do a morning assessment on a 24-hour postpartum patient. Which nursing intervention is *most* appropriate initially?
   1. Massage the fundus until it is firm.
   2. Instruct the mother to void prior to the assessment.
   3. Assess the lochia flow while massaging the fundus.
   4. Lower the head of the bed and have the mother lie flat.

7. A nurse is taking care of a G2P2 woman with a third-degree perineal tear during the fourth stage of labor. The nurse should include which intervention in the plan of care during her 12-hour shift?
   1. Assess vital signs every 4 hours.
   2. Keep patient NPO for first 12 hours.
   3. Catheterize patient prior to first ambulation.
   4. Prepare ice pack for application to perineal area.

8. The nurse is educating a postpartum woman on how to prevent engorgement. Which action of the patient indicates effective learning?
   1. Breastfeeding the infant every 2 to 3 hours
   2. Avoiding using soap on the breast when bathing
   3. Drinking 8 to 10 glasses of water during the day
   4. Binding the breast with a towel or stretch bandage

9. Which *best* represents the process of postpartum diuresis in a postpartum client?
   1. A nervous response to vasomotor changes
   2. Elimination of excess fluid through the skin
   3. Underarm perspiration that occurs after ambulation
   4. Loss of fluid from expulsion of the placenta and amniotic fluid

10. A nurse is providing postpartum care to a G4P4 woman who gave birth vaginally 48 hours ago to a 9 pound 10 ounce boy with only a pudendal block for anesthesia. The physician has written orders for the woman to have a sitz bath three times a day. Which information is *most* closely correlated with the order?
    1. The woman is multiparous.
    2. The woman has an episiotomy.
    3. The woman had a vaginal birth.
    4. The woman received a pudendal block for anesthesia.

11. The nurse receives a telephone call from a woman who has given birth 3 days ago. The woman states, "I am afraid that something is wrong because I have not had a bowel movement since I had my baby. I usually go every day." Which response by the nurse is appropriate?
    1. Instruct the woman to rest more often.
    2. Assure the woman that it will happen soon.
    3. Instruct the woman to come in to see the physician.
    4. Encourage the woman to add dried fruits to cereals, yogurts, and salads.

12. The nurse is educating the postpartum client on lactation suppression. Which instructions to the client regarding lactation suppression should be included? *Select all that apply.*
    1. "Take warm showers twice a day."
    2. "Pump each breast three times a day."
    3. "Apply a heating pad to each breast."
    4. "Apply ice packs to the axillary area of each breast."
    5. "Wear a well-fitting bra for the first 5 to 6 days."

13. The nurse is providing education to a postpartum woman about exercises to strengthen the pelvis musculature. Which instruction should be included?
    1. "Ambulate three times a day."
    2. "Perform Kegel exercises."
    3. "Enroll in an aerobics class after discharge."
    4. "Do passive range-of-motion exercises while lying in bed."

14. A breastfeeding postpartum woman tells the nurse, "I am not sure I want to breastfeed because I notice that when I feed my baby, I have strong contraction-like pain. Is something wrong?" Which response by the nurse is *most* appropriate?
    1. "I will call the doctor and let him know your concern."
    2. "You may be getting an infection and will have to stop breastfeeding."
    3. "This is normal because your uterus is shrinking back to the normal size."
    4. "The baby's sucking during breastfeeding releases the hormone oxytocin, which stimulates the uterus to contract."

15. A postpartum woman is having difficulty voiding for the first time after giving birth. Which actions should be effective to stimulate voiding? *Select all that apply.*
    1. Encourage ambulation.
    2. Pour cold water over her perineal area.
    3. Run water from faucet while woman is trying to void.
    4. Ensure that the woman has a bedpan within reach.
    5. Provide medications as prescribed by physician/midwife.

16. The nurse is educating a new postpartum woman about peri-care. Which action by the client indicates understanding?
    1. The woman applied her peri-pad from back to front.
    2. The woman performed peri-care three times a day.
    3. The woman washed her hands before and after performing peri-care.
    4. The woman mixed tap water and hydrogen peroxide in her peri-bottle.

17. Which statement should alert the nurse to the possibility of ineffective bonding between mother and newborn?
    1. "My baby has my eyes."
    2. "No one in my family has that big of a nose."
    3. "Where did he get those long fingers?"
    4. "Is it normal for him to sleep so much?"

18. Upon discharge on the fourth postpartum day, the nurse is assessing a postpartum woman. Which observations about the woman would the nurse be *most* likely to make?
    1. The woman states that she is very hungry and asking when she can eat.
    2. The woman wants to talk about her birth experience.
    3. The woman is crying and does not know why.
    4. The woman requests information about feeding and dressing her baby.

19. A G1P1 has just experienced a 24-hour labor that included a 3-hour second stage. The woman states to the nurse, "I just can't feed my baby now. All I want to do is sleep." What is the appropriate response from the nurse?
    1. Discuss with the woman that the needs of her infant should come first
    2. Recognize this as a behavior of the taking-hold stage
    3. Record the behavior as ineffective bonding/attachment
    4. Reassure the woman that it is okay for her to rest at this time

20. Which nursing care goal is the *highest priority* for a woman who had a vaginal delivery 3 hours earlier?
    1. The client will wear a well-supported bra.
    2. The client will eat 100% of her meals.
    3. The client will have a moderate lochia flow.
    4. The client will ambulate to the bathroom.

REVIEW QUESTIONS ANSWERS

1. ANSWER: 4

Rationale

1. There should be no evidence of lacerations. The cervix heals by the fourth to sixth week after delivery.
2. After delivery, the cervix constricts rapidly and regains its shape by the end of the first week. The os of the cervix never closes completely and usually remains about 1 cm dilated.
3. After birth, the mouth of the cervix will be somewhat wider, with a transverse slit shape.
4. Immediately after birth, the cervix appears soft and edematous and has little tone. However, by the end of the first week the cervix is firmer and thicker.

TEST-TAKING TIP: The cervix is the lowermost portion of the uterus. Cylindrical in shape, the cervix consists of the inner os (endocervix) and the outer os (ectocervix). The outer os is the portion of the cervix that is visible through the vaginal canal and is the area swabbed during a Pap smear. The inner os is the canal-like portion of the cervix that opens into the uterus. The size, shape, and color of the cervix depends on the woman's age, hormonal state, and whether or not she has given birth. For women who have not given birth, the cervix appears to have a small circular opening (external os). In women who have given birth, the cervix is thicker and the external os has a more slitlike shape.

Content Area: Cervix/Nursing Care of the Postpartum Woman
Integrated Process: Nursing Process—Assessment
Client Need: Health Promotion and Maintenance
Cognitive Level: Application
Concept: Pregnancy
Reference: London, M. L., Ladewig, P. A., Davidson, M. R., Ball, J. W., Bindler, R. C., & Cowen, K. J. (2014). Maternal & child nursing care. 4th ed. New Jersey: Pearson.

2. ANSWER: 3

Rationale

1. The nurse should lower the head and foot of the bed so that the woman is in a supine position with knees flexed prior to the assessment.
2. During the assessment, the nurse assesses the firmness of the fundus and should massage if the uterus is boggy or there is excessive bleeding.
3. Before assessing the uterine fundus, the nurse should encourage the patient to void before palpation of the uterine fundus because a full bladder displaces the uterus and can lead to excessive bleeding. Having the patient empty her bladder prior will provide a more accurate assessment.
4. During the assessment, the nurse should only massage the fundus if the uterus is boggy or there is excessive bleeding. The nurse should massage the fundus gently until firm.

TEST-TAKING TIP: Changes during pregnancy cause the bladder of postpartum women to have increased capacity and decreased muscle tone. During labor, the urethra, bladder, and tissue around the urinary meatus may become swollen and bruised as the presenting part (usually the fetal head) passes beneath the bladder. This may result in decreased sensitivity to pressure of a full bladder and no sensation of the need to void.

Content Area: Uterus/Nursing Care of the Postpartum Woman
Integrated Process: Nursing Process—Implementation
Client Need: Health Promotion and Maintenance
Cognitive Level: Analysis
Concept: Pregnancy
Reference: Perry, S. E., Hockenberry, M. F., Lowdermilk, D. L., & Wilson, D. (2014). Maternal child nursing care. 5th ed. St. Louis, MO: Elsevier.

3. ANSWER: 1

Rationale

1. Lochia after birth is rubra and usually scant to moderate for the first 1 to 3 days and then gradually decreases in amount and changes to serosa in color. A few small clots in the first 1 to 2 days after birth is normal and are a result from pooling of blood in the vagina. Saturating one pad in less than an hour, a constant trickle of lochia, or the presence of large (larger than a quarter) blood clots is an indication of more serious complications and should be investigated immediately.
2. Foul-smelling lochia typically indicates an infection and needs to be addressed as soon as possible.
3. These findings are normal.
4. Instructing the patient to increase her fluids is not an accurate nursing intervention for this assessment.

TEST-TAKING TIP: It is important for the nurse to understand and be able to educate the woman about the normal progression of lochia flow and uterine involution. These changes indicate the healing process.

Content Area: Lochia/Nursing Care of the Postpartum Woman
Integrated Process: Nursing Process—Assessment
Client Need: Management of Care
Cognitive Level: Analysis
Concept: Pregnancy
Reference: Durham, R. F., & Chapman, L. (2014). Maternal-newborn nursing: The critical components of nursing care. 2nd ed. Philadelphia: F.A. Davis.

4. ANSWER: 4

Rationale

1. Breastfeeding is not contraindicated because the virus is not transmitted in the breast milk.
2. The vaccine base is made of duck eggs, so an allergic reaction may occur if the woman has an egg allergy.
3. The woman does not have to be separated from her infant because there is no risk of the infant contracting the virus from her.
4. The woman should avoid becoming pregnant for 1 month after receiving the vaccine because of the vaccine's teratogenic effects on the fetus.

TEST-TAKING TIP: Pregnant women who become infected with rubella virus expose the fetus. Exposure can cause serious birth defects such as heart problems, hearing or vision loss, intellectual disability, and liver or spleen damage. Serious birth defects are more common if a woman is infected early in her pregnancy, especially in the first 12 weeks. Getting rubella infection during pregnancy can also cause a miscarriage or premature delivery.

Content Area: Immune System/Care of the Postpartum Woman
Integrated Process: Nursing Process—Intervention
Client Need: Physiological Integrity/Reduction of Risk Potential
Cognitive Level: Analysis
Concept: Infection
Reference: *Perry, S. E., Hockenberry, M. F., Lowdermilk, D. L., & Wilson, D. (2014). Maternal child nursing care. 5th ed. St. Louis, MO: Elsevier.*

5. ANSWER: 4
Rationale
1. Notifying the physician would not be an appropriate action because orthostatic hypotension is a known physiological occurrence during the immediate postpartum period.
2. Elevating the woman's legs will not alleviate the safety risk when she gets up out of bed.
3. Oxygenation is not the cause of orthostatic hypotension. Orthostatic hypotension can develop in the first 48 hours as a result of the splanchnic engorgement due to the pooling of blood within the blood vessels of the stomach cavity following the birth of the infant.
4. Orthostatic hypotension may be evident during the first 8 hours after delivery. The nurse should be aware that feelings of faintness and dizziness are signs that could indicate a safety risk for the woman. The nurse should instruct the woman to call for help the first few times she attempts to get out of bed.

TEST-TAKING TIP: Orthostatic hypotension symptoms include dizziness, faintness, or light-headedness that appears when standing. It is caused by low blood pressure.
Content Area: Cardiovascular/Postpartum Care of the Postpartum Woman
Integrated Process: Nursing Process—Intervention
Client Need: Physiological Integrity
Cognitive Level: Analysis
Concept: Pregnancy
Reference: *Perry, S. E., Hockenberry, M. F., Lowdermilk, D. L., & Wilson, D. (2014). Maternal child nursing care. 5th ed. St. Louis, MO: Elsevier.*

6. ANSWER: 3
Rationale
1. Massaging the fundus is not appropriate unless the fundus is boggy and soft.
2. Before starting the fundal assessment, the nurse should ask the woman when she last voided. If she has not voided recently, then the nurse should instruct her to empty her bladder so that an accurate assessment can be done.
3. The lochia flow should be assessed when checking the firmness and position of the fundus. However, to get an accurate assessment, the bladder must be empty.
4. Lowering the head of the bed and having the mother lie flat in the bed is the correct position for the nurse to accurately assess the fundus, but the woman should be placed in this position only when the nurse is about to do the assessment.

TEST-TAKING TIP: Nursing interventions are actions, based on clinical judgment and nursing knowledge, that nurses perform to achieve client outcomes. Interventions are also referred to as nursing actions, measures, strategies, and activities.

Content Area: Uterus/Care of the Postpartum Woman
Integrated Process: Nursing Process—Intervention
Client Need: Physiological Integrity/Reduction of Risk Potential
Cognitive Level: Analysis
Concept: Pregnancy
Reference: *London, M. L., Ladewig, P. A., Davidson, M. R., Ball, J. W., Bindler, R. C., & Cowen, K. J. (2014). Maternal & child nursing care. 4th ed. New Jersey: Pearson.*

7. ANSWER: 4
Rationale
1. This is a nursing assessment, not a nursing intervention.
2. Food and fluid intake is usually restricted during labor; however, it is not contraindicated for a woman after delivery.
3. Catheterization is performed only when the bladder is distended and the woman cannot void or is voiding only small amounts (less than 100 mL) frequently, or when she has not voided for 6 to 8 hours.
4. If a woman has an episiotomy or perineal tear, an ice pack is usually applied to the perineum to reduce edema. The application of ice also provides a numbing effect to the area.

TEST-TAKING TIP: Ice should be applied for the first 24 hours because this causes vasoconstriction, thereby reducing swelling and providing comfort. After the first 24 hours, a warm sitz bath should be used to increase circulation to tissues and promote healing.
Content Area: Perineum/Nursing Care of the Postpartum Woman
Integrated Process: Nursing Process—Intervention
Client Need: Physiological Integrity/Reduction of Risk Potential
Cognitive Level: Analysis
Concept: Pregnancy
Reference: *Durham, R. F., & Chapman, L. (2014). Maternal-newborn nursing: The critical components of nursing care. 2nd ed. Philadelphia: F.A. Davis.*

8. ANSWER: 1
Rationale
1. Engorgement can develop if the infant isn't nursing often enough. When the normal breast fullness is not relieved, fluid builds up and swelling occurs. The breasts become hard, and the skin is taut and shiny and becomes extremely tender and painful. Because the breast is so full and swollen, the nipple and areola may flatten out, making the tissue difficult for the infant to grasp.
2. Women should avoid using soap on the breasts while bathing to keep the skin of the nipple and areola intact and to avoid infection, not breast engorgement.
3. Adequate fluid intake is an important element of good nutrition. Women, especially those who are lactating, should be encouraged to drink enough to satisfy thirst and prevent constipation.
4. Bind the breast with a towel or stretch bandage to help suppress lactation.

TEST-TAKING TIP: Breast fullness is a normal part of lactation that nearly all women experience when their milk comes in, approximately 2 to 5 days after birth. This feeling of fullness, which may be accompanied by a feeling of heaviness, tenderness, and warmth, is caused by swelling of the breast tissue as blood, lymphatic fluid, and milk collect in the ducts as the process of milk production begins. With this normal fullness, the breast tissue is compressible, and the woman generally feels well.

Content Area: Breast/Nursing Care of the Postpartum Woman
Integrated Process: Nursing Process—Evaluation
Client Need: Health Promotion and Maintenance
Cognitive Level: Evaluation
Concept: Pregnancy
Reference: Durham, R. F., & Chapman, L. (2014). Maternal-newborn nursing: The critical components of nursing care. 2nd ed. Philadelphia: F.A. Davis.

9. ANSWER: 2
Rationale
1. Vasomotor changes refer to the response of a blood vessel that alters its diameter to a vasodilator action or a vasoconstrictor action. Vasomotor changes do not cause the diuresis noted during the postpartum period.
2. Sweating (especially night sweats) is a common physiological response observed in the postpartum period. This is one of the ways the body gets rid of the extra water retained during pregnancy.
3. This is a natural occurrence in everyone and not a response in the process of postpartum diuresis.
4. The fluid loss from the expulsion of the placenta is composed of the placenta, the amnion, the chorion, some amniotic fluid, blood, and blood clots.

TEST-TAKING TIP: Postpartum diuresis occurs within the first 12 hours and lasts about 2 to 3 days due to low estrogen levels and the body excreting excess water weight due to pregnancy.

Content Area: Cardiovascular/Nursing Care of the Postpartum Woman
Integrated Process: Nursing Process—Assessment
Client Need: Health Promotion and Maintenance
Cognitive Level: Application
Concept: Pregnancy
Reference: London, M. L., Ladewig, P. A., Davidson, M. R., Ball, J. W., Bindler, R. C., & Cowen, K. J. (2014). Maternal & child nursing care. 4th ed. New Jersey: Pearson.

10. ANSWER: 2
Rationale
1. *Multiparous* means a woman has been pregnant more than one time.
2. A sitz bath is used to decrease pain, promote circulation to tissues, promote healing, and reduce the incidence of infection. Usually prescribed for women who got an episiotomy or sustained a perineal tear during birth.
3. A vaginal birth alone is not an indication for using a sitz bath.
4. A pudendal block is a method of perineal anesthesia used in the latter transition stage, the second stage of labor, and in the repair of an episiotomy. However, just because the woman received a pudendal block is not an indication for a sitz bath during the postpartum period.

TEST-TAKING TIP: A question consists of the stem, the client's condition or the scenario, and distractors (choices that look correct but are actually wrong). Always analyze these parts to know exactly what the question is asking.

In a question, there is that one word or phrase that is the most important. Key words may relate to the client, the actual problem, and to specific aspects of the problem. In this question, the key words are *sitz bath*. So the student needs to think about the indications for a sitz bath.

Content Area: Perineum/Care of the Postpartum Woman
Integrated Process: Nursing Process—Intervention
Client Need: Physiological Integrity/Basic Care and Comfort
Cognitive Level: Application
Concept: Pregnancy
Reference: London, M. L., Ladewig, P. A., Davidson, M. R., Ball, J. W., Bindler, R. C., & Cowen, K. J. (2014). Maternal & child nursing care. 4th ed. New Jersey: Pearson.

11. ANSWER: 4
Rationale
1. Diet, fluids, and exercise are important factors in maintaining normal bowel patterns after giving birth.
2. This is being insensitive to the woman's feelings. She is upset and needs education.
3. This is not an issue where the physician should see the woman. It is more important that the nurse provide good education.
4. Good fiber sources include bran and other whole grains found in cereals, breads, and brown rice along with fresh fruits, such as dried fruits like raisins, apricots, and prunes.

TEST-TAKING TIP: Some women may experience constipation from the lack of fluid and food intake during labor. Bowel tone is sluggish because of elevated progesterone levels and anesthesia used during labor. Also, some women may be hesitant to have a bowel movement in the postpartum period due to pain in the perineal area resulting from an episiotomy, lacerations, or hemorrhoids. Health care providers may prescribe stool softeners and/or laxatives to treat constipation and provide perineal comfort during defecation.

Content Area: Gastrointestinal System/Nursing Care of the Postpartum Woman
Integrated Process: Nursing Process—Intervention
Client Need: Physiological Integrity/Basic Care and Comfort
Cognitive Level: Application
Concept: Bowel Elimination
Reference: Durham, R. F., & Chapman, L. (2014). Maternal-newborn nursing: The critical components of nursing care. 2nd ed. Philadelphia: F.A. Davis.

12. ANSWER: 4, 5
Rationale
1. When taking a shower, the woman should be instructed to turn her back to the running water. This action will decrease stimulation to the breasts.
2. Pumping the breasts will stimulate and cause more milk production.
3. Heat will stimulate the breasts and cause more milk production.
4. Ice packs to the axillary area of each breast or cold/gel packs placed in the bra will help to relieve pain and swelling.
5. A well-fitting bra for the first 5 to 6 days both day and night will support the breasts and provide comfort.

TEST-TAKING TIP: Be sure to understand the difference in breast care nursing interventions for the breastfeeding woman and the woman suppressing lactation.

Content Area: Breast/Nursing Care of the Postpartum Woman
Integrated Process: Nursing Process—Intervention
Client Need: Physiological Integrity/Reduction of Risk Potential
Cognitive Level: Application
Concept: Pregnancy
Reference: Perry, S. E., Hockenberry, M. F., Lowdermilk, D. L., & Wilson, D. (2014). Maternal child nursing care. 5th ed. St. Louis, MO: Elsevier.

13. ANSWER: 2
Rationale
1. Walking is an excellent exercise and the distance can be increased as strength and endurance resume while in the hospital; however, walking does not specifically strengthen the pelvic musculature.
2. Kegel exercises help to tone pelvic floor muscles.
3. The woman should be instructed that aerobic exercise should not be done until after she sees her physician/midwife after discharge. Aerobic exercise is usually not allowed until 6 weeks postpartum.
4. Passive range-of-motion exercises while resting in bed helps to improve peripheral circulation and to prevent thrombi but does not strengthen pelvic musculature.

TEST-TAKING TIP: All women should become familiar with Kegel exercises for strengthening the pelvis musculature. Kegel exercise involves contracting muscles around the vagina as though stopping the flow of urine and holding tightly for 10 seconds, and then relaxing for 10 seconds.
Content Area: Premium/Nursing Care of the Postpartum Woman
Integrated Process: Nursing Process—Intervention
Client Need: Physiological Integrity
Cognitive Level: Application
Concept: Pregnancy
Reference: London, M. L., Ladewig, P. A., Davidson, M. R., Ball, J. W., Bindler, R. C., & Cowen, K. J. (2014). Maternal & child nursing care. 4th ed. New Jersey: Pearson.

14. ANSWER: 4
Rationale
1. This is a normal physiological response. The nurse should document the education concerning afterbirth pains.
2. This is not a sign of infection.
3. This is a normal physiological response; however, the nurse should always provide the client with a rationale for her concerns.
4. Nipple stimulation by the infant causes the release of the hormone oxytocin from the posterior pituitary gland, which triggers the release of the hormone prolactin from the anterior pituitary. Oxytocin also causes the uterus to contract during involution.

TEST-TAKING TIP: Therapeutic communication should be goal oriented and directed at learning and growth promotion.
Content Area: Afterpain/Nursing Care of the Postpartum Woman
Integrated Process: Nursing Process—Intervention
Client Need: Physiological Integrity
Cognitive Level: Analysis
Concept: Pregnancy

Reference: Durham, R. F., & Chapman, L. (2014). Maternal-newborn nursing: The critical components of nursing care. 2nd ed. Philadelphia: F.A. Davis.

15. ANSWERS: 1, 3, 5
Rationale
1. Ambulation and using the bathroom to void is more natural and the patient is more likely to be successful.
2. Pouring warm water over the woman's perineal area helps to stimulate the sensation of needing to void.
3. Running water promotes relaxation of perineal muscles and stimulates the sensation of needing to void.
4. Using a bedpan decreases the sensation of voiding. If the woman is unable to get out of the bed and go to the bathroom, then the nurse should offer the bedpan and try pouring warm water over her perineum.
5. Medicating the woman for pain helps her to relax.

TEST-TAKING TIP: Urinary retention is common in the postpartum woman because of loss of bladder elasticity and tone due to trauma, medications, or anesthesia. Loss of bladder tone can cause uterine atony and displacement to one side, which lessens the ability of the uterus to contract and results in excessive bleeding. Urinary retention may also result in urinary stasis, allowing time for bacteria to multiply and causing a UTI.
Content Area: Urinary System/Nursing Care of the Postpartum Woman
Integrated Process: Nursing Process—Intervention
Client Need: Physiological Integrity
Cognitive Level: Analysis
Concept: Pregnancy
Reference: Durham, R. F., & Chapman, L. (2014). Maternal-newborn nursing: The critical components of nursing care. 2nd ed. Philadelphia: F.A. Davis.

16. ANSWER: 3
Rationale
1. The peri-pad should be applied from front to back.
2. Peri-care should be performed every time the woman voids, has a bowel elimination, and changes a peri-pad.
3. The nurse should emphasize the importance of thoroughly washing hands before touching her breasts, after diaper changes, after bladder and bowel elimination, and before and after handling peri-pads.
4. Warm water is used in the peri-bottle.

TEST-TAKING TIP: The student should concentrate while reading the question so details that make a difference are noted.
Content Area: Perineum/Nursing Care of the Postpartum Woman
Integrated Process: Nursing Process—Evaluation
Client Need: Physiological Integrity
Cognitive Level: Evaluation
Concept: Pregnancy
Reference: Durham, R. F., & Chapman, L. (2014). Maternal-newborn nursing: The critical components of nursing care. 2nd ed. Philadelphia: F.A. Davis.

17. ANSWER: 2
Rationale
1. Positive bonding/attachment signs shown by the mother can be touching, holding, kissing, cuddling, talking and singing, choosing the en face position, expressing pride,

attaching physical characteristics to other family members, and attempting to evoke a smile or vocal response.
2. Negative bonding/attachment signs shown by the mother can be refusing to look at the infant, refusing to touch or hold the infant, refusing to name the infant, finding the infant unattractive or ugly, or refusing to respond or responding negatively to infant cues such as crying or smiling.
3. Positive bonding/attachment signs shown by the mother can be touching, holding, kissing, cuddling, talking and singing, choosing the en face position, expressing pride, attaching physical characteristics to other family members, and attempting to evoke a smile or vocal response.
4. During the taking-hold phase, the woman's focus of concern is about her bodily function and taking care of her infant. This would be a normal question asked by the woman at this time.
TEST-TAKING TIP: The nurse needs to recognize and interpret the mother's behavior on an individual basis. Not all women act or react the same. The nurse should understand there may be underlying things influencing the mother's behavior that may not be apparent such as anesthesia, pain, a traumatic birthing experience, cultural beliefs, or current social situation.
Content Area: Psychological Postpartum Adaptations/ Nursing Care of the Postpartum Woman
Integrated Process: Nursing Process—Assessment
Client Need: Psychosocial Integrity
Cognitive Level: Analysis
Concept: Pregnancy
Reference: London, M. L., Ladewig, P. A., Davidson, M. R., Ball, J. W., Bindler, R. C., & Cowen, K. J. (2014). Maternal & child nursing care. 4th ed. New Jersey: Pearson.

18. ANSWER: 4
Rationale
1. The taking-in phase lasts approximately 1 to 2 days after birth. During this phase, the woman is focused primarily on her own needs, especially sleeping and eating.
2. During the taking-in phase, the woman will talk about her delivery experience, which enables her to integrate the birth of her infant with reality.
3. The letting-go phase is the last phase and usually starts 10 days postpartum. In this phase, the woman is trying to realize and accept the physical separation from the infant and to adjust her life to dependency of her infant and the additional workload. The woman may experience postpartum blues, caused by hormonal changes that occur postpartum. Common manifestations are irritability, tears, loss of appetite, and difficulty sleeping.
4. The taking-hold phase lasts from day 2 to 10. The woman is focused on her bodily functions and taking care of her infant.
TEST-TAKING TIP: A major psychological task for the parents is the process of bonding and attaching with their newborn. Nurses are in an exceptional position to observe and offer support and reassurance. Encouragement and education by the nurse can help in correcting negative bonding behaviors and reinforce the positive maternal–infant adaptations that are the basis for a strong and healthy family relationship.

Content Area: Psychological Postpartum Adaptations/ Nursing Care of the Postpartum Woman
Integrated Process: Nursing Process—Assessment
Client Need: Psychosocial Integrity
Cognitive Level: Analysis
Concept: Pregnancy
Reference: Durham, R. F., & Chapman, L. (2014). Maternal-newborn nursing: The critical components of nursing care. 2nd ed. Philadelphia: F.A. Davis.

19. ANSWER: 4
Rationale
1. The woman is experiencing the taking-in phase at this time and should be nurtured.
2. This is not the behavior observed during the taking-hold phase.
3. This behavior is typical during the taking-in phase and the nurse must take into consideration the difficult labor and delivery the woman has experienced.
4. This is an appropriate response for the nurse during the taking-in phase.
TEST-TAKING TIP: Recognize and interpret the mother's behavior on an individual basis. Not all women act or react the same. The nurse should understand there may be underlying things influencing the mother's behavior that may not be apparent such anesthesia, pain, a traumatic birthing experience, cultural beliefs, or current social situation.
Content Area: Psychological Postpartum Adaptations/Nursing Care of the Postpartum Woman
Integrated Process: Nursing Process—Assessment
Client Need: Psychosocial Integrity
Cognitive Level: Analysis
Concept: Pregnancy
Reference: Durham, R. F., & Chapman, L. (2014). Maternal-newborn nursing: The critical components of nursing care. 2nd ed. Philadelphia: F.A. Davis.

20. ANSWER: 3
Rationale
1. The client will wear a well-supported bra but this is not highest priority.
2. Eating 100% of her meals is important for nutrition and healing but is not highest priority.
3. Moderate lochia flow is appropriate for this woman and is the highest priority nursing goal.
4. Ambulating is important for bowel and bladder and circulation; however, it is not a priority.
TEST-TAKING TIP: The ABCs (airway, breathing, and circulation) should be used to prioritize the physiological needs. The function of the other vital organs comes next. Nutrition and gastrointestinal problems are low on the list when it comes to sustaining life. If excessive bleeding should occur, the circulatory system would be compromised.
Content Area: Lochia/Nursing Care of the Postpartum Woman
Integrated Process: Nursing Process—Evaluation
Client Need: Physiological Integrity/Reduction of Risk Potential
Cognitive Level: Evaluation
Concept: Pregnancy
Reference: Durham, R. F., & Chapman, L. (2014). Maternal-newborn nursing: The critical components of nursing care. 2nd ed. Philadelphia: F.A. Davis.

Chapter 18

Postpartum at Risk

Endometritis—Infection of the uterine endometrium

Estimated blood loss (EBL)—The total estimated blood loss after a delivery by visual estimation or by weight

Hemorrhagic shock—When the peripheral blood volume is insufficient to return enough blood and oxygen to the heart and vital organs, causing shock to ensue

Mastitis—A breast infection in one or both breasts. Mastitis typically originates from a milk duct and causes tenderness, swelling, and redness at the site with overall maternal flulike symptoms.

Postpartum depression (PPD)—Starts typically within 4 weeks after delivery and lasts longer than postpartum blues, interfering with activities of daily living and care of self and baby

Postpartum psychosis—A more severe syndrome, including postpartum depression, delusional thinking, and ideation of harming self, infant, or others

Thrombophlebitis—Vein inflammation with clot formation

I. Postpartum Hemorrhage

Postpartum hemorrhage (PPH) is the leading cause of maternal mortality and morbidity worldwide. Every 3.5 minutes, a mother somewhere in the world dies from postpartum hemorrhage. Tragically, this is 70% to 90% preventable. Nurses play a significant role in managing postpartum hemorrhage. Early recognition by the nurse and promptly calling in the entire health care team saves lives. Most often postpartum hemorrhage occurs early, shortly after delivery or within 24 hours of birth. Hemorrhage occurring more than 24 hours after delivery is considered a late postpartum hemorrhage.

A. Hemorrhage after vaginal delivery

The estimated blood loss (EBL) after a vaginal delivery is customarily more than 500 mL. However, the objective measurement of blood loss at delivery was found to be poorly estimated by most health care workers. They tend to overestimate small amounts of blood and underestimate large amounts of blood. Weighing blood-soaked items helps to accurately determine blood loss.

B. Hemorrhage after cesarean delivery

If the EBL after cesarean delivery is more than 1,000 mL, it is classified as a postpartum hemorrhage. This represents the blood lost from the surgical procedure itself combined with uterine blood loss from the placental site.

C. Accurate EBL

The most accurate way to estimate blood loss is to weigh blood-soaked linens, drapes, pads, and sponges and subtract the dry weight of the items from the total weight, thereby yielding the blood volume. Estimating blood loss using laboratory values and looking for the typical 10% drop in hemoglobin is difficult due to intrapartum intravenous fluid volume replacements.

D. Clinical symptoms

Some clinicians wait for the clinical symptoms of postpartum hemorrhage (PPH) to appear, like maternal dizziness, palpitations, tachycardia, and hypotension. However, the American College of Obstetricians and Gynecologists declares in their practice bulletin that this is unwise because with the expanded maternal blood volume, the increased cardiac output in pregnancy, and the youthful nature of the patient, mothers may lose 20% of their blood volume before becoming symptomatic. The nurse must remember that the patient's clinical symptoms can be a late sign. Postpartum hemorrhage is therefore an emergent situation that needs to be treated in real time rather than retrospectively on laboratory results.

E. Predisposing factors

It is crucial that nurses become aware of the common contributory and predisposing factors that lead to PPH:
- Overdistention of the uterus related to twins, triplets, a large infant, or large volume of amniotic fluid
- Prolonged labor
- Oxytocin augmentation or induction of labor
- Grand multiparity
- Use of magnesium sulfate or tocolytics

- Prolonged third stage of labor
- Preeclampsia
- Vacuum-assisted vaginal delivery
- Forceps-assisted vaginal delivery
- Retained placental fragments
- Placental previa
- Fetal malpresentation
- Macrosomia
- Episiotomy
- Precipitous delivery
- Prior cervical cerclage
- Shoulder dystocia
- Chorioamnionitis
- Extra placental lobes
- Blood-clotting disorders
- Low platelets
- Disseminated intravascular coagulation

Postpartum hemorrhage can also happen in the absence of any known risk factors.

F. Causes of postpartum hemorrhage

Postpartum hemorrhage is a symptom of a problem that is causing the blood loss; therefore, correctly discovering and addressing the problem should lead to the proper interventions to stop hemorrhaging.

1. **Uterine atony:** This is the failure of the uterus to contract after the placenta has been delivered. The uterine muscle remains flaccid and blood is allowed to continue to flow out through the site of the placenta. This is the most common cause of postpartum hemorrhage and usually begins within the first hour after delivery. After the placenta is delivered, the vascular area once connected to the placenta can hemorrhage if the uterine muscle does not clamp down to restrict vessel flow. If the smooth muscle of the uterus is able to contract, the muscle fibers act like a tourniquet to stop blood from hemorrhaging at the placenta site. Uterine contraction can be aided by medications and fundal massage.

   a) External fundal massage: The smooth muscle of the uterus has the propensity to contract when massaged. The uterus can be massaged externally by placing a hand just above the pubic bone and cupping the uterus to give it support. The other hand is placed on the fundus of the uterus and massaged in a circular fashion until it firms up and contracts. The uterus should feel firm after massage; if it does not contract, it will remain soft and boggy beneath the hands. External fundal massage is the primary nursing intervention when managing uterine atony (Fig. 18.1).

   b) Internal uterine massage or bimanual compression: The physician or midwife makes a fist with a gloved hand and places it against the uterus through the vagina. The other

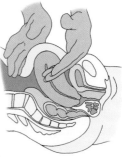

Fig 18.1 External fundal massage.

hand massages the uterus and compresses it against the internal hand, causing the uterus to contract.

2. Lacerations of the perineum, vagina, or cervix can also cause bleeding and postpartum hemorrhage. These lacerations can bleed slowly or rapidly and cause a large volume of accumulated blood loss over time. Usually these lacerations occur in the perineal area and are repaired immediately after delivery. If heavy bleeding continues in the presence of a firm fundus, look for lacerations. Causes of lacerations include the following:

   - Forceps-assisted vaginal delivery
   - Vacuum-assisted vaginal delivery
   - Prolonged second stage
   - Previous scarring
   - Fetal malpresentation

3. Retained placenta can be a significant source of bleeding. Usually the placenta is delivered within 30 minutes of the baby's birth. If the placenta fails to deliver, it continues to allow maternal blood to flow from it. A retained placenta will need to be manually removed by the licensed provider. This procedure is painful and the mother will need pain relief. Sometimes the placenta does not completely deliver and placental fragments remain in the uterus, causing excessive bleeding. These fragments will need to be removed manually or with uterine curettage. Occasionally the placenta imbeds itself into the uterine wall and is unable to detach. A hysterectomy may be performed for the following placental attachments:

   - Placenta accreta—the placenta has attached to the myometrium.
   - Placenta increta—the placenta invades deeply into the myometrium.
   - Placenta percreta—the placenta has perforated the myometrium and may be attached to other pelvic organs.

   a) Predisposing factors for abnormal placental attachment include the following:
      - Previous cesarean delivery
      - Previous uterine surgery

- Fibroids or other endometrial defects
- Advanced maternal age
- Placenta previa
- Multiparity

4. Blood clotting disorders are uncommon but can be the underlying cause of unmanageable postpartum bleeding. Abnormal coagulopathy may not have been identified before delivery. In the absence of other causes of bleeding, the mother's coagulation status must be assessed immediately. A variety of coagulation disorders could be present. More commonly a decreased number of platelets is the cause. Decreased fibrinogen levels, increased prothrombin time, or underlying abnormalities may be present, such as thrombocytopenic purpura, von Willebrand disease, or other hemophilia.

G. Late postpartum hemorrhage

Whereas early postpartum hemorrhage usually happens within the first few hours after delivery, late postpartum hemorrhage happens after the first 24 hours and up to 1 to 2 weeks after delivery. Late postpartum hemorrhage is less common and is typically slow and insidious, causing maternal fatigue and anemia.

1. Retained placental tissue
   a) Small pieces of placental tissue or an extra lobe of placenta can be unknowingly retained and still attached to the uterus. These fragments of placenta can cause a small but persistent bleeding that is cumulative over time. Curettage may be needed to remove remaining placental tissue.
2. Subinvolution
   a) The uterus does not return to normal size and continues to bleed from the placental site over time. Compounding factors to uterine subinvolution may be retained placenta, products of conception, or uterine infection. It is thought that subinvolution may be underdiagnosed. The underlying cause must be treated.

H. Prevention

It is important that nurses work together with other licensed providers as a team and take extra precautions and preventative measures when these risk factors exist. Staging the patient on admission as low, intermediate, or high risk for postpartum hemorrhage should be done.

1. Low risk: A "hold" tube should be sent to the blood bank on admission for a low-hemorrhage-risk patient.
2. Moderate risk: A type and screen should be ordered for a moderate-hemorrhage-risk patient.
3. High risk: A type and cross-match for 2 units of packed red blood cells to be held in the blood bank should be ordered and ready for a high-hemorrhage-risk patient.

I. Accurate estimation of blood loss

As previously discussed, the most accurate way to estimate blood loss is to weigh blood-soaked linens, drapes, pads, and sponges, and subtract the dry weight of these items from the total. Estimating blood loss using laboratory values and looking for the typical 10% drop in hemoglobin is difficult due to intrapartum intravenous fluid volume replacements.

DID YOU KNOW?

One gram of weight equals 1 mL of liquid volume. Weigh blood-soaked pads and linens in grams and then subtract the dry weight of the pads from the total to find mL of blood present. Another method is to zero the scale with a dry pad, remove that pad, and weigh the blood-saturated pad to determine the blood's weight.

J. Hypovolemic Shock

This is also sometimes called **hemorrhagic shock.** Shock happens when there is not enough blood volume to perfuse the body's tissues and organs. Hypovolemic shock is an emergency and can lead to death if not corrected. A patient in shock begins compensatory mechanisms and releases catecholamines, causing the remaining blood flow to be diverted to the brain and heart and away from extremities and other tissues.

1. Assessment of the patient in hypovolemic shock may reveal the following:
   - Tachycardia with a palpated radial pulse that is weak, irregular, or thready.
   - Respirations that are shallow and rapid.
   - Falling blood pressure and decreased central venous pressure.
   - Skin that is cool and clammy to the touch and is visually pale or mottled with a diminished capillary refill.
   - Anxiety and restlessness with a sense of impending doom, or confusion with lethargy.
   - Kidney function reduces or stops urine output.
   - Mucous membranes become pale or dusky.
2. Management of hypovolemic shock is focused on restoring the patient's blood volume and preventing further blood loss. Management can include the following medical and nursing interventions:
   - Activation of the hospital's obstetric hemorrhage response team.
   - Activation of the hospital's massive transfusion protocol.
   - Secondary IV access with a 16- or 18-gauge IV catheter.
   - IV fluid replacement with crystalloids such as Lactated Ringer's normal saline or Hetastarch, being careful not to fluid overload.

- Blood replacement with products such as packed red blood cells, platelets, and fresh frozen plasma.
- Placement of intermittent compression stockings and assessment for disseminated intravascular coagulation.
- Administration of oxygen with a nonrebreather face mask and monitored with a pulse oximeter.
- Placement of indwelling urinary catheter. This will prevent bladder distention, uterine displacement, and potential additional bleeding, as well as allow for monitoring of urine output.
- Central venous pressure or pulmonary artery catheter may be placed along with cardiac monitoring.
- Continued measuring of blood loss by weight.

ALERT Signs and symptoms of hypovolemic shock may not appear until 40% of the maternal blood volume has been lost. Therefore, diligent monitoring and assessment of the patient must be done to allow for early interventions.

K. Medications (Table 18.1)
  1. Oxytocin (Pitocin). Drug class: Hormone, oxytocic. Pitocin is the synthetic form of the endogenous hormone made in the hypothalamus and stored in the pituitary gland. This hormone stimulates the uterus to contract and stimulates the lacteal glands to contract during lactation. Oxytocin is used as the first line of defense in preventing and controlling postpartum bleeding. It is used to:
     - Induce or augment labor contractions.
     - Initiate or augment uterine contractions in the third stage of labor.

Table 18.1 Medications and Nursing Considerations for Postpartum Hemorrhage

Name	Classification/Action	Dosage/Route	Contraindications	Nursing Considerations
Oxytocin (Pitocin)	Oxytocic. Stimulates uterine smooth muscle and produces contractions similar to those that occur during spontaneous labor	10 units IM if no IV access; 10–40 units in 1,000 mL crystalloid IV fluid (Lactated Ringer's solution or normal saline)	Hypersensitivity	Monitor uterine response. DO NOT administer a bolus of undiluted oxytocin, as it can cause hypotension and cardiac arrhythmias. Consider administration of pain medication for uterine cramping.
Methylergonovine maleate (Methergine)	Ergot alkaloid. Causes uterine contractions by stimulating uterine and vascular smooth muscles.	0.1–0.2 mg IM every 2 to 4 h, followed by 0.2 mg PO every 4 to 6 h × 24 h (for 6 doses)	Hypersensitivity. History of or current elevation of blood pressure	Keep refrigerated. DO NOT add it to IV solutions or mix in a syringe with other medications. Take precautions to prevent inadvertent administration to the newborn.
Carboprost tromethamine (Hemabate)	Prostaglandin analogue. Stimulates contractions of the myometrium	0.25 mg (250 mcg) IM or directly into the uterus (by MD or CNM) q15–90 min; 8 doses maximum	Asthma, hepatic, renal, and cardiac disease	Do not administer if patient demonstrates shock, as it will not be well absorbed. Keep refrigerated. This medication is very expensive.
Misoprostol (Cytotec)	Prostaglandin analogue; stimulates powerful contractions of the myometrium	800–1,000 mcg rectally (single dose)	Hypersensitivity to prostaglandins	Stable at room temperature. Rectal absorption is likely slower than IV medication. Monitor uterine response.
Dinoprostone (Prostin E2)	Prostaglandin analogue; stimulates powerful contractions of the myometrium	20 mg suppository vaginally or rectally q2h	Hypersensitivity to prostaglandins. Avoid in severe hypotension	If vaginal bleeding is brisk, the use of vaginal suppositories is not likely to be effective. Fever is common. Stored frozen; it must be thawed to room temperature.

- Control postpartum bleeding.
  Controlling postpartum uterine bleeding involves administering 10 units deep intramuscular (IM) if no IV access, or mix 10 to 40 units in 500 to 1,000 mL of IV fluids. IV push should not be given; 30 units in 500 mL should be considered to avoid overhydration. The IV dose should be titrated based on uterine tone. Pitocin may be used continuously in conjunction with other oxytocic medications.

🛇 **ALERT** Use carefully in patients with renal deficiency, as oxytocin has an antidiuretic effect. Avoid fluid overload, especially in patients with hypertension, and carefully record intake and output.

2. Methylergonovine (Methergine). Drug class: oxytocic. Methergine is used to control postpartum hemorrhage. Administered deep IM, possibly using the deltoid, which is closer to the heart, for immediate circulation. Oral Methergine may be used for maintaining uterine tone after the postpartum hemorrhage has stopped. Blood pressure should be monitored closely because Methergine can cause hypertension.

🛇 **ALERT** Avoid Methergine use in hypertensive patients. Remember that blood pressure drops with blood volume loss, so base decisions on the patient's baseline blood pressure before postpartum hemorrhage.

3. Carboprost (Hemabate). Drug class: prostaglandin. Hemabate stimulates the uterus to contract. It is given deep IM and may be repeated every 15 to 90 minutes, not to exceed eight doses total. Hemabate may be given directly into the myometrium by a trained health care provider. This drug can cause immediate and severe diarrhea. Consider giving an antidiarrheal like Lomotil to help stop fluid and electrolyte losses from diarrhea.

🛇 **ALERT** Hemabate contracts smooth muscle and can cause bronchospasm. Use with extreme caution in patients with asthma.

4. Misoprostol (Cytotec). Drug class: prostaglandin. Misoprostol is a synthetic prostaglandin. This medication is inexpensive and can be given orally, sublingually, or rectally. If the patient is vomiting during postpartum hemorrhage, it should be administered rectally. Because this can be kept at room temperature, it can be brought to a high-risk delivery as a precaution.

II. Perineal Hematoma

Hematomas can occur in the perineum during delivery due to stretching and shearing of the blood vessels in the perineum (Fig. 18.2). Women with varicose veins of the labia are at a higher risk for hematomas. Sometimes hematomas develop around the site of a perineal laceration or an episiotomy. Typically they form under an intact layer of surface skin and appear as swollen, bruised tissue.

- The most common symptom is continuing pain and pressure and tenderness when touched.
- The patient should be assessed for increased bleeding.
- Usually hematomas are resolved within 1 week.
- A soft, dry, ice-filled pack can be applied to prevent further swelling.

III. Postpartum Infections

A. Mastitis
A breast infection in one or both breasts is called **mastitis.** This typically originates in lactating women from a milk duct and causes tenderness, swelling, and redness at the site, along with overall maternal flulike symptoms (Fig. 18.3). Frequently the mastitis is located under one breast, where it is not easily observed by the mother. The flulike symptoms, overall malaise, fever, and aches are usually the first symptoms she notices. Sometimes the infection is due to a plugged milk duct that allows the milk to back up. Sometimes the nipple becomes cracked and allows infection to enter. The bacteria that usually causes mastitis is *Staphylococcus aureus*. Occasionally there may be purulent nipple drainage. Rarely, untreated mastitis can develop into an abscess.

1. Treatment of mastitis
   - Antibiotic therapy to control the *S. aureus*.
   - Warm compresses for maternal comfort.
   - Analgesic and anti-inflammatory medications for pain control.
   - Continued breastfeeding or pumping during mastitis to prevent further milk stasis.

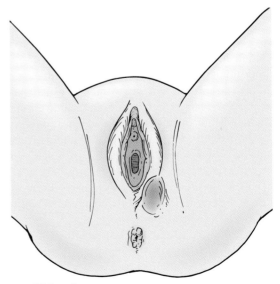

Fig 18.2 Vulvar hematoma.

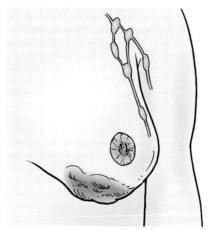

Fig 18.3 Mastitis.

2. Prevention teaching
   - Practice good hand-washing technique before breastfeeding.
   - Avoid engorgement by breastfeeding on each breast for each feeding.
   - Vary the position of the baby to avoid nipple breakdown.
   - Prevent nipple tissue cracks and fissures by massaging expressed colostrum or lanolin cream onto nipple.
   - Avoid harsh soaps that can break down the nipple tissue.
   - Pump or hand express excess breast milk if the baby misses a feeding.
   - Lean forward once during the feeding to express milk from the lower breast to allow complete emptying of the breast and avoid stagnation.
   - Feed every 2 to 4 hours and avoid going longer than 4 hours between feedings.
   - Recognize warning signs of mastitis before leaving the hospital.

B. Endometritis
Endometritis is an infection of the uterine endometrium. In postpartum women, it usually starts at the placental site and expands to include the entire endometrium and uterus. Bacteria typically enter the uterus from the vagina during labor and delivery or during postpartum. Rarely endometritis can spread to other tissues and develop into sepsis. Endometritis is more common in cesarean delivery; therefore, a single dose of an IV antibiotic preoperatively is typically given to prevent infection.
1. Predisposing risk factors for postpartum endometritis include the following:
   - Premature rupture of membranes
   - Prolonged rupture of membranes
   - Chorioamnionitis
   - Internal fetal or uterine monitoring devices
   - Multiple vaginal exams after rupture of membranes
   - Instrument-assisted delivery
   - Manual removal of the placenta or clots
   - Group B strep infection present during labor and delivery
   - Cesarean delivery
2. Symptoms of endometritis
   - Maternal fever
   - Uterine tenderness
   - Foul-smelling lochia
   - Elevated white blood count
3. Postpartum treatment of endometritis with a broad-spectrum antibiotic is usually sufficient.

C. Thrombophlebitis and thrombosis
Phlebitis is the inflammation of the vein that typically infiltrates into the vein wall. A thrombus is a clot in the vein, and **thrombophlebitis** is the inflammation of the vein after the clot forms. Thrombophlebitis can be limited to superficial veins, and formation could be at an IV site. The condition can be serious, developing in a deep vein of the leg. This is concerning because the clot can dislodge and travel to the lungs, causing a pulmonary embolism.

(!) ALERT Deep tissue massage of the area over a deep vein thrombosis (DVT) could cause a piece of the clot to break off and travel up through the heart and into the lungs, causing a pulmonary embolism.

1. Predisposing risk factors
   - Postpartum women may still have elevated fibrinogen levels from pregnancy.
   - Inactivity and bedrest after cesarean delivery.
   - Prolonged use of stirrups during second stage of labor.
   - Obesity.
   - History of thrombophlebitis.
   - Varicose veins.
   - Advanced maternal age.
   - Smoking.
   - Postpartum infection.
2. Prevention
   - Prenatal teaching and smoking cessation.
   - Avoiding the use of stirrups in the second stage of labor.
   - Encouraging reasonable and early ambulation after delivery.
   - Consistently using external sequential compression devices on all intraoperative and postoperative cesarean delivery patients.
3. Femoral thrombophlebitis
   Usually involves the saphenous or popliteal veins, and the femoral arterial flow may spasm in response

to the thrombophlebitis. The involved leg may be white and puffy with pitting edema or may be red and swollen with pitting edema.

4. Pelvic thrombophlebitis
Usually presents with fever and pelvic pain. The thrombophlebitis is usually found in the uterine, hypogastric, or ovarian veins. It may be a sequelae of endometritis. The leg below the affected site may become red, warm, and swollen. The edema may become so profound that the skin becomes stretched, shiny, and transparent white.

5. Diagnosis
Ultrasound is used to confirm the diagnosis of a DVT.

6. Treatment
Medical management involves using anticoagulant therapy along with elevating the affected leg to promote circulation. Moist warm compresses may help with circulation. Ongoing follow-up treatment involves the use of an anticoagulant like heparin or warfarin. Further testing will be needed to titer the anticoagulant therapy. Breastfeeding may continue with heparin but is contraindicated during the use of warfarin therapy.

IV. Postpartum Depression

Almost 20% of mothers develop **postpartum depression (PPD),** making it the most common maternal risk of childbirth. Mothers may feel shame about depressive feelings during a time when they are "supposed" to be happy. Origins of PPD are complex and compounding. There may be a maternal history of depression, but also interrelated are sleep deprivation, dissatisfaction with body image changes, a difficult pregnancy, a traumatic birth, having a baby with a disability or having twins or triplets, marital stress, being a teen mom, or having breastfeeding failure. Depression impacts the mother's sense of well-being, newborn attachment, and family welfare. For the safety of the mother and the newborn, all levels of PPD need to be assessed and investigated. Nurses should screen not just for depression but also for the cumulative sum of situational stress and overall life difficulties, rather than just the childcare tasks.

A. Postpartum blues
The "baby blues" occur commonly in postpartum mothers and is characterized by mild intermittent depression interspersed with happiness. Fifty to 80% of mothers report some transient baby blues. This is considered by some as an adjustment reaction after the birth of the baby and includes physical discomfort, anxiety about added caretaking responsibilities, and interrupted sleep lasting from birth through the first few weeks. The baby blues may be a response to the sudden hormonal alteration of estrogen, progesterone, and prolactin levels after

birth. Mothers may complain of fatigue, feeling overwhelmed, anxiety, and irritability along with episodes of intermittent crying.

1. Treatment
These women may need support with self-care and infant care. A follow-up appointment should be made to ensure the new mother is recovering. Single mothers will need help with the care of other children as well.

B. Postpartum major mood disorder
PPD without psychotic features is a severe and persistent sadness with unpredictable mood swings. Powerful feelings of anger, anxiety, fear, despondency, and hopelessness are present and persist beyond the baby's first few weeks. The prevalence is approximately 10% to 15% of new mothers and will usually require outside help for resolution. Teenagers are at a 50% higher risk for postpartum depression and are less likely to seek help. Women report an increased need for sleep along with intense irritability, including outbursts that may escalate to violence. Another common feature of PPD is that the mother may reject the infant and she may display an attitude of frustration with infant care demands. Intermittent and unwanted thoughts of hurting the baby are particularly disturbing to depressed mothers.

1. Treatment
Medication is typically needed in most cases of PPD. Antidepressants and counseling together provide the most comprehensive treatment. Assessment of suicidal or homicidal thoughts and monitoring progress are important, remembering that a common time for suicide is during the phase of improvement. Occasionally hospitalization is required.

DID YOU KNOW?
A person may be at highest risk for suicide during the recovery phase of a depressive episode, when they have more energy to carry out previously planned harmful actions. The depressed individual may not have enough energy to carry out a suicide during the depth of depression. The recovery phase is a time for the health care team and family members to stay on heightened awareness and assessment of the mother's condition.

C. Postpartum psychosis
Postpartum depression with psychotic features is rare, occurring after approximately 1% to 2% of births. With **postpartum psychosis,** typically symptoms of sadness, delusions, or hurting oneself or the baby begin within 3 weeks after delivery. Inability to perform activities of daily living, inability to work, agitation, and disorganized behavior are common. Untreated psychosis may progress to paranoia, detachment from reality, grandiose ideation, and visual or auditory hallucinations. Sensory input that

is not related to reality, like the sensation of bugs crawling on the skin, may also be present. Whenever mental illness occurs in the first year after childbirth, it is classified as a postpartum psychosis. Many women with postpartum psychosis have had a history of mental illness previous to the pregnancy or have had a family history of psychiatric problems; up to half of them will have a recurring episode with the next pregnancy.

1. Treatment

   Postpartum psychosis is a psychiatric emergency, and the mother will need at least a brief hospitalization. A mental health professional will evaluate her. Antipsychotic medication or mood stabilizers are usually effective treatment. Lactation consultation should be encouraged to determine the compatibility of medications and breastfeeding.

2. Ongoing follow-up should include:
   - Counseling.
   - Evaluation of medication efficacy over time.

- Close supervision and support with child care.
- Safe alternate care arrangements for the infant.
- Family support.
- Observation for ongoing cycles of depression throughout the first postpartum year.

DID YOU KNOW?

A mother who is clearly a danger to self, others, or property or who is unable to take care of basic safety or health needs will need a 72-hour emergency hospitalization for psychiatric evaluation and treatment. If she is unwilling to receive evaluation by designated mental health professionals, she can be committed involuntarily for a psychiatric evaluation at a treatment facility for up to 72 hours. States vary slightly as to the authorizing agent and circumstances for an involuntary 72-hour hold.

CASE STUDY: Putting It All Together

Subjective Data

The postpartum nurse is receiving handoff communication from the labor and delivery nurse about her new patient, Mrs. Miller. Mrs. Miller is a 30-year-old G4 T4 P0 A0 L4. She delivered by a vaginal-assisted forceps delivery of a 39-week-gestation newborn weighing 9 pounds 9 ounces. Pitocin was used to augment her labor. Mrs. Miller's second stage of labor lasted 2 hours and 30 minutes because of the infant's occipital posterior position. She also received a second-degree laceration, which was repaired. She received 1,000 mL of Lactated Ringer's (LR) with 20 units of Pitocin. She is currently on her second bag of LR with 20 units of Pitocin. She received an epidural for pain management while in labor.

After the postpartum nurse gets a report from the labor and delivery nurse, Mrs. Miller states that she needs help walking to the bathroom because she is dizzy and light-headed. She states that her pad needs to be changed because she has leaked all over the bed.

Objective Data

Nursing Assessment

Vital Signs
BP: 115/65
Pulse: 75
Respirations: 16
Temperature: 98.6°F
Pain score: 2/10. Denies the need for pain medication
Fundal exam: uterus midline at the umbilicus and boggy
Lochia: rubra heavy, pad saturated along with bed linens

Case Study Questions

1. As the nurse, what are your initial steps in this situation?

2. Is there sufficient information to make an analysis about what you as the nurse should do?

3. What oxytocic medications might be used to manage Mrs. Smith's bleeding and why?

REVIEW QUESTIONS

1. The nurse and provider estimate the blood loss at delivery to be 400 mL in the measuring drape; now when doing the initial perineal care, the nurse finds a large amount of blood underneath the patient. What action reflects safe and accurate nursing care?
   1. Estimate the amount of blood loss from the sheet and client clothing, and notify the physician.
   2. Encourage the mother to report any additional bleeding or clots.
   3. Draw the ordered hematocrit and notify the provider if the result is less than 28.
   4. Weigh the blood-soaked linens and notify the provider of the additional blood loss.

2. A patient delivered vaginally 20 minutes ago. Prophylactic Pitocin is infusing intravenously. During the initial postpartum assessment, the nurse notes a heavy amount of bleeding on the perineal pad. What are the priority nursing actions?
   1. Assess the perineum for lacerations and provide a clean peri-pad and ice pack.
   2. Assess the fundus and massage the uterus to determine uterine tone and location.
   3. Assess to see if the bladder is full and place an indwelling urinary catheter.
   4. Assess for clots, determine if this is a normal amount, and provide privacy during a pad change.

3. The nurse is performing an assessment of the uterus 30 minutes after a normal delivery and finds the fundus to be soft and boggy. IV Pitocin is infusing at 150 mL/hr. What is the priority nursing intervention?
   1. Increase the Pitocin, assess the fundus in 15 minutes, and update the licensed provider.
   2. Perform external massage of the uterus until it is firm, assess for additional bleeding on the pad, and update the licensed provider.
   3. Notify the provider of the increase in blood loss.
   4. Assist the patient to the bathroom and reassess the fundus after the patient voids.

4. The nurse is admitting a 38-year-old patient to triage in early labor with ruptured membranes. Her history includes a previous vaginal delivery 4 years ago and the presence of a uterine fibroid. What interventions are appropriate based on the hemorrhage risk for this patient?
   1. The patient is a moderate hemorrhage risk, so a type and screen should be ordered.
   2. The patient is a high hemorrhage risk, so 4 units of packed red blood cells should be ordered.
   3. The patient is a low hemorrhage risk, so a hold tube should be drawn.
   4. The patient is a moderate hemorrhage risk, but blood is not drawn at this time.

5. The nurse is caring for a postpartum woman and her 2-hour-old baby. The new mother has been preoccupied with breastfeeding and visitors, but suddenly she complains of dizziness and is light-headed. Which response by the nurse is appropriate?
   1. Explain that she needs to drink more fluids and eat because she needs to replace fluids and calories.
   2. Encourage the patient to rest, and ask a family member to watch the newborn in the crib.
   3. Tell the patient that the dizziness is probably caused by her pain medication and that it is normal.
   4. Obtain vital signs, assess fundal tone, and observe for excessive lochia.

6. A woman is 1 hour postcesarean delivery with nausea and an estimated blood loss of 1,200 mL. She is currently experiencing heavy vaginal bleeding and has a uterus that firms with massage. She has a history of asthma with a current O_2 saturation of 89%. The licensed provider has ordered Cytotec 800 mcg and Methergine 0.2 mg. What collaborative communication should occur between the nurse and provider?
   1. Since the total blood loss is under 1,500 mL, Cytotec and Methergine administration could be delayed for a time.
   2. Cytotec should be given rectally because the patient is already nauseated, and the Methergine route should be ordered.
   3. Recommend that the abdominal dressing be removed to inspect for incisional bleeding.
   4. Recommend that the patient not get Methergine because she has a history of asthma.

7. The nurse is caring for a woman who is 6 hours postpartum after a vaginal delivery. She has a history of labial varicose veins and is reporting perineal pain of 8 on a 10-point scale. What interventions should the nurse include in the plan of care?
   1. Provide the patient with an inflatable donut ring to sit on and administer her oral pain medication.
   2. Explain that this is normal after a vaginal delivery and assist her to a side-lying position.
   3. Assess the perineum for a hematoma or inflamed varicosities, and administer oral pain medication.
   4. Administer oral stool softeners and encourage fluids.

8. A postpartum patient calls the clinic 4 days after the birth of her newborn because she is extremely tired and her vaginal bleeding is heavier. Which does the nurse anticipate when advising her to come in to the office right now?
   1. A hematocrit will be drawn, and the licensed provider will check for retained placental fragments.
   2. Her stress level and sleep deprivation will be evaluated, and a prescription for sleeping medication will be given.
   3. The perineum will be evaluated for lacerations that were missed.
   4. Reassure the client that this is all normal and provide a prescription for slow-release iron tablets.

9. Hemabate has been ordered for a postpartum patient who has uncontrolled bleeding and uterine atony. Which is the appropriate nursing action?
   1. Check the patient's vital signs first for hypotension, and lower the head of the bed.
   2. Check the patient's blood glucose and increase the IV fluid rate.
   3. Check the patient's record for a history of asthma, and ask the licensed provider for an order of an antidiarrheal medication.
   4. Check the patient's record for a history of hypothyroid, and ask the licensed provider to order something for nausea.

10. The nurse is assessing a patient who is 12 hours postpartum. The uterus is firm to palpation, at midline, and is 1 cm below the umbilicus with continuous heavy vaginal bleeding. What is the nurse's first action?
    1. Massage the uterus and resume the IV Pitocin drip.
    2. Change the peri-pad and reassess the bleeding.
    3. Call the provider to check for a cervical laceration.
    4. Administer the ordered iron supplement and ibuprofen.

11. A breastfeeding patient who is 5 weeks postpartum calls the clinic and reports that she is achy all over, has a temperature of 100.2°F, and has pain and tenderness in her right breast. What is the nurse's best response?
    1. "You need to come to the clinic to be evaluated, as your symptoms indicate a possible breast infection."
    2. "You are having normal signs of engorgement with breastfeeding. More frequent breastfeeding will relieve your symptoms."
    3. "Please stop breastfeeding until you can come to see the clinic provider, as you may have a breast infection."
    4. "You may be experiencing sleep deprivation, which can make you feel achy and sore. Try to sleep when the newborn sleeps."

12. A postpartum cesarean patient comes into the rural health clinic at 1 week postdelivery for an incision check by the nurse. The vital signs reveal a temperature of 100.5°F, and the patient reports moderate foul-smelling lochia. The nurse determines that the skin incision is healing normally, but when palpating the uterus, she discovers the patient to have uterine and pelvic tenderness. What are the most appropriate nursing actions?
    1. Explain to the patient that the incision appears to be healing nicely. Have her take Tylenol for the elevated temperature and continue with the ordered pain medication until her next visit.
    2. Explain that the client should rest more to help the bleeding slow and that she should return to the clinic if she isn't feeling better in a few days.
    3. Explain to the patient that she is experiencing normal postoperative pain and bleeding and to come back for her scheduled 6-week postpartum checkup.
    4. Explain to the patient that she may have an infection of her uterus, and blood will need to be drawn to determine if this is the cause of her pain and excess bleeding.

13. The postpartum nurse notices that the last dose of IV Cefazolin is not running well. The patient's IV site appears red, inflamed, and swollen. The patient states that the IV is tender and sore. What are the nurse's next actions?
    1. Flush the IV with normal saline to improve the flow rate.
    2. Put the IV antibiotic on a pump for more accurate infusion of the correct dose.
    3. Remove the IV, restart it in a new location, and complete the antibiotic administration.
    4. Allow the IV to continue to drip slowly since it is her last dose.

14. A patient who has been on prolonged bedrest for bleeding associated with placenta previa was taken to the operating room for an emergency cesarean delivery. Sixteen hours postoperatively, the patient complains that her left leg is hurting. The nurse finds that the entire left leg is swollen and has pitting edema, while the right leg appears to be normal. Which order does the nurse anticipate when paging the health care provider to the room?
    1. White blood cell count (WBC)
    2. Ultrasound of the leg
    3. X-ray of the leg
    4. Serum creatinine

15. The postpartum nurse receives handoff communication from the postanesthesia care unit on a postoperative cesarean patient. Medical history includes smoking, obesity, history of thrombophlebitis, and varicose veins. The patient reports abdominal pain of 3 on a 10-point scale and is restless. What is the highest priority nursing action?
    1. Provide the patient with clear liquid to assist with hydration.
    2. Administer the ordered nicotine patch to prevent agitation from nicotine withdrawal.
    3. Administer pain medication and reassess the pain level in 1 hour.
    4. Apply external sequential compression devices to her legs.

16. A patient with no prenatal care arrives to the labor and delivery unit via ambulance because she has no transportation. She is in labor and has multiple bruises; she denies domestic violence. After a normal delivery over an intact perineum of a healthy baby, who appears to be term, she is comfortably breast-feeding. The fundus remains firm at the umbilicus and the placenta was found to be intact. The nurse evaluates the vaginal flow of bleeding over the first 2 hours and determines that over time she has slowly but persistently lost a total of 500 mL of blood. Which is the most important initial step for the bedside nurse to perform?
    1. Obtain a new set of vital signs, change her peri-pad, and move her to postpartum care.
    2. Obtain a new set of vital signs, increase the rate of her Pitocin drip, and massage the fundus.
    3. Obtain a new set of vital signs, page the licensed provider to the room for a postpartum hemorrhage, and draw laboratory work for platelets and clotting factors.
    4. Obtain a new set of vital signs, move her to a secure postpartum room, and notify the social worker that she is a victim of domestic violence.

17. What is the priority risk factor for the health care team to assess related to postpartum depression?
    1. A previous pregnancy and birth
    2. A history of postpartum or other depression
    3. Attendance at prenatal classes
    4. Employment status

18. During the immediate postpartum period, the nurse should assess risk factors for postpartum depression. Which of the following signs and symptoms should be monitored to verify this condition? *Select all that apply.*
    1. Decreased level of consciousness
    2. Disorganized behavior
    3. Hopelessness
    4. Unpredictable mood swings
    5. Increased need for sleep

19. A postpartum client's handoff communication revealed forceps-assisted delivery resulting in vaginal lacerations. What would the nurse identify if the client's bleeding was from the lacerations?
    1. Boggy uterus and heavy lochia
    2. Boggy uterus with fundus above umbilicus and deviated to the right
    3. Firm, contracted uterus with vaginal bleeding
    4. Firm, contracted uterus with scant lochia

20. A nurse is caring for a client who has a history of DVT. Instructions to the client should include which of the following? *Select all that apply.*
    1. Early ambulation
    2. Use compression hose
    3. Sit in a cross-legged position
    4. Elevate the leg as much as possible
    5. Massage the leg

21. When may a depressed mother be at the highest risk for actually committing suicide?
    1. When she discovers that she is unexpectedly pregnant during a busy and active time in her life.
    2. When she is in the depths of depression and can't get out of bed or complete any activities of daily living.
    3. During the recovery phase of depression, when she is starting to have more energy to carry out a previously planned suicide.
    4. Mothers don't usually carry out suicidal plans because they love their babies too much.

22. The nurse is assessing a postpartum client who has just given birth 1 hour ago. Which of the following would be most important to assess for at this time?
    1. Postpartum hemorrhage
    2. Postpartum infection
    3. Postpartum depression
    4. Postpartum mastitis

23. The physician has given the nurse an order to administer Methylergonovine (Methergine) to a postpartum client. What priority nursing assessment should the nurse do?
    1. Check the client's pulse
    2. Check the client's deep tendon reflexes
    3. Check the client's blood pressure
    4. Check the client's fundus

24. The postpartum nurse notes in the client records that she received Carboprost (Hemabate). The nurse understands that this medication was administered for which of the following?
    1. Breast engorgement
    2. Hypotension from epidural administration
    3. Excessive postpartum bleeding
    4. Cervical laceration

25. A 2-week postpartum client reports that her breast is very painful when she nurses. She states that she feels like she has the flu and has an elevated temperature. Which of the following statement made by the nurse is accurate?
    1. "I think that your breast is engorged. Increase breastfeeding time to empty your breast completely."
    2. "You may have an infection and will need to start bottle-feeding your baby."
    3. "You may have an infection and will need to be started on an antibiotic."
    4. "The flu is going around. You need to drink plenty of fluids and rest."

REVIEW QUESTIONS ANSWERS

1. ANSWER: 4
Rationale
1. Lifting the sheets and pads does not give an accurate estimation of blood loss volume.
2. Nurses and doctors tend to underestimate large volumes of blood loss; therefore, it is not as accurate, which is important in this case because she has already lost 400 mL of blood.
3. A laboratory draw will take too long to get back and the patient plan of care needs to be revised now; this hematocrit may not be accurate because of IV fluids that the patient may have received. A hematocrit the following day could be useful for ongoing care but not for immediate postdelivery care.
4. Weighing the blood-soaked linens and pads from under the patient and subtracting the dry weight of the items gives an accurate blood loss. This should be added to the total estimated blood loss, and the licensed provider should be informed and the plan of care appropriately revised.
TEST-TAKING TIP: One gram of weight equals 1 mL of liquid volume. Weigh blood-soaked pads and linens in grams, subtract the dry weight of the pads from the total to find mL of blood present. Another method is to zero the scale with a dry pad, remove that pad, and weigh the saturated pad to determine the blood's weight.
Content Area: Postpartum Hemorrhage
Integrated Process: Nursing Process—Implementation
Client Need: Safe and Effective Care
Cognitive Level: Application
Concept: Perfusion
Reference: *Alvarez-Ramirez, P., Trial, J., Hoff, B., & Scott, A. (2015). Quantifying blood loss at birth saves lives: Proceedings of the 2015 AWHONN convention. Journal of Obstetric, Gynecologic & Neonatal Nursing, 44(6), 45.*

2. ANSWER: 2
Rationale
1. The most common cause of heavy postpartum bleeding is uterine atony, so that should be checked immediately.
2. The most common cause of heavy postpartum bleeding is uterine atony, so checking the uterus first is correct.
3. The uterus needs to be assessed first. In an effort to reduce patient infection, it is better to assist the patient to the bathroom to void when safe to do so.
4. Moderate to heavy bleeding after 15 minutes always needs to be investigated as to the cause, to appropriately control excessive bleeding.
TEST-TAKING TIP: If uterine atony is found, immediately providing external fundal massage causes the uterus to contract. This is an important first step in preventing postpartum hemorrhage.
Content Area: Postpartum Hemorrhage
Integrated Process: Nursing Process—Assessment
Client Need: Safe and Effective Care
Cognitive Level: Application
Concept: Perfusion
Reference: *Durham, R. F., & Chapman, L. (2016). Maternal-child nursing care. 2nd ed. Philadelphia: F.A. Davis.*

3. ANSWER: 2
Rationale
1. Turning up the Pitocin may be an appropriate future action, but the first action should be to perform external fundal massage in an effort to firm the uterus and lessen bleeding from the placental site. Turning up the Pitocin may not be necessary if the uterus becomes firm with massage.
2. The nurse's priority action is to perform external fundal massage.
3. The nurse must first provide direct care to the patient with uterine atony in an attempt to immediately firm the fundus; next the nurse will update the provider.
4. If the boggy uterus can be firmed with massage, then having the patient empty the bladder may assist in keeping the fundus firm, but emptying the bladder does not cause the fundus to become firm, and it is not the first nursing action.
TEST-TAKING TIP: If the uterine fundus is atonic, soft, and boggy, it is the responsibility of the bedside nurse to first perform external massage and check to see if additional bleeding is present and then update the licensed provider. If the uterus does not firm up, then secondary measures are taken.
Content Area: Postpartum Hemorrhage
Integrated Process: Nursing Process—Assessment and Implementation
Client Need: Safe and Effective Care
Cognitive Level: Application
Concept: Perfusion
Reference: *Durham, R. F., & Chapman, L. (2016). Maternal-child nursing care. 2nd ed. Philadelphia: F.A. Davis.*

4. ANSWER: 1
Rationale
1. The patient is a moderate hemorrhage risk because of the fibroid and advanced maternal age. At minimum, a type and screen should be ordered.
2. The patient is not a high hemorrhage risk, and blood does not need to be ordered yet.
3. The patient is a moderate hemorrhage risk because of the fibroid and advanced maternal age.
4. It is important to assess the patient's hemorrhage risk on admission to the hospital and order a type and screen for a moderate-risk patient at that time. Later if blood is actually needed, valuable time will be lost waiting for blood typing and screening.
TEST-TAKING TIP: Predisposing factors for abnormal placental attachment leading to postpartum hemorrhage include previous cesarean delivery, previous uterine surgery, fibroids or other endometrial defects, advanced maternal age, placenta previa, or multiparity.
Content Area: Postpartum Hemorrhage
Integrated Process: Nursing Process—Planning
Client Need: Safe and Effective Care
Cognitive Level: Analysis
Concept: Perfusion
Reference: *Holt, J. (2015). Multidisciplinary care of a woman experiencing obstetric hemorrhage. Journal of Obstetric, Gynecologic & Neonatal Nursing, 44(6), 85-86.*

5. ANSWER: 4
Rationale
1. Clinical symptoms of dizziness may be a sign of postpartum hemorrhage, so it is important to assess the patient for bleeding.
2. Clinical symptoms of dizziness may be a sign of postpartum hemorrhage, so it is important to assess the patient for bleeding; however, it is okay to lower the head of the bed and allow a family member to hold the baby while assessing blood loss. The patient needs to be awake to communicate symptoms to the nurse.
3. Clinical symptoms of dizziness may be a sign of postpartum hemorrhage, so it is important to assess the patient for bleeding first; do not assume symptoms are due to medications.
4. This answer shows good situational awareness; a new set of vital signs will reveal if the patient is now hypotensive or has tachycardia and consider a manual radial pulse to assess quality of pulse.
TEST-TAKING TIP: Assessment for obvious bleeding or occult bleeding is mandatory in the presence of clinical symptoms.
Content Area: Postpartum Hemorrhage
Integrated Process: Nursing Process—Assessment
Client Need: Safe and Effective Care
Cognitive Level: Analysis
Concept: Perfusion
Reference: Cooper, S., Bulle, B., Endacott, R., et al. (2012). Managing women with acute physiological deterioration: Student midwives performance in a simulated setting. Women & Birth, 25(3), 27-36.

6. ANSWER: 2
Rationale
1. Cytotec and Methergine should be given now to keep the uterus firm and control further bleeding. Situational awareness would reveal that with the bleeding over 1,000 mL, the patient is already in an active postpartum hemorrhage.
2. This would be the correct medication to discuss and administer.
3. The abdominal dressing should not be removed at this time, considering the patient has a uterus that firms with massage; medication should be given to keep the uterus firm.
4. Methergine is not contraindicated in asthmatics; however, Hemabate should be given with extreme caution with asthmatic patients.
TEST-TAKING TIP: The nurse knows that in the nauseated patient, vomiting may ensue, hypotension from hemorrhage can cause vomiting, and Cytotec may cause vomiting; therefore, the best route is rectal. Methergine should also be given deep IM during active bleeding, and a site closer to the heart will disperse the medication more quickly. Oral Methergine may be given later to prevent bleeding after the initial hemorrhage is controlled.
Content Area: Postpartum Hemorrhage
Integrated Process: Nursing Process—Implementation
Client Need: Safe and Effective Care
Cognitive Level: Analysis
Concept: Perfusion
Reference: American College of Obstetricians and Gynecologists ACOG. (2006). Postpartum hemorrhage. ACOG Practice Bulletin No.76. Washington DC: ACOG.

7. ANSWER: 3
Rationale
1. Sitting on a donut ring may further compromise circulation to the perineal hematoma and is not recommended.
2. Perineal pain is normal after a vaginal delivery, but it should be assessed as to the source and be treated accordingly.
3. A perineal hematoma can be soothed with a soft perineal ice pack and oral medications.
4. The pain is coming from a perineal hematoma, not hemorrhoids, and although stool softeners may be important, they do not directly care for this problem.
TEST-TAKING TIP: Teaching the mother to breastfeed in a side-lying position will diminish the amount of time she has to sit directly on the hematoma.
Content Area: Perineal Hematoma
Integrated Process: Nursing Process—Assessment
Client Need: Safe and Effective Care; Patient Education
Cognitive Level: Application
Concept: Clotting
Reference: Oliveira, S., Silva, F., Riesco, M., Latorre, M., & Nobre, M. (2012). Comparison of application times for ice packs used to relieve perineal pain after normal birth: A randomized clinical trial. Journal of Clinical Nursing, 21(23), 3382-3391.

8. ANSWER: 1
Rationale
1. The patient is tired and has had continued blood loss, so a hematocrit will reveal her current status on which to base a plan of care. The most likely cause of increased bleeding is retained placental fragments, so this needs to be investigated first.
2. Sleeping medication does not address the increased bleeding and potential anemia as the root cause of the fatigue.
3. Evaluation of the uterus is the priority.
4. This action shows a lack of assessment by the nurse concerning the cause of increased bleeding.
TEST-TAKING TIP: Late postpartum hemorrhage happens after the first 24 hours and up to 1 or 2 weeks after delivery. Late postpartum hemorrhage is less common and is typically slow and insidious, causing maternal fatigue and anemia.
Content Area: Late Postpartum Hemorrhage
Integrated Process: Nursing Process—Assessment
Client Need: Safe and Effective Care
Cognitive Level: Analysis
Concept: Perfusion
Reference: Debost-Legrand, A., Riviere, O., Dossou, M., & Vendittelli, F. (2015). Risk factors for severe secondary postpartum hemorrhages: A historical cohort study. Birth: Issues in Perinatal Care, 42(3), 235-241.

9. ANSWER: 3
Rationale
1. Blood pressure does not affect the use of Hemabate.
2. Blood glucose does not affect Hemabate use.
3. The nurse correctly double-checks for a history of asthma.
4. The thyroid status does not affect the use of Hemabate, although an annoying side effect can be nausea.
TEST-TAKING TIP: Hemabate should be used with extreme caution in patients with asthma. It can also cause immediate and severe diarrhea, so an antidiarrheal medication is preventative.

Content Area: Postpartum Hemorrhage
Integrated Process: Nursing Process—Planning
Client Need: Safe and Effective Care
Cognitive Level: Application
Concept: Perfusion
Reference: California Maternal Quality Care Collaborative, CMQCC. (2014). Planning for and responding to obstetric hemorrhage. Obstetric hemorrhage toolkit, version 2. California Department of Public Health.

10. **ANSWER: 3**
Rationale
1. The uterus does not need fundal massage because it is already firm. The next step is to have the provider investigate for a laceration.
2. The nurse first needs to investigate the cause of the increased seepage of blood so that it can be controlled.
3. Continued heavy seepage from the vagina may indicate a cervical laceration; the provider needs to assess the patient for this.
4. The patient needs to be diagnosed as to the cause of the increased seepage so that it can be controlled.
TEST-TAKING TIP: Causes of lacerations include the use of forceps-assisted vaginal delivery, use of a vacuum-assisted vaginal delivery, a prolonged second stage, previous scarring, or fetal malpresentation.
Content Area: Postpartum Hemorrhage
Integrated Process: Nursing Process—Assessment
Client Need: Safe and Effective Care
Cognitive Level: Application
Concept: Perfusion
Reference: California Maternal Quality Care Collaborative, CMQCC. (2014). Planning for and responding to obstetric hemorrhage. Obstetric hemorrhage toolkit, version 2. California Department of Public Health.

11. **ANSWER: 1**
Rationale
1. With a temperature of 100.2°F and pain in the right breast, the patient probably does have mastitis. She needs to be brought into the office for an exam of the breast, and if it is mastitis, she needs antibiotics and to continue with the breastfeeding. Tylenol can be used for pain control in many cases.
2. The underlying cause of the pain needs to be identified and treated, not just medicated. She should be past the normal phase of engorgement at 5 weeks postpartum.
3. Mastitis needs to be treated and breastfeeding should continue.
4. Aches and a temperature of 100.2°F is not normal; the patient needs to come in for an examination of the breast.
TEST-TAKING TIP: Treatments for mastitis include antibiotic therapy to control the *S. aureus,* warm compresses for maternal comfort, analgesic and anti-inflammatory medications for pain control, and continued breastfeeding or pumping to prevent further milk stasis.
Content Area: Mastitis
Integrated Process: Nursing Process: Implementation
Client Need: Safe and Effective Care; Teaching/Learning
Cognitive Level: Application
Concept: Infection
Reference: Lowdermilk, D. L., Perry, S. E., Cashion, K., & Alden, K. R. (2016). Maternity & women's health care. 11th ed. St. Louis, MO: Elsevier.

12. **ANSWER: 4**
Rationale
1. The source of the pain, fever, and foul-smelling lochia needs to be diagnosed and treated, remembering to treat the source of the pain not just the pain.
2. This answer shows no situational awareness; yes, the incision was checked but the overall situation of endometritis was missed.
3. This answer shows no situational awareness; yes, the incision was checked but the overall situation of endometritis was missed.
4. The nurse correctly suspects endometritis with maternal fever, uterine and pelvic tenderness, and foul-smelling lochia. She draws a complete blood count because an elevated white blood count will help establish the diagnosis. She correctly communicates to the licensed provider that the patient needs to be assessed and prescribed a broad-spectrum antibiotic. The patient needs a follow-up appointment to ensure treatment is effective.
TEST-TAKING TIP: Endometritis is more common in cesarean delivery; therefore, a single dose of an IV antibiotic preoperatively is typically given to prevent infection.
Content Area: Endometritis
Integrated Process: Nursing Process—Implementation
Client Need: Safe and Effective Care
Cognitive Level: Application
Concept: Infection
Reference: Meaney-Delman, D., Bartlett, L., Gravett, M., & Jamieson, D. (2015). Oral and intramuscular treatment options for early postpartum endometritis in low-resource settings: A systematic review. Obstetrics & Gynecology, 125(4), 789-800.

13. **ANSWER: 3**
Rationale
1. The patient has developed phlebitis. Do not flush it with normal saline; remove it.
2. Do not pump IV fluids into an IV site that has developed phlebitis.
3. The initial steps for discovering an IV site that has developed phlebitis with a nontoxic medication is to stop the infusion and remove the IV. Restarting the antibiotic in a new site is correct.
4. Do not continue to administer IV fluids into a site that has developed phlebitis.
TEST-TAKING TIP: Predisposing risk factors for developing phlebitis include elevated fibrinogen levels from pregnancy, inactivity and bedrest, prolonged use of stirrups during second stage of labor, obesity, history of thrombophlebitis, varicose veins, advanced maternal age, smoking, or postpartum infection.
Content Area: Phlebitis
Integrated Process: Nursing Process—Assessment
Client Need: Safe and Effective Care
Cognitive Level: Application
Concept: Critical Thinking
Reference: Ogston-Tuck, S. (2014). Patient safety and pain in IV therapy. British Journal of Nursing, 23(2), 23.

14. **ANSWER: 3**
Rationale
1. The WBC does not diagnose DVT.
2. The nurse should anticipate getting an order for an ultrasound of the leg.

3. X-ray is not used to diagnose DVT.

4. The edema in the leg is caused by DVT, not poor kidney function.

TEST-TAKING TIP: Ultrasound of the leg is used to diagnose DVT before anticoagulant therapy is started.

Content Area: Thrombosis
Integrated Process: Nursing Process—Implementation
Client Need: Safe and Effective Care
Cognitive Level: Comprehension
Concept: Clotting
Reference: Burgazli, K., Bilgin, M., Ertan, A., et al. (2011). Diagnosis and treatment of deep-vein thrombosis and approach to venous thromboembolism in obstetrics and gynecology. Journal of the Turkish-German Gynecological Association, 12(3), 168-175.

15. ANSWER: 4

Rationale

1. The most important initial step is to apply external sequential compression devices to her legs to prevent DVT because she has seven (postpartum, postoperative, pain from surgery, history of smoking, obesity, thrombophlebitis, and varicose veins) risk factors identified. Advance the diet as tolerated with liquids first.

2. The most important initial step is to apply external sequential compression devices to her legs to prevent DVT because she has seven (postpartum, postoperative, pain from surgery, history of smoking, obesity, thrombophlebitis, and varicose veins) risk factors identified.

3. The most important initial step is to apply external sequential compression devices to her legs to prevent DVT because she has seven (postpartum, postoperative, pain from surgery, history of smoking, obesity, thrombophlebitis, and varicose veins) risk factors identified.

4. The nurse correctly applies the external sequential compression devices to her legs because the patient has seven (postpartum, postoperative, pain from surgery, history of smoking, obesity, thrombophlebitis, and varicose veins) identifiable risk factors for a DVT.

TEST-TAKING TIP: Prevention for DVT includes prenatal teaching and smoking cessation, avoiding the use of stirrups in the second stage of labor, encouraging reasonable and early ambulation after delivery, and consistently using external sequential compression devices on all intraoperative and postoperative cesarean delivery patients.

Content Area: Thrombosis
Integrated Process: Nursing Process—Implementation
Client Need: Safe and Effective Care
Cognitive Level: Analysis
Concept: Clotting
Reference: Brady, M., Carroll, A., Cheang, K., Straight, C., & Chelmow, D. (2015). Sequential compression device compliance in postoperative obstetrics and gynecology patients. Obstetrics & Gynecology, 125(1), 19-25.

16. ANSWER: 4

Rationale

1. This patient needs to remain in one-on-one care until the source of the persistent vaginal bleeding is identified.

2. The uterine fundus is already firm; increased Pitocin and fundal massage is not needed.

3. The nurse correctly assesses and communicates to the licensed provider the urgency of the problem and draws laboratory work to look for the source of the bleeding, which may be due to a clotting disorder or low platelets.

The patient's bruises may also represent a symptom of this problem.

4. This patient needs to remain in one-on-one care until the source of the persistent vaginal bleeding is identified. The patient's bruises may be due to a clotting disorder instead of domestic violence.

TEST-TAKING TIP: Decreased fibrinogen levels, increased prothrombin time, or underlying abnormalities may be present, like thrombocytopenic purpura, von Willebrand disease, or other hemophilia disorders.

Content Area: Postpartum Hemorrhage
Integrated Process: Nursing Process—Implementation
Client Need: Safe and Effective Care
Cognitive Level: Application
Concept: Perfusion
Reference: Lagana, A. S., Sofo, V., Salmeri, F. M., Chiofalo, B., Ciancimino, L., & Triolo, O. (2015). Postpartum management in a patient affected by thrombotic thrombocytopenic purpura: Case report and review of literature. Clinical and Experimental Obstetrics and Gynecology, 42(1), 90-94.

17. ANSWER: 2

Rationale

1. A previous pregnancy and birth does not increase a client's risk for postpartum depression.

2. Maternal history of depression put a client at an increased risk of developing postpartum depression.

3. Attending prenatal classes is not a risk factor for developing postpartum depression.

4. Employment status is not a risk factor for developing postpartum depression.

TEST-TAKING TIP: Other risk factors include sleep deprivation, dissatisfaction with body image changes, a difficult pregnancy, traumatic birth, having a baby with a disability, having twins or triplets, marital stress, being a teen mom, or having a breastfeeding failure.

Content Area: Postpartum Depression
Integrated Process: Nursing Process—Assessment
Client Need: Physiological Integrity—Reduction of Risk Potential
Cognitive Level: Comprehension
Concept: Mood
Reference: Liu, C., & Tronick, E. (2013). Rates and predictors of postpartum depression by race and ethnicity: Results from the 2004 to 2007 New York City PRAMS survey (Pregnancy Risk Assessment and Monitoring System). Maternal & Child Health Journal 17(9), 1599-1610.

18. ANSWER: 3, 4, 5

Rationale

1. With postpartum depression, the client does not have a decreased level of consciousness.

2. Disorganized behavior is associated with postpartum psychosis.

3. Hopelessness is a reported symptom of postpartum depression.

4. Unpredictable mood swings are a reported symptom of postpartum depression.

5. Increased need for sleep is a reported symptom of postpartum depression.

TEST-TAKING TIP: Medication is typically needed in most cases of PPD. Antidepressants and counseling together provide the most comprehensive treatment.

Content Area: Postpartum Depression
Integrated Process: Nursing Process—Assessment

Client Need: Physiological Integrity—Reduction of Risk Potential
Cognitive Level: Comprehension
Concept: Mood
Reference: *Lowdermilk, D. L., Perry, S. E., Cashion, K., & Alden, K. R. (2016). Maternity & women's health care. 11th ed. St. Louis, MO: Elsevier.*

19. ANSWER: 3
Rationale
1. This would be uterine atony.
2. This would be from a distended bladder.
3. This would indicate that the blood is coming from the vaginal laceration.
4. This is a normal finding and does not indicate active bleeding.
TEST-TAKING TIP: Lacerations of the perineum, vagina, or cervix can cause bleeding and postpartum hemorrhage. Lacerations can bleed slowly or rapidly and cause a large volume of accumulated blood loss over time.
Content Area: Postpartum Hemorrhage
Integrated Process: Nursing Process—Assessment
Client Need: Physiological Integrity
Cognitive Level: Comprehension
Concept: Perfusion
Reference: *Lowdermilk, D. L., Perry, S. E., Cashion, K., & Alden, K. R. (2016). Maternity & women's health care. 11th ed. St. Louis, MO: Elsevier.*

20. ANSWERS: 1, 2
Rationale
1. Early ambulation promotes good circulation and decreases clotting.
2. Compression hose help to promote good circulation and decrease clotting.
3. Legs should not be crossed and both feet should be on floor.
4. This does not help to promote circulation.
5. Deep-tissue massage of the area over a DVT can cause a piece of the clot to break off and travel up through the heart and into the lungs, causing a pulmonary embolism.
TEST-TAKING TIP: When answering a "select all that apply" question, first you must understand what the question is asking by identifying the topic and stem. Take each option separately and read as a true/false answer.
Content Area: Deep Vein Thrombosis
Integrated Process: Nursing Process—Assessment
Client Need: Physiological Integrity
Cognitive Level: Comprehension
Concept: Clotting
Reference: *Lowdermilk, D. L., Perry, S. E., Cashion, K., & Alden, K. R. (2016). Maternity & women's health care. 11th ed. St. Louis, MO: Elsevier.*

21. ANSWER: 3
Rationale
1. This is not an indication that the client is at a high risk for committing suicide.
2. The depressed individual may not have enough energy to carry out a suicide during the depth of depression.
3. This is the time the client would be at the highest risk.
4. Severely depressed mothers may commit suicide.
TEST-TAKING TIP: A client may be at highest risk for suicide during the recovery phase of a depressive episode, when they have more energy to carry out previously planned harmful actions.

Content Area: Postpartum Depression
Integrated Process: Nursing Process—Assessment
Client Need: Psychosocial Integrity
Cognitive Level: Comprehension
Concept: Mood
Reference: *Liu, C., & Tronick, E. (2013). Rates and predictors of postpartum depression by race and ethnicity: Results from the 2004 to 2007 New York City PRAMS survey (Pregnancy Risk Assessment and Monitoring System). Maternal & Child Health Journal 17(9), 1599-1610.*

22. ANSWER: 1
Rationale
1. Early postpartum hemorrhage can be assessed at this time.
2. Postpartum infection would be noted after the first 24 hours postdelivery.
3. Postpartum depression is noted several weeks following delivery.
4. Mastitis would be noted several weeks following delivery.
TEST-TAKING TIP: Uterine atony is the failure of the uterus to contract after the placenta has been delivered. The uterine muscle remains flaccid, and blood is allowed to continue to flow out through the site of the placenta. This is the most common cause of postpartum hemorrhage and usually begins within the first hour after delivery.
Content Area: Postpartum Hemorrhage
Integrated Process: Nursing Process—Assessment
Client Need: Physiological Integrity—Reduction of Risk Potential
Cognitive Level: Application
Concept: Perfusion
Reference: *Ward, S. L., & Hisley, S. M. (2016). Maternal-child nursing care. 2nd ed. Philadelphia: F.A. Davis.*

23. ANSWER: 3
Rationale
1. Methergine is not contraindicated if the client has a high or low pulse. The pulse should be checked if Procardia had been ordered.
2. If the client was receiving magnesium sulfate, the deep tendon reflexes should be assessed.
3. A priority assessment before administration of methylergonovine is blood pressure.
4. This is not a priority prior to giving methylergonovine. The fundus would be checked after administering to check for the drug's effect.
TEST-TAKING TIP: Note the key word *priority*. Always think about airway, breathing, circulation when considering priority options.
Content Area: Postpartum Hemorrhage
Integrated Process: Nursing Process—Assessment
Client Need: Physiological Integrity
Cognitive Level: Application
Concept: Perfusion
Reference: *Lowdermilk, D. L., Perry, S. E., Cashion, K., & Alden, K. R. (2016). Maternity & women's health care. 11th ed. St. Louis, MO: Elsevier.*

24. ANSWER: 3
Rationale
1. Carboprost does not treat breast engorgement.
2. Ephedrine is given for hypotension caused by epidural administration.
3. Carboprost is administered to prevent uterine atony.
4. Carboprost is not effective for cervical laceration.

TEST-TAKING TIP: Hemabate stimulates the uterus to contract. It is given deep IM and may be repeated every 15 to 90 minutes, but do not exceed eight doses total. Hemabate may also be given directly into the myometrium.

Content Area: Postpartum Hemorrhage
Integrated Process: Nursing Process—Assessment
Client Need: Physiological Integrity
Cognitive Level: Application
Concept: Perfusion
Reference: Ward, S. L., & Hisley, S. M. (2016). Maternal-child nursing care. 2nd ed. Philadelphia: F.A. Davis.

25. **ANSWER: 3**
Rationale
1. Breast engorgement does not cause flulike symptoms.
2. The client should be instructed to continue to breastfeed on both breasts.
3. Antibiotics will be prescribed for mastitis.
4. Flu does not affect the breast.

TEST-TAKING TIP: Mastitis typically originates in lactating women from a milk duct and causes tenderness, swelling, and redness at the site, along with overall maternal flulike symptoms.

Content Area: Mastitis
Integrated Process: Nursing Process—Implementation
Client Need: Physiological Integrity
Cognitive Level: Application
Concept: Infection
Reference: Durham, R. F., & Chapman, L. (2016). Maternal-child nursing care. 2nd ed. Philadelphia: F.A. Davis.

Newborn

Chapter 19

Newborn Adaptation

KEY TERMS

Acrocyanosis—Decrease in the amount of oxygen delivered to the extremities. The hands and feet turn blue because of the lack of oxygen. Decreased blood supply to the affected areas is caused by constriction or spasm of small blood vessels. It may appear intermittently for the first 10 days as a normal finding.

Brown fat—A type of fat present in newborns and rarely found in adults. This is a unique source of heat energy for the infant because it has greater thermogenic activity than ordinary fat. Brown fat deposits occur around the kidneys, neck, and upper chest.

Caput succedaneum—Diffuse edema of fetal scalp that crosses the suture lines. Head compression against the cervix impedes venous return, forcing serum into the interstitial tissues. The swelling reabsorbs within 1 to 3 days.

Cephalohematoma—A mass composed of clotted blood, located between the periosteum and the skull of a newborn. It is confined between suture lines and usually is unilateral. The cause is rupture of periosteal bridging veins due to pressure and friction during labor and delivery. The blood reabsorbs gradually within a few weeks of birth. Incidence is 1.5% to 2.5% of all deliveries. The overlying scalp is not discolored. If the lesion is extensive, hyperbilirubinemia may develop.

Conduction—The transfer of electrons, ions, heat, or sound waves through a conductor or conducting medium. This state of excitation affects adjacent portions of tissue or cells so that the disturbance is transmitted to remote points. This occurs in the fibers of muscles and the nervous system.

Convection—Loss of body heat by means of transfer to the surrounding cooling air

Evaporation—Loss in volume due to conversion of a liquid into a vapor; evaporative cooling occurs when reducing the body temperature of a patient with fever or heat stroke by spraying his or her skin with mist and then fanning the patient.

Hyperbilirubinemia—an excessive amount of bilirubin in the blood. It is seen in any illness causing jaundice, including diseases in which the biliary tree is obstructed, blood formation is ineffective, or severe hemolysis is present.

Insensible losses—The amount of fluid lost on a daily basis from the lungs, skin, respiratory tract, and water excreted in feces. The exact amount cannot be measured, but it is estimated to be between 40 and 600 mL in an adult under normal circumstances.

Lanugo—Fine downy hair over the face, shoulders, and back of the term infant that decreases with fetal age and serves as an indicator of gestational age

Pseudomenstruation—Thin, white or blood-tinged mucus may be present due to withdrawal of maternal hormones.

Radiation—The process by which energy is propagated through space or matter or the emission of rays in all directions from a common center

Surfactant—Protein that lowers surface tension and aids in lung expansion

Thermogenesis—Production of heat

Vernix caseosa—Thick, whitish substance fused with epidermis and serves as a protective covering for the infant

Vitamin K—In the newborn, the colon is sterile until food is ingested and bacteria colonize the site. Because this bacterial source of vitamin K is not immediately available, an intramuscular injection of 1 mg of water-soluble vitamin K (phytonadione) is recommended for all newborns.

I. The Newborn Period

The newborn period is a transition time that occurs immediately following birth until the 28th day of life. During this time, the newborn undergoes a series of transitional events that allows them to adjust to extrauterine life (life outside the womb) (Table 19.1). These changes happen when the umbilical cord is cut during the delivery period. Changes that occur during this time set the stage for later growth and development milestones. These adaptations are based on a full-term delivery of a newborn without complications.

II. Normal Physical Changes of the Newborn

A. Vital Signs
  Heart rate: 120–160 beats per minute (bpm). Heart rate may drop to 80 to 90 bpm during deep sleep and reach 170 to 180 bpm during excitability.
  Respiratory rate: 30 to 60 breaths per minute; rate may drop to 20 during stages of deep sleep.
  Blood pressure: 60 to 80 mm Hg systolic and 40 to 50 mm Hg diastolic; may drop by 15 mm Hg systolic during first hour of life.
B. Measurements
  Length: 7 to 22 in. (44 to 55 cm)
  Weight: 5 lb 8 oz to 8 lb 14 oz (2,500 to 4,000 g)
  Head circumference: 13 to 15 in. (32 to 38 cm) measured at the widest diameter (occipitofrontal circumference) of the head
  Chest circumference: 12 to 14 in. (30 to 36 cm), measured at the nipple line

III. The Neonatal Period (Birth to 28 Days of Life)

The neonatal period occurs from birth through the first 28 days of life. The transition from intrauterine life to extrauterine life occurs as the newborn tries to adjust to life in a new atmosphere. This transition begins when the umbilical cord is clamped and the neonate takes the first breath. The respiratory and cardiovascular systems undergo the most dynamic changes at this time, while other systems will also respond to significant changes. Supporting neonates as they transition into their new world is critical as they experience various physiological adaptations. Offering protection to the neonate at this time is equally important.

IV. Behavioral Stages During Newborn Transition

A. Transitional period
  1. The time frame occurring between intrauterine and extrauterine life; this occurs in phases. Apgar scoring uses five physiological signs the nurse can use to evaluate the physiological status of the newborn during the transitional period following delivery. Scoring includes heart rate, respiratory rate, skin color, reflex irritability, and muscle tone.
     Scoring: Infants will be given a score of 0 to 10 at 1 minute and 5 minutes after delivery, using the parameters indicated in Table 19.2. Each parameter will be given a separate score of 0, 1, or 2.
     a) Apgar scores 0 to 3: indicate that the neonate is in severe distress
     b) Scores of 4 to 6: indicate moderate difficulty with transition to extrauterine life
     c) Scores of 7 to 10: indicate stability; monitoring of the infant for potential changes or distress should still continue

ALERT The neonatal intensive care unit should be called to the bedside of the delivery if a baby is known or thought to be at risk for a traumatic delivery.

DID YOU KNOW?
Apgar scores provide the health care provider (HCP) with a way to assess how well the baby is tolerating the transition from intrauterine to extrauterine life.

B. General assessment
  In addition to measuring Apgar, the infant should be assessed for temperature, heart and respiratory rates,

Table 19.1 Comparison of Fetus and Newborn

System Changes	Fetus	Newborn
Respiratory	Fluid-filled, high-pressure system leads to blood shunting from lungs through ductus arteriosus to remainder of the body.	Air-filled, low-pressure system allows blood flow through lungs; increased oxygen content of blood leads to closing of ductus arteriosus.
Gas exchange	Placenta	Lungs
Circulatory	Right atrium pressure is greater than left, allowing blood flow through foramen ovale.	Left atrium pressure is greater than right, leading to foramen ovale closure.
Thermoregulation	Body temperature maintained by maternal body through intrauterine environment	Body temperature maintained through flexed posture and brown fat.

Table 19.2 The Apgar Scoring System

Physiological Parameter	Score		
	0	1	2
Heart rate	Absent	Slow: below 100	Above 100
Respiratory effort	Absent	Slow: irregular, weak cry	Good; strong cry
Muscle tone	Flaccid	Some flexion of extremities	Well flexed
Reflex irritability	No response	Grimace	Vigorous cry
Color	Blue, pale	Pink body, blue extremities	Completely pink

Range of Apgar Score: from 0 to 10

A 5-minute Apgar score of 7 to 10 is considered normal. Scores of 4, 5, and 6 are intermediate and not markers of increased risk of neurological dysfunction because such scores may be the result of physiological immaturity, maternal medications, the presence of congenital malformations, and other factors.

American Academy of Pediatrics and American College of Obstetricians and Gynecologists (2007). *Guidelines for perinatal care* (6th ed.). Elk Grove Village, IL: AAP.

skin color, adequacy of peripheral circulation, respiration effort, level of consciousness, muscle tone, and activity at least every 30 minutes until the infant remains stable for 2 hours.

C. Phase 1 of transition period
   1. First period of reactivity: lasts up to 30 minutes following delivery. Heart rate will increase to 160 to 180 bpm, then falls during the next 30 minutes to a baseline of 100 to 120 bpm. Respirations are irregular and range from 60 to 80 breaths per minute.
   2. These changes should resolve by the end of the first hour of life. Infants should be alert and startle to sound and touch; they may also display tremors, crying, and movement of the head from side to side. Upon auscultation, fine crackles and audible bowel sounds should be heard. Grunting, nasal flaring, and retractions may also be seen. The passage of urine and/or meconium may occur. The infant will then show decreased activity levels for the next 60 to 100 minutes.

   ALERT Oxygen and suction should always be readily available at the bedside regardless of whether the delivery is seen as high or low risk.

D. System changes during the transition to extrauterine life
   1. Respiratory system: Changes occurring in the respiratory system are critical for the infant as they begin their transition from fetus to neonate. The changes occur as a result of compression from the thorax, lung expansion, increase in alveolar oxygen concentration, and vasodilation of the pulmonary vessels. Changes can be impacted by sensory, mechanical, and chemical stimuli. While in utero, the infant's lungs are filled with amniotic fluid, which is forced out during delivery.

Surfactant, a phospholipid within the alveoli, helps to establish functional residual capacity. This lipoprotein allows the alveolar sacs to stay partially open at the end of exhalation, thereby decreasing the amount of pressure and energy the infant requires during inspiration. If decreased surfactant levels occur, usually related to immature lung development, then this transition to extrauterine life can be negatively affected.

DID YOU KNOW?

The signs of respiratory distress are cyanosis, apnea or tachypnea, retractions of the chest wall, grunting, nasal flaring, or hypotonia.

   2. Circulatory system: The transition from fetal to neonatal circulation occurs when the clamping of the umbilical cord is performed and the neonate takes his first breath. The respiratory system strongly impacts the transition to successful circulation. The ductus venosus, foramen ovale, and the ductus arteriosus undergo major circulatory changes.
   3. Ductus venosus: connects the umbilical vein to the inferior vena cava and closes by the third day of life. When the umbilical cord is clamped, blood flow to the umbilical vein ceases.
   4. Foramen ovale: opening between the right atrium and left atrium that should close after birth when the left atrial pressure is higher than the right atrial pressure. Any form of significant hypoxia can result in the reopening of the foramen ovale. However, it does not always close after birth and may not result in any significant problems.
   5. Ductus arteriosus: connects the pulmonary artery with the descending aorta and closes within the first day of life. When the infant takes the first breath, the pulmonary vascular resistance becomes less than systemic vascular resistance, causing a

left to right shunt. If the lungs do not expand effectively, the ductus arteriosus will remain open.

E. Phase 2 of transition period
   1. Occurs between 4 and 8 hours after birth and lasts 10 minutes to several hours.
   2. During this time, tachycardia and tachypnea are common, along with improved muscle tone, skin color changes, and mucus production. Meconium and/or urine may again be passed at this time.

V. Nursing Interventions During the Transition to Extrauterine Life

A. Safety measures
   The overall goal is to maintain airway patency, ensure that proper identification protocols have occurred, administer prescribed medications, and maintain thermoregulation measures. Abide by facility policy and procedures on properly identifying the newborn and parents. At this time, footprints may be done. Suction mouth and nose to remove fluid and mucus to prevent aspiration into the lungs by a sudden gasp of air.

   🛈 **ALERT** Suction the mouth first so that if the newborn takes a deep breath, secretions are not aspirated into the lungs.

B. Medication administration
   1. Medications are administered. **Vitamin K** does not cross the placenta of the newborn. The newborn's bowel is sterile, so inadequate amounts of vitamin K are produced and can lead to bleeding. Vitamin K is given to promote blood clotting.
   2. An eye prophylaxis (erythromycin or tetracycline) is administered to prevent ophthalmia neonatorum, which can lead to blindness.
   3. At some facilities, triple dye or bacitracin will be applied on the umbilical cord to prevent bacterial overgrowth.
   4. Hepatitis B vaccine may be given at this time as well and requires parental consent.

DID YOU KNOW?

Parents may refuse the eye prophylaxis and the hepatitis B treatments. Be sure to provide education to them before administering and obtain consent if warranted by the facility.

C. Gestational age/physical assessments
   1. Body temperature: not easily controlled by the infant and is of high priority during extrauterine transition. Assessment of body temperature is performed every 30 minutes for the first 2 hours of life until the temperature is stable, and then it is repeated every 4 to 8 hours, depending on facility protocol and nursing judgment.
   2. Heart rate and respiratory rate: taken immediately after birth, again on admission to the nursery, and once every 30 minutes for 2 hours if stable, after which they are taken once every 4 to 8 hours until discharge, depending on facility protocol and nursing judgment. Blood pressures are not routinely checked after the initial reading unless the infant's condition warrants it.

D. Gestational age assessment
   This is done after the baby is stable in the newborn nursery, generally within the first 2 hours of life.

E. Newborn classification
   Once the score is obtained, newborns are classified according to the following description:
   • Preterm or premature: born prior to 37 completed weeks gestation, regardless of birth weight
   • Term: can be further classified as early, full, and late, based on the following guidelines by the American Colleges of Obstetrics and Gynecology:
   • Early term: born between 37 weeks and 38 weeks plus 6 days
   • Full term: born between 39 weeks and 40 weeks plus 6 days
   • Late term: born between 41 weeks and 41 weeks plus 6 days
   • Post-term or postdates: born after completion of week 42 of gestation and beyond
   • Postmature: born after 42 weeks and demonstrating signs of placental aging

F. Weight and gestational age
   Once gestational age has been determined, birth weight will now be considered and newborns will be classified as the following:
   • Small for gestational age (SGA): weight less than the 10th percentile on standard growth charts
   • Appropriate for gestation age: weight between 10th and 90th percentiles

MAKING THE CONNECTION

Understanding the Dubowitz and Ballard System

This assessment will determine the stage of maturity based on physical signs and neurological characteristics. The tool that is most commonly used to determine gestational age assessment is the Dubowitz/Ballard system. Points are given for each assessment parameter with a low score of –1 or –2, indicating early gestational age and a high score of 4 or 5, indicating late gestational age or postmaturity. The total score will correspond to a specific gestational age in weeks. The assessment tool will allow the nurse to determine whether there is a possible growth and development problem resulting from prematurity or postmaturity.

- Large for gestational age (LGA): weight more than the 90th percentile on standard growth charts
G. General head-to-toe assessment
A general assessment of the infant should occur within a couple hours after the baby is born and may be performed in same room as the mom, in the newborn nursery, or during the transitional period. It is important that the room be well lit. The nurse should assess each system systematically, beginning with the head and then moving from head to toe. Generally this assessment should be done with the infant resting in the crib or under the radiant warmer. Abnormal findings within each system are discussed later in this chapter and in Chapter 21.
1. **Integumentary:** With the gloved hand, examine the skin, starting with the scalp and body hair. Assess nail color, textures, distribution, disruptions, eruptions, and birthmarks. Skin should appear pink, which indicates adequate cardiac perfusion. The nurse can assess bony prominences by blanching the skin, making sure that it returns from white to pink in less than 3 seconds. The nurse should note any changes and any marks in the skin related to birth injuries.
2. **Head:** The nurse should next examine the head, eyes, ears, nose, and throat. In general, the face should appear symmetrical throughout. Shape and size of eyes, coordination of eyelids, and placement in relationship to the forehead should all be assessed. Fontanels should be assessed along with suture lines. The anterior fontanel is palpated and is diamond shaped and is about 1 inch (2.5 cm) in size. The posterior fontanel is triangular in shape and 0.4 inches (1 cm) in size. Closures of fontanels vary in time; the posterior fontanel closes within 2 months or 8 weeks, although it can occasionally be closed at the time of birth. The anterior fontanel should stay open until the infant is 12 to 18 months of age. Any swelling should be assessed and determined if it crosses or does not cross suture lines.
   Lip movement should be symmetrical. Location of the ears should be assessed for placement and symmetry, although it is common for one ear to lie slightly lower than the other.
   The infant's nostrils should be patent and open bilaterally. Lip and tongue should be similar in color, and both upper and lower lip should be uniform in size. The chin/jaw should be easily visible in a profile position, as a small chin may impede tooth development, sucking, or swallowing. Movement of the tongue can also be hindered by a jaw that is too small.
   a) Palpation: The eyes, ears, and nose should be palpated for shape and size. The nurse needs to look at the iris, sclera, and conjunctiva and note any scleral hemorrhages that could occur

secondary to birth trauma. It is a good idea to perform a thorough exam of the eyes before eye prophylaxis is performed so the ointment does not obscure any findings. Nurses may use an ophthalmoscope to check for red reflexes in the eyes. If the red eye reflex is not seen, the nurse should notify the practitioner immediately. Mouth and gums should be palpated next to determine if neonatal teeth or cleft palate are present. While palpating the gums, the nurse should note the strength of the sucking and gag reflex.
3. **Respiratory system:** Symmetrical chest movement should be observed along with respiratory effort. Respiratory rate should be counted for 1 full minute; use of accessory muscles must be assessed and noted if seen. Placement and size of the breast tissue should be noted. Nasal patency should also be assessed by occluding one nare and closing the infant's mouth. This action should elicit rise of the infant's chest and then repeated to check the other side.
4. **Gastrointestinal system:** The infant's abdomen should appear round and symmetrical bilaterally. The nurse should pay particular attention to the cord, ensuring that it is free of signs of infection, active bleeding, or oozing. The inspection should ensure the cord has three vessels: two arteries and one vein. If inspection reveals anything abnormal, the nurse should document findings and notify the practitioner, as this finding could be associated with a congenital abnormality. Auscultation of the abdomen should reveal bowel sounds in all four quadrants, noting the gastric bubble in the upper abdominal area and heart sounds of the abdominal aorta.

DID YOU KNOW?
If an infant has not passed any meconium stool yet, the abdomen may appear to be distended. Wharton's jelly, a gelatinous substance found within the umbilical cord to provide cushion and support to the arteries and vein, may also be present.

   a) Palpation: light to deep palpation should be used to assess the abdomen. The nurse should start with light palpation at the lower sternal border; move midline to the umbilicus, assessing for an umbilical hernia; then move toward the symphysis pubis out toward the ribs. Deep palpation should reveal liver borders that are smooth and firm and located right below the right costal margin. The spleen is located below the left costal margin, and the nurse should only be able to palpate the tip of it. Palpation of any more than a tip of the spleen should be reported to the practitioner because it could indicate enlargement of the spleen. Kidneys may be difficult to palpate because of their small size, but if they are palpated, they should be 1 to 2 cm above the umbilicus. The bladder may also be palpated and should be smooth; it is located just below the umbilicus in a midline position.

DID YOU KNOW?

If a hernia is present, the nurse should determine the size as small or large. Small hernias may close without surgery, but if the hernia extends into the midline toward the symphysis pubis area, surgical intervention may be needed. Diastasis rectus, or thinning of the abdominal wall, may be found upon palpation of the abdomen. It will be felt as a long, raised midline lump that may be more easily identified if the infant is crying. Both conditions should be documented and reported to the practitioner.

5. **Genitourinary system:** In the male infant, the scrotum should be examined while hips are abducted to confirm that both testicles have properly descended. A testis that is undescended will reveal a flat or depressed area. The nurse should palpate the scrotum by using the second finger at the posterior scrotal midline while the thumb is on the anterior midline. Palpation should detect presence of a testis on both sides. Undescended testicles in infants born at 35 weeks gestation or more should receive a urological consultation. The nurse can stroke the inguinal canal or apply warm soapy water to this area to more easily examine the testicles.

   Female inspection starts with assessment of the labia majora. In a term or near term infant, examination should reveal that the borders touch and cover the clitoris completely. Infants with delayed development of the genitalia will reveal labia minora and exposed clitoris.

   a) Anus/anal opening: assessment should reveal only one opening. The nurse should document the passage of stool if possible, which confirms patency. Palpation should be done gently by touching the tissue surrounding the anal opening and assessing the muscle structures. Any rectal tears should be documented. Next, the nurse can place the infant in a prone position to observe for the wink reflex. This reflex can be assessed by stroking the buttocks from side to side, which should make the buttocks press together, producing a wink reflex at the opening. The reflex confirms correct anatomical position.

6. **Musculoskeletal system:** Assessment of the musculoskeletal system starts through observation of the infant's movements in the crib or under the warmer. The nurse should observe for flexion and extension of the extremities, head movements from side to side, and any sucking on the fingers or hands. Upon closer inspection, the nurse should document any difference in size and length of extremities that could be indicative of congenital conditions such as achondroplasia, more commonly known as *dwarfism*.

   a) Muscle tone and strength: with the infant in a supine position, the nurse should assess for any asymmetrical movements that could result from birth trauma, such as floppy tone, or hypotonia or hypertonia, which can be seen as tremors, twitches, or jerky movements. These findings should be documented and reported to the practitioner and may be related to problems associated with the pregnancy or birthing process.

   b) Palpation: the nurse should begin with the shoulders and then move slowly downward to the legs. Symmetry and passive range of motion should be assessed to reveal joint movement of the neck and upper and lower extremities. Head lag can be assessed by pulling the infant up while observing the head, which should gently fall back. It should be easy for the nurse to detect any bulging of the neck related to the thyroid gland and overall tone of the upper body and extremities.

DID YOU KNOW?

Congenital torticollis can occur as a result from positioning in utero or from the blood supply to the neck being compromised during injury to the infant. The condition produces limited range of motion and can also reveal one shoulder that is higher than the other and stiffness or swelling of the neck. The infant should be able to easily turn toward sound, but if this condition is present, the ability to rotate the neck may be hindered.

   c) Hip dysplasia: Ortolani and Barlow maneuvers are done during the assessment period to test for congenital developmental dysplasia of the hip (DDH). A trained HCP should perform this maneuver on the newborn. A "clicking" or "clucking" sound heard during the Ortolani maneuver will be heard when legs are abducted, indicating the femoral head is hitting the acetabulum; this is highly suggestive of DDH. During the Barlow maneuver, the provider may feel the femoral head slipping out of the acetabulum, while also listening for the "click" sound, again indicating DDH.

DID YOU KNOW?

If the baby has DDH, treatment will be initiated immediately upon discharge. The typical treatment for DDH is a Pavlik harness that is worn a minimum of 23 hours a day for several weeks.

7. **Neurological system:** assessment of the neurological system will also reveal reflexes.

Therefore, it is helpful if the nurse separates these findings by *major* reflexes, which include gag, Moro or startle, Babinski, and Galant, while *minor* reflexes include the grasp, toe grasp, rooting, sucking, head righting, stepping, and tonic neck. Table 19.3 will demonstrate proper technique in eliciting these reflexes.

Table 19.3 Newborn Reflexes

Palmar grasp	The infant curls his fingers around an object.
Toe or plantar grasp	The infant curls his toes around an object that has been placed at the sole of the foot.
Rooting and sucking reflexes	Stroke the infant's cheek and watch him turn toward the finger, open his mouth, and suck on an object placed in his mouth.
Extrusion reflex	Touch the tip of the infant's tongue and the tongue will protrude outward.
Stepping reflex 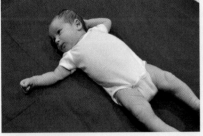	Hold the infant in an upright position with the legs flexed. The soles of the feet are lightly brushed against a flat surface. In response to the stimulation, the infant lifts his feet and then places them back down in a stepwise pattern that imitates walking.
Tonic neck or fencing reflex	Observe the infant in a supine position, extend his arm and leg on the side to which his head and jaw is turned while flexing his arm and leg on the opposite side.
Glabellar reflex	Tap on infant's forehead and observe him blink for the first few taps.
Babinski reflex	Lightly stroke the plantar surface of the foot from the heel toward the toes. The infant responds to this stimulation by first incurving the toes, then uncurling and stretching them out.
Moro reflex	Observe the infant's head as it is lifted while the nurse mimics a release and watches for extension of both arms along with flexion of the legs.
Galant reflex or trunk incurvation reflex 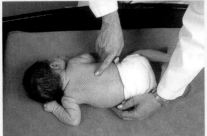	Observe the infant while supported in a prone position. Stroke one side of the vertebral column. The infant responds to this stimulus by moving his buttocks in a curving motion toward the side that is being stroked.
Crawling reflex	Place infant on his abdomen; observe him attempt to crawl.

VI. Normal Variations Seen in the Extrauterine Transition

A. Normal physical variations seen in the newborn (see Table 19.4)
   1. Cardiopulmonary changes: those arising during the delivery as a result of the squeezing of lung fluid from the newborn's trachea and lungs. This process is typically not seen during a cesarean section and therefore may create respiratory distress for the newborn.
   2. Breathing: The infant will typically be regarded as an abdominal breather. Chest size is relatively smaller in comparison to the abdomen; therefore, respirations are often better seen by watching the abdomen rise and fall.
      a) Transient tachypnea of the newborn (TTN) typically occurs in infants who are full or near term delivery. The condition generally lasts less than 24 hours and is more common among babies delivered via cesarean section, born to diabetic mothers, or born before 38 weeks gestational age. TTN can cause cyanosis of the skin, rapid breathing, grunting, nasal flaring, and/or retractions.
   3. Heart sounds: These should be auscultated for 1 full minute and may be irregular following delivery, lasting for the first few hours of life.
      a) Oftentimes, a murmur can be heard, and as long as it is not accompanied by any other physical changes, including respiratory distress, increased heart rate, or respiratory rate, it is disregarded as a normal variation.
      b) **Vernix caseosa** will cover the infant and offers protection to the skin. Although this thick, white substance does not need to be removed from the skin due to natural absorption, it will likely be removed postdelivery and during the first bath.

MAKING THE CONNECTION

Feeding Considerations

Infants with TTN may need oxygen to maintain stable blood-oxygen levels. It is common for the infant to appear in the most distress within the first few hours after delivery. Improvements are usually seen within 12 to 24 hours. The infant may not feed well during this time due to the rapid breathing pattern. Therefore, it may be necessary to support fluid and nutrition intravenously until improvements are seen. Antibiotics may also be administered until an infection is ruled out. Full recovery is typical within 1 week of the delivery.

---

   4. Acrocyanosis: Infants have vasomotor instability and capillary stasis, which produces a state of **acrocyanosis** for the newborn.
   5. **Lanugo:** The infant may have lanugo present at the time of delivery. The amount of lanugo will vary, depending on whether the infant was born term or preterm.
   6. Elongation of the head: this is typically seen as sutures override to accommodate passage through the birth canal. It will resolve within 1 week of delivery.
   7. **Caput succedaneum:** This is a generalized, edematous area of the scalp due to pressure of the presenting vertex on the cervix. The swelling will cross suture lines of the skull and disappear within approximately 3 to 4 days of birth. It is also common after a vacuum-assisted delivery.
   8. **Cephalohematoma:** This is a collection of blood between the skull bone and the periosteum. It does not cross the suture lines and may occur with or without caput succedaneum. This normal variation may not appear until the second or third day after delivery and may take up to 3 to 6 weeks for complete resolution.
      a) **Hyperbilirubinemia** and jaundice may occur as the destroyed red blood cells are reabsorbed, warranting further follow-up. See Chapter 22 for more details on this condition and treatment.

B. Heat loss
   1. Body temperature regulation: Due to an infant's immature ability to regulate their own body temperature, limited use of voluntary muscle activity, large body surface areas in comparison to body weight, and lack of subcutaneous fat, it is important to protect the infant from heat loss. Newborns have nonshivering **thermogenesis,** which occurs from **brown fat** and from their increased metabolic activity of vital organs. Interventions that can help to protect heat loss include keeping a cap on the baby's head, swaddling with warm blankets, and getting skin-to-skin contact with the mother's body. It is of equal importance to avoid overheating the infant, since they are not able to sweat and have an immature central nervous system to regulate their own body temperature. Therefore, body temperature should be maintained at 97.9°F to 99.7°F.
   2. Heat loss mechanisms can occur in the following ways:
      • **Convection:** flow of heat from body surface to cooler ambient air. Keep infants away from drafts.
      • **Radiation:** loss of heat from the body surface to a cooler solid surface that is near but not in direct contact with the infant (e.g., windows).
      • **Evaporation:** loss of heat occurring when a liquid is converted to vapors (e.g., after a bath or insensible losses).

- **Conduction:** loss of heat from the body surface to cooler surfaces in direct contact with the infant (e.g., a baby scale).

  Table 19.4 highlights the normal system changes during the transition to extrauterine life.

C. Stool patterns of the newborn
1. Meconium: The infant's first stool contains amniotic fluid, intestinal secretions, and ingested maternal blood (possible). This is passed within the first 24 to 48 hours after birth and is very sticky.
2. Transitional stools: appear by day 3 after feeding is established. It is greenish brown to yellowish brown and is thin, less sticky, and may contain milk curds.
3. Milk stool: appear by day 4. If the infant is breast-fed, the stools will be yellow to golden, pasty, and smell similar to sour milk. If the infant is formula-fed, the stools will be pale yellow to light brown and will be firmer in consistency and have a more pungent smell.
   a) Frequency: infants who are breastfed will have more frequent stools because the breast milk is more easily digested.

DID YOU KNOW?
Female newborns will sometimes have a bloody vaginal discharge during the first few weeks of life, called **pseudomenstruation.** This phenomenon requires no treatment and occurs as a result of the maternal hormones.

D. Primitive reflexes seen during the newborn period
   Absence or presence will alert the HCP as to whether the infant's development is normal or abnormal based on the response (see Table 19.3).

DID YOU KNOW?
If the caregiver continues to see the primitive reflexes after the expected disappearance time, he or she should notify the HCP. Persistence of primitive reflexes could be indicative of cerebral palsy.

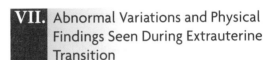

VII. Abnormal Variations and Physical Findings Seen During Extrauterine Transition

If any of the following behaviors are seen, immediate follow-up should be performed:
- Nasal flaring, intercostal or subcostal retractions, grunting, stridor, or gasping for air as a result of an airway obstruction.
- Respiratory rate less than 30 breaths per minute.
- Respiratory rate greater than 60 breaths per minute during rest.

Table 19.4 Normal System Changes During the Transition to Extrauterine Life

System Changes	Comments
Gastrointestinal	Hypoactive to normal bowel sounds heard. Bacterial colonization of gut within 24 hours of delivery allowing for vitamin K production. Stomach is size of a marble and can only hold small amounts of food for the first few days of life. Weight loss of 10% during first 2 weeks of life.
Genitourinary	Passage of meconium.
Renal	Maintains normal acid-base balance; body mass is 75% water, inability to concentrate urine until 3 months of age.
Immune	Receive antibodies/immunity from the mother in utero (passive acquired immunity), offering protection for the first 3 months of life. Infant immunoglobulin production will not be mature until later in infancy and childhood.
Integumentary	Thin epidermis; therefore can tear easily.
	Stork bites or salmon patches: superficial vascular areas found on the nape of the neck, eyelids, and in between eyes or upper lip; they disappear within first year. Milia: unopened sebaceous glands on the nose, chin, or forehead; disappear with 1 month of birth. Mongolian spots: blue/gray macules located on the lower back and buttocks, occurring more in African American, Asian, and Indian newborns; disappear within first 4 years of life.
	Erythema toxicum (newborn rash): small papules or pustules on skin resembling flea bites. It is a benign, idiopathic, generalized, transient rash during first week. Harlequin sign: dilation of blood vessels on one side of the body, common in low-birth-weight newborns, lasting less than 30 minutes. Nevus flammeus (port-wine stain): red/purple area with clear demarcation appearing on the face that does not fade or resolve spontaneously. Nevus vasculosus (strawberry mark/hemangioma): benign capillary hemangioma that appears raised, rough, dark red, with clearly identified demarcation marks found in the head within a few weeks to months of life; more common in premature infants, resolving by 3 years.
Neurological	Development is cephalocaudal and proximal-distal. Hearing is the only sense that is fully mature at birth; all others (vision, smell, taste, and touch) will mature over time. Primitive reflexes present at birth (discussed later).

- Apnea, rhonchi, crackles, wheezing, or stridor.
- Hypothermia—infants with a body temperature below 97.7°F may be at risk. Symptoms include shivering and cold, pale to blue skin. Infants will need immediate intervention for this condition. It is common for SGA infants to be more prone to hypothermia than term babies due to less brown fat and subcutaneous tissue, which offers protection against cold.
- Hypoglycemia—this condition can appear asymptomatically or along with symptoms of lethargy, irritability, poor feeding habits, pale to blue skin color, high-pitched or weak crying, jitteriness or tremors, floppy muscles, eye rolling, or seizures. Blood glucose levels will be below 40 mg/dL. The infant may be at increased risk of hypoglycemia if they are born to a diabetic mother or if they are LGA, post-term or preterm, SGA, hypothermic, or have an infection, respiratory distress, or birth trauma.
- Murmur along with poor feeding, apnea, cyanosis or pallor, tachycardia more than 160 bpm or bradycardia less than 100 bpm.
- Abnormal newborn size, either SGA or LGA.
- Subgaleal hemorrhage occurs when there is bleeding into the subgaleal compartment from forces that compress and drag the head through the pelvic outlet. The bleeding will extend beyond the bone, continues after birth, and can lead to hypovolemic shock or anemia. Early detection is imperative.
- Sepsis—although rare in the newborn, it can result in infant mortality. Common causes of sepsis in this age group may result from preterm birth, prolonged labor, rupture of membranes occurring over 18 hours prior to birth, maternal fever or positive group B streptococcal infection present at time of delivery, or if amniocentesis was performed. Sepsis will be categorized based on the specific time of onset. Although the infant may be asymptomatic, some signs and symptoms the nurse should be aware of include change in behavior, hypothermia or hyperthermia, lethargy, low blood sugar, and poor oral intake.

The nurse should notify the physician or practitioner immediately if any of these findings are seen.

MAKING THE CONNECTION

Recognizing Signs of Deterioration

Because some conditions can occur quickly in newborns, it is important that continuity of care occurs in areas such as the newborn nursery or neonatal intensive care unit so subtle changes can be recognized quickly. When sepsis is suspected in the newborn, laboratory work will be need to be drawn and may include C-reactive protein, complete blood count, and blood cultures. A spinal tap and/or urinalysis may also be performed.

VIII. Common Problems Found in the Newborn Period

A. Birth trauma during labor and delivery
Physical injury to the newborn can occur. Injuries may require specific interventions, while others are minor, requiring no intervention. The causes of injury may be related to the following:
- Maternal factors: uterine dysfunction leading to a prolonged labor process, a preterm or postdate delivery, and cephalopelvic disproportion.
- Intrauterine factors: macrosomia, multiple fetuses, abnormal presentation, congenital anomalies.
- Birthing methods: births that require forceps, vacuum extraction, external version or cesarean birth.

B. Birth trauma resulting in soft tissue injuries
Subconjunctival and/or retinal hemorrhages are a result of increased pressure occurring during birth and should disappear within 1 week of delivery. Skin changes may occur as a result of the use of forceps or vacuum and can appear in the form of bruising, petechiae, abrasions, lacerations, or edema. Be sure to explain to the parents why these may be present.

ALERT Parents must be told about any possible or sustained injuries during delivery and follow-up care that may be necessary.

CASE STUDY: Putting It All Together

Subjective Data

A 36-year-old African American female delivers a small for gestational age baby at the local women's hospital 1 hour ago, via a spontaneous vaginal delivery. The mother was afebrile at the time of delivery, and no other family members were present. The mother was 41 weeks gestational age and has had prenatal care since 6 weeks gestation. The mother has two other children, who were delivered before 37 weeks gestational age. After delivery, Apgar scores were assessed, a head-to-toe assessment was performed by the labor and delivery nurse, and the baby was transferred to the newborn nursery for further monitoring. Upon arrival to the nursery, the newborn was placed under the radiant warmer. The mother reports taking the following medications during pregnancy:

- Prenatal vitamin starting around 12 weeks gestational age until delivery, 1 cap by mouth once a day
- Acetaminophen (Tylenol) 500 mg by mouth when necessary for headaches and cramping

Objective Data

Nursing Assessment of Newborn

1. Apgar scores: reported as 9 at 1 minute and 10 at 5 minutes
2. Heart sounds: regular rate and rhythm
3. Respirations: clear, equal, and bilateral
4. Bowel sounds: absent
5. Pulses: 2+ brachial, 2+ pedal
6. Anterior and posterior fontanels: soft and flat
7. Acrocyanosis: noted, all other skin pink and warm to touch
8. Reflexes noted: Babinski+, rooting +, palmar grasp+, plantar grasp+, sucking+

Vital Signs

Heart rate: 155 bpm
Respiratory rate: 42 breaths per minute
Temperature: 98°F axillary

Laboratory results not performed at this time

Health Care Provider Orders

1. Obtain vital signs every 30 minutes for 2 hours; if stable, every 4 hours for 24 hours, then every 8 hours until discharge. Notify provider if vital signs outside normal parameters for age.
2. Transfer to newborn nursery once stable in labor and delivery.
3. Apply erythromycin eye ointment and triple dye to umbilical cord per hospital policy.
4. Administer vitamin K IM per hospital policy.
5. Administer hepatitis B vaccine if parental consent obtained.
6. Perform hearing screen on day of discharge.
7. Notify pediatrician or practitioner upon arrival to newborn nursery.
8. Allow mother to breastfeed or bottle feed immediately upon transfer to nursery and then every 3 hours as needed.
9. Notify practitioner if meconium not passed within 24 hours after delivery.
10. Await further orders per pediatric services.

Case Study Questions

1. What subjective and objective data are most important for the labor and delivery nurse to report to the newborn nursery nurse upon transfer?

2. What factors are most concerning regarding the patient and/or mother?

3. What interventions will be provided for the infant during the hospital stay?

4. What nursing diagnoses should take priority for this newborn after delivery?

Continued

CASE STUDY: Putting It All Together (Continued)

Continuing Case Study

The newborn has been in the newborn nursery for 3 hours. The mother has also been transferred to the postpartum floor located across from the newborn nursery. An assessment has been performed by the newborn nursery nurse, Dubowitz/Ballard screening has been performed, and vital signs are being assessed every 4 hours. The newborn has transferred to the open crib after reaching a stable temperature. The mother breastfed the baby one time in the nursery and is currently sleeping. She has requested that the baby stay in the nursery until she has more sleep. No one is in the room with the mother at this time. The mother has just received antibiotics because her temperature was recorded at 101.5°F upon arrival to the postpartum floor.

Objective Data

Physical Assessment of the Newborn

1. Sleep: sleeping quietly in an open crib
2. Cardiovascular: regular rate and rhythm
3. Respiratory: clear, equal bilateral breath sounds
4. Bowel sounds: active in all four quadrants
5. Stool: voided once; dark, tarry, green stool; passed 15 minutes ago
6. Skin: pink, warm, capillary refill time less than 3 seconds; blue/gray discoloration noted on buttocks area
7. Fontanels: soft and flat

Vital Signs
Heart rate: 146 bpm at rest
Respiratory rate: 38 breaths per minute
Temperature: 98.2°F axillary

Case Study Questions

5. What data are concerning regarding the mother at this time?

6. What education should the newborn nursery provide to the mother at this time?

REVIEW QUESTIONS

Be sure to read the Introduction for valuable test-taking tips.

1. Which assessment findings would the nurse expect to find on a newborn who delivered 24 hours ago?
   1. Blood pressure of 120/80
   2. Heart rate of 145 beats per minute
   3. Temperature of 96.8°F
   4. Respiratory rate: 62 breaths per minute

2. Which interventions should the nurse perform following the delivery of the newborn?
   1. Place the infant on the mother's chest after wrapping in a sterile blanket
   2. Measure the Apgar score at 5 and 10 minutes after delivery, report findings to the physician
   3. Remove vernix caseosa that is covering the infant's body while stimulating the infant to cry
   4. Transfer the infant to the newborn nursery after securing in warm blankets and an open crib

3. What is the Apgar score for the infant whose findings are heart rate 120 bpm, crying vigorously, actively moving extremities, blue hands and feet, and sneezed upon suctioning with bulb suction?
   1. Score of 7
   2. Score of 8
   3. Score of 9
   4. Score of 10

4. Why is the Dubowitz/Ballard assessment tool used on newborns following delivery?
   1. To determine whether the infant is transitioning to extrauterine life
   2. To predict any growth and development problems that the infant may have
   3. To determine the neuromuscular and physical maturity of the infant
   4. To compare the newborn with other newborns born at the same gestational age

5. A new mother and father are inspecting their baby after the nurse brings the infant to them. The mother wants to know why her baby has bruises on the buttocks area. Which statement should be made by the nurse?
   1. "Bruises are common after a traumatic delivery. I will ask the physician to come discuss the delivery."
   2. "These areas are called blue/gray macules and are common in certain ethnic groups, but will disappear around 3 years of age."
   3. "These are not bruises; these spots are birthmarks and are usually a permanent impairment."
   4. "The previous nurse did not report these findings. Who else has been in the room with the baby?"

6. The nursing student checks the newborn baby's temperature and finds the temperature to be 96°F axillary. What is the *next* action that should be taken?
   1. Notify the physician.
   2. Document the findings on the flow sheet.
   3. Swaddle the newborn and place a cap on the baby's head.
   4. Educate the mother on heat loss mechanisms in infants.

7. Which statement is the *most* accurate regarding suctioning of the oral and nasal passages of a newborn?
   1. The bulb syringe should be compressed after it is inserted into the baby's nose to suction.
   2. Suction the nose and then the mouth of the newborn to prevent aspiration.
   3. Saline should be placed in the baby's nose and mouth prior to suctioning.
   4. Place the bulb syringe on the side of the infant's cheek while suctioning the mouth.

8. Which step is *most* appropriate following delivery of a healthy newborn?
   1. Assess the newborn's temperature rectally following delivery.
   2. Place the newborn skin to skin in the mother's arms after the baby is dry.
   3. Clothe the baby and place the newborn under the radiant warmer until the temperature is stable.
   4. Wrap the baby in warm blankets; apply a cap to the bed and place open crib near the window.

9. Which condition of a newborn should the nurse further investigate?
   1. Temperature of 97.5°F axillary
   2. Respirations of 60 breaths per minute while soundly sleeping
   3. Acrocyanosis in a baby born 6 hours ago
   4. Fontanels that feel soft and flat

10. Which finding would indicate a baby who may be considered preterm?
    1. Labia minora are larger than labia majora
    2. Plantar creases cover two-thirds of foot
    3. Lanugo is mostly absent
    4. Ears with instant recoil

11. The newborn nursery nurse walks into the mother's room and notices the patient next to the window. What is the nurse's *next* course of action?
    1. Ask the mom to hold the infant using skin-to-skin contact.
    2. Nothing; infants are encouraged to be near the windows for sun exposure.
    3. Place the infant near the door on the other side of the room.
    4. Position the baby on the baby scale to obtain a weight.

12. Parents of an infant born 3 hours ago ask the nurse what medicine had to be given to their newborn. What is the *most* appropriate statement made by the nurse?
    1. "Clindamycin was given to prevent eye infections from sexually transmitted infections."
    2. "Vitamin K was given to prevent hemorrhagic disease."
    3. "Haemophilus influenzae vaccine was given to prevent the flu."
    4. "Rotateq was given to prevent gastrointestinal illness."

13. Which statement is *most* accurate regarding delivery of a newborn?
    1. Infants delivered via cesarean section are at lower risk of transitional problems.
    2. Vaginal deliveries increase the risk of infants aspirating lung fluid.
    3. Cesarean deliveries do not allow for thoracic squeeze of fluid.
    4. Vaginal deliveries are often avoided in term infants.

14. The nurse is teaching a student nurse about some of the differences between a term and preterm infant. Which statement is *most* accurate?
    1. Infants born at 32 weeks gestational age have sufficient alveolar stability to maintain adequate lung expansion.
    2. Surfactant may need to be given to the infant born less than 34 to 36 weeks of age to assist with alveolar stability.
    3. Women with gestational diabetes have larger babies; therefore, there are fewer issues with lung maturity when born preterm.
    4. Mothers carrying multiples fetuses will increase the surfactant production naturally in utero.

15. Which assessment indicates that the neonate is not transitioning to extrauterine life?
    1. The infant is maintaining breathing patterns with brief periods of periodic breathing for no longer than 10 seconds.
    2. Skin remains blue in color in hands and feet and pink centrally.
    3. Respiratory rate is 50 breaths per minute at rest.
    4. There are moderate retractions at rest.

16. Which finding should be *most* concerning immediately following delivery of a newborn?
    1. Capillary refill time of 3 seconds
    2. Heart rate of 180 bpm
    3. Respiratory rate of 65 breaths per minute
    4. Apgar score of 8 at 5 minutes

17. Which infant is at risk for heat loss? *Select all that apply.*
    1. Infant born at 38 weeks gestational age on a baby scale
    2. Preterm infant lying extended in the warmer
    3. Term infant who is lying in an open crib next to the door
    4. Infant born at 41 weeks swaddled in the open crib of the nursery

18. Which situation places the infant at *greatest* risk for developing hypothermia?
    1. Maternal fever
    2. Neutral ambient environment
    3. Large for gestational age infant
    4. Jaundice

19. Parents of a newborn are asking the nurse why their baby has to have a shot. Which is the nurse's *best* response?
    1. "We are trying to prevent any risk of infection in the eyes that could lead to blindness."
    2. "The umbilical cord is a site for infection. This shot will prevent illness."
    3. "Hospital policy states that all babies must receive a shot after delivery."
    4. "Clotting problems can occur in infants because they don't receive food right away."

20. An infant has just been admitted to the newborn nursery after an uncomplicated delivery. Upon assessment, the nurse notes poor muscle tone and a temperature of 96°F axillary. What is the *next* course of action?
    1. Obtain a blood glucose reading
    2. Prepare for resuscitation needs
    3. Call for a transfer to the neonatal intensive care unit
    4. Place warm blankets around the newborn in the open crib

21. A mother is concerned that her infant was very awake and alert immediately after birth for about 45 minutes but has now been asleep for 3 hours. Which statement by the nurse is *most* appropriate to address the mother's concerns?
    1. "Babies will go in and out of sleep constantly; this is nothing to be concerned about."
    2. "This behavior is concerning. I will call the practitioner and take the baby back to the nursery."
    3. "When was the last time the baby has had anything to eat? It may be time to offer another feeding."
    4. "This is common; babies will have periods of activity and inactivity following delivery."

22. Which diagnosis should the newborn nursery nurse consider for a baby during the second period of reactivity?
    1. Altered health maintenance related to maternal infant bonding
    2. Risk for infection related to immature status of the newborn's immunological system
    3. Risk for ineffective airway clearance related to increased oral mucus and gagging episodes
    4. Altered nutrition, less than body requirements related to limited nutritional and fluid intake, decreasing caloric intake

23. The first period of reactivity is a great time for the nurse to do which action for the baby?
    1. Allow for maternal and infant bonding
    2. Perform a thorough head-to-toe assessment
    3. Initiate the hearing screen on the baby
    4. Bathe the baby in the nursery

24. During the first period of reactivity, the nurse should provide which action for the baby?
    1. Feed the infant in the nursery
    2. Assess vital signs every 15 minutes
    3. Obtain a blood glucose reading on the baby
    4. Encourage skin-to-skin contact or wrap the baby in blankets

25. A mother has just given birth to her infant. Which intervention should be made *next* by the nurse for the infant?
    1. Place the infant in the mother's arms after swaddling in the blanket provided by the parents.
    2. Dry the infant before placing unclothed under the warmer.
    3. Feed the infant 1 ounce of glucose water.
    4. Suction the infant's nose and then mouth.

REVIEW QUESTIONS ANSWERS

1. **ANSWER: 2**
Rationale
1. Normal blood pressure parameters are 50 to 75 mm Hg systolic and 30 to 45 mm Hg diastolic.
2. Normal heart rate for a newborn is 120 to 160 bpm.
3. Normal temperature parameters are 97.9°F to 99.5°F.
4. Normal respiratory rate is 30 to 60 breaths per minute.
TEST-TAKING TIP: Recognize that a blood pressure is not typically taken on a healthy newborn with an uncomplicated delivery. Recall that the other findings are not within the normal vital sign parameters for a newborn.
Content Area: Newborn
Integrated Processes: Caring; Nursing Process—Assessment
Client Need: Physiological Integrity; Reduction of Risk Potential; Changes/Abnormalities in Vital Signs
Cognitive Level: Analysis
Concept: Assessment
Reference: *Ward, S. L., & Hisley, S. M. (2009).* Maternal-child nursing care: Optimizing outcomes for mothers, children & families. *Philadelphia: F.A. Davis.*

2. **ANSWER: 1**
Rationale
1. The nurse should receive the infant in a sterile blanket and place on the mother's abdomen to provide comfort, which allows the mother's body temperature to keep the infant warm.
2. Apgar scores should be measured within 1 minute and 5 minutes after delivery. Waiting until 5 minutes and then again at 10 minutes is too long of a time frame to know whether the infant is making a safe transition from intrauterine to extrauterine life.
3. The vernix caseosa serves as a protective covering for the infant and does not need to be removed after birth because it will be absorbed into the skin.
4. Although the infant may eventually be transferred to the newborn nursery in warm blankets and an open crib, this is not the first priority. The first priority is to make sure transition from intrauterine to extrauterine life is safe.
TEST-TAKING TIP: Recall that Apgar scores should be taken at 1 minute, 5 minutes, and 10 minutes and that nurses want to promote the infant and mother bonding relationship immediately after delivery.
Content Area: Newborn
Integrated Processes: Caring; Nursing Process—Analysis
Client Need: Physiological Integrity; Reduction of Risk Potential; Therapeutic Procedures
Cognitive Level: Application
Concept: Critical Thinking
References: *Ricci. S. S. (2013).* Essentials of maternity, newborn and women's health nursing. *3rd ed. Philadelphia: Lippincott, Williams and Wilkins; Ward, S. L., & Hisley, S. M. (2009).* Maternal-child nursing care: Optimizing outcomes for mothers, children & families. *Philadelphia: F.A. Davis.*

3. **ANSWER: 3**
Rationale
1. This score is too low; the infant is missing 2 points. Points are allocated as follows: 2 points for heart rate greater than 100 bpm, crying vigorously (respiratory effort), sneezing upon stimulation (reflex), actively moving (activity), and 1 point for having acrocyanosis (color).

2. This score is too low; the infant is missing 1 point. Points are allocated as follows: 2 points for heart rate greater than 100 bpm, crying vigorously (respiratory effort), sneezing upon stimulation (reflex), actively moving (activity), and 1 point for having acrocyanosis (color).
3. The infant received a score of 2 points for heart rate greater than 100 bpm, crying vigorously (respiratory effort), sneezing upon stimulation (reflex), actively moving (activity), and 1 point for having acrocyanosis (color).
4. This score is too high for the infant; 1 point was lost for color of blue hands and feet.
TEST-TAKING TIP: Recall that Apgar scores are assessed by measuring activity level, respiratory effort, reflex, color, and crying in the infant.
Content Area: Newborn
Integrated Processes: Caring; Nursing Process—Assessment
Client Need: Physiological Integrity; Reduction of Risk Potential; Changes/Abnormalities in Vital Signs
Cognitive Level: Analysis
Concept: Assessment
Reference: *American Academy of Pediatrics (2012). Ages and stages: Apgar score. Retrieved from www.healthychildren.org/English/ages-stages/prenatal/delivery-beyond/Pages/Apgar-Scores.aspx?nfstatus=401&nftoken=00000000-0000-0000-0000-000000000000&nfstatusdescription=ERROR%3a+No+local+token.*

4. **ANSWER: 3**
Rationale
1. The Apgar score is used to determine transition to extrauterine life.
2. The Dubowitz/Ballard screening tool is not used to determine growth and development problems.
3. The screening tool does determine physical and neuro-muscular maturity.
4. The screening tool is not used as a comparison with any other infants.
TEST-TAKING TIP: Recognize the purpose of the Dubowitz/Ballard assessment tool for screening newborns through the transitioning process.
Content Area: Newborn
Integrated Processes: Caring; Nursing Process—Analysis
Client Need: Physiological Integrity; Reduction of Risk Potential; Potential for Alterations in Body Systems
Cognitive Level: Analysis
Concept: Assessment
Reference: *Ward, S. L., & Hisley, S. M. (2009).* Maternal-child nursing care: Optimizing outcomes for mothers, children & families. *Philadelphia: F.A. Davis.*

5. **ANSWER: 2**
Rationale
1. Although a traumatic delivery can cause injury, these spots are most likely a result of blue/gray macules or Mongolian spots, which resemble bruises and are commonly found on the back and buttocks.
2. Blue/gray macules or Mongolian spots are common in newborns of Mediterranean, Latin American, Asian, or African descents and will commonly disappear in early childhood. The nurse should point out that although they appear as bruises, they are not painful and no interventions are necessary.
3. These spots are not birthmarks, so this answer is not true.

4. This answer is accusatory in nature and assumes that someone else has inflicted bruises on the infant.
TEST-TAKING TIP: Recognize what the common skin variations are in newborns based on ethnicities.
Content Area: Newborn
Integrated Processes: Communication & Documentation; Nursing Process—Planning
Client Need: Psychosocial Integrity; Therapeutic Communication
Cognitive Level: Analysis
Concept: Promoting Health
Reference: *Ward, S. L., & Hisley, S. M. (2009). Maternal-child nursing care: Optimizing outcomes for mothers, children & families. Philadelphia: F.A. Davis.*

6. ANSWER: 3
Rationale
1. Notifying the physician would be necessary only if the baby's temperature continues to stay low after interventions have been initiated.
2. Documenting this information is important but is not the first step.
3. This is the first intervention that should be done to raise the baby's temperature.
4. Educating the mother is important but should be done after the baby's temperature is stable.
TEST-TAKING TIP: Recognize first if the temperature in the stem is a normal or abnormal finding, then determine what the next best course of action would be.
Content Area: Newborn
Integrated Processes: Caring; Nursing Process—Implementation
Client Need: Safe and Effective Care Environment; Management of Care; Continuity of Care
Cognitive Level: Analysis
Concept: Critical Thinking
Reference: *Ward, S. L., & Hisley, S. M. (2009). Maternal-child nursing care: Optimizing outcomes for mothers, children & families. Philadelphia: F.A. Davis.*

7. ANSWER: 4
Rationale
1. The bulb syringe should always be compressed before it is inserted into the mouth or nose to prevent secretions from entering the respiratory tract.
2. The mouth should always be suctioned before the nose in a newborn to prevent aspiration of contents farther into the respiratory tract.
3. Saline is not routinely used in suctioning of a newborn following delivery; the nurse should check with the facility's policies on using saline while suctioning.
4. Placing the bulb syringe on the newborn's cheek will prevent stimulation of the gag reflex, thereby preventing aspiration into the respiratory tract.
TEST-TAKING TIP: Recall the *most* correct technique for using a bulb syringe.
Content Area: Newborn
Integrated Processes: Caring; Nursing Process—Implementation
Client Need: Safe and Effective Care Environment; Safety and Infection Control; Safe Use of Equipment

Cognitive Level: Application
Concept: Nursing
Reference: *Ward, S. L., & Hisley, S. M. (2009). Maternal-child nursing care: Optimizing outcomes for mothers, children & families. Philadelphia: F.A. Davis.*

8. ANSWER: 2
Rationale
1. The baby's temperature should be checked using an axillary method or by attaching a thermoprobe to the skin. Rectal temperatures are not recommended.
2. Placing the baby skin to skin on the mother after the newborn is dry will help to maintain the baby's temperature.
3. The baby should not be placed under the warmer with clothes on because there will be no benefit of the radiant heat to the baby.
4. Placing warm blankets on the baby and a cap is helpful to prevent heat loss, but placing the baby next to a window will allow for heat loss by radiation.
TEST-TAKING TIP: Recall how to maintain a stable temperature in a newborn following delivery using the word *most* in the stem as the priority.
Content Area: Newborn
Integrated Processes: Caring; Nursing Process—Implementation
Client Need: Safe and Effective Care Environment; Management of Care; Establishing Priorities
Cognitive Level: Application
Concept: Assessment
Reference: *Ward, S. L., & Hisley, S. M. (2009). Maternal-child nursing care: Optimizing outcomes for mothers, children & families. Philadelphia: F.A. Davis.*

9. ANSWER: 2
Rationale
1. Temperature of a newborn will range from 97.5°F to 99°F axillary.
2. Normal respirations are between 30 and 60 breaths per minute. While at rest, a patient who is breathing at 60 breaths per minute should be watched more closely, as this is a sign of potential respiratory distress.
3. Acrocyanosis is common in newborns and does not warrant any further investigation.
4. Fontanels should remain soft and flat; this does not warrant any further investigation.
TEST-TAKING TIP: Recognize which descriptor is normal or abnormal and then decide which answer is the most concerning.
Content Area: Newborn
Integrated Processes: Teaching and Learning; Nursing Process—Assessment
Client Need: Physiological Integrity; Reduction of Risk Potential; Potential for Alterations in Body Systems
Cognitive Level: Analysis
Concept: Critical Thinking
Reference: *Ward, S. L., & Hisley, S. M. (2009). Maternal-child nursing care: Optimizing outcomes for mothers, children & families. Philadelphia: F.A. Davis.*

10. ANSWER: 1
Rationale
1. In a preterm infant, the labia minora and clitoris will be larger than the labia majora.

2. A full-term infant is expected to have plantar creases on two-thirds of the foot.
3. In a full-term infant, lanugo should have bald areas.
4. Ear recoil in a full-term infant should be instant with thick cartilage or stiffness.
TEST-TAKING TIP: Recall normal findings in a preterm infant upon physical exam.
Content Area: Newborn
Integrated Processes: Teaching and Learning; Nursing Process—Assessment
Client Need: Health Promotion and Maintenance; Developmental Stages and Transitions
Cognitive Level: Comprehension
Concept: Assessment
Reference: Ward, S. L., & Hisley, S. M. (2009). Maternal-child nursing care: Optimizing outcomes for mothers, children & families. Philadelphia: F.A. Davis.

11. **ANSWER: 1**
Rationale
1. Placing the infant in the mother's arms using skin to skin contact will help warm the newborn.
2. Windows are often drafty and can create heat loss through convection.
3. Placing the infant near the door will allow for heat loss through convection and is therefore not the best choice.
4. Placing the baby on the baby scale can create more heat loss through conduction.
TEST-TAKING TIP: Recognize which action in the descriptors would not interfere with heat loss in the newborn.
Content Area: Newborn
Integrated Processes: Teaching and Learning; Nursing Process—Implementation
Client Need: Health Promotion and Maintenance; Principles of Teaching and Learning
Cognitive Level: Comprehension
Concept: Promoting Health
Reference: Ward, S. L., & Hisley, S. M. (2009). Maternal-child nursing care: Optimizing outcomes for mothers, children & families. Philadelphia: F.A. Davis.

12. **ANSWER: 2**
Rationales
1. Erythromycin not clindamycin is given to prevent eye infections related to sexually transmitted illness.
2. This is true; vitamin K is given to prevent hemorrhagic disease.
3. A flu vaccine is only given to infants older than 6 months of age, so this is incorrect.
4. Rotateq is not given until the infant reaches 4 months of age.
TEST-TAKING TIP: Recognize the priority word in the stem is *most* to determine which statement is most appropriate for the nurse to make.
Content Area: Newborn
Integrated Processes: Teaching and Learning; Nursing Process—Implementation
Client Need: Health Promotion and Maintenance; Principles of Teaching and Learning
Cognitive Level: Assessment
Concept: Nursing Roles

Reference: Ward, S. L., & Hisley, S. M. (2009). Maternal-child nursing care: Optimizing outcomes for mothers, children & families. Philadelphia: F.A. Davis.

13. **ANSWER: 3**
Rationale
1. Infants born via cesarean delivery are at increased risk of transitional problems because they do not have the thoracic squeeze that the babies born vaginally receive; therefore, the transition to extrauterine life and risk of pulmonary complications can be increased.
2. Vaginal deliveries decrease the risk of aspirating lung fluid because the infant will go through the thoracic squeeze in the birth canal.
3. This answer is true and therefore places the infant at a higher risk of pulmonary complications.
4. This is not true; each delivery is unique and the term status of an infant would not warrant a cesarean delivery.
TEST-TAKING TIP: Recognize the priority word in the stem is *most* to determine which statement is most accurate in correlation with delivery of a newborn.
Content Area: Newborn
Integrated Processes: Teaching and Learning; Nursing Process—Analysis
Client Need: Health Promotion and Maintenance; Developmental Stages and Transitions
Cognitive Level: Comprehension
Concept: Critical Thinking
Reference: Ward, S. L., & Hisley, S. M. (2009). Maternal-child nursing care: Optimizing outcomes for mothers, children & families. Philadelphia: F.A. Davis.

14. **ANSWER: 2**
Rationale
1. Infants will not have alveolar stability because their lungs are not fully mature at 32 weeks.
2. Premature infants are at risk to have respiratory distress syndrome because of low surfactant production if born less than 36 weeks gestational age.
3. While newborns born to women with gestational diabetes may be larger, that doesn't necessarily decrease their risk for full lung maturity. They are at risk for transient tachypnea of the newborn.
4. Surfactant production will not increase due to multiple gestation. There is an increased risk for multiple gestational pregnancies to deliver early, increasing the risk of respiratory problems.
TEST-TAKING TIP: Recall when full lung maturity occurs in a newborn and risk factors that newborns have for respiratory distress.
Content Area: Newborn
Integrated Processes: Teaching and Learning; Nursing Process—Analysis
Client Need: Physiological Integrity; Physiological Adaptation; Body Systems
Cognitive Level: Analysis
Concept: Critical Thinking
Reference: Ward, S. L., & Hisley, S. M. (2009). Maternal-child nursing care: Optimizing outcomes for mothers, children & families. Philadelphia: F.A. Davis.

15. ANSWER: 4
Rationale
1. Periodic breathing lasts between 5 and 15 seconds and is not concerning. Any apnea lasting more than 20 seconds should be immediately reported.
2. Acrocyanosis is common in the infant for up to 24 hours postdelivery.
3. The respiratory rate should be between 40 and 60 breaths per minute.
4. Moderate retractions and/or grunting would be concerning in the infant.
TEST-TAKING TIP: Determine which statement is a normal transition to extrauterine life and which statement is not, as the neonate who is not transitioning to extrauterine life.
Content Area: Newborn
Integrated Processes: Caring; Nursing Process—Analysis
Client Need: Physiological Integrity; Physiological Adaptation; Alterations in Body Systems
Cognitive Level: Analysis
Concept: Critical Thinking
Reference: Ward, S. L., & Hisley, S. M. (2009). Maternal-child nursing care: Optimizing outcomes for mothers, children & families. Philadelphia: F.A. Davis.

16. ANSWER: 3
Rationale
1. Capillary refill time would be concerning if it were greater than 3 seconds.
2. The heart rate following delivery can be as high as 160 to 180 beats per minute but should then decline to 120 to 160 beats per minute within 30 minutes; this is still a normal finding.
3. A respiratory rate of 40 to 60 breaths per minute is within the normal range for newborns; therefore, 65 breaths per minute is concerning.
4. An Apgar score of 8 does not warrant immediate action; this is still a normal finding.
TEST-TAKING TIP: Recognize the priority words in the stem are *most* and *immediately* following delivery.
Content Area: Newborn
Integrated Processes: Caring; Nursing Process—Assessment
Client Need: Physiological Integrity; Physiological Adaptation; Illness Management
Cognitive Level: Analysis
Concept: Critical Thinking
Reference: Ward, S. L., & Hisley, S. M. (2009). Maternal-child nursing care: Optimizing outcomes for mothers, children & families. Philadelphia: F.A. Davis.

17. ANSWER: 1, 3
Rationale
1. The risk factor for heat loss in this infant is that they are lying on the baby scale, which is an example of conduction.
2. Although the infant is preterm, they are in a neutral thermal environment of the warmer, so heat loss should not be present.
3. The infant is at risk of convection heat loss because of the draft from the door.
4. This infant is not at risk of heat loss because they are swaddled, conserving heat and minimizing loss.
TEST-TAKING TIP: Recall how an infant loses heat through radiation, evaporation, conduction, or convection, and

recognize which factors the newborns in the examples are most at risk for.
Content Area: Newborn
Integrated Processes: Caring; Nursing Process—Assessment
Client Need: Physiological Integrity; Physiological Adaptation; Hemodynamics
Cognitive Level: Analysis
Concept: Assessment
Reference: Ward, S. L., & Hisley, S. M. (2009). Maternal-child nursing care: Optimizing outcomes for mothers, children & families. Philadelphia: F.A. Davis.

18. ANSWER: 3
Rationale
1. Maternal fever is not a factor for an infant's maintenance of body temperature; this is not a risk factor.
2. The neutral ambient temperature can be a factor in helping to keep the infant warm but it is the large body surface area compared to the body weight that serves as a greater risk factor.
3. Infants have an inability to regulate their own body temperature, and their limited use of voluntary muscle activity, large body surface areas in comparison to body weight, and lack of subcutaneous fat make it important to protect the infant from heat loss. This answer is correct.
4. Jaundice does not serve as the greatest risk factor to protect the infant from heat loss.
TEST-TAKING TIP: Recall how infants lose heat from their bodies and what contributes as the greatest risk factors.
Content Area: Newborn
Integrated Processes: Caring; Nursing Process—Evaluation
Client Need: Physiological Integrity; Reduction of Risk Potential; Potential for Alterations in Body Systems
Cognitive Level: Synthesis
Concept: Critical Thinking
Reference: Ward, S. L., & Hisley, S. M. (2009). Maternal-child nursing care: Optimizing outcomes for mothers, children & families. Philadelphia: F.A. Davis.

19. ANSWER: 4
Rationale
1. Eye infection is something that can occur after birth, but the treatment for that is erythromycin ointment, not a shot.
2. Although the umbilical cord can be a site of infection, a purple dye is used for it, not a shot.
3. Policy may state that it is to be given but this does not answer the parents' question or help them to understand why it is done.
4. Clotting problems can occur in newborns because until they have food and normal flora in their gut, vitamin K is not present to help with clotting problems.
TEST-TAKING TIP: Recognize the word *best* in the stem as the priority to determine which statement by the nurse best addresses the parents' concern.
Content Area: Newborn
Integrated Processes: Teaching and Learning; Nursing Process—Implementation
Client Need: Physiological Integrity; Pharmacological and Parenteral Therapies; Medication Administration
Cognitive Level: Analysis
Concept: Critical Thinking

Reference: Ward, S. L., & Hisley, S. M. (2009). Maternal-child nursing care: Optimizing outcomes for mothers, children & families. *Philadelphia: F.A. Davis.*

20. **ANSWER: 1**
Rationale
1. Poor muscle tone and temperature instability are signs of hypoglycemia and therefore a blood glucose level should be checked.
2. Resuscitation is not needed at this time; there is no information that states the infant is having difficulty breathing or maintaining a normal heart rate.
3. Transfer to the neonatal intensive care unit is not necessary at this time.
4. Placing warm blankets may be necessary, but the nurse would not leave the infant in the open crib. Typically upon delivery, the newborn would be placed under the radiant warmer for assessment.

TEST-TAKING TIP: Recognize the priority words *next* and *uncomplicated* delivery as important in this stem to determine which action should be next.
Content Area: Newborn
Integrated Processes: Caring; Nursing Process—Implementation
Client Need: Safe and Effective Care Environment; Management of Care; Establishing Priorities
Cognitive Level: Analysis
Concept: Critical Thinking
Reference: Ward, S. L., & Hisley, S. M. (2009). Maternal-child nursing care: Optimizing outcomes for mothers, children & families. *Philadelphia: F.A. Davis.*

21. **ANSWER: 4**
Rationale
1. This answer does not really address the mother's concern.
2. This answer may make the mother believe there is something wrong, when in fact this is a normal finding in a newborn.
3. This answer implies that the mother is not doing a good job responding to her baby's needs and does not address her concerns.
4. Babies do go through periods of activity and inactivity, so this is common and normal.

TEST-TAKING TIP: Recognize the priority word *most* in the stem. Recall what the normal patterns of reactivity and rest are in the newborn phase.
Content Area: Newborn
Integrated Processes: Teaching and Learning; Nursing Process—Implementation
Client Need: Health Promotion and Maintenance; Principles of Teaching and Learning
Cognitive Level: Analysis
Concept: Promoting Health
Reference: Ward, S. L., & Hisley, S. M. (2009). Maternal-child nursing care: Optimizing outcomes for mothers, children & families. *Philadelphia: F.A. Davis.*

22. **ANSWER: 3**
Rationale
1. There is no data to support that maternal/infant bonding is a concern for this baby.
2. Risk for infection may be a concern but it doesn't increase during this second phase of reactivity for any specific reason.

3. During the second phase of reactivity, the infant's bowel sounds are usually present and the infant may begin to have oral mucus and transient episodes of gagging and even vomiting. Therefore, the infant is at increased risk of ineffective airway clearance.
4. There is no evidence of insufficient feeding during this time period.

TEST-TAKING TIP: Recognize the stem is asking the nurse specifically about the *second* period of reactivity. Recall the information related normal patterns of reactivity in a newborn.
Content Area: Newborn
Integrated Processes: Teaching and Learning; Nursing Process—Implementation
Client Need: Health Promotion and Maintenance; Principles of Teaching and Learning
Cognitive Level: Analysis
Content Areas: Behavioral Stages During Newborn Transition; Phase 2 of Transition Period; Nursing Process; Evaluation: Analysis Level
Concept: Critical Thinking
Reference: Ward, S. L., & Hisley, S. M. (2009). Maternal-child nursing care: Optimizing outcomes for mothers, children & families. *Philadelphia: F.A. Davis.*

23. **ANSWER: 1**
Rationale
1. Since the baby is active and alert, this is prime time for the mother and baby to bond and for the mother to inspect her baby and/or provide skin-to-skin contact.
2. Because it is the prime time for bonding, this is not the ideal time for the nurse to perform a head-to-toe assessment.
3. The hearing screen is not done while the baby is active and alert, but rather when quiet.
4. The baby can wait to have the bath until after the mother has a chance to bond with the baby.

TEST-TAKING TIP: Be alert to the stem when it asks the nurse to answer the question based on the *first* period of reactivity.
Content Area: Newborn
Integrated Processes: Teaching and Learning; Nursing Process—Implementation
Client Need: Safe and Effective Care Environment; Management of Care; Continuity of Care
Cognitive Level: Analysis
Content Areas: Behavioral Stages During Newborn Transition; Phase I of Transition Period; Nursing Process—Evaluation; Analysis Level
Concept: Nursing
Reference: Ward, S. L., & Hisley, S. M. (2009). Maternal-child nursing care: Optimizing outcomes for mothers, children & families. *Philadelphia: F.A. Davis.*

24. **ANSWER: 4**
Rationale
1. This time frame is when the parents will get to know their infant because the infant is active and alert; therefore, taking the infant back to the nursery for a feeding is not encouraged. The mother can be encouraged to breastfeed her infant at this time.

2. Vital signs do not need to be assessed every 15 minutes at this time unless the infant is having an issue outside of normal parameters.
3. A blood glucose reading is not necessary unless other evidence is provided to suggest blood sugar levels are being monitored.
4. Because the infant is alert and active, it is a great time for the parents to bond with the baby. The temperature will naturally drop during this time, so providing skin-to-skin contact is encouraged or wrapping the baby in a blanket.

TEST-TAKING TIP: Recognize the stem is asking the nurse to provide an action during the *first* period of reactivity. Consider how alert the infant is at this time and what priorities are essential.

Content Area: Newborn
Integrated Processes: Caring; Nursing Process—Implementation
Client Need: Health Promotion and Maintenance; Developmental Stages and Transitions
Cognitive Level: Analysis
Concept: Nursing
Reference: *Ward, S. L., & Hisley, S. M. (2009).* Maternal-child nursing care: Optimizing outcomes for mothers, children & families. *Philadelphia: F.A. Davis.*

25. **ANSWER: 2**
Rationale
1. The problem with this answer is that sterile blankets are needed for the infant who was just delivered.
2. The infant should be dried completely and placed under the warmer without any clothes; this answer is correct.
3. The infant should not be immediately fed.
4. The infant would need to be suctioned in the mouth first and then the nose to prevent the infant from taking a breath and breathing in any secretions.

TEST-TAKING TIP: Recognize the key priority in the stem is asking what the nurse should do following delivery of the infant.

Content Area: Newborn
Integrated Processes: Caring; Nursing Process—Implementation
Client Need: Safe and Effective Care Environment; Management of Care; Establishing Priorities
Cognitive Level: Application
Concept: Critical Thinking
Reference: *Ward, S. L., & Hisley, S. M. (2009).* Maternal-child nursing care: Optimizing outcomes for mothers, children & families. *Philadelphia: F.A. Davis.*

General Assessment and Care of the Newborn

KEY TERMS

Circumcision—Surgical removal of the genital foreskin of the penis usually performed at the request of the parents, in some cases for religious reasons

Epstein's pearls—Benign retention cysts resembling small pearls, which are sometimes present on the infant's palate and disappear at 1 to 2 months of age

Maternal–infant bonding—The emotional and physical attachment between infant and mother that is initiated in the first hour or two after normal delivery of a baby

who has not been dulled by anesthetic agents or drugs. It is believed that the stronger this bond, the greater the chances of a mentally healthy infant–mother relationship in both short- and long-term periods after childbirth. For that reason, the initial contact between mother and infant should be in the delivery room and the contact should continue for as long as possible in the first hours after birth. It is also called *mother–infant attachment.*

I. Assessment of the Newborn

A. General assessment and measurements after transition to extrauterine life
  1. Transfer to nursery: The labor and delivery nurse is typically the first provider to perform an assessment on the newborn. This may occur while the newborn rooms with the mother in the labor and delivery suite. Once the mother is stable, she may be transferred to a postpartum room, while some facilities continue to care for the mother in the same room throughout the hospitalization. The newborn will then be transferred to the nursery for further assessment. After the newborn has successfully transitioned to extrauterine life, it is important for the nurse to perform an in-depth assessment as part of the admission process. It is important for the delivery nurse to report an accurate history to the nursery nurse and report time of birth, Apgar scores, delivery type, birth weight, gestational age, and complications including use of forceps, vacuum, or medications during delivery. If the mother was febrile at the time of delivery, this would also be important to note during the report.

Measurements of the newborn's head, chest, length, and weight will need to be recorded. In addition, the gestational age may be estimated using a standardized tool that looks at physical and neuromuscular maturity. The preferred method used is the Ballard Gestational Age by Maturity Rating tool, which is further explained below.

ALERT The nurse should always protect him- or herself against the transmission of viruses from maternal blood and amniotic fluid that may also be bloodstained. Therefore, standard precautions should be used when handling the newborn until after the bath has taken place. Viruses transmitted may include hepatitis B and HIV.

  2. Weight: If the newborn has not already been weighed, a weight needs to be recorded in grams. Weight of a normal newborn ranges from 2,500 to 4,300 grams (5 pounds, 8 ounces to 9 pounds, 8 ounces), with 3,400 grams (7 pounds, 8 ounces) being the average weight.
  3. Length: The newborn's recumbent length, measured from crown to heel, is generally recorded next in centimeters. For the most accurate recording, the newborn should be placed in a supine

position. This process is used to measure the newborn until 24 months of age. The typical newborn length is 18 to 22 inches (45 to 55 cm).

4. Head circumference: Next, the head circumference can be obtained by recording the frontal-occipital circumference. The tape measure is placed just above the eyebrows and pinna of the ears and then is carefully wrapped around the occipital prominence of the head. The head measurement is usually performed three times to ensure accuracy and is recorded in centimeters. The average measurement is 13 to 15 inches (33 to 38 cm).

5. Chest circumference: The chest circumference is assessed by placing the tape measure on the nipple line and wrapping it around the thoracic areas. During the first several days of life, the head and chest circumference may be equal in size.

6. Abdominal circumference: It is not usually necessary to measure the abdominal circumference, but if it is, the tape measure should be placed directly above the umbilicus and the recording should be similar to the chest size.

DID YOU KNOW?

It is important for the nurse to plot all (except abdominal circumference unless necessary) of these measurements on the chart to determine if the newborn is small, average, or large for gestational age. If the physical measurements recorded are outside the normal parameters for growth, the health care practitioner (HCP) should be notified for further assessment and follow-up.

B. Gestational age assessment
   1. Ballard Gestational Age Maturity Rating tool: Some hospitals will use this tool to assess the gestational age of all newborns transferring to the newborn nursery, while other facilities utilize this assessment for premature newborns only. Refer to your hospital's policies for use of this screening tool.

   The tool looks at the newborn's physical and neuromuscular maturity. It will help identify decreased levels of muscle and joint flexibility that is typically exhibited in the premature newborn. Likewise, the tool will determine if the newborn is able to return to an original position after movement, demonstrating characteristics of a mature newborn.

   It is recommended this assessment be performed within the first 36 hours after delivery and yields the best results within the first 12 hours of life. The scoring system of the tool ranges from –1 (premature) to 5 (postmature); half scores are also observed. The scoring system is indirectly related to gestational age and may show slight variations among observers. The score the newborn receives is compared to the gestational age recorded in the chart and may be further

evaluated if the differences are greater than 2 weeks above or below the recorded gestational age. The examiner should refer to the hospital policy on using this tool and notification of the physician (refer to the Dubowitz/Ballard system in Chapter 19).

2. Physical assessment and body position: After conducting the assessment using the Ballard tool, a physical assessment of each system should be done using a head-to-toe approach. The newborn can be assessed under the radiant warmer to maintain temperature, in the mother's room, or in an open crib if temperature is stable. Observing the newborn in the mother's room allows the mother to see the nurse explore the newborn's body and allows the opportunity for the nurse to educate the mother on normal variations of her newborn. This also presents a great time for the mother to ask questions about her newborn. While performing the assessment, the newborn may attempt to seek comfort in the in utero position. Most newborns will demonstrate flexion of the upper and lower extremities and extension or flexion of the legs. However, newborns born prematurely will remain more floppy in position.

🛑 **ALERT** Nurses must pay particular attention to the newborn's body position during the assessment and immediate transition phase. Newborns exhibiting asymmetrical positioning during the assessment or failure to move one or more extremity should be further examined by the HCP. This abnormal presentation may be the result of injury from birth trauma.

II. Assessment by Systems: Normal Findings

A. Integumentary system
   1. General assessment: The assessment should always occur in a well-lit room and begin with the skin.

MAKING THE CONNECTION

Importance of Body Temperature

Newborns should be placed under the radiant warmer while the assessment is being conducted to prevent heat loss. A diaper can be placed on the newborn at this time, but it is not necessary to do so initially. The nurse will want to apply a skin temperature probe on the newborn's stomach to ensure that the newborn's temperature is being recorded while the warmer is on. Never wrap the newborn in blankets while the warmer is on, or the newborn's temperature will rise. In addition, the skin temperature probe will not record the temperature accurately if clothing or blankets are covering the site because the warmer works by heating only the outer surface of the newborn.

DID YOU KNOW?

The lighting and conditions of the room can alter the assessment findings of the newborn, in particular the skin assessment. Pink walls and rooms with artificial light can mask some conditions, such as jaundice, or interfere with the ability to perform a more accurate assessment. Therefore, the nurse should observe the newborn in natural light when possible.

With gloved hands, the nurse should begin by examining the newborn's skin, scalp, body hair, and nails for color, texture, distribution, disruptions, eruptions, and birthmarks. Findings should indicate pink skin, which signifies adequate peripheral cardiac perfusion. The nurse should check for blanching over bony prominences, which would reveal a pink-white color before return to normal pigmentation. Acrocyanosis, a bluish discoloration of the hands and feet, is a normal finding related to vasomotor instability and poor peripheral circulation that should resolve when the newborn cries or if the sole of the foot turns pink when rubbed vigorously.

🛑 **ALERT** If the newborn's foot remains white during vigorous rubbing or while crying, this is a sign of true cyanosis that should be reported immediately.

2. Skin variations: Upon assessment, the nurse might discover some variations in the skin (Table 20.1). Although not all of these findings are alarming, it is important to record the findings daily or as soon as the change in the assessment is noted.
3. Umbilical cord: The umbilical cord must also be evaluated. It should contain two arteries and one vein.

MAKING THE CONNECTION

Proper Lighting for Assessments Is a Priority

To obtain the most accurate assessment, it is recommended that the nurse use an assortment of light sources to examine the newborn's skin and body. It is important to note the ethnicity of the newborn to ensure the nurse is observing the true skin color. Skin color that appears yellow may be a result of jaundice, while areas that are white may be a result of pallor. Areas that should be inspected in detail should include the palms, soles of the feet, lips, and behind the ears. Other areas that need special attention include bony prominences such as the nose, sternum, wrists, ankles, and sacrum. The nurse should apply only slight pressure to these sites and observe for blanching of the skin.

Table 20.1 Common Skin Variations Seen During the Newborn and Infant Period	
Variation	**Description**
Plethora	Deep, purple color related to number of circulating RBCs.
Petechiae	Pinpoint hemorrhagic areas.
Milia	Small, white papules or sebaceous cysts on the face; may resemble pimples.
Erythema toxicum	Transient rash that is small and irregular with flat red patches on the cheeks that then develop into singular small, yellow pimples on the chest, abdomen, and extremities; also called *erythema neonatorum*, *newborn rash*, or *flea-bite dermatitis*.
Mongolian spots or macular gray-blue discoloration	Gray, dark blue or purple areas on the back and buttocks, but can also be found on the shoulders, wrists, forearms, and ankles; most common in Mediterranean, Latin American, Asian, and African ethnicities.
Nevi	Brown skin marks that may vary to deep black.
Nevus flammeus	Capillary angioma below the epidermis, nonelevated, red to purple areas of dense capillaries most commonly appearing on the face; blanching does not occur.
Telangiectatic nevus	Red birthmark seen usually at the nape of the neck; commonly called a *stork bite* or *angel kiss* and may also appear on the face.
Nevus vasculosus	Red, raised capillary hemangioma occurring anywhere on the body; referred to as a *strawberry mark*.

🛑 **ALERT** If the cord has only one artery and one vein, the HCP must be notified immediately. This may be a sign of renal or cardiac abnormalities. Further investigation is warranted for this finding. Likewise, if fewer than three vessels are seen during the assessment, the nurse should document the findings and notify the HCP, as this may be associated with a congenital anomaly.

B. Newborn's head

The assessment of the head follows the skin assessment and includes eyes, ears, nose, and throat.

1. General assessment: Assess for symmetrical placement of the eyes, nose, lips, mouth, and ears. Movements of the eyelids and lips should be observed. Ears should be observed to shape, size, and placement. If one ear is positioned slightly lower than the other, there is generally no reason for alarm. The newborn's nostrils should display bilateral openings and a centrally placed nasal

bridge and should be free of deviations. Lip color should be congruent with the tongue and buccal mucosa, and the upper and lower lips should be relatively similar in size. The nurse should inspect the lips for position and note any deviations from normal development.

DID YOU KNOW?

Damage to the facial nerve (7th cranial nerve) can result in drooping of the tongue or mouth, a unilateral appearance, or unequal movement of the cheeks. Inappropriate eyelid movement may be a reason for concern. Ears that are low set may need further evaluation for chromosomal abnormalities, such as trisomy 21, or Down syndrome. Newborns with a small jaw or micrognathia may later display problems with tooth development, sucking, swallowing, and tongue movements inside the mouth that occur while speaking. All of these signs need to be further evaluated.

a) Eyes: Eyes should be opened to observe the iris, sclera, and conjunctiva. Scleral hemorrhage can be normal in the outer canthus of the eyes as a result of birth trauma. If the eye prophylaxis has already been instilled in the newborn's eyes, they may appear swollen and produce a yellow discharge.

b) Mouth: The newborn's mouth should be opened and visually inspected. Gums should be palpated for the presence of neonatal teeth (Fig. 20.1). If teeth are emerging through the gums, the examiner must check for looseness because these teeth may need to be extracted.

🛑 **ALERT** Presence of natal teeth can be alarming because the newborn can aspirate any teeth that may be loose. In addition, this condition may be present if another congenital defect exists; therefore, further evaluation is necessary.

c) Variations: **Epstein's pearls** are whitish, hard nodules that appear or are palpated on the roof of the mouth or the newborn's gums. This finding can be common and should disappear within a few weeks (Fig. 20.2).

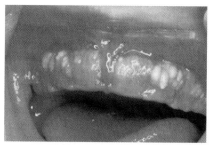

Fig 20.2 Epstein's pearls usually disappear within a few weeks.

d) Reflexes and cleft lip/palate: With gloves, the nurse should insert a finger into the newborn's mouth and record the presence and strength of the sucking motion, a normal reflex should be exhibited. At the same time, the nurse should note the hard and soft palate for size, shape, and any presence of cleft formation. This defect would be felt as an open space or notched bridge. Newborns with a high, arched palate or open space may have difficulty with swallowing or develop speech problems later in life. Surgery would be indicated to fix the cleft palate typically before it has a chance to affect speech patterns, but will be left at the discretion of the HCP after discharge.

e) Fontanels: The head should be palpated and assessment made of the anterior and posterior fontanels, cranial suture lines, and areas of edema resulting from birth trauma. The anterior fontanel is diamond shaped and approximately 2.5 to 4 cm in size. Closure of the anterior fontanel does not typically occur until 12 to 18 months of life. The posterior fontanel is located at the back of the cranium and is smaller and triangular in shape. It is typically 0.4 inches (1 cm) in size and might be closed initially. Both fontanels should be open, soft to the touch, and slightly depressed. Upon a newborn's crying, the fontanels may bulge slightly.

MAKING THE CONNECTION

Assessment of Fontanels

It is important for the anterior fontanel to remain open during the first year of the newborn's life to accommodate normal brain growth. The fontanels should be a part of the newborn's ongoing assessment during the first year of life during normal well-child visits. Any deviation outside the normal patterns should be further assessed for proper development of the skull and brain.

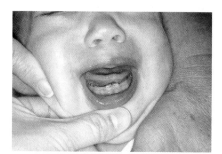

Fig 20.1 Natal teeth.

2. Neck: The neck should move freely from side to side. The nurse may have to check for neck rotation by carefully turning the newborn's head.

3. Ears: The thickness of the earlobe and pinna should be determined. Normal ear malformations can occur and result in ear pits or tiny pinholes and tags, which are fleshy bulb-shaped growths. Ear tags are removed by plastic surgeons to avoid any cosmetic concerns. The patency of ear canals should also be assessed.

4. Nose: Symmetrical placement of the nose is important to check. The nurse can begin the assessment by forming an imaginary line from the center of the bridge of the nose down to the upper lip notch. Either side of the nose should be symmetrical and vertical to this line.

DID YOU KNOW?

It is important to be aware of ethnic differences when assessing the nose. Newborns of African American or Asian descent may have a flattened nasal bridge, which is a normal finding.

C. Respiratory system
The newborn's respiratory efforts, chest movement, and placement and size of breast tissue should all be examined at this time.

1. Respiratory effort: It is important to observe for symmetrical movement of the chest. In addition, the nurse must observe for nasal patency by occluding one nare while ensuring that the newborn's mouth remains closed. The nurse should observe for a rise in the newborn's chest. Then, repeat with the same technique on the other nostril. The respiratory rate should remain between 30 and 60 breaths per minute. A newborn's pattern of breathing tends to be slightly irregular as they adjust to extrauterine life and may have periods of increases with crying and decreases with sleeping.

2. Respiratory rate: The nurse should count the respirations and the pattern or use of accessory muscles at this time. It is common for newborns to exhibit slight sternal retractions. Occasionally, the xiphoid process is prominent in some newborns and does not indicate a reason to be alarmed, as this finding usually diminishes over time. Normal breathing patterns will be irregular with periods of apnea lasting 15 to 20 seconds. The rate should be between 30 and 60 breaths per minute or less. Observe and record the rate during different intervals of the assessment process for a more accurate estimate of the newborn's respiratory rate.

(!) ALERT A respiratory rate that remains greater than 60 breaths per minute during rest or if the newborn displays nasal flaring; retractions between the ribs, below the rib cage, or above the sternum and/or clavicles; or grunting with expirations is abnormal and warrants further investigation. A newborn who has weak chest wall musculature may also exhibit respiratory distress.

3. Placement and size of chest: The breast tissue should be observed for symmetry and size. Enlargement of the breast tissue in males is a normal finding due to the excretion of maternal hormones. The nurse should assess if breast tissue and nipples lie in the midclavicular line, which is determined by drawing an imaginary line that is half the distance from the midline to the lateral border of the chest wall. If the tissue is between the midclavicular line and lateral chest wall, the nipples are documented as wide spaced. Nipples that are wide spaced can be a sign of other congenital findings, such as Down syndrome. Also noteworthy is the documentation of any accessory nipples, which can be removed later and is not necessarily suggestive of any abnormality.

DID YOU KNOW?

A newborn born prematurely is at risk of developing respiratory distress because of the inability to produce adequate levels of surfactant, which improves lung compliance. Inadequate levels are a result of early gestational age because these levels normally rise during the last few weeks of pregnancy.

D. Cardiovascular system
The cardiovascular system inspection should include the skin, lips, gums, and buccal mucosa, which can reveal important information about perfusion.

1. Skin and pulses: Skin should remain pink but occasionally progress to red with crying or moving. Capillary refill is determined in extremities by gently pinching the newborn's finger or toe and counting the number of seconds it takes for the skin to return to its original color; a normal finding is 3 seconds or less. Peripheral pulses should reveal symmetry, strength, and rate. Femoral pulses are compared to brachial pulses; any decrease in strength should be reported to the HCP, as this may indicate a condition known as *coarctation of the aorta,* which will be further detailed in the next chapter.

2. Normal heart rate: The newborn's normal heart rate should remain between 110 and 160 beats per minute (bpm). Heart rates above 160 bpm are referred to as *tachycardia,* while heart rates lower than 100 bpm are referred to as *bradycardia* and should be reported for additional follow-up.

3. Heart murmur: It is not uncommon to hear a murmur in newborns who are less than 24 hours old. Typically this murmur will resolve by the newborn's second or third day of life when the ductus closes. If the murmur is still present after this time, further follow-up may be necessary, as this may be indicative of an underlying heart condition. See Chapter 21 for further details on normal and abnormal patterns of the cardio-vascular system.

E. Gastrointestinal system

With the newborn in the supine position, inspection should reveal a round and bilaterally symmetrical abdomen. Umbilical cord should be free of bleeding or oozing, and two arteries and one vein should be present.

1. Bowel sounds: All four quadrants should be auscultated. The gastric bubble should be heard in the upper abdomen, and heart sounds may be heard near the abdominal aorta. Absence of bowel sounds may be a sign of a bowel obstruction and may warrant additional assessment.

2. Palpation: Light palpation should be performed at the lower sternal border and proceed down to the umbilicus. Any thinning of the abdominal wall or lump along the midline that is more prominent while the newborn is crying may be indicative of diastasis rectus. If an umbilical hernia is present around the umbilicus, it should be assessed for size. Small hernias are often common and require nothing further than a watchful eye.

MAKING THE CONNECTION

Maintaining Body Temperature

The nurse can reduce the effects of cold stress by doing the following:

• Maintain a neutral thermal environment, slowly warming the newborn up (warming a newborn too quickly can lead to apnea or hypotension)

• Increase the temperature hourly by 0.5 to 1° until the newborn has reached a stable temperature (keep room temperature at 70 to 75°)

• Apply a skin temperature probe to the newborn so temperatures can be monitored at least every 15 to 30 minutes

• Avoid trapping cool air by removing plastic wrap, caps, or heat shields during the rewarming process

• Use warm IV fluids for infusion

• Allow for skin-to-skin contact with the mother after the newborn is completely dried after birth

• Avoid heat loss through evaporation, convection, conduction, or radiation

F. Genitourinary system

This assessment should begin in the supine position with the hips abducted.

1. Males: The scrotum should reveal that both testicles have descended. A flattened or depressed area may reveal an undescended testicle. Palpate the scrotum's left side with the index finger and thumb to determine the presence of the testis and then use the third finger and thumb to feel for the testis on the right side. Assessment should occur in this fashion to ensure that each testis is only counted once (Fig. 20.3). To palpate the testes, the inguinal canal can be softly stroked, which will help determine if an undescended testicle is present. Newborns greater than 35 weeks gestation with undescended testicles should receive a urological consult.

a) Visual inspection and palpation: This is important to detect swelling. The bowel can become trapped in the scrotum, causing swelling. The nurse should auscultate for bowel sounds and apply a light source (penlight or ophthalmo-scope) against the scrotum to determine if a reddish yellow reflection is present. If no reflection is present, it could be indicative of a mass and needs to be reported immediately. Newborns of various ethnic backgrounds can have dark-colored scrotal skin.

b) Penis: The length should be estimated; a full-term newborn's penile length is approximately 0.8 inches (2 cm). The prepuce of the foreskin should be retracted by the nurse to inspect for the urethral opening and visualize the location. A waxy substance called *smegma* may be present on the foreskin, which is a normal finding.

2. Females: Begin with the labia majora and note the maturity of the newborn by determining the degree to which the labia cover the surrounding tissues. The term newborn's labia majora will fully cover the clitoris.

a) Visual inspection of the female genitalia may reveal the presence of vernix caseosa, which is a normal finding. A hymenal tag, a small

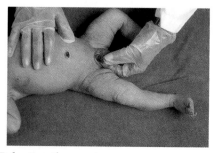

Fig 20.3 Palpating the scrotum.

triangle-shaped piece of tissue, is sometimes present between the labia, which are often palpated during the exam of the labia majora and labia minora.

b) Pseudomenstruation may be present from maternal hormone circulating throughout the newborn's body and is described as whitish mucoid discharge in the vaginal area; blood-tinged discharge may also be present and is not uncommon or a reason for alarm.

3. Males and females: Inspection should be done of the anus and opening. Anal patency is confirmed with the passing of stool; therefore, it is advantageous for the nurse to see the passage of meconium to ensure that stool is being passed from only one opening.

a) Palpation: Touch the anal opening tissue to assess the muscles around the opening. Any rectal tears from passing stool should be noted. The nurse should place the newborn in the prone position and stroke the buttocks from side to side to ensure that the buttocks draw together and "wink" at the point of the anal opening.

G. Musculoskeletal system

Observation of the newborn's movement marks the beginning steps of the musculoskeletal assessment. The nurse should note the flexion and extension of arms and legs, head rotation from side to side, and any movement involving sucking of fingers or hands. Lack of movement or asymmetry in movement may be related to fractures or nerve damage secondary to birth trauma. The general appearance or position of the newborn is equally important in the assessment. Newborns should *not* appear floppy, which could indicate hypotonia. On the contrary, newborns should also not display increased muscle tone, or hypertonia, which can cause tremors, twitches, or jerky movements.

1. Length and size and skin folds: It is important to assess the symmetry of length and size of extremities and to observe for symmetry of skin folds. Any asymmetry in skin folds may be a result of possible birth trauma injuries.

2. Tone and strength: Placing the newborn supine and then prone will help the nurse to evaluate for muscle tone and strength. Symmetry should be noted in all movements.

3. Range of motion: This is assessed by rotating the neck in both directions. At this time, also assess head lag by pulling the newborn up slightly while watching for the head to fall gently back. The display of head lag is a common finding in newborns and will begin to disappear within a few months as the newborn gains strength (Fig. 20.4).

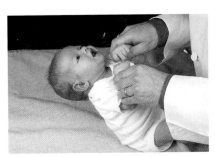

Fig 20.4 To assess head lag, the infant is gently pulled up as the nurse observes his head fall back.

H. Neurological system

The features of the newborn's nervous system and reflexes are the focus of this assessment and serve as indicators of appropriate neurological function. The nurse will assess for major and minor reflexes during this assessment. Proper major reflexes (Babinski, Moro, and gag) indicate correct neurological function, while issues with minor reflexes (grasp, rooting, sucking, stepping, and tonic neck) indicate problems of a lesser concern. The gag reflex must be documented to confirm that the newborn can eat and swallow food appropriately without choking. Typically when the nurse suctions the newborn's mouth, this reflex is noted. (See Table 19.3 for detailed information on newborn reflexes.)

III. Nursing Care During the Newborn Period

A. Bathing

The first bath is usually done in the nursery; some facilities will allow parents to observe or even participate in this experience. At some facilities, the bath may be recommended before the first set of vaccines are administered.

Upon discharge, education for the parents should focus on when to bathe the newborn, how to bathe, and how to observe the newborn after the bath. During the first year of life, it is not necessary to bathe the newborn daily. Bathing should occur two to three times a week to avoid overdrying the skin. If the umbilical cord has not fallen off, then only a sponge bath is required. This process may take up to 2 full weeks. Likewise, if the male newborn had a **circumcision**, the parents should sponge bathe the newborn for only approximately 1 to 2 weeks until full healing has occurred. Steps to bathing the newborn are as follows:

1. Choose a room in which to bathe the newborn that is warm and has a flat surface that is easily accessible to the parent.

2. Gather all supplies that are needed: towels, washcloths, newborn soap, small tub or basin to support newborn in while bathing.

3. Always support the newborn's head and never leave the newborn unattended.

4. A blanket or towel can be placed underneath the newborn to help support the newborn and provide comfort.

5. Bathe the newborn by moving from the cleanest areas to the dirtiest areas. Start with the eyes and only use water to wipe from the inner to outer corner. Avoid using the same area of the cloth to wash both eyes in case an infection is present. Then proceed with the rest of the face, avoiding soap in these areas. Next wash the hair using newborn shampoo/soap, and move down to the remainder of the body. Be sure to get all creases and dry thoroughly and cover the newborn as you move down the body. Be sure to wash the diaper area last and pay particular attention to any skin irritation or rashes. Rinse the newborn with warm water and pat dry thoroughly.

B. Diapering

The use of cloth or disposable diapers may be used and is based on the parents' decision. Parents should be instructed to count the number of diapers a day that their newborn has and what the stool consistency is like. Newborns typically have 6 to 10 wet diapers a day; stools will depend on whether the newborn is breastfeeding or formula feeding. Breastfeeding babies may have a stool with each diaper change until about 1 month of age, at which time it may decrease to one stool per day or every other day, whereas bottle-fed babies will typically pass one to two stools per day. Stools that are green or loose are not normal findings and should be reported to the HCP. Likewise, any sign of constipation or inability to pass stool easily should also be reported.

DID YOU KNOW?

Parents should avoid applying lotions, oils, and powders on their newborn's skin. Lotions and oils may promote skin irritation and rashes, and powder may be inhaled and lead to respiratory distress. If a parent insists on using a lotion or oil, it should be applied sparingly.

MAKING THE CONNECTION

Preventing Heat Loss

Newborns born prematurely or who are small for gestational age can be at risk for increased heat loss or cold stress. This phenomenon occurs when the newborn maintains a higher respiratory rate and nonshivering thermogenesis or use of brown fat stores in order to keep their core temperature at 98.6°F (37°C). This type of heat loss can also be seen with evaporation, convection, conduction, and radiation. Because of their small body size, they have decreased adipose tissue, brown fat reserves, and glycogen to use.

C. Cord care

Although the cord will begin to dry several hours after delivery, it will not be ready to fall off for up to 2 weeks. The cord should never be removed by anyone. Parents should be taught to observe for bleeding, redness, foul odors, or drainage around the cord stump and should notify their primary care provider (PCP) immediately if noted. Tub baths should also be avoided until the cord falls off. The cord stump should be exposed to air as much as possible; therefore, parents should be instructed to fold the top of the diaper down to avoid rubbing the area. Some facilities may instruct parents to wipe the base of the cord stump with alcohol to assist in drying out the cord more quickly. It is important for parents to know that the cord will change from yellow to brown to black before falling off (if a triple dye was not applied in the hospital), and this is a normal finding.

D. Clothing

It is important to avoid overheating the newborn, especially at times of sleep, to decrease the risk of sudden infant death syndrome (SIDS). Newborns should be dressed in one layer more than what an adult is comfortable wearing.

DID YOU KNOW?

If the newborn exhibits sweating, a rash, restlessness, damp hair, or an increased respiratory rate, he or she may be overheating. It is easy to overheat newborns by applying too many blankets or bundling them too tightly, especially indoors.

Hats are often encouraged when the newborn is outside during colder weather. Newborns should not remain outside for extended periods of time because it is important to protect their skin from the sun.

E. Feeding

Newborns should be fed on demand or at a minimum of every 2 to 4 hours during the day and when the newborn wakes up at night for the first days of life. Parents should pay particular attention to hunger cues such as crying, sucking on fingers or fists, rooting, and sucking. A breastfeeding mother may breastfeed between 10 and 20 minutes on each breast, while formula-fed babies may take up to 30 minutes to finish a bottle. To determine if the newborn is eating the appropriate amount of food, the nurse should instruct the parents to count the number of wet diapers in a 24-hour period. Newborns should produce at least 6 to 10 wet diapers per day. Likewise, weight gain should be obvious and the newborn should sleep well.

1. Iron storage: Initially, red blood cells (RBCs) undergo destruction after birth, and the liver houses the iron until it is needed for new RBCs

to be created. As long as the maternal iron stores are adequate, these iron stores will be sufficient until the newborn is about 5 months of age. Therefore, iron supplementation will be needed around this age to compensate for the natural loss of iron stores.

DID YOU KNOW?

Breast milk can be frozen and kept for up to 3 months. Once thawed, it is good for 24 hours. It should never be placed in the back of the freezer. Each bottle should be labeled with date and time. Milk should never be heated in the microwave.

F. Maternal–Infant Bonding

While **maternal–infant bonding** is important to a healthy newborn's growth and development, both parents are encouraged to bond with their newborn. These behaviors are best demonstrated by role modeling of proper nurturing behaviors. Behaviors that can be promoted upon discharge include gentle ways to wake up the newborn prior to feeding, explaining what and why you are performing certain actions, encouraging ways to soothe the newborn, and assisting parents with understanding hunger cues. Caution parents that the only form of communication the newborn has is crying, so they will need to try to eliminate what may be the causative factor. Some of these factors may include temperature, hunger, diaper needs, gas, or the need for nurturing.

G. Safety

1. Bulb syringe: Proper use of the bulb syringe should begin upon admission to the postpartum area, prior to discharge. Bulb syringes should be compressed before insertion into the nose or mouth to remove drainage. Once in place, pressure should be released from the bulb syringe to allow for expelling of the drainage directly into the device. Drainage can then be expressed into a towel or tissue by compressing the device. This can be repeated until all drainage is removed from the newborn's passageways. Once complete, the parents should be instructed to clean the bulb syringe with warm, soapy water and let it dry.

2. Nonnutritive sucking: This is a helpful way for the newborn to self-soothe. Parents may choose to offer the newborn a pacifier, or the newborn may try to suck on their fingers or thumb as a way to calm themselves and can be a pleasurable behavior. It is recommended the breastfed newborns avoid the use of a pacifier for the first month of life until breastfeeding patterns are well established.

ⓘ **ALERT** Feedings should not be delayed or avoided as a result of the newborn sucking on a pacifier. A pacifier should never be secured to newborn's neck. Pacifiers should be washed frequently with soap and water.

IV. Routine Procedures Occurring in the Newborn Period

A. Circumcision

This surgical procedure removes the skin covering the end of the penis and is performed prior to discharge. The American Academy of Pediatrics (AAP) believes that although the procedure does pose risks, the medical benefits outweigh them. However, parents should still make the ultimate decision if they would like to have a circumcision performed.

ⓘ **ALERT** Newborns experience pain and physiological stress associated with circumcision; therefore, analgesic can be provided as a safe and effective way to manage pain symptoms.[1] Check with your facility on the administration of an analgesic prior to a circumcision.

1. Postprocedure care of the circumcision site: care after the procedure should include the following:
   a) Nursing observation: This should be done every hour for the first 4 to 6 hours following the procedure to ensure bleeding is not occurring and voiding is normal.
   b) Bleeding: If bleeding is present, gentle pressure should be applied with sterile gauze or sprinkles of powdered gel foam should be administered.
   c) Cleaning and dressings: Following diaper changes, the penis should be cleansed with water and petrolatum should be applied to protect the penis from adhering to the diaper.
   d) Discharge teaching: Inspect the penis every 4 hours, cleanse the area with water only, and avoid soap for at least 6 to 7 days until the circumcision area has healed completely. Notify the PCP if redness, swelling, or discharge is present. After circumcision, if bleeding continues after gentle pressure is applied, then the nurse should notify the physician immediately and continue to apply pressure until the physician arrives.

V. Laboratory and Diagnostic Tests

A. During hospitalization and at discharge
1. Laboratory and diagnostic tests are often done during the hospitalization and immediately following discharge during the newborn period. These tests will often detect whether adaptation is occurring appropriately and will determine if any disorders are present that impact the child indefinitely. These tests are typically done by collecting blood specimens

[1]Brady, M. T. (2016). Newborn male circumcision with parental consent, as stated in the AAP circumcision policy statement, is both legal and ethical. *Journal of Law, Medicine and Ethics, 44*, 256-262. DOI: 10.1177/1073110516654119.

through a heel stick. The newborn's heel should be warmed with a damp cloth or disposable heel warmer approximately 5 to 10 minutes prior to the heel stick. The nurse should cleanse the area and use a spring-loaded automatic puncture device to stick the heel. The heel stick is best accomplished when done on the outer aspect of the heel. Pressure is applied immediately following the puncture to minimize bleeding (Fig. 20.5). The area should not be cleansed again because this will promote further bleeding. Venipuncture may be performed but is rare in the newborn period.

B. Specific laboratory results assessed
Nurses should check facility protocol on which tests should be performed prior to discharge or in the outpatient setting, as these vary by state. Blood levels are performed to assess for the following laboratory results:
- Bilirubin levels: detection of jaundice
- Blood glucose: detects for hypo- or hyperglycemia
- Newborn screening tests (phenylketonuria, hypothyroidism, sickle cell disease, and galactosemia)

C. Hearing screen
Healthy Children, a division of the AAP, advocates for universal hearing screening in all newborns by 3 months.[2] Screenings are generally done prior to discharge and may be repeated in an outpatient setting. Healthy Children reported newborns may be at increased risk of problems if:
- There is a positive family history of hearing loss.
- Congenital infections are present.
- Craniofacial anomalies are present.
- The newborn has been in the neonatal intensive care unit for more than 2 days.
- The newborn has had a postnatal infection, trauma, drug exposure, or hyperbilirubinemia

ⓘ ALERT If a problem is suspected, then early intervention services may be initiated after the screening is repeated and verified by an audiologist.

[2]Healthy Children. (2015). Purpose of newborn hearing screening. Retrieved from https://www.healthychildren.org/English/ages-stages/baby/Pages/Purpose-of-Newborn-Hearing-Screening.aspx.

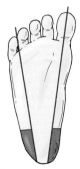

Fig 20.5 Heel stick of foot.

VI. Discharge Planning of the Newborn

A. Car seat safety
Parents should not be allowed to take their newborn home unless a car seat is in place in the vehicle. HCPs should never place the newborn in the car seat for the parents. According to Parents Central, a rear-facing car seat is recommended up until age 2.[3] The National Highway Traffic Safety Administration reported that car accidents account for a large number of deaths in children aged 1 to 12; therefore, parents should refer to the user manual as well as current recommendations for when to change car seats for their child based on the age, height, weight, and guidelines of the car seat itself.[4]

B. Sleeping
Newborns usually sleep for about 15 hours a day, in 2- to 4-hour intervals.
1. Teach parents that newborns have a hard time regulating their body temperature and therefore require one additional layer of clothing than what the parent is wearing. At night, it is important that the newborn be swaddled in blankets; the use of loose blankets is avoided to prevent SIDS. However, parents want to avoid overheating their newborn, which can increase the risk of SIDS. More information for SIDS can be found in Chapter 23.

C. Immunizations
Although the newborn will have some maternal protection passed on through active acquired immunity, their immunological system remains immature. Active acquired immunity occurs as a direct result of the mother's exposure to illness or immunizations, creating antibody formation in the newborn. Passive acquired immunity also occurs through antibodies that are transferred through the placenta in the form of IgG immunoglobulins. At birth, the full-term newborn has acquired immunity to tetanus, diphtheria, smallpox, measles, mumps, poliomyelitis, and bacterial and viral diseases. However, premature newborns born at 34 weeks gestation have not acquired this protection, creating a risk potential. Regardless, this protection will begin to cease around 6 months of age. Illness and infection can therefore be hard to identify in the newborn due to subtle changes exhibited. It is highly encouraged to immunize newborns for certain illnesses, beginning at birth.

[3]American Academy of Pediatrics. (2016). Healthy children: Car seat checkup. Retrieved from: https://www.healthychildren.org/English/safety-prevention/on-the-go/Pages/Car-Safety-Seat-Checkup.aspx.
[4]Parents Central. (n.d.) From car seats to car keys: Keeping kids safe. Retrieved from http://www.safercar.gov/parents/CarSeats/Right-Car-Seat-Age-Size.htm?view=full.

The Centers for Disease Control and Prevention (CDC) recommends that newborns receive a hepatitis B vaccine at birth.[5] By the age of 1 year, a newborn should have received at least 10 different types of vaccines. There may be slight variations about when the newborn will receive each vaccine based on their birth weight, time of the year, and current health status; most newborns should follow the recommended schedule. For a complete list of recommended vaccines, visit the CDC or AAP websites, as these schedules may change slightly from year to year.

DID YOU KNOW?

IgA helps the newborn fight gastrointestinal and respiratory infections and can be found in the mother's breast milk. The infant's own levels of immunoglobulin won't be found until 2 to 3 weeks of age. IgM is usually found in the newborn by 30 weeks of gestation and may increase dramatically after birth if intrauterine infection is present.

D. Assessing temperature
If a parent feels that their newborn is sick, it is important for them to call their HCP. However, they should determine the newborn's temperature by rectal measurement for children under 3 years of age. If the child is older than 3 months, an axillary temperature can be taken, although it is not regarded as the most accurate. Rectal temperatures can be taken by using a clean thermometer and lubricating the end of it with petroleum jelly. Once the probe is lubricated, the newborn should be placed

on the back and legs held in a flexed position while the thermometer is inserted approximately 0.5 inches into the anal opening and left until the temperature is recorded. Axillary temperatures can be assessed by placing the thermometer in the axillae area and holding the newborn's arm against their side until the thermometer records the temperature. The thermometer should always be cleansed after each use with soap and cold water.

E. Swaddling
This is a technique of wrapping blankets snugly around the newborn's body to offer warmth. It can also create a feeling of security and calmness to the newborn.

F. Soothing methods
Parents should be instructed that newborns will cry when hungry, if they are in pain or uncomfortable, or sick. Some newborns may cry when a diaper needs to be changed. Therefore, newborns should be fed if hungry, changed if dirty or wet diapers are noted, repositioned, swaddled, or held for comfort and taken on a walk to help calm them.

G. Skin care
Inspection of the skin should be performed on a daily basis. Parents should be instructed to avoid bathing their newborn with soap; using any form of adhesive, which may remove the delicate top layer of the skin (epidermis); and avoiding any ointments containing perfumes, dyes, and/or preservatives. Petroleum-based ointments can be applied to the skin but should be done so sparingly, and caution should be taken to avoid the head and face.
1. Uncircumcised male: Newborns who are uncircumcised need special care of the foreskin to avoid infection. The penis should be cleansed during bathing or changing the diaper. Foreskin should never be forced over the penis.

[5]Centers for Disease Control and Prevention. (2014). Hepatitis B and the vaccine (shot) to prevent it. Retrieved from http://www.cdc.gov/vaccines/parents/diseases/child/hepb.html.

CASE STUDY: Putting It All Together

Subjective Data
A couple presents to the emergency room with the mother stating, "I am leaking green fluid." Immediately, the patient is rushed to the labor and delivery unit. Upon arrival, vital signs are taken.

Vital Signs
Temperature: 99.1°F
Heart rate: 110 bpm
Respiratory rate: 22 breaths/min
Blood pressure: 140/85 mm Hg

The mother is placed on monitors to detect contractions and the baby's heart rate. After assessment, the mother is having strong contractions, is 100% effaced, and is dilated 7 cm. The nurse tells her she will deliver soon.

Joseph was born at 08:07 a.m. to Caucasian parents with prenatal care beginning at 8 weeks gestational age. She was 37+5, and this is their first child. They have already signed consent for hepatitis B vaccines and a circumcision. They have a supportive family, but Mom suffers from occasional depressive episodes.

Continued

CASE STUDY: Putting It All Together (Continued)

_____ **Case Study Questions** _____

1. What are at least five possible nursing diagnoses for this newborn?

2. What education should be provided for the parents regarding their newborn's care during the hospitalization?

3. Describe some discharge instructions related to the following topics: bathing, feeding, swaddling, taking a temperature, maternal–infant bonding, using a bulb syringe, practicing car seat safety, and having the newborn receive immunizations.

4. What medications will the newborn receive while in the hospital?

5. When should the parents initially return to the PCP following discharge from the hospital?

REVIEW QUESTIONS

Be sure to read the Introduction for valuable test-taking tips.

1. A nurse is planning discharge needs to a family whose baby has just been born. Which statement is the *most* accurate regarding care of the umbilical cord?
   1. Wash the newborn every day in a shallow tub of water.
   2. Rinse the umbilical cord with water and soap until it falls off.
   3. Notify the practitioner if the umbilical cord is still in place after 1 week.
   4. Swab the umbilical cord with alcohol or water daily until it falls off.

2. The nurse enters the room of a patient who just gave birth 2 days ago to a healthy newborn. The nurse asks her what her newborn's name is and she shrugs and says, "I haven't thought about a name yet." What priority is the nurse *most* concerned about with this patient?
   1. The patient has not transitioned from the fourth stage of labor.
   2. Parent-to-newborn attachment may be a concern.
   3. The mother may be contemplating suicide.
   4. Different cultural practices.

3. What information should be documented during the admission process to the newborn nursery following the delivery of the newborn? *Select all that apply.*
   1. Time of birth
   2. City and state of birth location
   3. Apgar scores at 1 and 5 minutes
   4. Birth weight
   5. Mother's emotional status
   6. Family present during delivery

4. Which behaviors should be alarming to the newborn nursery nurse and reported to the practitioner for further assessment?
   1. The newborn's upper and lower extremities are flexed, bringing the arms toward the face.
   2. A newborn actively moves more on one side of the body.
   3. The newborn cries while being bathed.
   4. The newborn passes a sticky, thick greenish black stool.

5. A mother brings her 4-week-old newborn into the clinic for a well-child check. She reports to the nurse that the newborn developed small white marks on her nose. What are these small white marks commonly called?
   1. Milia
   2. Mongolian spots
   3. Erythema toxicum
   4. Port-wine stain

6. A newborn was born over 3 days ago and has not passed any meconium stools. What should the nurse be *most* concerned about at this time?
   1. Jaundice
   2. Constipation
   3. Bowel obstruction
   4. Gastrointestinal infection

7. Which diagnosis is *most* appropriate for a newborn who has not voided within 24 hours after delivery?
   1. Hypovolemia related to insufficient fluid intake
   2. Altered growth and development related to gestational age of 36 weeks
   3. Altered nutrition, less than body requirements related to failure to properly latch onto the breast
   4. Constipation related to failure to pass a meconium stool and possible bowel obstruction

8. Upon assessment, the RN notices that the newborn remains red at rest. Which laboratory value is *most* important for the nurse to evaluate?
   1. Glucose
   2. Bilirubin
   3. Sodium
   4. Hematocrit

9. As an effort to reduce cold stress and respiratory depression, which intervention is *most* important for the nurse to perform?
   1. Maintain the temperature in the room at or below 70°F to stimulate respirations in the newborn.
   2. Place the newborn immediately in the mother's arms following delivery and allow for breastfeeding to occur.
   3. Bathe the newborn shortly after delivery and wrap the newborn in warm blankets in the mother's arms.
   4. Dry the newborn with warm blankets and place the newborn under a radiant warmer.

10. Which method is correct for obtaining a blood glucose reading on a newborn?
    1. Placing a tourniquet on the newborn's wrist and obtaining a blood sample from a venipuncture to be sent to the laboratory.
    2. Warming the hand and obtaining a sample from the thumb.
    3. Warm the foot, clean it with an alcohol pad, and puncture the side of the heel.
    4. Elevate the foot and obtain a blood sample from the heel.

11. The nurse is preparing a new mother and newborn for discharge. Which statement indicates learning has occurred in the mother?
    1. "I will feed my newborn every 3 hours while awake."
    2. "I will exclusively breastfeed my newborn every 2 to 3 hours."
    3. "I will supplement feedings with formula until my breast milk comes in."
    4. "Iron-fortified formula will be needed after my newborn is 6 months of age."

12. Which statement indicates that learning has occurred in a new mother regarding iron storage in her newborn?
    1. "My iron stores have been passed to my newborn, so my newborn doesn't need iron-fortified formula."
    2. "I will add iron to my breast milk after I pump so my newborn's iron levels don't drop too low."
    3. "Iron is not needed unless I stop breastfeeding before 6 months of age."
    4. "I will add iron to the formula to be sure that my newborn has enough."

13. A mother asks the newborn nursery RN why her newborn's eyes are yellow. Which offers the mother the *most* accurate explanation?
    1. "Your newborn may have kernicterus; I will notify the doctor immediately."
    2. "A newborn's liver is immature and can't conjugate bilirubin; this is nothing to worry about."
    3. "Jaundice sometimes occurs in newborns because of increased levels of bilirubin; we may need to do some laboratory work."
    4. "Because your newborn was premature, he is at a higher risk of having jaundice or hypobilirubinemia."

14. Which assessment finding of a newborn in the newborn nursery warrants further investigation and notification to the physician?
    1. Absent bowel sounds 15 minutes after delivery
    2. Bluish discoloration on the buttocks area
    3. Regurgitation of small amounts of feedings
    4. Absent meconium stool on day 2 of life

15. Which of the following newborn assessment findings is the *most* concerning to the newborn nursery nurse?
    1. Newborn who has not voided in 24 hours
    2. Meconium passage with every bowel movement
    3. Small, retractable protrusion next to the umbilicus
    4. Extra digit next to the fifth digit on the left foot

16. Which baby is at *highest* risk of skin infection upon discharge?
    1. Newborn with scabs forming over heels where blood has been drawn
    2. Newborn with a new circumcision
    3. Newborn with jaundice
    4. Newborn with milia

17. What is the proper method for cleaning the bulb syringe?
    1. Boil the syringe after each use
    2. Microwave in warm water for 1 minute after use
    3. Wash in warm soapy water daily or after each use
    4. Wipe with alcohol prep each day and after each use

18. You are receiving report from the nightshift nurse. Which newborn should you assess *first*?
    1. Newborn born 12 hours ago with reported acrocyanosis
    2. Newborn with bilateral breath sounds and nasal flaring
    3. Term newborn born 36 hours ago, currently breastfeeding
    4. Preterm newborn who failed the hearing screen test recently taken

19. Upon discharge, parents of a newborn reveal their plans to take their newborn to the beach with them on a vacation when the newborn is 3 months old. Which statement by the nurse is the *most* appropriate?
    1. "Newborns are encouraged to get at least 2 hours of sun each day for vitamin D synthesis."
    2. "You should make plans to leave your newborn with a relative or a babysitter while you are on vacation."
    3. "Sunscreen should be applied to your newborn every hour to prevent sunburn."
    4. "It is best to place your newborn in lightweight clothing and in the shade when outdoors."

20. Which of the following findings would be *most* concerning to the infant nursery nurse performing an initial assessment on an infant born minutes ago?
    1. Umbilical cord with one artery and two veins
    2. Respiratory rate of 35 breaths per minute
    3. Pink body, blue extremities
    4. No retractions of grunting

REVIEW QUESTIONS ANSWERS

1. ANSWER: 4
Rationale
1. The newborn should not be bathed in a tub of water until after the cord falls off. Newborns should be sponge bathed until the cord falls off.
2. It is recommended to cleanse the umbilical cord area with water or a neutral-based cleanser until it falls off.
3. The cord will take approximately 10 to 14 days to completely fall off; 1 week is not enough time to allow the cord to fall off.
4. Umbilical cords should be cleansed with a neutral cleanser or water for 10 to 14 days or until it falls off.
TEST-TAKING TIP: Identify the word in the stem that sets a priority. The word *most* in the stem sets a priority. Recall the appropriate way to bathe a newborn when the umbilical cord is still intact.
Content Area: Newborn
Integrated Processes: Nursing Process—Implementation
Client Need: Physiological Integrity; Basic Care and Comfort
Cognitive Level: Application
Concept: Nursing
Reference: Ward, S. L., & Hisley, S. M. (2009). Maternal-child nursing care: Optimizing outcomes for mothers, children & families. Philadelphia: F.A. Davis.

2. ANSWER: 2
Rationale
1. The fourth stage of labor is from the time the placenta is delivered until about 1 to 2 hours after birth. The baby in this scenario is 2 days old, so this answer is incorrect.
2. The mother should have time to think about naming the baby. The mother's behavior indicates that there may be a problem with maternal–infant bonding.
3. Attempting suicide cannot be determined with this information.
4. Cultural practices are not a factor in this question.
TEST-TAKING TIP: Recognize the normal and abnormal patterns of maternal/newborn attachment and the word in the stem that sets a priority; the word *most* sets the priority.
Content Area: Newborn
Integrated Processes: Nursing Process—Assessment
Client Need: Health Promotion and Maintenance; High-Risk Behaviors
Cognitive Level: Synthesis
Concept: Family
Reference: Ward, S. L., & Hisley, S. M. (2009). Maternal-child nursing care: Optimizing outcomes for mothers, children & families. Philadelphia: F.A. Davis.

3. ANSWER: 1, 3, 4
Rationale
1. The time of birth is essential to the newborn assessment.
2. Although the location of the birth is important, this is documented throughout the chart and is not part of the immediate assessment of the newborn.
3. The Apgar scores are important to record to allow the nurse to understand the current status of the newborn.
4. The birth weight should always be indicated on the immediate newborn assessment.

5. The emotional state of the mother is not part of the newborn assessment, but should be noted on the postpartum assessment.
6. Documenting who was present for the delivery is not part of the newborn assessment.
TEST-TAKING TIP: Recognize the appropriate information to be included during the admission process.
Content Area: Newborn
Integrated Process: Nursing Process—Evaluation
Client Need: Health Promotion and Maintenance; Developmental Stages and Transitions
Cognitive Level: Comprehension
Concept: Safety
Reference: Ward, S. L., & Hisley, S. M. (2009). Maternal-child nursing care: Optimizing outcomes for mothers, children & families. Philadelphia: F.A. Davis.

4. ANSWER: 2
Rationale
1. Newborns' upper and lower extremities often remain in a flexed position following delivery; this is a normal behavior.
2. Newborns should move both sides of their body; moving only one side of the body may indicate injury and needs further assessment.
3. Crying during the bath is normal and does not warrant any further investigation by the practitioner.
4. Following birth, newborns are expected to pass meconium, which is thick, sticky, and greenish to black in color; this is a normal finding.
TEST-TAKING TIP: Recognize the normal and abnormal movements or behaviors of a newborn following delivery.
Content Area: Newborn
Integrated Processes: Nursing Process—Evaluation
Client Need: Physiological Integrity; Reduction of Risk Potential; System-Specific Assessments
Cognitive Level: Application
Concept: Critical Thinking
Reference: Ward, S. L., & Hisley, S. M. (2009). Maternal-child nursing care: Optimizing outcomes for mothers, children & families. Philadelphia: F.A. Davis.

5. ANSWER: 1
Rationale
1. Milia are small, white papules or sebaceous cysts on the newborn's face that resemble pimples.
2. Mongolian spots are gray, dark blue, or purple discolorations typically found on the back and buttocks; this is not correct.
3. Erythema toxicum is a rash covering the face and chest and can spread to the entire body; this is not correct.
4. Port-wine stain is a nevus flammeus caused by a capillary angioma located below the dermis of the skin; this is not correct.
TEST-TAKING TIP: Recognize normal skin variations on newborns, when and where they appear.
Content Area: Newborn
Integrated Processes: Nursing Process—Assessment
Client Need: Physiological Integrity; Physiological Adaptation
Cognitive Level: Analysis
Concept: Promoting Health
Reference: Ward, S. L., & Hisley, S. M. (2009). Maternal-child nursing care: Optimizing outcomes for mothers, children & families. Philadelphia: F.A. Davis.

6. ANSWER: 3

Rationale

1. Jaundice is caused by high levels of bilirubin.
2. A bowel obstruction is generally the cause of failure to pass meconium.
3. This answer is correct; a bowel obstruction prevents meconium stool to pass.
4. Typically a gastrointestinal illness will cause diarrhea, not failure to pass meconium.

TEST-TAKING TIP: Recognize the word in the stem that sets a priority. The word *most* sets the priority, so you can determine which condition is most concerning for the newborn.

Content Area: Newborns at Risk
Integrated Processes: Nursing Process—Assessment
Client Need: Physiological Integrity; Reduction of Risk Potential; Potential for Alteration in Body Systems
Cognitive Level: Application
Concept: Critical Thinking
Reference: Ward, S. L., & Hisley, S. M. (2009). Maternal-child nursing care: Optimizing outcomes for mothers, children & families. *Philadelphia: F.A. Davis.*

7. ANSWER: 1

Rationale

1. This is correct; hypovolemia is related to a decrease in fluid intake.
2. We do not have enough information to make this diagnosis at this time. Prematurity does not necessarily affect the ability to void.
3. Nutrition might be a concern, but the fact that the newborn has voided is priority.
4. The question does not state any problems related to failure to pass meconium; therefore, this diagnosis is not appropriate.

TEST-TAKING TIP: Recognize the word in the stem that sets a priority is *most* and which diagnosis correlates with a patient who has not voided.

Content Area: Newborns
Integrated Processes: Nursing Process—Assessment
Client Need: Physiological Integrity; Reduction of Risk Potential; Potential for Alteration in Body Systems
Cognitive Level: Application
Concept: Critical Thinking
Reference: Ward, S. L., & Hisley, S. M. (2009). Maternal-child nursing care: Optimizing outcomes for mothers, children & families. *Philadelphia: F.A. Davis.*

8. ANSWER: 4

Rationale

1. Glucose is not the most concerning at this time in the newborn.
2. Bilirubin is not the most concerning at this time in the newborn.
3. Sodium levels are not the most concerning at this time in the newborn.
4. Hematocrit levels are the most concerning and are usually 60 or more in the newborn with polycythemia vera.

TEST-TAKING TIP: Recognize the priority word in the stem as *most* to determine which laboratory value correlates with a newborn remaining red at rest.

Content Area: Newborns
Integrated Processes: Nursing Process—Evaluation
Client Need: Physiological Integrity; Hemodynamics
Cognitive Level: Application
Concept: Hematologic Regulation
Reference: Ward, S. L., & Hisley, S. M. (2009). Maternal-child nursing care: Optimizing outcomes for mothers, children & families. *Philadelphia: F.A. Davis.*

9. ANSWER: 4

Rationale

1. The room temperature needs to be maintained between 70°F and 75°F so the transition to extrauterine life will be smooth and the initiation of respirations can occur without distress.
2. The newborn will need to dry completely before allowing the mother to hold her newborn.
3. Bathing the newborn will not occur immediately following delivery. It is important for the newborn to be dried completely first.
4. The newborn will need to be dried completely and placed under a radiant warmer or directly on the mother's skin to provide for skin-to-skin contact.

TEST-TAKING TIP: After recognizing the priority word in the stem is *most,* determine which intervention is critical for the nurse to do.

Content Area: Newborns
Integrated Processes: Nursing Process—Implementation
Client Need: Physiological Integrity; Reduction of Risk Potential; Therapeutic Procedures
Cognitive Level: Application
Concept: Nursing
Reference: Ward, S. L., & Hisley, S. M. (2009). Maternal-child nursing care: Optimizing outcomes for mothers, children & families. *Philadelphia: F.A. Davis.*

10. ANSWER: 3

Rationale

1. Blood samples are generally not taken via venipuncture on a newborn; only a small sample is needed, so a heel stick would be a sufficient place to obtain the sample.
2. Blood samples are generally not taken from the hand; only a small sample is needed, so a heel stick would be a sufficient place to obtain the sample.
3. This is the proper technique to obtain a blood glucose reading. Some facilities do not have heel warmers, so a warm washcloth can be used.
4. The foot should not be elevated, as this would impede blood flow.

TEST-TAKING TIP: Recognize which step is most accurate in obtaining a blood glucose reading on a newborn.

Content Area: Newborns
Integrated Processes: Nursing Process—Planning
Client Need: Physiological Integrity; Reduction of Risk Potential; Diagnostics Tests
Cognitive Level: Analysis
Concept: Safety
Reference: Ward, S. L., & Hisley, S. M. (2009). Maternal-child nursing care: Optimizing outcomes for mothers, children & families. *Philadelphia: F.A. Davis.*

11. ANSWER: 2
Rationale
1. Newborns need to eat often, so only feeding the newborn every 3 hours while awake is not enough. Even if the newborn is asleep, they must be woken up to eat every 3 to 4 hours for newborns being formula-fed and every 2 to 3 hours for newborns being breastfed.
2. Feeding the newborn every 2 to 3 hours indicates that learning has occurred.
3. The mother should not supplement formula for breast milk. She should offer the breast with each feeding; even if her milk supply has not come in yet, the newborn will still benefit from the colostrum.
4. In formula-fed infants, iron-fortified formula is needed right after birth due to insufficient iron stores.
TEST-TAKING TIP: Recall what the normal patterns for feeding are in a newborn.
Content Area: Newborns
Integrated Processes: Nursing Process—Evaluation
Client Need: Psychosocial Integrity; Therapeutic Communication
Cognitive Level: Analysis
Concept: Nursing Roles
Reference: Ward, S. L., & Hisley, S. M. (2009). Maternal-child nursing care: Optimizing outcomes for mothers, children & families. Philadelphia: F.A. Davis.

12. ANSWER: 3
Rationale
1. Iron stores are passed to the baby, but if the baby is term and on formula, then an iron-fortified formula is needed.
2. Iron does not need to be added to breast milk if the baby is breastfed and the mother should be encouraged to put the baby directly to the breast.
3. This is a true statement; iron does not need to be added unless the newborn begins to take formula before 6 months of age.
4. Formulas have added iron in them, so there is no need to add extra iron to the formula.
TEST-TAKING TIP: Recall how iron is stored in a newborn to determine which statement by the mother summarizes these findings.
Content Area: Newborns
Integrated Processes: Nursing Process—Evaluation
Client Need: Physiological Integrity; Physiological Adaptation; Pathophysiology
Cognitive Level: Analysis
Concept: Nursing Roles
Reference: Ward, S. L., & Hisley, S. M. (2009). Maternal-child nursing care: Optimizing outcomes for mothers, children & families. Philadelphia: F.A. Davis.

13. ANSWER: 3
Rationale
1. Kernicterus is a life-threatening condition caused by increased levels of unconjugated bilirubin in the brain and spinal cord. This is a result of jaundice, so this statement would not fully explain what is happening and could create anxiety in the mother.
2. Although part of this statement is true, jaundice can be a very serious condition, so it would be not correct to tell the mother it is nothing to worry about.
3. This statement is true and laboratory work may be warranted to see what exact levels are so the proper interventions can be done.
4. Although babies who are born prematurely are at risk of having jaundice, it is a result of increased levels of bilirubin, not lower levels.
TEST-TAKING TIP: Recall the symptoms of jaundice and what interventions are done if this condition is diagnosed.
Content Area: Newborns
Integrated Processes: Nursing Process—Evaluation
Client Need: Psychosocial Integrity; Therapeutic Communication
Cognitive Level: Analysis
Concept: Promoting Health
Reference: Ward, S. L., & Hisley, S. M. (2009). Maternal-child nursing care: Optimizing outcomes for mothers, children & families. Philadelphia: F.A. Davis.

14. ANSWER: 4
Rationale
1. Bowel sounds are usually absent in the newborn for the first 15 to 30 minutes following delivery because of air entering the stomach and small intestine.
2. This bluish discoloration is likely the result of Mongolian spots, a common finding in some children.
3. Regurgitation of small amounts of feeding is normal in a newborn during the first 3 months of life due to the immaturity of the cardiac sphincter.
4. Babies should pass meconium during the first days of life. Failure to do so could be the result of an intestinal obstruction.
TEST-TAKING TIP: Recognize which descriptor is an abnormal or concerning finding in a newborn.
Content Area: Newborns
Integrated Processes: Nursing Process—Implementation
Client Need: Physiological Integrity; Reduction of Risk Potential; Potential for Alterations in Body Systems
Cognitive Level: Analysis
Concept: Critical Thinking
Reference: Ward, S. L., & Hisley, S. M. (2009). Maternal-child nursing care: Optimizing outcomes for mothers, children & families. Philadelphia: F.A. Davis.

15. ANSWER: 1
Rationale
1. The inability to pass urine may be a result of a urinary obstruction.
2. Meconium passage during the first few days of life is expected.
3. A small protrusion next to the umbilicus could be an umbilical hernia, and as long as it is retractable, it is not an emergency.
4. Although an extra digit may need to be removed, it is not as concerning as the inability to pass urine.
TEST-TAKING TIP: Recognize which descriptor is the *most* concerning finding in a newborn, based on the priority word in the stem set, which is *most*.
Content Area: Newborn
Integrated Processes: Nursing Process—Implementation
Client Need: Physiological Integrity; Reduction of Risk Potential; Potential for Alterations in Body Systems
Cognitive Level: Analysis
Concept: Assessment

Reference: Ward, S. L., & Hisley, S. M. (2009). Maternal-child nursing care: Optimizing outcomes for mothers, children & families. *Philadelphia: F.A. Davis.*

16. **ANSWER: 2**

Rationale

1. Although heel sticks can be a source of infection, these are scabbed over, which means they are healing and are thus at a lower risk than the circumcision site.
2. This baby has a new circumcision, so he is at a high risk of infection.
3. The baby with jaundice is not at a higher risk of a skin infection than the baby with the circumcision.
4. Milia is a common finding in a newborn and does not place the newborn at an increased risk of skin infection.

TEST-TAKING TIP: Recognize the priority word in the stem to determine which descriptor is either normal or places the newborn at *highest* risk. It may be helpful to rank the findings in order of most risk.

Content Area: Newborns
Integrated Processes: Nursing Process—Assessment
Client Need: Physiological Integrity; Reduction of Risk Potential; Potential for Alterations in Body Systems
Cognitive Level: Analysis
Concept: Critical Thinking
Reference: Ward, S. L., & Hisley, S. M. (2009). Maternal-child nursing care: Optimizing outcomes for mothers, children & families. *Philadelphia: F.A. Davis.*

17. **ANSWER: 3**

Rationale

1. This is not the correct technique to clean the bulb syringe.
2. This is not the correct technique to clean the bulb syringe.
3. This is the correct technique to clean the bulb syringe.
4. This is not the correct technique to clean the bulb syringe.

TEST-TAKING TIP: Recognize the proper technique for cleaning a bulb syringe.

Content Area: Newborns
Integrated Processes: Nursing Process—Assessment
Client Need: Safe and Effective Care Environment; Safety and Infection Control
Cognitive Level: Comprehension
Concept: Safety
Reference: Ward, S. L., & Hisley, S. M. (2009). Maternal-child nursing care: Optimizing outcomes for mothers, children & families. *Philadelphia: F.A. Davis.*

18. **ANSWER: 2**

Rationale

1. This finding is normal and does not warrant immediate investigation.
2. This finding is concerning; the nurse should assess this patient first.
3. This newborn should be assessed after the mother is done breastfeeding.
4. Although this finding is important, it does not require immediate attention.

TEST-TAKING TIP: Determine if each behavior of the newborn is normal or abnormal and prioritize which is most concerning.

Content Area: Newborns
Integrated Processes: Nursing Process—Assessment
Client Need: Safe and Effective Care Environment; Management of Care; Establishing Priorities
Cognitive Level: Analysis
Concept: Critical Thinking
Reference: Ward, S. L., & Hisley, S. M. (2009). Maternal-child nursing care: Optimizing outcomes for mothers, children & families. *Philadelphia: F.A. Davis.*

19. **ANSWER: 4**

Rationale

1. The amount of sun exposure a newborn should receive is minimal; 2 hours would be too long.
2. Telling them to get a babysitter does not help them understand why sun exposure can be harmful to their newborn.
3. Sunscreen is not recommended for newborns less than 6 months.
4. When babies are going to be outside, they should be dressed appropriately for the climate. Lightweight clothing should be applied in warmer areas and newborns should be kept cool in the shady areas.

TEST-TAKING TIP: Recall that newborns should not be placed directly in the sun for longer than 2 hours a day and what methods are appropriate for them in terms of clothing and skin protection.

Content Area: Newborns
Integrated Processes: Teaching/Learning
Client Need: Health Promotion and Maintenance; Principles of Teaching and Learning
Cognitive Level: Synthesis
Concept: Safety
Reference: Ward, S. L., & Hisley, S. M. (2009). Maternal-child nursing care: Optimizing outcomes for mothers, children & families. *Philadelphia: F.A. Davis.*

20. **ANSWER: 1**

Rationale

1. Newborns should be born with two arteries and one vein.
2. A respiratory rate of 35 breaths per minute is normal for a newborn and should range at rest between 20 and 40 breaths/minute.
3. Newborns are commonly born with acrocyanosis, which means their bodies will be pink, with slightly blue extremities.
4. Newborns should not present with grunting or retractions, because this would be indicative of respiratory distress.

TEST-TAKING TIP: Recall that newborn assessment of the gastrointestinal system will reveal a three-cord vessel with two arteries and one vein. Congenital anomalies can be associated with fewer than three vessels.

Content Area: Newborns
Integrated Processes: Nursing Process—Implementation
Client Need: Physiological Integrity; Physiological Adaptation
Cognitive Level: Application
Concept: Critical Thinking
Reference: Ward, S. L., & Hisley, S. M. (2009). Maternal-child nursing care: Optimizing outcomes for mothers, children & families. *Philadelphia: F.A. Davis.*

Chapter 21

The At-Risk Newborn

KEY TERMS

Bilirubin—Orange-colored or yellowish pigment in bile derived from the hemoglobin of red blood cells that have completed their life span and are destroyed and ingested by the macrophage system of the liver, spleen, and red bone marrow. It is excreted in the bile. Pathological accumulation of bilirubin leads to jaundice in many cases such as physiological jaundice of the newborn.

Direct or conjugated bilirubin—Bilirubin conjugated by the liver cells, which is water soluble and excreted in urine

Down syndrome—The clinical consequence of having three copies of chromosome 21, marked by mild to moderate mental retardation and physical characteristics that include a sloping forehead, low-set ears with small canals, and short, broad hands with a single palmar crease known as a *simian crease.*

Epispadias—A congenital opening of the urethra on the dorsum of the penis

Hypospadias—An abnormal congenital opening of the male urethra upon the undersurface of the male penis

Indirect or unconjugated bilirubin—Unconjugated bilirubin that is present in the blood and is fat soluble

Jaundice—Yellow staining of body tissues and fluids, due to excessive levels of bilirubin in the bloodstream; usually not visible until the total bilirubin level rises above 3 mg/dL

Petechiae—Small, purplish, hemorrhagic spots on the skin that may appear in patients with platelet deficiencies and in many febrile illnesses

Phototherapy—Exposure to sunlight or to ultraviolet light for therapeutic purposes. Can be used to treat neonatal jaundice in which the jaundiced infant is exposed to UV light to decrease bilirubin levels in the blood, reducing the risk of bilirubin depositing in the brain.

I. Abnormal findings by systems

Some of the findings presented in this chapter place the newborn at risk for more individualized care. As such, some facilities will continue to monitor for changes in the newborn nursery, while others may require more specialized care in the neonatal intensive care unit. Nurses should be familiar with the policies and protocols within their institution.

A. General assessment

The nurse should record the location of any birth injuries such as forceps marks, fetal monitoring lesions, or bruising. Particular attention should be paid to areas around the scalp, face, shoulders, arms, legs, and feet. Larger newborns often have marks associated with birth trauma from a difficult vaginal birth. Newborns with a nuchal cord or umbilical cord around the neck may have bruising of the neck and face. If the newborn was born with a presenting part such as a leg, feet, or buttocks, then edema or bruising may be seen in the

lower extremities. If any of these conditions are noted, a thorough assessment should be performed while the newborn is prone and supine, which allows for visual inspection of the area.

DID YOU KNOW?

Nurses can help improve the infant's survival by minimizing risk of infection by following strict hand-washing protocols and minimizing risks of contamination during any necessary invasive procedures. Nurses should promote attachment with the parents and provide education regarding developmental and supportive care of the preterm or premature infant based on each infant's unique needs. Infants may be sent home on monitoring devices or with other hospital equipment that will require specific education by the nurse.

1. Appropriate for gestational age (AGA): Newborns who plot between the 10th and 90th percentile in weight, length, head

circumference, and gestational age may be categorized as AGA.

2. Small for gestational age (SGA): A newborn who is plotted below the 10th percentile on the growth chart may be labeled as SGA. Birth weight, length, head circumference, and gestational age will further help classify a newborn. A term or preterm infant can be SGA because of intrauterine growth restriction (IUGR); this can occur during pregnancy when there are advanced gestational weeks but limited growth of the fetus.

   a) Risk factors: Maternal factors such as multiparity, lack of prenatal care, age, low socioeconomic factors, smoking, high blood pressure during pregnancy, maternal heart disease, substance abuse, sickle cell disease, phenylketonuria, and lupus may predispose the newborn to this condition. Environmental factors such as high altitudes, exposure to x-rays or toxins, hyperthermia, placental variations, and fetal factors such as congenital infections, chromosome syndromes, umbilical cord anomalies, and inborn errors of metabolism can also increase the risk factors of IUGR.

   b) Complications: As a result, newborns may then be at a higher risk of polycythemia, hypoglycemia, perinatal asphyxia, fetal hypoxia, aspiration syndrome, or perinatal mortality.

   c) Care of the infant: The nurse will need to monitor the infant's respiratory rate and airway patency. Any sign of respiratory distress should be reported immediately, and protocols regarding oxygen administration should be followed.

MAKING THE CONNECTION

Asymmetrical and Symmetrical SGA

In infants who are considered SGA, there is a report of a nutritional or oxygenation deficit occurring in utero that may have resulted from fetal or maternal causes or a placental or cord compression. If the problem was present during the first trimester, the infant is usually symmetrically SGA, but when the problem is present after the 20th week of gestation, the infant is more likely to have asymmetrical SGA. The difference between symmetrical and asymmetrical SGA infants is related to their head size. If the infant is below the 10th percentile for weight but the head circumference measures between the 10th and 90th percentile, then the infant is considered asymmetrical SGA. If both the head circumference and weight are below the 10th percentile, then the infant is considered symmetrical SGA.

The body temperature, glucose levels, and blood gases should all be monitored according to practitioner order or hospital protocol. Reflexes for sucking, swallowing, gagging, and coughing should be assessed; upon normal findings, feedings or IV intake may be initiated per protocol.

3. Large for gestational age (LGA): Newborns who plot at or above the 90th percentile on the growth chart are considered LGA in relationship to weight, length, head circumference, and gestational age.

   a) Risk factors: Some conditions that may increase the chance of a newborn being LGA may be related to the mother's weight gain above recommendations during pregnancy or maternal obesity prior to pregnancy, multiparous women, male gender, erythroblastosis fetalis, Beckwith-Wiedemann syndrome (genetic condition with omphalocele and neonatal hypoglycemia and hyperinsulinemia), and transposition of the great vessels.

   b) Complications: birth trauma related to cephalopelvic disproportion (CPD). Other complications associated with hypoglycemia, polycythemia, and hyperviscosity may be directly related to a diabetic mother or a newborn with erythroblastosis fetalis, or Beckwith-Wiedemann syndrome.

   c) Care of the infant: Based on the risks and complications associated with an infant who is LGA, the nurse should monitor vital signs, screen for hypoglycemia and polycythemia, and observe for any birth-related trauma markings. Specific facility protocols should be followed in regard to how often the vital signs and blood glucose monitoring should be recorded. Special care should be provided to the parents of this infant in regard to attachment, whether any visual marks are noted as a result of birth trauma, proper handling of the infant, and how to arouse and console the infant to further enhance bonding.

DID YOU KNOW?

Hypoglycemia should be considered in any newborn born to a diabetic mother or if the newborn is SGA or premature, LGA, smaller than their twin, male, or is considered a late preterm birth.

   d) Care of the infant of a diabetic mother: Infants who are born to diabetic mothers may be LGA; however, mothers with severe diabetes or long-term diabetes may have SGA infants; these infants will require close monitoring at least for several hours and up to the first few days of life. Infants who are born LGA as a result of a diabetic mother will generally be ruddy in color, macrocosmic, and have more adipose tissue. The larger size of the infant is a result of the infant's exposure to the maternal glucose, which crosses the placenta. In utero, these increased glucose levels cause the fetus to increase insulin production, which inhibits the breakdown of fat to free fatty acids.

e) Feedings: When serum glucose levels are below 40 mg/dL, early feedings should occur; formula or breast milk may be offered based on the mother's preference. An infant who does not maintain normal glucose levels with oral feedings may require IV placement for glucose administration.

DID YOU KNOW?

Growth charts are based on the patient's gender and ethnicity. Charts can vary slightly among developers. The nurse should measure and plot the newborn based on the chart that best represents the patient population.

4. Post-term or post dates: A newborn born after 42 weeks gestational age is considered post-term or post dates. Although the exact cause is unknown, this occurrence may be the result of an inaccurate estimate of the due date. Newborns may be of normal size and health while some may grow to be over 4,000 grams at birth.

   a) Complications: CPD and shoulder dystocia may result in a newborn larger in size; hypoglycemia, meconium aspiration, polycythemia, congenital anomalies, seizures, and cold stress may also occur.

   b) Care of the infant: The nurse should monitor for hypoglycemia based on the hospital protocol and accordingly place the infant on IV glucose infusion or start on oral feedings. Close monitoring of respiratory distress is warranted due to increased risk of asphyxia within the first

---

MAKING THE CONNECTION

Monitoring Infant's Blood Sugar Levels

Infants born to a mother with diabetes will typically have hypoglycemia begin 1 to 3 hours after delivery and then rise to more normal levels about 4 to 6 hours later. Initially the blood glucose is determined by examining the cord blood after delivery or by heel stick on an hourly basis during the first 4 hours. The hospital may then go to a 4-hour interval to check blood glucose levels for the next 48 hours; the nurse should verify the hospital's policy.

---

24 hours of life. If the infant was SGA and post dates, then checking for polycythemia might be indicated via peripheral or central hematocrit levels, which are dependent on the hospital's protocol. Oxygen may need to be applied if respiratory distress is noted.

5. Postmaturity: a newborn born after 42 weeks of gestation who exhibits postmaturity syndrome.

   a) Causes: advanced gestational age, placental aging and decreased function, continued exposure to amniotic fluid

   b) Complications: hypoglycemia, meconium aspiration, polycythemia, congenital anomalies, seizure activity, cold stress

   c) Care of the postmature infant: The nurse should monitor the infant in the same manner as discussed previously for the post dates infant.

6. Prematurity: newborns born at or before 37 weeks gestational age. Infants born prematurely are at risk for many conditions due to their immaturity of systems; these will be further discussed in Chapter 22.

   a) Complications: inadequate surfactant amounts; left to right shunting of blood through the ductus arteriosus, thereby increasing blood flow to the lungs; hypoxia; heat loss; insensible water losses; feeding difficulties; altered immune responses; anuria or oliguria, fluid retention; apnea of prematurity; patient ductus arteriosus; respiratory distress syndrome; and intraventricular hemorrhage; these complications can lead to long-term problems that will be further discussed in Chapter 22.

   b) Care of the infant: Care of the infant may have slight variations based on the hospital policy, but a thorough assessment should consider the following:

   (1) Early feedings and/or maintenance of fluid and electrolyte status may be initiated for the premature infant, and the specific protocols should be instituted based on each hospital's policy.

   (2) General appearance: The nurse should carefully assess and monitor for color, which may be pink or ruddy with acrocyanosis. Any sign of cyanosis, pallor, or jaundice should be reported to the practitioner immediately. Skin is typically red and somewhat transparent so that blood vessels are readily seen and the presence of subcutaneous fat is minimal; lanugo is often readily present and distributed throughout the body.

   (3) Head size may appear large in relationship to their overall body size, and the skull

bones are more pliable than those of full-term infants, with a smooth, flat fontanel. The ears are also more pliable and may fold over.

(4) Genitals: The infant's genitals will be smaller; males may have undescended testes and a nonrugated scrotum while females will have a more noticeable labia minora and clitoris.

(5) Musculoskeletal: The infant appears more floppy in nature or may position himself or herself similar to that of a frog while showing more jerky movements. Reflexes, in particular sucking and swallowing, may be weak. Any seizure activity is abnormal and should be reported immediately.

B. Integumentary

1. Skin color: A newborn with skin that remains deep pink or red in color while at rest may have an excessive number of red blood cells, known as *plethora*.

2. Hair distribution: Newborns with variations in their hair patterns may have underlying problems. The pattern of hair distribution should be examined. Texture, color, distribution, and any area of asymmetry should be noted. Hair that covers the forehead may occur in newborns born prematurely. Any hair that is lighter in color or whiter than other hair or grows in a circular pattern or hair whorl should be noted. These could all be signs of congenital syndromes and may warrant further investigation.

3. Lesions or other abnormalities: Any newborn who displays a hairy pigmented skin lesion with two different areas of color should be seen by a

---

MAKING THE CONNECTION

Improving Respiratory Function in the Infant

Premature infants will be at an increased risk of respiratory distress and obstruction. To help improve respiratory function, the nurse may want to elevate the head slightly (avoid hyperextension) to maintain the airway. This may be done by placing a small roll under the shoulders of the infant while the infant is lying supine. The infant should be closely monitored for signs of respiratory distress or compromise: cyanosis, tachypnea, retractions, expiratory grunting, nasal flaring, apnea, rales, rhonchi, or shallow airway sounds upon auscultation. If any of these signs are noted, the practitioner should be notified immediately and the hospital protocol should be followed, which may include applying oxygen, sampling blood gas, enforcing NPO, and ensuring a neutral thermal environment.

---

dermatologist, as it may signify a structural defect. An ultrasound is typically performed to examine the tissue beneath the skin. Any individual hairs or tufts of hair found along the spinal column could be an indicator of a vertebral defect and also warrant further investigation.

a) Petechiae: Any newborn with **petechiae** that is widespread over the body or unrelated to the birthing process should be further assessed by the health care practitioner (HCP) to determine if infection, low platelets, or congenital problems such as rubella are present.

4. Infection: may be present if discharge is noted at the site of the umbilical cord; redness at the site may be from omphalitis, which can be treated with antibiotics.

a) Cord: The cord should be pale yellow unless the bacteriostatic dye was previously placed. A cord that is gray-green in color may be the result of meconium passing in utero. The nurse should ensure that the cord remains clean and dry during the diaper changes.

C. Head, eyes, ears, mouth

1. Caput succedaneum: This occurs when there is swelling or soft tissue edema of the head as a result of trauma or prolonged pressure of the newborn's head against the maternal cervix during the birthing process. This swelling crosses the cranial sutures and disappears within a few days without any medical intervention.

2. Cephalohematoma: This is a more concerning condition that results from a subperiosteal hemorrhage. This swelling does not cross the suture lines and appears more localized on one side of the newborn's head in a well-defined outline. This condition can result from birth trauma to the head and may take several weeks to months to fully resolve as the fluid from the tissue is broken down and absorbed. **Jaundice** can result from this condition due to red blood cell damage from the hemorrhage.

3. Down syndrome: This can be identified during the early assessment of the newborn. The occiput may appear flat instead of round, and there may be a broad nasal bridge, an upward slant of the eyes, epicanthic folds, low-set ears, enlarged tongue, high arched palate, and a small chin. Infants with Down syndrome may also have other anomalies, so each body system should be carefully monitored for any unusual findings. All abnormal findings should be reported immediately to the practitioner. Further explanation of the condition will be detailed in Chapter 23.

4. Cleft palate (CP) or cleft lip (CL): These conditions can occur as an isolated case or in combination

with one another. Risk factors include family history, smoking during pregnancy, maternal use of alcohol or certain drugs, and possible deficiency in folate.

a) CP occurs during the 5th to 12th week of gestation when the tongue fails to move downward, which will in turn prevent the palates from fusing properly. This condition may be felt with a gloved finger during assessment of the mouth and can be unilateral or bilateral and involve either the hard palate, soft palate, or both.

b) CL occurs approximately during the 6th week of gestation, when the maxillary process and the frontal prominences fail to fuse properly. This condition is visible at birth and can be unilateral or bilateral, which will impact the degree of nasal deformity that may also be associated with CL.

   (1) Care of the infant: Surgical intervention of CL may occur as early as 6 months while CP repair will frequently occur during the toddler years.
   (2) Feeding: Proper sucking of a bottle or nipple during breastfeeding may be impacted and will require special bottles/nipples or feeding techniques.

DID YOU KNOW?

Infants with CL or CP have a tendency to swallow air and therefore may need to be burped more frequently. Infants should be fed in an upright position to prevent aspiration. Thickened formulas may also help provide extra calories and may be ordered for the infant. The nurse should communicate this to the parents.

   (3) Oral care: Proper cleansing of the cleft is important to minimize the chance of infection.
   (4) Positioning: Infants should be placed in the prone or side-lying position if they have CP to help prevent aspiration and facilitate drainage. Infants with CL may be discouraged from the prone position to prevent unintentional rubbing and irritation of the CL.
   (5) Bonding: The nurse should allow for parents to express their feelings and concerns with the health care team; parental bonding and attachment can sometimes be an issue with a child who has a visible defect such as CP.

D. Respiratory effort
   1. General assessment: Any newborn who exhibits signs of respiratory distress will need further monitoring and evaluation. These signs can be marked

by sternal or intercostal retractions, nasal flaring, or grunting.

a) Retractions: These occur as a result of excess negative pressure, which is required to increase the depth of respirations. They may be seen as intercostal or sternal in the newborn.

b) Nasal patency
   (1) Flaring: This presents as a widening of the nares during inspiration.
   (2) Choanal atresia: This condition is found if the newborn exhibits any difficulty while the nurse checks for nasal patency. Similarly, this condition is also present if cyanosis is noted when the nurse closes the newborn's mouth, but cyanosis is absent when the mouth is open. The head should be positioned to maximize airway entry. A feeding tube may be inserted to assess for patency and help to confirm diagnosis, which may require the nurse's assistance as the practitioner checks for patency.

ALERT The inability to pass a small catheter through the nares of the newborn is considered a positive diagnosis of choanal atresia; the practitioner must be notified immediately.

c) Grunting: This commonly occurs before exhalation as air is expelled through the larynx.
d) Birth injuries: Palpate the lung fields to more accurately assess for fractures of the clavicle or ribs that may cause increased respiratory rate secondary to pain. Asymmetry of the chest wall during respirations can also be a sign of a rib fracture.
   (1) Anatomical deformities: Pectus carinatum (pigeon chest) and pectus excavatum (funnel chest) may be present from abnormal development of the ribs and sternum. Both of these conditions can impact proper lung expansion.
e) Respiratory distress syndrome (RDS): This will affect preterm newborns due to a lack of sufficient surfactant production. The signs of RDS will be first seen soon after birth. Premature infants may even be cyanotic at birth and need oxygen supplementation. Tachypnea with retractions may also be present. If so, the health care team should be notified; orders for pulse oximetry, arterial blood gas, and oxygen are probable and will help determine the diagnosis.

DID YOU KNOW?

Infants may require oxygenation via an endotracheal tube (ETT) and receive synthetic surfactant within 15 to 30 minutes of birth, which can also be administered through the ETT. Infants weighing less than 1,000 g are given surfactant to coat the alveoli, which will help keep their alveoli open. Infants weighing greater than 1,000 g will be given surfactant within the first 6 hours of life. Both may require continuous oxygenation via ETT.

MAKING THE CONNECTION

Educating Parents About Recognizing Respiratory Distress

Prior to discharge, parents should be taught how to recognize the signs of respiratory distress in their newborn: above normal respirations (greater than 60, initially), prolonged periods of apnea (greater than 15 seconds), sucking in or seesaw movements of the rib cage (intercostal retractions), nasal flaring, or grunting sounds. Parents should proceed immediately to the nearest hospital or call 911 if they suspect any of these conditions. Respiratory obstruction may also occur. Any newborn exhibiting signs of choking, coughing, gagging, or blue discoloration should be assessed immediately. Parents should dial 911 if these symptoms occur.

E. Cardiovascular system
Several conditions may warrant additional assessment by the HCP. More common low-risk defects will be discussed in this chapter. Defects requiring specialized care will be discussed in Chapter 22.
1. Ventricular septal defect (VSD): This occurs when there is a small hole in the ventricle wall between the right and left heart chambers. This defect is one of the most common among newborns. Although the defect is small, the murmur is loud because of the increased pressure in the chambers. Most VSDs are small and will close naturally. Typically, closure occurs by the first year of birth without further intervention. Larger VSDs may cause congestive heart failure and require surgical intervention.
2. Atrial septal defect: This condition occurs when there is an opening in the atrial septum creating a left to right shunt of blood flow. The level of defect can range from small to large. Initially infants may not have visible symptoms, thereby creating a late diagnosis in later years. Some openings may close within the first few years of life. Surgical closure may be necessary when increased pulmonary blood flow causes congestive heart failure or if closure does not occur on its own by 2 or 3 years.
3. Patent ductus arteriosus: This condition is a persistence after birth of a communication between the main pulmonary artery and the aorta. It can be common among preterm infants who also have respiratory distress syndrome. Some patients will be asymptomatic. Medications such as indomethacin and IV ibuprofen may be used when congestive heart failure is not present or when surgical intervention may be necessary to treat this condition.
4. Care of the infant with a heart condition: Early identification and referral is a priority in the care of the infant with an underlying cardiac condition. If the infant is stable, routine care may continue in the newborn nursery and further follow-up may occur upon discharge. If the infant is unstable, then he or she may be transferred to the neonatal intensive care unit for additional monitoring. The nurse should follow the hospital's protocol for further monitoring procedures or orders.
F. Gastrointestinal system
Abdominal distention, absent bowel sounds, umbilical cord discharge, or a palpable abdominal mass are uncommon, and the nurse should notify the practitioner immediately.

G. Genitourinary system

The nurse should examine for any bruising or swelling in the genitalia that may result from a breech presentation or birth trauma. Meconium stool should be noted during the assessment or within 8 to 24 hours of life.

1. Hypospadias: This is diagnosed when the opening of the urethra is on the ventral side of the penile surface.
2. Epispadias: This is diagnosed when the urinary opening is on the dorsal surface.

DID YOU KNOW?

Hypospadias and **epispadias** require surgical intervention. The foreskin is used to construct the meatus. Circumcision is contraindicated in all male newborns with known hypospadias or epispadias because the foreskin will be used in the surgical correction of these conditions.

3. Urates: This is a common finding among newborns, which will be noted as a pink stain in the diaper. If urates are present after two diaper changes, it could be a sign of dehydration or weight loss and should be reported to the HCP.
4. Ambiguous genitalia: This is a condition where the male has genital structures that look similar to labia or the female has features similar to that of a penis.
5. Imperforate anus: This occurs when there is no opening of the anal ring. It is considered a medical emergency because the passage of stool is not possible.
6. Females: Rectovaginal fistula is an opening between the rectum and vagina. This condition is a possibility when stool is present in the vagina.

H. Musculoskeletal system

1. Developmental dysplasia of the hip (DDH): This is a congenital condition that can affect walking in later years and must be assessed for at this time.

MAKING THE CONNECTION

Recognizing Gender Ambiguity

Newborns with an undetermined gender are further evaluated for genetic studies and adrenal gland insufficiency. This diagnosis can be troubling for the parents. It is important that the nurse avoid referring specifically to the newborn as a "boy" or "girl," which may only add to the parents' emotional stressors and confusion. Care for the newborn must be implemented in a delicate and compassionate manner. Parents should focus their efforts on getting to know their newborn. The idea of naming their newborn might need to wait until the doctor (typically a specialist) has the chance to assess the newborn and determine how to proceed.

Breech presentation increases the risk of DDH. After assessing the skin folds for symmetry in both prone and supine positions, leg length and size, and knee height for evenness, the nurse should perform the Ortolani and Barlow maneuvers.

2. Joint positions: It is important for the nurse to assess for passive range of motion (ROM) in all other joints as well while also noting spontaneous movements. The foot is a common area that may have unusual presentations, usually secondary to in utero positioning. Pronation or a turning inward of

---

MAKING THE CONNECTION

Ortolani and Barlow Maneuvers

Some hospitals require that the Ortolani and Barlow maneuvers be performed only by the experienced staff and/or physicians. Check the hospital policy before doing these maneuvers. The nurse can assess for DDH while the newborn is in the supine position. Assessment begins by placing the thumb on the newborn's inner thigh with a finger on the outside of the greater trochanter of the hip. First, pressure will be applied in a downward movement on the head of the femur to see if the femur can be dislocated from the acetabulum. Next, a circular turning of the femoral head in an inward to outward movement will attempt to position the head if it was displaced by the previous movement—the Barlow maneuver. If the development is abnormal, there will be a slight "clicking" sound and then a "clunk" as the head of the femur pops out of socket.

MAKING THE CONNECTION

Developmental Hip Dysplasia

Any child who is suspected of having DDH will need to have confirmation of the diagnosis by x-ray exam. Then the newborn's legs and hips will be maintained in an abducted position (frog-leg) by a splint, commonly referred to as a Pavlik harness. This harness is worn continuously 24 hours a day for about 3 to 6 months until newer bone growth occurs around the head of the femur, forming a normal cup-shaped hip joint. Parents should thoroughly understand that this condition is not life-threatening but will need constant monitoring and follow-up appointments with specialists. Surgery is generally not necessary, unless improvement is not achieved by 6 months of age. Special considerations are needed for holding, car seat positioning, proper clothing, bathing, traveling, and playing with the newborn in a Pavlik harness and can be found at the International Hip Dysplasia Institute's website: http://hipdysplasia.org/.

one or both feet is common and ranges from mild to severe positioning problems. In mild cases, the foot can be gently manipulated back to the original position over time through exercises performed by the parents. However, for more severe positioning, medical management might be necessary.

a) Clubfoot: Although this condition does not have an exact cause, clubfoot can be related to intrauterine positioning, neurovascular problems, genetics or chromosomal anomalies, or family history. The condition occurs either unilaterally or bilaterally when the midfoot is turned downward, the hindfoot turns inward, and the forefoot curls in toward the heel. This condition involves muscles, tendons, and bones and varies in degree of deformity. Diagnosis is made at birth by visual inspection, and severity is confirmed by radiograph. Treatment will vary depending on degree of severity. Parents should receive a diagnosis soon after delivery and will be further instructed on timing of follow-up appointments prior to discharge or with their pediatrician.

3. Fractures: The nurse must determine whether any fractures exist anywhere in the body. The clavicle needs to be thoroughly examined, as this is a common fracture site of the newborn because the newborn's shoulders do not rotate easily during the birthing process. Other common sites include ribs, skull, and humerus. Signs and symptoms of fractures may include swelling at the site, bruising, discoloration, or obvious signs of pain and discomfort. An x-ray will confirm the diagnosis. Fractures of the clavicle will heal over time, while others may need more specialized care in the ICU.

⓵ ALERT Nurses will need to ensure parents are aware of all the special handling that accompanies any of these musculoskeletal conditions. Special techniques on diapering, bathing, holding, swaddling, and car seat safety will need to be thoroughly discussed prior to discharge.

4. Torticollis: This condition results from a deviation of the neck to one side. It is caused by a spasmodic

---

MAKING THE CONNECTION

Recognizing Clubfoot

Newborns may have a condition known as clubfoot, which is a result of shorter tissues that connect muscles to bone, causing a clubbed appearance of the foot similar to the shape of a golf club. An x-ray will confirm the diagnosis. Treatment involves serial casting to restore proper alignment. Parents will need to be reassured that this is not a life-threatening condition and over time can be corrected.

---

contraction of the neck muscles and is seen when the head is positioned on one side and the chin points to the opposed side. Neck movement may be limited and should be reported immediately.

⓵ ALERT The treatment involves passive ROM or stretching exercises typically within 3 months of birth.

5. Other anomalies: Some newborns are born with extra digits on hand or feet, commonly referred to as *polydactyl*. In this occurrence, it is important to note whether a bone can be palpated. When bones are absent, typical management includes tying off the extra digit with suture silk, which occludes blood flow and results in necrosis and loss of the digit. However, when bone is present, the digit will be surgically removed. Webbing of the skin between fingers and toes can also occur and is known as *syndactyly*. It is commonly removed through surgical procedures.

DID YOU KNOW?

Polydactyl may be a familial trait, and parents should be asked if any other family members have a history of this condition. The surgical release of the webbing of toes may be refused by some families since it does not impact balance or walking. Surgical correction of the fingers does help with dexterity and is typically corrected for other cosmetic concerns as well.

a) Simian crease: This crease appears as a single, straight line in the middle of the palm on either or both hands. If this finding is in association with other specific symptomology, the condition may be diagnosed as Down syndrome. See Figure 21.1 for a comparison of a normal palmar crease and a simian crease.

I. Neurological system
Some abnormalities seen during the neurological assessment are common and involve the brachial plexus associated with shoulder rotation difficulty during delivery. This injury must be compared to another similar injury referred to as *shoulder dystocia*, which results in a short-term decrease in movement and muscle

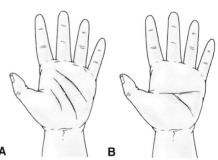

A   **B**

Fig 21.1 How to properly distinguish between normal palmar crease and simian crease.

tone in the shoulder and upper extremity. Shoulder dystocia should begin to improve soon after delivery.

1. Erb's palsy: This is a form of brachial plexus that can be quickly identified in the supine position due to the specific arrangement of the newborn's arm. This injury results in either or both of the arms remaining in an extended position; flexion of the extremities is not present. Decreased muscle tone, grasp reflex, and absent arm recoil will also be noted on the affected side of the newborn.

DID YOU KNOW?

Injuries that involve the brachial plexus will typically resolve within 2 weeks without any further interventions or treatment. Arm position should be maintained in a gently flexed position when held. The affected arm should be supported during the healing process. Gentle exercises to strengthen the extremities involve flexion and extension and can be taught to the parents. These exercises will help foster the bonding relationship and should be encouraged and approached as such.

2. Severe injuries or those that may have occurred during the development stage or as a result of the birthing process, or any damage that involves brain or muscle movement associated with anoxia should be more thoroughly examined in the neonatal ICU.
   a) Cerebral palsy: This may result from oxygen deprivation and involves problems specifically with motor development. In infancy, the problems seen involve swallowing, breathing, and/or moving and are dependent on the length of time the newborn went without oxygen. Other problems may also be seen as the child ages. This diagnosis ranges from mild to severe impairments and is a lifelong condition for the child.

II. Variations of the Newborn

A. Jaundice

Jaundice is yellowing of the skin and eyes by the second day of life and appears as a result of **bilirubin** levels above 5 mg/dL. This condition arises when bilirubin begins to build up in the newborn's blood. To determine if the newborn has jaundice, bilirubin levels must be drawn. Assessment may be helpful initially but will not provide accurate findings of jaundice. If jaundice is present, applying pressure over a bony prominence (nose, forehead) will reveal a yellowish appearance when the pressure is removed. Causes of jaundice may include fetal or neonatal asphyxia, use of indomethacin, hypothermia, hypoglycemia, maternal drug exposure to sulfa drugs and aspirins, prematurity, history of sibling with jaundice, cephalohematoma, significant bruising (can be in association with breech presentation), or being of East Asian, American Indian, or Greek descent.

🛑 **ALERT** Excessive bruising can elevate the bilirubin levels and lead to a condition known as jaundice in the newborn. Therefore, it is important to pay particular attention to bilirubin levels in all newborns, but in particular in newborns with excessive bruising.

1. Physiological jaundice: This occurs as a result of increased red blood cell (RBC) destruction, a defective ability for bilirubin to conjugate, and acceleration of bilirubin reabsorption in the gastrointestinal tract. It is a normal process the newborn undergoes.
2. Breastfeeding jaundice: Also called *breast milk jaundice,* this typically appears in the first few days of life and can occur at a higher incidence in newborns who are exclusively breastfed. The breast milk can make certain proteins in the liver more difficult to break down, which then increases bilirubin levels. When these levels accelerate above 20 mg/dL, it may be advised to halt breastfeeding to determine the cause; resuming breastfeeding is usually allowed after bilirubin levels are less than 20 mg/dL.
   a) Risk factors: This may be associated with maternal diabetes, ABO incompatibility, Rh incompatibility, prematurity, delayed feeding, birth trauma, liver immaturity, newborn stress, Pitocin administration during labor, cultural background, and family history.

B. Therapies for jaundice

1. Therapy includes special lighting referred to as bili lights or **phototherapy.** The HCP should place the newborn under the lights for the majority of the day, allowing the mother to feed the newborn when needed. It is important to cover the eyes to prevent overexposure and cover the genitals to prevent long-term damage. See Figure 21.2 for proper placement of lights during phototherapy.

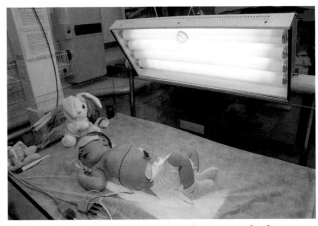

Fig 21.2 Phototherapy and proper placement of infant to prevent eyes and genitalia injury.

🛑 **ALERT** Phototherapy can alter the newborn's temperature and increase the risk of fluid loss or dehydration. Special precautions should be taken to monitor for these changes.

C. Physiological anemia of infancy

This occurs in correlation with the normal drop in hemoglobin levels at 8 to 12 weeks of age and the decrease in fetal hemoglobin. The amount of hemoglobin will vary in the term and preterm newborn: 10 to 11 g/dL at 6 to 12 weeks and 7 to 9 g/dL at 5 to 10 weeks; the bone marrow will then resume RBC production, causing the anemia to resolve.

D. Hypoglycemia

This may occur in the newborn because maternal glucose stores immediately cease when the umbilical cord is clamped. During the first 3 hours of life, the blood glucose levels will remain low and slowly rise to normal levels. Glucose levels in newborns should remain between 40 and 65 mg/dL in term newborns. Low blood sugar levels may result in the following manifestations: jitteriness, respiratory distress, cyanosis, apnea, high-pitched crying, feeding problems, lethargy, and seizures. Babies born to mothers who have experienced gestational diabetes, gestational hypertension, or terbutaline administration may be at a higher risk of experiencing hypoglycemia. Newborns who have been subjected to infection, hypothermia, hypoxic events, congenital anomalies, or fetal hydrops may also be at an increased risk. Even the length of labor, early or late feeding of the newborn and blood sugar level of the mother at the time of birth can affect the blood glucose level of the newborn.

DID YOU KNOW?

Newborns experiencing consistently low blood sugar levels will require close observation and monitoring of blood sugar levels every 2 to 3 hours. Specific interventions, close monitoring, and practitioner awareness may be necessary for those newborns who have blood glucose levels less than 40 mg/dL or who are elevated above the normal levels.

MAKING THE CONNECTION

Neonatal Jaundice

Neonatal jaundice may occur within the infant's first week of life because of excessive levels of **unconjugated bilirubin.** The signs of jaundice are usually first seen on the infant's face and sclera after serum bilirubin levels are at least 4 to 6 mg/dL. When bilirubin is present in higher amounts, the yellow discoloration will progress on the infant's body. Jaundice that occurs within the infant's first 24 hours of life is referred to as *pathological jaundice.* Total serum bilirubin levels usually are in excess of 12.9 mg/dL in term infants but can be greater than 15 mg/dL in preterm infants.

E. Illness

The HCP should be notified if the newborn exhibits any of the following: rectal temperature higher than 100.4°F (38°C), skin rash, oozing, bloody discharge, or foul odor from circumcision or cord site, vomiting or watery green stools, fewer than six wet diapers per day, increased sleepiness, or diminished appetite.

1. Care of the infant: Although the newborn may not experience illness in the hospital setting, parents will need to be instructed on how to care for their infant if illness arises. There are many types of thermometers available, and proper instruction on the correct use is imperative. Nurses should discuss the thermometer types and directions for use with parents before discharge. Although Tylenol and ibuprofen drops are available for infants, the dosages and administration of these medicines should always be discussed with and approved by the practitioner first.

III. Laboratory or Other Diagnostic Findings

A. Pulse oximetry

This measures arterial oxygen saturation. Be sure to change the disposable sensor every 8 hours or more to prevent skin breakdown or burns associated with longer use.

B. Transcutaneous oxygen monitor ($TcPO_2$)

This measures oxygen diffusion across the skin.

C. Cardiorespiratory monitors

Electrodes are placed on the newborn to measure the heart rate (HR) and respiratory rate (RR). These are used in the hospital or at home. Alarms can be set to sound when specified numbers are reached.

D. Blood glucose monitoring. May be performed if the newborn is LGA. A newborn with a blood glucose reading less than 60 mg/dL is in need of immediate action. Nurses should be prepared to feed the newborn 5% glucose, formula, or breast milk. Check the facility for specific policies regarding protocols to check blood glucose levels.

E. Bilirubin levels

Bilirubin is an orange or yellow pigment found in bile from hemoglobin of RBCs that are destroyed and found in the liver, spleen, and red bone marrow. Bilirubin is excreted in the bile via the duodenum and later in stool. When accumulation of bilirubin occurs, the result can lead to jaundice.

1. Conjugated (direct) bilirubin: conjugated bilirubin by liver cells to form bilirubin, which is water soluble and excreted in urine
2. Unconjugated (indirect) bilirubin: fat soluble, present in blood as unconjugated bilirubin
3. Total bilirubin: sum of conjugated and unconjugated bilirubin

F. ABO incompatibility

This hemolytic disease of the newborn can occur when the mother has type O blood and newborn has type A or B. The Rh factor is not significant when this occurs because type O blood carries no antigens. The problem occurs if the child is born with type A or B blood because the mother has anti-A and anti-B antibodies present with her first pregnancy. If the newborn is affected, the IgG antibodies can cross the placenta, causing destruction of fetal RBCs.

1. Cord blood: Blood will be taken from the umbilical cord after delivery and evaluated for bilirubin levels.

G. Erythroblastosis fetalis

When an Rh-negative mother is pregnant and the fetus is Rh-positive, maternal antibodies cross the placenta and enter fetal circulation, destroying the RBCs of the fetus. The fetus will react by making more RBCs, resulting in jaundice, anemia, and compensatory erythropoiesis. As a result, immature RBCs or erythroblasts are increased. This condition has decreased over recent years because of the administration of RhoGAM.

H. Urine collection

1. Drug levels: Urine from the newborn may be screened to determine if drugs are present that may have been passed onto the newborn during pregnancy.

CASE STUDY: Putting It All Together

Subjective Data

As a nurse on the labor and delivery unit, you are beginning to make rounds on each of your patients. You begin your shift by assessing a patient of Chinese descent named Mrs. Wong. She delivered her baby 1 hour before your shift and had a vaginal delivery with forceps assistance at 6:02 a.m. History is reported as follows:

G: 38 weeks P: 0

Maternal blood type: A +

Prenatal care: since 7 weeks gestation

Vital Signs
Heart rate: 115 bpm
Respiratory rate: 16
Temperature: 101°F
Blood pressure: 142/85

General Findings: Mother is awake, alert, and oriented x3; has voided x1; and is asking about breast-feeding. Pitocin was given for 12 hours prior to delivery.

Family history: Mrs. Wong's husband has been deployed with the military. Her sister is staying with them while Mr. Wong is on active duty, and she has 3 children younger than 6 years of age.

Newborn Assessment

Apgar scores were 9 and 10 at 1 and 5 minutes, respectively. The infant is under a radiant warmer and is awake and moving arms and legs spontaneously. HR is 155 bpm, RR is 35, temperature is 99.5°F.

Case Study Questions

1. What are some possible risk factors that this newborn may have based on the scenario presented?

2. List at least five possible nursing diagnoses that would apply to this case.

3. What education should be provided to the mother prior to discharge?

4. What are some expected interventions possibly needed during the hospitalization?

REVIEW QUESTIONS

Be sure to read the Introduction for valuable test-taking tips.

1. Which intervention should the nurse instruct the parents to do for their newborn who has acute diaper rash?
   1. Apply the diaper loosely to infant, allowing for better air circulation.
   2. Change the newborn every 4 hours to prevent a moist environment.
   3. Wash the newborn's diaper area with an antibacterial soap and newborn wipes.
   4. Wipe off the diaper cream thoroughly between diaper changes.

2. A newborn's blood glucose level is recorded at 42 mg/dL. What is the *next* step the nurse should take?
   1. Record the number in the chart.
   2. Immediately ask the mother to feed the newborn.
   3. Report the blood glucose level to the practitioner.
   4. Observe for hypoglycemia in the newborn.

3. Which rationale is true regarding jaundice in newborns?
   1. Jaundice can result in a newborn when the mother and newborn have the same blood type.
   2. A mother who breastfeeds her newborn who develops jaundice may have to begin formula temporarily.
   3. Bilirubin levels will drop in newborns who have jaundice and may cause brain abnormalities.
   4. Keeping a newborn with jaundice below 98.7°F is essential in lowering bilirubin levels.

4. A newborn born 72 hours ago was diagnosed with jaundice, requiring phototherapy. Which is *most* important to educate the family on at this time?
   1. Anticipatory guidance regarding immunization schedules
   2. Covering the newborn's eyes during phototherapy.
   3. Proper clothing for the newborn during seasonal changes
   4. How to accurately measure the newborn's temperature

5. Which characteristics are typically found in a patient diagnosed with Down syndrome? *Select all that apply.*
   1. Low-set ears
   2. Broad nasal bridge
   3. Round occiput
   4. Small tongue
   5. Upward slanted eyes
   6. Epicanthic folds

6. As the newborn nursery nurse, you are assessing your patients. Which assessment warrants further investigation?
   1. Irregular patterns of breathing with periods of apnea lasting 5 seconds
   2. Periodic episodes of grunting during expiration
   3. Breathing at a rate of 45 breaths per minute
   4. Mild sternal retractions

7. Which diagnosis is *most* common in a newborn born at 35 + 3 gestational age?
   1. Hyperglycemia
   2. Respiratory distress syndrome
   3. Infection
   4. Altered nutrition, more than body requirements

8. Which are risk factors for a newborn developing hypoglycemia? *Select all that apply.*
   1. Prematurity
   2. Large for gestational age
   3. Cold stress
   4. Breastfeeding
   5. Maternal diabetes
   6. Respiratory distress syndrome

9. Which factor does *not* influence bilirubin levels in the infant?
   1. Prematurity
   2. Maternal diabetes
   3. Exclusively breastfeeding
   4. Birth trauma

10. The RN in the newborn nursery is reviewing the newborn's chart and notices that the bilirubin levels are elevated. What intervention should the nurse perform next?
    1. Place the patient NPO and notify a physician.
    2. Weigh the patient to see if weight loss has occurred.
    3. Take the newborn's vital signs and report to the physician.
    4. Apply phototherapy according to the hospital protocol, then notify the physician.

11. Which laboratory value is important to check on a newborn with excessive bruising following delivery?
    1. White blood cells
    2. Glucose
    3. Bilirubin
    4. Potassium

12. The nurse is reviewing a chart in the newborn nursery. An RN was ordered to take blood glucose (BG) recordings on a newborn delivered that morning. BG readings are as follows: 50 mg/dL at 7:00 a.m.; 57 mg/dL at 10:00 a.m.; 62 mg/dL at 12:00 p.m.; 67 mg/dL at 2:00 p.m.; and 68 at 4:00 p.m. What action should the nurse perform with these recordings?
    1. Notify the physician immediately that the BG readings on this newborn are low.
    2. Immediately give the newborn glucose water.
    3. Confirm the readings with the laboratory.
    4. Review orders for the timing of next BG reading.

13. Whose baby is at *highest* risk of developing jaundice based on risk factors?
    1. A 16-year-old mother who labored with Pitocin and had an uncomplicated delivery
    2. A 23-year-old mother who made it to the hospital after a delivery at home, umbilical cord cut at the hospital
    3. A 28-year-old mother with type A blood and a father with O+ blood type delivered a newborn with nuchal cord x2; forceps used
    4. A 30-year-old mother who delivered twins via cesarean section; newborn A was breech; father unknown

14. Which baby is *most* at risk for developing physiological jaundice?
    1. Newborn with bilirubin levels of 10 mg/dL on the 9th day of life, bottle feeding only.
    2. A 5-day-old term newborn with bilirubin levels of 13 mg/dL exclusively breastfeeding
    3. Premature newborn with bilirubin levels of 5 mg/dL on day 7 of life who has passed meconium for 3 days
    4. Term newborn with bilirubin levels of 15 mg/dL on day 4 of life who is breastfed every 6 hours around the clock

15. Which sign will the newborn experiencing respiratory obstruction often exhibit *first*?
    1. Gagging
    2. Vomiting
    3. Decreased heart rate
    4. Increased respiratory rate

16. Which laboratory results might be expected if the mother's Rh has type O blood and the newborn's Apgar score is low?
    1. Cardiac enzymes
    2. Blood glucose
    3. Electrolyte panel
    4. Cord blood gas

17. Which patient should be assessed *first*?
    1. Infant with a blood glucose level of 45 mg/dL, maternal history of gestational diabetes
    2. Infant who is plotted on the growth chart between the 75th and 85th percentile for weight and length and the 50th percentile for head circumference
    3. Infant born at 42 weeks gestation to 40-year-old mother who was otherwise healthy during pregnancy and at the time of delivery
    4. Infant born at 38 weeks gestation with a green stain and bruising noted on initial assessment at delivery

18. You are the nurse educator of the newborn nursery. Which behavior indicates a need for further education?
    1. Nurse obtaining blood for a blood glucose level using the heel stick method
    2. Infant placed on phototherapy after being swaddled
    3. Obtaining weight by placing the infant directly on the scale
    4. Placing the infant in the supine position to perform Ortolani and Barlow maneuvers

19. An infant weight is documented as being in the 90th percentile. What does the RN understand about this measurement?
    1. The infant's weight is appropriate or average.
    2. The infant's weight is less than 90% of all other infants' weights.
    3. The 90th percentile indicates LGA.
    4. Infants in the 90th percentile will be overweight as adults.

20. The parents of an infant have just been told that their infant has physiological anemia of infancy. Which serves as an important rationale to support why this occurred?
    1. Gestational diabetes in the mother leading to LGA in the infant
    2. Hypervolemia as a result of maternal bleeding, which accumulates in the fetal circulation
    3. Red blood cell death, which occurs every 15 days in the infant
    4. Decline in fetal erythrocytes around 2 months of age

REVIEW QUESTIONS ANSWERS

1. ANSWER: 1

Rationale

1. Allowing the skin to dry completely between diaper changes will help allow the skin to heal.
2. Diapers should be changed as soon as they become soiled; newborns should be changed approximately every 2 hours; waiting 4 hours would be too long.
3. The baby's diaper area should be cleansed with a mild soap and water.
4. The diaper cream serves as a barrier to the skin and should not be removed between diaper changes unless the area is visibly soiled.

TEST-TAKING TIP: Recall the interventions necessary for treating diaper rash.

Content Area: Newborn
Integrated Process: Teaching/Learning
Client Need: Physiological Integrity; Basic Care and Comfort
Cognitive Level: Application
Concept: Skin Integrity
Reference: *Ward, S. L., & Hisley, S. M. (2009).* Maternal-child nursing care: Optimizing outcomes for mothers, children & families. *Philadelphia: F.A. Davis.*

2. ANSWER: 1

Rationale

1. Hypoglycemia in newborns does not occur unless the blood glucose level is below 40 mg/dL; this newborn's blood glucose level is normal, so no action is necessary.
2. The newborn's blood glucose level is normal, so immediate feeding is not necessary.
3. Because the newborn's blood glucose level is normal, the first step would be to record the reading in the chart. It would not be necessary to immediately report this number to the practitioner.
4. The first action to take would be to record the reading in the chart since the value is within normal limits.

TEST-TAKING TIP: Recognize the priority in the stem as the *next* step to be taken for normal blood glucose levels and interventions for monitoring.

Content Area: Newborn
Integrated Process: Nursing Process; Planning
Client Need: Physiological Integrity; Physiological Adaptation; Fluid and Electrolyte Imbalances
Cognitive Level: Application
Concept: Metabolism
Reference: *Ward, S. L., & Hisley, S. M. (2009).* Maternal-child nursing care: Optimizing outcomes for mothers, children & families. *Philadelphia: F.A. Davis.*

3. ANSWER: 2

Rationale

1. Jaundice results when the mother and newborn have blood incompatibility issues, so the blood types would be different.
2. It may be encouraged to stop breastfeeding or supplement temporarily with formula to promote bowel elimination, thus lowering the bilirubin levels.
3. Bilirubin levels will increase in newborns with jaundice and can cause brain abnormalities and disabilities.

4. It is important to keep temperatures above 98.7°F to prevent cold stress in a newborn, which can increase bilirubin levels.

TEST-TAKING TIP: Recall why jaundice occurs, the effects of prolonged jaundice, and how to promote bilirubin levels to drop.

Content Area: Newborn at Risk
Integrated Process: Nursing Process; Assessment
Client Needs: Physiological Integrity; Physiological Adaptation; Pathophysiology
Cognitive Level: Analysis
Concept: Hematologic Regulation
Reference: *Ward, S. L., & Hisley, S. M. (2009).* Maternal-child nursing care: Optimizing outcomes for mothers, children & families. *Philadelphia: F.A. Davis.*

4. ANSWER: 2

Rationale

1. Although immunization schedules are important, it is not the most critical factor at this point. Concerns about how jaundice may delay the hospital stay and affect nutrition and bonding are of the utmost importance.
2. Covering the newborn's eyes is important to prevent retinal and tissue damage.
3. Proper clothing is important but can be addressed at a later time.
4. It is important that the mother know how to properly take a baby's temperature, but this is not the time to stress this point; the mother needs to know how to care for the baby while undergoing phototherapy.

TEST-TAKING TIP: Recognize the priority in the stem as *most* and determine why bonding can be a concern during phototherapy in a baby diagnosed with jaundice and the steps on minimizing attachment issues.

Content Area: Newborn Nursing Process
Integrated Process: Teaching/Learning
Client Need: Psychosocial Integrity; Coping Mechanisms
Cognitive Level: Analysis
Concept: Promoting Health
Reference: *Ward, S. L., & Hisley, S. M. (2009).* Maternal-child nursing care: Optimizing outcomes for mothers, children & families. *Philadelphia: F.A. Davis.*

5. ANSWER: 1, 2, 5, 6

Rationale

1. This is a typical finding in a patient diagnosed with Down syndrome.
2. This is a typical finding in a patient diagnosed with Down syndrome.
3. The occiput is typically flat, not round.
4. The tongue usually protrudes and is larger, not smaller.
5. This is a typical finding in a patient diagnosed with Down syndrome.
6. This is a typical finding in a patient diagnosed with Down syndrome.

TEST-TAKING TIP: Recognize normal findings of a newborn diagnosed with trisomy 21, or Down syndrome.

Content Area: Newborn at Risk
Integrated Process: Nursing Process; Assessment
Client Need: Physiological Integrity; Physiological Adaptation; Pathophysiology

Cognitive Level: Comprehension
Concept: Assessment
Reference: Ward, S. L., & Hisley, S. M. (2009). Maternal-child nursing care: Optimizing outcomes for mothers, children & families. Philadelphia: F.A. Davis.

6. **ANSWER: 2**
Rationale
1. It is common for newborns to have irregular patterns of breathing and apneic episodes that last as long as 15 to 20 seconds. Any further signs of respiratory distress should be noted.
2. Grunting is not a normal finding in a newborn's breathing pattern and should be examined further as a sign of potential respiratory distress.
3. Normal respiratory rate of a newborn is between 30 and 60 breaths per minute.
4. It is common for newborns to have slight or mild sternal retractions while breathing. Retractions between ribs, above the sternum, or below the ribs are a sign of respiratory distress and should be investigated further.

TEST-TAKING TIP: Recognize abnormal patterns of breathing in a newborn upon physical assessment by ruling out which of the descriptors are normal.
Content Area: Newborn at Risk
Integrated Process: Nursing Process; Assessment
Client Need: Physiological Integrity; Physiological Adaptation; Alterations in Body Systems
Cognitive Level: Analysis
Concept: Critical Thinking
Reference: Ward, S. L., & Hisley, S. M. (2009). Maternal-child nursing care: Optimizing outcomes for mothers, children & families. Philadelphia: F.A. Davis.

7. **ANSWER: 2**
Rationale
1. A preterm newborn is not always at risk of high blood sugar levels but rather hypoglycemia.
2. A preterm newborn is at risk of developing respiratory distress because of lower levels of surfactant production in newborns less than 36 weeks.
3. Infection may or may not be present in this newborn, but the gestational age does not necessarily affect this diagnosis.
4. The patient would likely exhibit altered nutrition, less than body requirements at this young gestational age.

TEST-TAKING TIP: Recognize the possible risk factors associated with a preterm newborn delivery using the priority word *most* in the stem.
Content Area: Newborn at Risk
Integrated Process: Nursing Process; Analysis
Client Need: Physiological Integrity; Reduction of Risk Potential; System Specific Assessments
Cognitive Level: Application
Concept: Assessment
Reference: Ward, S. L., & Hisley, S. M. (2009). Maternal-child nursing care: Optimizing outcomes for mothers, children & families. Philadelphia: F.A. Davis.

8. **ANSWER: 1, 2, 3, 5**
Rationale
1. Prematurity is a risk factor for hypoglycemia.
2. Large for gestational age and small for gestational age are risk factors for hypoglycemia.

3. Cold stress is a risk factor for hypoglycemia.
4. Breastfeeding is not a risk factor for hypoglycemia.
5. Maternal diabetes is a risk factor for hypoglycemia.
6. Respiratory distress syndrome is not a risk factor for hypoglycemia.

TEST-TAKING TIP: Recall the risk factors associated with hypoglycemia in a newborn.
Content Area: Newborn
Integrated Process: Nursing Process; Assessment
Client Need: Physiological Integrity: Reduction of Risk Potential; Potential for Alterations in Body Systems
Cognitive Level: Application
Concept: Assessment
Reference: Ward, S. L., & Hisley, S. M. (2009). Maternal-child nursing care: Optimizing outcomes for mothers, children & families. Philadelphia: F.A. Davis.

9. **ANSWER: 3**
Rationale
1. Prematurity is a risk factor that can influence bilirubin levels in the neonate.
2. Maternal diabetes is a risk factor that can influence bilirubin levels in the neonate.
3. Exclusively breastfeeding may not raise bilirubin levels, but delayed feedings may influence bilirubin levels.
4. Traumatic births, including those with use of forceps or vacuum extraction, may lead to destruction of the erythrocytes.

TEST-TAKING TIP: Recognize the priority word in the stem as *not* and determine which descriptor does not affect bilirubin levels.
Content Area: Newborns at Risk
Integrated Process: Nursing Process; Analysis
Client Need: Physiological Integrity; Reduction of Risk Potential; Therapeutic Procedures
Cognitive Level: Comprehension
Concept: Hematologic Regulation
Reference: Ward, S. L., & Hisley, S. M. (2009). Maternal-child nursing care: Optimizing outcomes for mothers, children & families. Philadelphia: F.A. Davis.

10. **ANSWER: 4**
Rationale
1. Fluids are encouraged and should not be limited. In some facilities, it may be common practice to switch the patient from exclusively breastfeeding to formula feeding until bilirubin levels return to normal.
2. Weighing the patient would not be helpful in the treatment of this condition.
3. Taking the newborn's vital signs is not necessary unless other conditions suggest there is a problem with their vital signs.
4. Applying phototherapy would help to reduce bilirubin levels.

TEST-TAKING TIP: Recognize the priority word *next* in the stem to determine which action is priority.
Content Area: Newborns at Risk
Integrated Process: Nursing Process; Implementation
Client Need: Physiological Integrity; Reduction of Risk Potential; Therapeutic Procedures
Cognitive Level: Application
Concept: Critical Thinking

Reference: *Ward, S. L., & Hisley, S. M. (2009). Maternal-child nursing care: Optimizing outcomes for mothers, children & families. Philadelphia: F.A. Davis.*

11. **ANSWER: 3**
Rationale
1. White blood cells are not the most concerning at this time in this newborn.
2. Glucose is not the most concerning at this time in the newborn.
3. Bilirubin levels are concerning because the newborn should be observed for jaundice, which may occur after excessive bruising.
4. Potassium is not the most concerning laboratory value at this time in the newborn.
TEST-TAKING TIP: Recognize which laboratory value correlates directly with bruising.
Content Area: Newborns
Integrated Process: Nursing Process; Evaluation
Client Need: Physiological Integrity; Reduction of Risk Potential; Potential for Complications From Surgical Procedures and Health Alterations
Cognitive Level: Application
Concept: Hematologic Regulation
Reference: *Ward, S. L., & Hisley, S. M. (2009). Maternal-child nursing care: Optimizing outcomes for mothers, children & families. Philadelphia: F.A. Davis.*

12. **ANSWER: 4**
Rationale
1. The blood glucose recordings are normal; no need to notify the physician.
2. The recordings are within normal range for the newborn, so no glucose water is needed.
3. The readings do not need to be confirmed with the laboratory.
4. The results are normal, so the nurse needs to determine if any new BG readings are needed.
TEST-TAKING TIP: Determine if the blood glucose readings in the stem of the question are normal so the best action can be determined.
Content Area: Newborns
Integrated Process: Nursing Process; Planning
Client Need: Physiological Integrity; Physiological Adaptation; Fluid and Electrolyte Imbalances
Cognitive Level: Analysis
Concept: Critical Thinking
Reference: *Ward, S. L., & Hisley, S. M. (2009). Maternal-child nursing care: Optimizing outcomes for mothers, children & families. Philadelphia: F.A. Davis.*

13. **ANSWER: 3**
Rationale
1. The only risk factor for this baby is that the mother had Pitocin.
2. The only risk factor for this baby is that the mother may have had a delayed umbilical cord cut since the baby was delivered at home and the cord was cut at the hospital.
3. This baby has two known risk factors: ABO incompatibility and nuchal cord x2, placing the baby at risk for asphyxia and birth trauma with use of forceps.
4. The only risk factor that this baby has is that the baby was breech.

TEST-TAKING TIP: Recognize the priority word in the stem as *highest* risk factors. Determine how many risk factors are in each descriptor.
Content Area: Newborns at Risk
Integrated Process: Nursing Process; Evaluation
Client Need: Physiological Integrity; Reduction of Risk Potential; Potential for Alterations in Body Systems
Cognitive Level: Analysis
Concept: Hematologic Regulation
Reference: *Ward, S. L., & Hisley, S. M. (2009). Maternal-child nursing care: Optimizing outcomes for mothers, children & families. Philadelphia: F.A. Davis.*

14. **ANSWER: 4**
Rationale
1. This baby has a lower risk than the breastfed babies, and the levels are normal for the 9th day of life, as the bilirubin levels are usually highest at 72 hours of life and reported to be above 15 mg/dL.
2. This baby is term, which places him at a lower risk than the premature newborn, and has levels of only 13 mg/dL, which is an acceptable level on the 5th day of life.
3. This baby is premature, placing her at a higher risk than the term baby, and is passing meconium regularly.
4. This term baby is only feeding every 6 hours on the 4th day of life, placing him at a greater risk because the caloric intake for him may not be sufficient. Also, this level of bilirubin is high for day 4 of life.
TEST-TAKING TIP: Recognize the priority word in the stem as *most* at risk. Decide which individual descriptor has the most risk factors.
Content Area: Newborns at Risk
Integrated Process: Nursing Process; Evaluation
Client Need: Physiological Integrity: Reduction of Risk Potential; System Specific Assessments
Cognitive Level: Analysis
Concept: Assessment
Reference: *Ward, S. L., & Hisley, S. M. (2009). Maternal-child nursing care: Optimizing outcomes for mothers, children & families. Philadelphia: F.A. Davis.*

15. **ANSWER: 4**
Rationale
1. Gagging is not the first sign of a newborn with respiratory obstruction because the baby won't be able to move air.
2. Vomiting is not the first sign of a newborn with a respiratory obstruction.
3. A decreased heart rate would not be the first sign; it may be a later sign if the problem is not addressed in a timely manner.
4. Increased respiratory rate is the first sign of a newborn with a respiratory obstruction.
TEST-TAKING TIP: Realize which symptoms occur *first* in a newborn with respiratory obstruction.
Content Area: Newborns at Risk
Integrated Process: Nursing Process; Assessment
Client Need: Physiological Integrity; Reduction of Risk Potential; System Specific Assessments
Cognitive Level: Comprehension
Concept: Oxygenation
Reference: *Ward, S. L., & Hisley, S. M. (2009). Maternal-child nursing care: Optimizing outcomes for mothers, children & families. Philadelphia: F.A. Davis.*

16. ANSWER: 4

Rationale

1. Cardiac enzymes would not be taken on the newborn at this time.

2. Blood glucose levels would not be taken on the newborn at this time.

3. An electrolyte panel would not be taken initially on the newborn at this time.

4. The cord blood gas would be one of the first laboratories taken on this newborn to detect newborn blood type and Rh factor.

TEST-TAKING TIP: Recall what interventions are performed for a newborn with a low Apgar score.

Content Area: Newborns

Integrated Process: Nursing Process; Implementation

Client Need: Physiological Integrity; Physiological Adaptation; Pathophysiology

Cognitive Level: Application

Concept: Hematologic Regulation

Reference: *Ward, S. L., & Hisley, S. M. (2009). Maternal-child nursing care: Optimizing outcomes for mothers, children & families. Philadelphia: F.A. Davis.*

17. ANSWER: 4

Rationale

1. The blood glucose findings are normal, and at this time the infant should be monitored closely but does not require immediate assessment.

2. These are normal findings for an appropriate gestational age infant.

3. Although the infant's gestational age is considered post dates and can be concerning, there is no other indication that this infant is in immediate distress.

4. This infant has the most immediate risk because the green stain is likely from meconium and bruising is related to birth trauma during delivery. This infant is at risk of red blood cell destruction and respiratory distress.

TEST-TAKING TIP: Recall which finding poses an immediate risk for respiratory distress among the infants.

Content Area: Newborn at Risk

Integrated Process: Nursing Process; Assessment

Client Need: Physiological Integrity; Reduction of Risk Potential

Cognitive Level: Application

Concept: Critical Thinking

Reference: *Ward, S. L., & Hisley, S. M. (2009). Maternal-child nursing care: Optimizing outcomes for mothers, children & families. Philadelphia: F.A. Davis.*

18. ANSWER: 2

Rationale

1. Nurses should obtain blood from an infant using the heel stick method; this procedure is correct.

2. Infants should not be swaddled while under phototherapy lights. An opaque cover should be placed on the infant's eyes and genitals, but all other areas of the body should be exposed.

3. When measuring an infant, the scale should be covered with a protective pad or blanket, zeroed, and then the infant can be placed on the protective cover.

4. Infants should be in the supine position before performing Ortolani and Barlow maneuvers.

TEST-TAKING TIP: Recall the proper procedures for blood draws, phototherapy, weighing, and checking the Ortolani and Barlow maneuvers.

Content Area: Newborn at Risk

Integrated Process: Caring

Client Need: Physiological Integrity; Reduction of Risk Potential for Complications of Diagnostic Tests; Treatments; Procedures

Cognitive Level: Analysis

Concept: Critical Thinking

Reference: *Ward, S. L., & Hisley, S. M. (2009). Maternal-child nursing care: Optimizing outcomes for mothers, children & families. Philadelphia: F.A. Davis.*

19. ANSWER: 3

Rationale

1. A patient would need to plot within the 10th to 90th percentile to be considered normal or average.

2. A patient who plots above the 90th percentile means that the patient plots higher than the general population of the same age plotted.

3. Patients who plot above the 90th percentile are considered LGA.

4. A patient's growth at birth does not necessarily predict their measurement in adulthood.

TEST-TAKING TIP: Recall the percentiles on the growth chart and know when a patient falls under, over, or within the normal or average parameters for body measurements.

Content Area: Newborns at Risk

Integrated Process: Nursing Process; Assessment

Client Need: Health Promotion and Maintenance; Health Screening

Cognitive Level: Comprehension

Concept: Assessment

Reference: *Ward, S. L., & Hisley, S. M. (2009). Maternal-child nursing care: Optimizing outcomes for mothers, children & families. Philadelphia: F.A. Davis.*

20. ANSWER: 4

Rationale

1. Gestational diabetes typically leads to an LGA infant, but this is not the cause of physiological anemia in the infant.

2. Low volume occurs as a result of maternal bleeding, not higher volumes.

3. Red blood cell death does occur at a faster rate than in the adult, but death occurs in these cells every 35 to 50 days; 15 days is too short of a time.

4. This is correct. Fetal erythrocytes will decline around 2 or 3 months of age as adult hemoglobin begins to form.

TEST-TAKING TIP: Recognize which statement causes an infant to be diagnosed with physiological anemia.

Content Area: Conjugation of Bilirubin; Development of Physiological Jaundice

Integrated Process: Nursing Process; Diagnosis

Client Need: Physiological Integrity; Physiological Adaptation

Cognitive Level: Comprehension

Content Area: Hematologic Regulation

Reference: *Ward, S. L., & Hisley, S. M. (2009). Maternal-child nursing care: Optimizing outcomes for mothers, children & families. Philadelphia: F.A. Davis.*

Newborn at High Risk

Apnea of prematurity (AOP)—Apnea in the premature newborn, marked by repeated episodes of apnea lasting longer than 20 seconds. The diagnosis of AOP is one of exclusion, arrived at when no treatable cause can be found. Increased frequency of apneic episodes directly relates to the degree of prematurity. AOP is not an independent risk factor for sudden infant death syndrome. Apneic episodes may result in bradycardia, hypoxia, and respiratory acidosis.

Asystole—Cardiac standstill; absence of electrical activity and contractions of the heart evidenced on the surface of the electrocardiogram as a flat (isoelectric) line during cardiac arrest. In most instances, asystole is an electrographic confirmation that a patient has died.

Cyanosis—A bluish discoloration of the mucous membranes in the mouth, indicating hypoxemia and respiratory failure

Grunting—An abnormal sound heard during labored exhalation that indicates a need for high chest pressures to keep the airways open. It is caused by closing of the glottis at the end of expiration.

Hypoglycemia—Blood sugar of less than 40 mg/dL in infants during the first hours of life

Hypoxia—An oxygen deficiency in body tissues. May be due to reduced oxygen supply, respiratory obstruction, reduced pulmonary function, or inadequate ventilation.

Periventricular leukomalacia—White matter brain injury characterized by necrosis around the ventricles

Pneumatosis intestinalis—The presence of thin-walled gas-filled cysts in the intestines. The cause is unknown. The cysts usually disappear but occasionally rupture and cause pneumoperitoneum.

Rales—Crackles

Surfactant—A lipoprotein secreted by type II alveolar cells that decrease the surface tension of the fluid lining the alveoli, permitting expansion. Synthetic lung surfactant is available for treating patients with respiratory distress syndrome.

Transient tachypnea of the newborn—A self-limited condition often affecting newborns who have experienced intrauterine hypoxia resulting from aspiration of amniotic fluid, delayed clearance of fetal lung fluid, or both. Signs of respiratory distress commonly appear within 6 hours after birth, improve within 24 to 48 hours, and resolve within 72 hours of birth, without respiratory assistance. May also be referred to as *tachypnea*.

I. Preterm Neonates

Infants less than 37 weeks gestation are considered premature.[1,2]

A. Maturity ratings

Determining gestational age is imperative for providers to assess growth and development, identify risks, and establish morbidity and mortality rates when advising families on best treatment options.[3] The Ballard gestational age assessment tool may be used for determining gestational age for infants ranging from 20 to 44 weeks gestation. The Ballard score assesses neuromuscular and physical maturity signs, which may be totaled to determine a maturity rating equaling gestational age in weeks.[4] The Ballard score is most authentic if performed between 30 and

[1]Fanaroff, A., & Fanaroff, J. (2013). *Klaus & Fanaroff's care of the high-risk neonate*. Philadelphia: Elsevier Saunders.

[2]Gomella, T., Cunningham, D., & Eyal, F. (2013). *Neonatology: Management, on-call problems, diseases, and drugs*. 6th ed. New York, NY: McGraw Hill Education.

[3]Tappero, & E. & Honeyfield, M. (2015). *Physical assessment of the newborn: A comprehensive approach to the art of physical examination*. 5th ed. Petaluma, CA: NICU Ink.

[4]Nagtalon-Ramos, J. (2014). *Best evidence-based practices: Maternal-newborn nursing care*. Philadelphia: F.A. Davis Company.

42 hours of life, correctly identifying gestational age ± 2 weeks.[5]

1. Birth weight
   - Low birth weight is defined as less than 2,500 grams.
   - Very low birth weight is less than 1,500 grams.
   - Extremely low birth weight is less than 1,000 grams.[6]

2. Assessment findings

   Assessment findings will vary depending on the gestational age of the preterm infant:
   - Skin may be thin, transparent, and sticky to pink and smooth.
   - Lanugo may be completely absent with early preterm infants to more prominent in later gestational ages until term, when the lanugo tends to disappear.
   - A smooth plantar surface.
   - Eyes may be fused, depending on the infant's gestational age. Extremely premature infants are more likely to have tightly fused eyes.
   - Pinna of the ear may be flat, soft, and folded to formed with spontaneous recoil.
   - Genitalia: males may have a flat, smooth scrotum to testes palpable in the upper inguinal canal with few rugae. Females may have a prominent clitoris with flattened labia to equally prominent labia majora and minora.[7]

3. Medical management
   a) Cardiopulmonary support: Establishing adequate cardiopulmonary support is crucial to the premature infant in the first minutes of life. Respiratory rate, heart rate, and skin color should be assessed.

DID YOU KNOW?

The *Textbook of Neonatal Resuscitation* (7th ed., 2016) is the national standard of care for neonatal resuscitation.

   (1) Respiratory rate may be observed or auscultated in order to identify breath sounds. If breath sounds are not observed or respiratory effort is inadequate, positive pressure ventilation should be given.
   (2) Heart rate is determined by palpating the umbilical cord at the base or auscultating heart sounds. If the heart rate is less than 100 beats per minute (bpm), positive pressure ventilation (40 to 60 breaths per minute) should be given. If the heart rate is less than 60 bpm, the provider should consider intubation, provide chest compressions, and administer epinephrine (1:10,000) via the endotracheal tube (ETT) or, preferably, the IV.
   (3) Skin color is best evaluated by assessing the mucous membranes (lips, mouth, and tongue). **Cyanosis** indicates the need for supplemental oxygen. Pulse oximetry provides the most accurate evaluation of oxygen saturations.[8,9]

   b) Medications
   (1) Epinephrine (1:10,000) is given during **asystole** and/or severe bradycardia. Dose is 0.3 to 1 mL/kg via ETT and 0.1 to 0.3 mL/kg via IV.
   (2) Volume expanders include normal saline, 5% albumin, and whole blood. Dose is 10 mL/kg given slowly via IV over 5 to 10 minutes for hypotension secondary to intravascular volume depletion.
   (3) Narcan (Naloxone; 0.4 mg/mL) is given for narcotic depression. Dose is 0.1 to 0.2 mg/kg and is given intravenously, intramuscularly (IM), or subcutaneously.[10]

🛑 **ALERT** Narcan should not be ordered if maternal history is significant for narcotic addiction because the infant can experience withdrawal, potentially causing seizures.[11,12] Sodium bicarbonate (0.5 mEq/mL) is rarely given in the delivery room—without adequate ventilation, it can increase the risk of intracranial hemorrhage by increasing P_{CO_2} if given rapidly, creating cerebral acidosis. Sodium bicarbonate may improve metabolic acidosis during lengthened resuscitation.[13] Dose is 1 to 2 mEq/kg given via IV at a rate of less than 10 mL/minute.[14]

[5]Gomella, T., Cunningham, D., & Eyal, F. (2013). *Neonatology: Management, on-call problems, diseases, and drugs.* 6th ed. New York, NY: McGraw Hill Education.

[6]Cloherty, J., Eichenwald, E., & Stark, A. (2012). *Manual of neonatal care.* 8th ed. Philadelphia: Lippincott Williams & Wilkins.

[7]Tappero, E., & Honeyfield, M. (2015). *Physical assessment of the newborn: A comprehensive approach to the art of physical examination.* 5th ed. Petaluma, CA: NICU Ink.

[8]Cloherty, J., Eichenwald, E., & Stark, A. (2012). *Manual of neonatal care.* 8th ed. Philadelphia: Lippincott Williams & Wilkins.

[9]Gomella, T., Cunningham, D., & Eyal, F. (2013). *Neonatology: Management, on-call problems, diseases, and drugs.* 6th ed. New York, NY: McGraw Hill Education.

[10]NeoFax and Pediatrics. (2016). Retrieved from http://micromedex.com/neofax-pediatric.

[11]Cloherty, J., Eichenwald, E., & Stark, A. (2012). *Manual of neonatal care.* 8th ed. Philadelphia: Lippincott Williams & Wilkins.

[12]Gomella, T., Cunningham, D., & Eyal, F. (2013). *Neonatology: Management, on-call problems, diseases, and drugs.* 6th ed. New York, NY: McGraw Hill Education.

[13]Gomella, T., Cunningham, D., & Eyal, F. (2013). *Neonatology: Management, on-call problems, diseases, and drugs.* 6th ed. New York, NY: McGraw Hill Education.

[14]NeoFax and Pediatrics. (2016). Retrieved from http://micromedex.com/neofax-pediatric.

4. Nursing management

a) Making assessment of systems: perform a head-to-toe assessment on the neonate, utilizing the same methods discussed in Chapter 20.

b) Monitoring the newborn: assess vital signs, including temperature, heart rate, respirations, blood glucose, and pulse oximetry.

🛑 **ALERT** Supplemental oxygen should always be available at the infant's bedside. If the infant's oxygen saturations are low, supplemental oxygen should be given. According to the American Academy of Pediatrics, "there is not a specific plasma glucose concentration or duration of **hypoglycemia** that can predict permanent neurologic injury in high-risk infants".[15] If an infant is symptomatic with a plasma glucose below 40 g/dL, dextrose 10% in water (D10W) 2 mL/kg is given via slow-push IV.

c) Assessing interventions: continually evaluate the infant's condition and response to interventions, and adjust as indicated.

d) Laboratory assessments and findings: arterial blood gas, blood culture, and complete blood count (CBC) with differential are obtained on admission. Follow-up CBC with differential, C-reactive protein (CRP), and electrolytes are collected at 24 hours of life.

🛑 **ALERT** The gold standard for diagnosing sepsis is peripheral blood cultures. At least 1 mL of blood is needed per culture bottle. CRP is another test used to diagnose infants with sepsis. Serial CRPs are more predictive. Elevated CRP levels are indicative of sepsis. If the CRP is normal, it is rare that the infant is septic.[16]

e) Medication administration: erythromycin ointment is placed in the eyes (if they are open), vitamin K is given to promote clotting, and hepatitis B is given with parental consent if the infant is heavier than 2,000 grams.

f) Skin care: high-risk infants are not bathed until they are in stable condition. A mild, tear-free baby shampoo and warm water are used to bathe the infant. Tape, adhesives, and adhesive remover are not recommended for use on the premature infant's skin.

g) Cardiovascular support: leads should be placed on the infant at admission to monitor cardiac status and should remain there until discharge.

h) Fluid and electrolyte balance: IV fluids are started on admission. Parental nutrition is started on infants weighing less than 1,500 grams or those who are unstable and unable to start enteral nutrition.

i) Meeting nutritional requirements: Most infants receive nothing by mouth (NPO) on admission until respiratory status is assessed and they are deemed stable. Feeds may be started if the infant is in stable condition. The amount of feeds to be given is based on feeding protocols guided by weight and gestational age. Breast milk is best.

j) Pain management: Pain is often overlooked in the neonate but can be considered the fifth vital sign. The Neonatal Infant Pain Scale (NIPS) may be used to measure pain in preterm and full-term infants.

k) Developmental concerns: Sick premature infants often fall behind full-term infants in meeting developmental milestones. Developmental milestones should be carefully assessed as the infant grows to determine if further intervention is needed.

II. Acquired and Congenital Disorders

A. Respiratory distress syndrome (RDS)
RDS is characterized by **surfactant** deficiency. Physiologically, diffuse atelectasis and pulmonary edema reduce lung compliance, decreasing oxygenation.[17]
1. Risk factors
- Prematurity
- Low birth weight
- Maternal history of diabetes

MAKING THE CONNECTION

Developmental Delays

According to the AAP (2008), the physician should be notified if the child does not crawl, stand with support, say single words, learn simple gestures, point, or look for things that you hide by 1 year of age. Assessing for developmental delay early is essential to provide interventions necessary to promote appropriate developmental milestones. Parents of sick or preterm infants often have many questions and concerns. Anticipatory guidance may be given based on gestational age of the infant, condition, and medical diagnosis.

[15]American Academy of Pediatrics, Committee on Fetus and Newborn. (2011). Postnatal glucose homeostasis in late-preterm and term infants. *Pediatrics*, *127*, 575–579. DOI: 10.1542/peds.2010-3851.

[16]Gomella, T., Cunningham, D., & Eyal, F. (2013). *Neonatology: Management, on-call problems, diseases, and drugs.* 6th ed. New York, NY: McGraw Hill Education.

[17]Ward, S., & Hisley, S. (2009). *Maternal-child nursing care enhanced.* Philadelphia: F.A. Davis.

- Perinatal hypoxia-ischemia
- Elective delivery without labor[18,19]
2. Assessment findings
   - Increased work of breathing
   - Nasal flaring
   - Tachypnea
   - Intercostal and subcostal retractions.
   - Expiratory **grunting**
   - Cyanosis
   - Apnea
   - Edema[20,21]
3. Medical management
   - Correct acidosis and hypoxemia.
   - Minimize metabolic requirements.
   - Prevent lung injury.
   - Enhance fluids and nutrition.[22]
   - Perform chest x-ray; will show a reticulogranular pattern with air bronchograms present.[23,24]
   - Use surfactant administration for prophylaxis and rescue.

DID YOU KNOW?

Exogenous surfactant is a lipoprotein containing phosphatidylcholine, which reduces surface tension in the lungs. Surfactant given through the endotracheal tube is standard of care for premature infants requiring intubation and mechanical ventilation. Administration of surfactant decreases the incidence of bronchopulmonary dysplasia and mortality.

a) Respiratory support may be provided by mechanical ventilation with endotracheal intubation, continuous positive airway pressure (CPAP), and oxygen administration through nasal cannula. Utilize the least invasive method to maintain adequate oxygenation in order to minimize lung injury. Ideally, target oxygen saturations range from 88% to 92% in infants less than 30 weeks, and 88% to 95% in infants greater than 30 weeks gestation.[25,26]

b) Blood gas monitoring to correct acidosis and prevent alkalosis while improving arterial oxygen tension (Table 22.1).

c) Septic workup, including blood cultures, CBC with differential, and CRP. Antibiotics may be ordered based on laboratory results and clinical presentation.

d) Electrolyte management should include an order for laboratory work (chemistry panel) to be followed every 12 to 24 hours in order to optimize parental nutrition, prevent hypocalcemia, and stabilize serum glucose levels.

e) Echocardiogram to determine the presence of a patent ductus arteriosus (PDA) may be ordered.[27]

4. Nursing management
   a) Maintain adequate oxygenation by utilizing pulse oximetry, keeping oxygen saturations within the targeted range.
   b) Provide a thermoneutral environment to assist in the process of thermoregulation, minimizing the incidence of cold stress (increasing oxygen demand). Efforts should be made to minimize insensible water loss by placing infants less than 2,000 grams in an incubator, assessing ambient temperature and humidity, increasing total intravenous fluids when appropriate, and providing humidified oxygen.
   c) Continuously monitor vital signs (temperature, heart rate, respirations, blood pressure, and oxygen saturations).
   d) Provide cluster care, minimizing stimulation, which tends to decrease PaO_2.
   e) Maintain strict urinary output.[28]
   f) In mechanically ventilated infants, watch for deterioration, which could indicate ventilator malfunction, air leak syndrome, or a dislodged endotracheal tube.[29]

5. Complications
   - Air leak syndromes, including pneumothorax, pneumopericardium, and/or interstitial emphysema.
   - Pulmonary hemorrhage after surfactant administration, often in the presence of a patent ductus arteriosus.
   - Intracranial hemorrhage.
   - PDA, contributing to acidosis, oliguria, hypotension, and decreased tissue perfusion.

[18]Cloherty, J., Eichenwald, E., & Stark, A. (2012). *Manual of neonatal care.* 8th ed. Philadelphia: Lippincott Williams & Wilkins.

[19]Martin, R., Fanaroff, A., & Walsh, M. (2015). *Fanaroff & Martin's neonatal-perinatal medicine: Diseases of the fetus and infant.* 10th ed. Philadelphia: Elsevier Saunders.

[20]Martin, R., Fanaroff, A., & Walsh, M. (2015). *Fanaroff & Martin's neonatal-perinatal medicine: Diseases of the fetus and infant.* 10th ed. Philadelphia: Elsevier Saunders.

[21]Fanaroff, A., & Fanaroff, J. (2013). *Klaus & Fanaroff's care of the high-risk neonate.* Philadelphia: Elsevier Saunders.

[22]Cloherty, J., Eichenwald, E., & Stark, A. (2012). *Manual of neonatal care.* 8th ed. Philadelphia: Lippincott Williams & Wilkins.

[23]Cloherty, J., Eichenwald, E., & Stark, A. (2012). *Manual of neonatal care.* 8th ed. Philadelphia: Lippincott Williams & Wilkins.

[24]Gomella, T., Cunningham, D., & Eyal, F. (2013). *Neonatology: Management, on-call problems, diseases, and drugs.* 6th ed. New York, NY: McGraw Hill Education.

[25]Cloherty, J., Eichenwald, E., & Stark, A. (2012). *Manual of neonatal care.* 8th ed. Philadelphia: Lippincott Williams & Wilkins.

[26]Gomella, T., Cunningham, D., & Eyal, F. (2013). *Neonatology: Management, on-call problems, diseases, and drugs.* 6th ed. New York, NY: McGraw Hill Education.

[27]Gomella, T., Cunningham, D., & Eyal, F. (2013). *Neonatology: Management, on-call problems, diseases, and drugs.* 6th ed. New York, NY: McGraw Hill Education.

[28]Fanaroff, A., & Fanaroff, J. (2013). *Klaus & Fanaroff's care of the high-risk neonate.* Philadelphia: Elsevier Saunders.

[29]Cloherty, J., Eichenwald, E., & Stark, A. (2012). *Manual of neonatal care.* 8th ed. Philadelphia: Lippincott Williams & Wilkins.

Table 22.1 The Relationship Between pH and Concentration of Arterial Blood

	pH	Pco$_2$	Pao$_2$	Phco$_3^-$
	Measures blood acidity	Partial pressure of carbon dioxide in blood	Partial pressure of oxygen in blood	Partial pressure of bicarbonate (alkaline or base) in blood
Normal neonatal values	pH = 7.25–7.45	Pco$_2$ = 35–40 mm Hg	Pao$_2$ = 50–80 mm Hg	Phco$_3^-$ = 20–22 mEq/L
Respiratory acidosis (caused by poor ventilation)	↓ pH	↑ Pco$_2$	WNL	WNL
Metabolic acidosis (anaerobic metabolism from hypoxia, diarrhea, or kidney disease)	↓ pH	WNL	WNL	↑ Phco$_3^-$
Respiratory alkalosis (hyperventilation)	↑ pH	↓ Pco$_2$	↑ Pao$_2$	WNL
Metabolic alkalosis (vomiting, diarrhea, or hypocalcemia)	↑ pH	WNL	WNL	↑Phco$_3^-$

WNL = within normal limits.
Adapted from Noerr, B. (2000). Neonatal respiratory disease and management strategies, May 18. A continuing education service of Penn State's College of Medicine at the Milton S. Hershey Medical Center. Hershey, PA.

- Bronchopulmonary dysplasia.
- Retinopathy of prematurity.[30]

DID YOU KNOW?
Administration of antenatal steroids given to infants younger than 34 weeks reduces the prevalence and severity of RDS, necrotizing enterocolitis, and intraventricular hemorrhage.[31]

B. Bronchopulmonary dysplasia (BPD)
BPD is characterized by the need for supplemental oxygen at 36 weeks postconceptional age for those infants born less than 32 weeks gestation. BPD, also termed *chronic lung disease,* ranges in severity from mild to severe. Infants diagnosed with mild BPD may have no oxygen requirement after 36 weeks; moderate is characterized by an oxygen need of less than 30%; and severe necessitates supplemental oxygen greater than 30%.[32,33]
1. Risk factors
The prevalence of BPD is highest in extremely low birth weight infants, secondary to the need for mechanical ventilation longer than the first week of life. The combination of fragile underdeveloped lungs, surfactant deficiency, and inflammation in the presence of mechanical ventilation creates acute lung injury.[34,35]
2. Assessment findings
Include tachypnea, mild to moderate retractions, and **rales**. Radiographic abnormalities may include diffuse haziness, hyperinflation, and bubbly lucencies.[36,37]
3. Medical management
This is aimed at decreasing oxygen toxicity and acute lung injury caused by mechanical ventilation; avoid using mechanical ventilation, utilizing CPAP if possible after delivery.
a) Supplemental oxygen: provides oxygen to the tissues and prevents the occurrence of pulmonary hypertension.
b) Frequent blood gas monitoring: prevents **hypoxia** and hypercarbia.
c) Surfactant administration: to prevent or minimize respiratory distress syndrome.
d) Chest x-rays: use to diagnose and follow changes.
e) Caffeine: decreases the occurrence of apnea, reducing time on mechanical ventilation. Decreases the risk of BPD and improves survivability with better neurodevelopmental

[30]Cloherty, J., Eichenwald, E., & Stark, A. (2012). *Manual of neonatal care.* 8th ed. Philadelphia: Lippincott Williams & Wilkins.
[31]Martin, R., Fanaroff, A., & Walsh, M. (2015). *Fanaroff & Martin's neonatal-perinatal medicine: Diseases of the fetus and infant.* 10th ed. Philadelphia: Elsevier Saunders.
[32]Cloherty, J., Eichenwald, E., & Stark, A. (2012). *Manual of neonatal care.* 8th ed. Philadelphia: Lippincott Williams & Wilkins.
[33]Gomella, T., Cunningham, D., & Eyal, F. (2013). *Neonatology: Management, on-call problems, diseases, and drugs.* 6th ed. New York, NY: McGraw Hill Education.
[34]Cloherty, J., Eichenwald, E., & Stark, A. (2012). *Manual of neonatal care.* 8th ed. Philadelphia: Lippincott Williams & Wilkins.
[35]Gomella, T., Cunningham, D., & Eyal, F. (2013). *Neonatology: Management, on-call problems, diseases, and drugs.* 6th ed. New York, NY: McGraw Hill Education.
[36]Cloherty, J., Eichenwald, E., & Stark, A. (2012). *Manual of neonatal care.* 8th ed. Philadelphia: Lippincott Williams & Wilkins.
[37]Gomella, T., Cunningham, D., & Eyal, F. (2013). *Neonatology: Management, on-call problems, diseases, and drugs.* 6th ed. New York, NY: McGraw Hill Education.

outcomes in infants less than 1,250 grams if given during the first 10 days of life.[38]

🛑 **ALERT** Caffeine may be given IV or PO. A loading dose of 20 to 25 mg/kg/dose is give initially; then 24 hours later a maintenance dose of 5 to 10 mg/kg per dose is given every 24 hours.[39]

   f) Diuretics: (Lasix and/or chlorothiazide) provide diuresis of retained fluid.
   g) Postnatal steroids: (controversial) decrease oxygen requirements and weaning of mechanical ventilation.
   h) Inhaled nitric oxide: (controversial) decreases pulmonary vascular resistance and improves oxygenation. It is administered in infants with persistent pulmonary hypertension (PPHN). Inhaled nitric oxide given to premature infants remains controversial; further clinical trials are needed to determine effectiveness.
   i) Fluid management: prevents fluid retention and pulmonary edema.[40,41]

DID YOU KNOW?

Infants experiencing **apnea of prematurity** are given caffeine citrate to reduce the incidence of apnea and BPD. A loading dose of 20 mg/kg is given initially, followed by a maintenance dose of 5 to 10 mg/kg every 24 hours. Caffeine may be given IV or PO.

   4. Nursing management
      a) Pulse oximetry—keep oxygen saturations in targeted range.
      b) Vital signs—watch for decomposition (tachypnea, apnea, bradycardia, tachycardia, hypotension, hypothermia, decrease in oxygen saturations) and increased oxygen requirements.
      c) Proper fluid administration and nutrition.
      d) Discharge planning and teaching parents and caregivers signs of deterioration, such as proper nutrition, hand washing, equipment usage, medication administration, smoke-free environment, and cardiopulmonary resuscitation.[42]

   5. Complications
      Complications include impaired growth, retinopathy of prematurity, neurodevelopmental impairment, sepsis, and reactive airway disease.[43,44]
C. Patent ductus arteriosus
   The ductus arteriosus provides a passage that blood can follow away from fetal lungs while in utero. During the transition to extrauterine life, the ductus should close within the first 96 hours of life.[45] A PDA remains open after birth, causing oxygenated blood to mix with unoxygenated blood.[46]
   1. Risk factors: Preterm infants are at higher risk for developing a PDA than full-term infants. The shorter the gestation, the higher the incidence of PDA.[47] Respiratory distress syndrome, sepsis, fluid overload, high altitude, congenital heart defects, and genetic syndromes all increase the prevalence of PDA.[48]

🛑 **ALERT** The prostaglandin synthetase inhibitor indomethacin may be administered to premature infants in the first weeks of life to facilitate ductal closure in the presence of a PDA.

   2. Assessment findings
      Infants with a PDA (left to right shunt) often have respiratory decompensation, tachypnea, rales, and apnea. They present with bounding peripheral pulses, an active precordium, heart murmur, widened pulse pressures, and hypotension. PDA can contribute to heart failure.
   3. Medical management
      The following may be ordered by the health care team:
      • Chest x-ray and echocardiogram to visualize blood flow
      • Mechanical ventilation due to respiratory distress may be started
      • Blood gas monitoring
      • Fluid restriction
      • Administration of indomethacin or ibuprofen in an effort to close a symptomatic duct
      • Surgery in infants who are hemodynamically unstable[49]

[38]Cloherty, J., Eichenwald, E., & Stark, A. (2012). *Manual of neonatal care.* 8th ed. Philadelphia: Lippincott Williams & Wilkins.

[39]NeoFax and Pediatrics. (2016). Retrieved from http://micromedex.com/neofax-pediatric.

[40]Cloherty, J., Eichenwald, E., & Stark, A. (2012). *Manual of neonatal care.* 8th ed. Philadelphia: Lippincott Williams & Wilkins.

[41]Gomella, T., Cunningham, D., & Eyal, F. (2013). *Neonatology: Management, on-call problems, diseases, and drugs.* 6th ed. New York, NY: McGraw Hill Education.

[42]Cloherty, J., Eichenwald, E., & Stark, A. (2012). *Manual of neonatal care.* 8th ed. Philadelphia: Lippincott Williams & Wilkins.

[43]Cloherty, J., Eichenwald, E., & Stark, A. (2012). *Manual of neonatal care.* 8th ed. Philadelphia: Lippincott Williams & Wilkins.

[44]Gomella, T., Cunningham, D., & Eyal, F. (2013). *Neonatology: Management, on-call problems, diseases, and drugs.* 6th ed. New York, NY: McGraw Hill Education.

[45]Gomella, T., Cunningham, D., & Eyal, F. (2013). *Neonatology: Management, on-call problems, diseases, and drugs.* 6th ed. New York, NY: McGraw Hill Education.

[46]Nagtalon-Ramos, J. (2014). *Best evidence-based practices: Maternal-newborn nursing care.* Philadelphia: F.A. Davis Company.

[47]Martin, R., Fanaroff, A., & Walsh, M. (2015). *Fanaroff & Martin's neonatal-perinatal medicine: Diseases of the fetus and infant.* 10th ed. Philadelphia: Elsevier Saunders.

[48]Gomella, T., Cunningham, D., & Eyal, F. (2013). *Neonatology: Management, on-call problems, diseases, and drugs.* 6th ed. New York, NY: McGraw Hill Education.

[49]Gomella, T., Cunningham, D., & Eyal, F. (2013). *Neonatology: Management, on-call problems, diseases, and drugs.* 6th ed. New York, NY: McGraw Hill Education.

4. Nursing management
   a) Monitor vital signs and respiratory status.
   b) Observe for physical signs of symptomatic PDA, such as heart murmur, bounding pulses, increased pulse pressure, respiratory distress, and hypotension. If untreated, the PDA can cause heart failure, pulmonary edema, and hepatomegaly.[50]
   c) Protect the airway, providing improved oxygenation; follow pulse oximetry to provide targeted oxygen saturations.
   d) Administer IV fluids, nutrition, and medication as ordered.
   e) Monitor strict intake and output.
   f) Support family, be a patient advocate.[51]
5. Complications
   - Respiratory distress and/or failure.
   - Congestive heart failure.
   - Shock/hypotension.
   - Hypoxemia.
   - Acid-base imbalance.[52]
   - Infants are also at risk for intracranial hemorrhage, retinopathy of prematurity, and necrotizing enterocolitis.[53]

DID YOU KNOW?

The subsequent administration of dexamethasone and indomethacin are contraindicated. If given together, the neonate is at increased risk for spontaneous perforation.

D. Periventricular/intraventricular hemorrhage
This happens when the fragile subependymal germinal matrix, a vascular area of the brain that exists during maturation, ruptures, causing blood to flow into the ventricular space. It contributes to ventriculomegaly and possible hydrocephalus. [54]
1. Risk factors
   a) Preterm infant
      - Ischemia and reperfusion
      - Alternations in cerebral blood flow
      - Platelet dysfunction and coagulopathy
   b) Trauma
   c) Perinatal asphyxia[55]

2. Assessment findings
   a) In some infants, intraventricular hemorrhage is undetected and only found on routine cranial ultrasound.
   b) Larger hemorrhage may present with spastic movement, hypotonia, atypical eye movement, and posturing.
   c) Preterm infants may have increased head circumference, lethargy, protuberant fontanelle, split sutures, abnormal eye movement, and decomposition in clinical status.
   d) Term infants may have apnea, lethargy, full fontanelles, and/or seizures.[56]
3. Medical management
   The following may be ordered by the health care team:
   a) Cranial ultrasounds should be performed on infants less than 32 weeks gestation. They may also be performed in infants with perinatal asphyxia, trauma, pneumothorax, or impaired neurological assessments. MRI may also be ordered.
   b) Maintenance of adequate electrolyte balance, acid-base status, and volume.
   c) Correction of anemia and/or thrombocytopenia.
   d) Maintain normal blood pressure and cerebral profusion (inotropes, hydrocortisone, and vasopressors may be indicated).
   e) Perform ventricular taps and/or surgery for shunt placement if indicated.[57]
4. Nursing management
   - Monitor vital signs.
   - Identify infants at risk.
   - Observe for decreased level of consciousness and impaired neurological exam (e.g., full fontanelle, abnormal eye movements, seizure-like activity).
   - Position to maintain an open neutral airway.
   - Monitor for signs of complications (e.g., hypotension, hypoglycemia, anemia, jaundice).
   - Provide support for the family.
   - Administer IV fluids as ordered (slowly in preterm infants).[58]
5. Complications
   Complications can include hydrocephalus and possible hemorrhagic venous infarction.[59] Infants are also at risk for cerebral palsy, poor neurodevelopmental outcomes, and **periventricular leukomalacia**.[60]

[50]Gomella, T., Cunningham, D., & Eyal, F. (2013). *Neonatology: Management, on-call problems, diseases, and drugs.* 6th ed. New York, NY: McGraw Hill Education.

[51]Nagtalon-Ramos, J. (2014). *Best evidence-based practices: Maternal-newborn nursing care.* Philadelphia: F.A. Davis Company.

[52]Gomella, T., Cunningham, D., & Eyal, F. (2013). *Neonatology: Management, on-call problems, diseases, and drugs.* 6th ed. New York, NY: McGraw Hill Education.

[53]Fanaroff, A., & Fanaroff, J. (2013). *Klaus & Fanaroff's care of the high-risk neonate.* Philadelphia: Elsevier Saunders.

[54]Fanaroff, A., & Fanaroff, J. (2013). *Klaus & Fanaroff's care of the high-risk neonate.* Philadelphia: Elsevier Saunders.

[55]Cloherty, J., Eichenwald, E., & Stark, A. (2012). *Manual of neonatal care.* 8th ed. Philadelphia: Lippincott Williams & Wilkins.

[56]Cloherty, J., Eichenwald, E., & Stark, A. (2012). *Manual of neonatal care.* 8th ed. Philadelphia: Lippincott Williams & Wilkins.

[57]Cloherty, J., Eichenwald, E., & Stark, A. (2012). *Manual of neonatal care.* 8th ed. Philadelphia: Lippincott Williams & Wilkins.

[58]Cloherty, J., Eichenwald, E., & Stark, A. (2012). *Manual of neonatal care.* 8th ed. Philadelphia: Lippincott Williams & Wilkins.

[59]Fanaroff, A., & Fanaroff, J. (2013). *Klaus & Fanaroff's care of the high-risk neonate.* Philadelphia: Elsevier Saunders.

[60]Cloherty, J., Eichenwald, E., & Stark, A. (2012). *Manual of neonatal care.* 8th ed. Philadelphia: Lippincott Williams & Wilkins.

E. Necrotizing enterocolitis (NEC)

NEC is a life-threatening gastrointestinal disease process with unknown etiology. NEC with bowel perforation is considered a surgical emergency in the neonate.[61] Diagnosis is made based on physical exam and radiographic studies showing **pneumatosis intestinalis**, portal venous gas, and/or bowel perforation.[62]

1. Risk factors
   - Prematurity
   - Enteral feeds
   - Sepsis
   - Ischemia/hypoxemia and reperfusion
   - Maternal drug abuse (e.g., cocaine)
   - Intrauterine growth restriction with impaired intrauterine end diastolic flow.[63,64,65]

2. Assessment findings

   Overall, the assessment will find clinical decompensation with respiratory distress, apnea, bradycardia, hypothermia, hypotension, acidosis, decreased urine output, feeding intolerance, increase of abdominal girth, distention, and bloody stools.[66,67]

3. Medical management

   The following may be ordered by the health care team:
   - Bowel rest for 7 to 14 days
   - Replogle placement (a tube placed in the stomach to drain fluid and vent air) to suction
   - Serial abdominal x-rays (every 6 hours)
   - Septic workup, including blood culture, CBC with differential, and CRP
   - Provide and maintain respiratory support as indicated
   - Antibiotics (ampicillin, gentamicin, clindamycin)
   - Parental nutrition
   - Follow electrolytes (basic metabolic profile)
   - Surgery; indicated for fixed loop, portal venous gas, and pneumoperitoneum.[68]

4. Nursing management
   - Continuously monitor vital signs and abdominal circumference.
   - Maintain thermoregulation.
   - Provide IV therapy and maintain nutritional status.
   - Promote breastfeeding and the use of pumped breast milk for first feedings or once feedings are restarted.
   - Introduce feeding slowly; use feeding protocols for premature infants.
   - Monitor for signs of feeding intolerance (e.g., vomiting, increased abdominal distention, bloody stools). If feeding intolerance is present, stop feeds and immediately notify the practitioner.
   - Strict intake and output.
   - Maintain a comfortable environment for the infant to promote healing and rest.
   - Support the family.[69]

5. Complications

   Complications include neurodevelopmental delay, strictures, and short bowel syndrome.[70]

DID YOU KNOW?

NEC is essentially diagnosed in premature infants after introduction of enteral feeds. However, 10% of NEC cases occur in term infants.

F. Retinopathy of prematurity

This disease process affects the developing vasculature in the retina of premature infants. Normal migration of retinal vessels is interrupted secondary to an insult (e.g., decreased blood pressure, over- or underoxygenation of the tissues), creating neovascularization.[71] Neovascularization can ultimately lead to fibrosis of the tissues, resulting in blindness.

1. Risk factors
   - Prematurity
   - Birth weight less than 1,500 grams (highest risk is less than 1,000 grams)
   - Length of mechanical ventilation
   - Intraventricular hemorrhage
   - Bronchopulmonary dysplasia
   - Numerous blood transfusions
   - Vitamin E deficiency
   - Infection[72]

2. Assessment findings

   The International Classification of Retinopathy of Prematurity has developed a staging system portraying the progressive disease:
   - Stage I: A line of demarcation evolves between the avascular zone and the vascularized region of the retina.
   - Stage II: The line of demarcation forms a protruding ridge into the vitreous.

[61]Fanaroff, A., & Fanaroff, J. (2013). *Klaus & Fanaroff's care of the high-risk neonate.* Philadelphia: Elsevier Saunders.

[62]Cloherty, J., Eichenwald, E., & Stark, A. (2012). *Manual of neonatal care.* 8th ed. Philadelphia: Lippincott Williams & Wilkins.

[63]Cloherty, J., Eichenwald, E., & Stark, A. (2012). *Manual of neonatal care.* 8th ed. Philadelphia: Lippincott Williams & Wilkins.

[64]Gomella, T., Cunningham, D., & Eyal, F. (2013). *Neonatology: Management, on-call problems, diseases, and drugs.* 6th ed. New York, NY: McGraw Hill Education.

[65]Fanaroff, A., & Fanaroff, J. (2013). *Klaus & Fanaroff's care of the high-risk neonate.* Philadelphia: Elsevier Saunders.

[66]Cloherty, J., Eichenwald, E., & Stark, A. (2012). *Manual of neonatal care.* 8th ed. Philadelphia: Lippincott Williams & Wilkins.

[67]Nagtalon-Ramos, J. (2014). *Best evidence-based practices: Maternal-newborn nursing care.* Philadelphia: F.A. Davis Company.

[68]Gomella, T., Cunningham, D., & Eyal, F. (2013). *Neonatology: Management, on-call problems, diseases, and drugs.* 6th ed. New York, NY: McGraw Hill Education.

[69]Nagtalon-Ramos, J. (2014). *Best evidence-based practices: Maternal-newborn nursing care.* Philadelphia: F.A. Davis Company.

[70]Gomella, T., Cunningham, D., & Eyal, F. (2013). *Neonatology: Management, on-call problems, diseases, and drugs.* 6th ed. New York, NY: McGraw Hill Education.

[71]Cloherty, J., Eichenwald, E., & Stark, A. (2012). *Manual of neonatal care.* 8th ed. Philadelphia: Lippincott Williams & Wilkins.

[72]Cloherty, J., Eichenwald, E., & Stark, A. (2012). *Manual of neonatal care.* 8th ed. Philadelphia: Lippincott Williams & Wilkins.

- Stage III: Fibrovascular proliferation occurs along the ridge.
- Stage IV: Fibrosis of the tissues occurs as the proliferation develops into the vitreous, possibly leading to partial detachment of the retina.
- Stage V: Retinal detachment occurs.
- Plus disease: Vessels behind the established ridge become tortuous.[73]

3. Medical management

An ophthalmoscopic examination establishes the diagnosis. At 4 to 6 weeks of age, infants who were born at less than 32 weeks gestation and/or who weighed less than 1,500 grams at birth should have an eye exam performed by a pediatric ophthalmologist with experience in retinopathy of prematurity (ROP). Other orders or therapies may include the following:
- Maintain oxygen tension between 50 and 80 mm Hg.[74]
- Cryotherapy to scar the peripheral retina.
- Laser photocoagulation to scar the peripheral retina.
- Retinal reattachment, scleral buckling, or vitrectomy.
- Follow-up eye exams based on the severity of the disease.[75]

4. Nursing management
- Titrate oxygen to keep saturations within the targeted range.
- Support and educate the family.

5. Complications
- Retinal detachment
- Blindness[76,77]

III. Postmature Neonates

Postmature neonates are infants born after 42 weeks gestation.

A. Risk factors

Risk factors include macrosomia and placental insufficiency.[78]

B. Assessment findings
- Dry, cracked, and/or peeling skin.
- Decreased or absent vernix

- Ample scalp hair
- Sparse or absent lanugo
- Thick formed cartilage of pinna
- Creases cover the entire sole of the foot[79]

C. Medical management
- C-section, in the case of fetal distress, cephalopelvic disproportion.
- Induction to stimulate labor and delivery; as the infant reaches postdates, the placenta does not work as efficiently.
- Supportive care.[80]

D. Nursing management
- Evaluate for birth trauma.
- Maintain thermoregulation.
- Perform Ballard score.
- Assess for problems secondary to placental insufficiency and transition to extrauterine life.
- Monitor and maintain blood sugar homeostasis.[81]

E. Complications
- **Transient tachypnea of the newborn**
- Meconium aspiration
- Perinatal depression
- Persistent pulmonary hypertension
- Hypoglycemia
- Polycythemia[82]

(!) **ALERT** Postmature infants are at increased risk for developing meconium aspiration.

IV. Meconium Aspiration Syndrome

Meconium is present in approximately 10% of all births. The presence of meconium at delivery suggests a possible hypoxic event in utero.[83] Meconium aspiration syndrome happens when the infant gasps for air and aspirates meconium into the lungs, creating blockage, pneumonitis, and atelectasis.[84]

A. Risk factors
- Asphyxia
- Stress
- Postdates[85,86]

[73]Gomella, T., Cunningham, D., & Eyal, F. (2013). *Neonatology: Management, on-call problems, diseases, and drugs.* 6th ed. New York, NY: McGraw Hill Education.

[74]Fanaroff, A., & Fanaroff, J. (2013). *Klaus & Fanaroff's care of the high-risk neonate.* Philadelphia: Elsevier Saunders.

[75]Gomella, T., Cunningham, D., & Eyal, F. (2013). *Neonatology: Management, on-call problems, diseases, and drugs.* 6th ed. New York, NY: McGraw Hill Education.

[76]Cloherty, J., Eichenwald, E., & Stark, A. (2012). *Manual of neonatal care.* 8th ed. Philadelphia: Lippincott Williams & Wilkins.

[77]Gomella, T., Cunningham, D., & Eyal, F. (2013). *Neonatology: Management, on-call problems, diseases, and drugs.* 6th ed. New York, NY: McGraw Hill Education.

[78]Martin, R., Fanaroff, A., & Walsh, M. (2015). *Fanaroff & Martin's neonatal-perinatal medicine: Diseases of the fetus and infant.* 10th ed. Philadelphia: Elsevier Saunders.

[79]Fanaroff, A., & Fanaroff, J. (2013). *Klaus & Fanaroff's care of the high-risk neonate.* Philadelphia: Elsevier Saunders.

[80]Nagtalon-Ramos, J. (2014). *Best evidence-based practices: Maternal-newborn nursing care.* Philadelphia: F.A. Davis Company.

[81]Nagtalon-Ramos, J. (2014). *Best evidence-based practices: Maternal-newborn nursing care.* Philadelphia: F.A. Davis Company.

[82]Cloherty, J., Eichenwald, E., & Stark, A. (2012). *Manual of neonatal care.* 8th ed. Philadelphia: Lippincott Williams & Wilkins.

[83]Fanaroff, A., & Fanaroff, J. (2013). *Klaus & Fanaroff's care of the high-risk neonate.* Philadelphia: Elsevier Saunders.

[84]Nagtalon-Ramos, J. (2014). *Best evidence-based practices: Maternal-newborn nursing care.* Philadelphia: F.A. Davis Company.

[85]Fanaroff, A., & Fanaroff, J. (2013). *Klaus & Fanaroff's care of the high-risk neonate.* Philadelphia: Elsevier Saunders.

[86]Nagtalon-Ramos, J. (2014). *Best evidence-based practices: Maternal-newborn nursing care.* Philadelphia: F.A. Davis Company.

B. Assessment findings
- Meconium-stained cord, skin, and nails
- Visualization of meconium below the vocal cords with laryngoscopy
- Yellow, green, or brown amniotic fluid
- Respiratory acidosis and/or failure
- Tachypnea, rales, rhonchi, and/or wheezing
- Chest x-ray consistent with patchy infiltrates, hyperexpansion of the lungs, pulmonary interstitial emphysema, and/or pneumothorax[87,88]

C. Medical management
The following may be ordered by the health care team:
- At delivery, follow the most current Neonatal Resuscitation Program (NRP) guidelines. If the infant is vigorous, suction the mouth and nose with a bulb syringe. If the infant is not vigorous, intubate and suction meconium from below the cords. Provide positive-pressure ventilation as needed.
- Provide oxygen therapy and assisted ventilation, and nitric oxide if indicated.
- Surfactant therapy.
- Perform a septic workup and start antibiotics until cultures are negative.
- Provide volume expansion and vasopressors to correct hypotension.[89,90,91]

D. Nursing management
1. Assess for the following:
   - Meconium-stained fluid.
   - Whether the infant is vigorous or nonvigorous at delivery. A vigorous infant with meconium-stained fluid will be treated much differently than a nonvigorous infant. Always follow NRP guidelines.
   - Respiratory status: Are breath sounds present bilaterally, clear, or are rales and rhonchi present? Is there tachypnea? Apnea? Grunting? Retractions? These are indications that the infant may be experiencing hypoxia.
   - Vital signs: Heart rate can increase (tachycardia) as the infant attempts to compensate for hypoxia or decrease (bradycardia) as the infant decompensates. Blood pressure can decrease (hypotension) and poor perfusion can occur as shock sets in.[92,93]

2. Interventions
   - Maintain a patent airway.
   - Administer oxygen as indicated.
   - Follow blood gases to determine respiratory and/or metabolic acidosis, hyper- or hypoxia, hyper- or hypocapnia.
   - Chest x-ray to determine lung pathophysiology. Looking for atelectasis, pulmonary interstitial emphysema, air leaks, patchy infiltrates.
   - Provide antibiotics to decrease risk of infection from meconium aspiration and pneumonitis.
   - Maintain a neutral thermal environment.
   - Bundle hands-on care to minimize stress.
   - Minimize ventilator pressures to prevent airway trauma and air-leak syndrome.
   - Provide support and education to the family.[94,95]

DID YOU KNOW?
Meconium aspiration causes a chemical pneumonitis. At the alveolar level, surfactant may be inactivated. Therefore, infants with meconium aspiration syndrome may be treated with surfactant to help prevent respiratory failure.

V. Persistent Pulmonary Hypertension of the Newborn (PPHN)

PPHN is characterized by an interruption in an infant's ordinary adaption from fetal circulation to that of a neonatal circulation.[96] Physiologically, the pulmonary vascular resistance and pulmonary arterial pressures remain elevated postbirth, thus leading to an abnormally persistent right-to-left shunting at the atrial or ductal levels. The resultant of PPHN is an overall decrease in pulmonary perfusion leading to intrinsic hypoxemia.[97,98,99]

A. Risk factors
1. Term or post-term deliveries (most common finding), late preterm and intrauterine growth restrictive infants
   a) Maladaptation: normal pulmonary development but pulmonary resistance remains elevated[100]
      - Asphyxia: prolonged delivery stress, causing pulmonary vasospasm

[87]Fanaroff, A., & Fanaroff, J. (2013). *Klaus & Fanaroff's care of the high-risk neonate*. Philadelphia: Elsevier Saunders.
[88]Nagtalon-Ramos, J. (2014). *Best evidence-based practices: Maternal-newborn nursing care*. Philadelphia: F.A. Davis Company.
[89]Fanaroff, A., & Fanaroff, J. (2013). *Klaus & Fanaroff's care of the high-risk neonate*. Philadelphia: Elsevier Saunders.
[90]Gomella, T., Cunningham, D., & Eyal, F. (2013). *Neonatology: Management, on-call problems, diseases, and drugs*. 6th ed. New York, NY: McGraw Hill Education.
[91]Nagtalon-Ramos, J. (2014). *Best evidence-based practices: Maternal-newborn nursing care*. Philadelphia: F.A. Davis Company.
[92]Fanaroff, A., & Fanaroff, J. (2013). *Klaus & Fanaroff's care of the high-risk neonate*. Philadelphia: Elsevier Saunders.
[93]Nagtalon-Ramos, J. (2014). *Best evidence-based practices: Maternal-newborn nursing care*. Philadelphia: F.A. Davis Company.

[94]Fanaroff, A., & Fanaroff, J. (2013). *Klaus & Fanaroff's care of the high-risk neonate*. Philadelphia: Elsevier Saunders.
[95]Nagtalon-Ramos, J. (2014). *Best evidence-based practices: Maternal-newborn nursing care*. Philadelphia: F.A. Davis Company.
[96]Verklan, M., & Walden, M. (2010). *Core curriculum for neonatal intensive care nursing*. 5th ed. St. Louis, MO: Elsevier Saunders.
[97]Cloherty, J., Eichenwald, E., & Stark, A. (2012). *Manual of neonatal care*. 8th ed. Philadelphia: Lippincott Williams & Wilkins.
[98]Gomella, T., Cunningham, D., & Eyal, F. (2013). *Neonatology: Management, on-call problems, diseases, and drugs*. 6th ed. New York, NY: McGraw Hill Education.
[99]Martin, R., Fanaroff, A., & Walsh, M. (2015). *Fanaroff & Martin's neonatal-perinatal medicine: Diseases of the fetus and infant*. 10th ed. Philadelphia: Elsevier Saunders.
[100]Verklan, M., & Walden, M. (2010). *Core curriculum for neonatal intensive care nursing*. 5th ed. St. Louis, MO: Elsevier Saunders.

- Pulmonary parenchymal disease processes: respiratory disease syndrome, meconium aspiration, pneumonia, causing pulmonary vasospasm and remodeling of pulmonary vasculature
- Sepsis: overabundant toxin release causing pulmonary vasospasm
- Postdelivery resuscitation/hypoxia
- Premature closure of ductus arteriosus: caused by maternal use of aspirin, phenytoin, lithium, indomethacin, SSRIs
- Hypothermia, hypoglycemia postbirth: causes increased acidosis leading to pulmonary vasoconstriction
- Hyperviscosity
  b) Maldevelopment: abnormal development of pulmonary structures and vasculature[101]
  - Intrauterine asphyxia: prolonged intrauterine stress causing pulmonary structure remodeling
  - Fetal closure of ductus arteriosus: abnormal intrauterine blood flow to pulmonary system
  - Congenital myocardial dysfunction or heart disease: abnormal pulmonary vessels
  - Genetic predisposition (questionable)
  c) Underdevelopment: abnormal development of lung tissue and pulmonary vessels present, causing blood to be diverted away from the pulmonary system[102]
  - Pulmonary hypoplasia
  - Diaphragmatic hernia
  - Cystic adenomatoid malformation
  - Pulmonary or tricuspid atresia

B. Assessment findings
- Presents in first 24 hours with persistent and intractable severe cyanosis.
- Respiratory distress: tachypnea, Pao_2 less than 50 mm Hg (despite high levels of O_2 delivery), labile oxygenation, differentiation in preductal saturations greater than postductal saturations, especially with handling (greater than 10% difference suggests PPHN if there is no cardiac disease process).
- Presence of loud audible systolic murmur, single second heart sound, active pericardium, rarely hepatomegaly.
- Chest x-ray reveals normal to decreased pulmonary markings unless aspiration or pneumonia is present (then infiltrates will be present); normal to increased heart silhouette.

- Thrombocytopenia (60% of cases unknown etiology).
- Echocardiogram study (evaluation of pulmonary vascular resistance, hemodynamic shunting, congenital anomalies, function, and structure).[103,104,105]

C. Medical management

Management is aimed at correcting the severe hypoxia, hypoxemia, and acidotic state the infant is currently in, as well as improving pulmonary vasculature dilation, allowing for an increase in pulmonary and systemic perfusion. Management will be based mostly on the etiology of the disease state.[106] The following may be ordered by the health care team:
- Supplementation of oxygen (most potent pulmonary vasodilator)
- Monitor preductal and postductal oxygen saturations
- Maintain postductal oxygen saturations greater than 95%
- Arterial blood gas (ABG) to maintain Pao_2 greater than 80 mm Hg (allow pulmonary vasodilation)
- Arterial access via umbilical/peripheral arterial line
- Obtain echocardiogram to rule out cardiac defects

1. Ventilation
- Intubation (provide best route for oxygenation)
- Chest x-rays (assess underlying issues)
- Treat any underlying lung disease
- Conventional mechanical or high-frequency ventilation (whichever mode allows for the best oxygenation and correction of acidosis)
- Hyperoxygenation (allow for vasodilation affect)—ABG to maintain Pao_2 greater than 80 mm Hg
- Mild hyperventilation—maintain $Paco_2$ 35 to 45 mm Hg (reduction in acidosis)
- Surfactant administration (may aid in decreasing pulmonary vascular resistance and assisting with surfactant deficiencies)
- Inhaled nitric oxide (iNO) (selective pulmonary vasodilator)
  - Start after 35 weeks gestational age on 20 ppm (lack of evidence to start and increased risk of methemoglobinemia at higher dosing)
  - ABG 30 to 60 minutes after initiation of iNO (Pao_2 should increase substantially after initiation)
  - Monitor methemoglobin level every 12 hours (to prevent toxicity)

[101]Verklan, M., & Walden, M. (2010). *Core curriculum for neonatal intensive care nursing.* 5th ed. St. Louis, MO: Elsevier Saunders.
[102]Verklan, M., & Walden, M. (2010). *Core curriculum for neonatal intensive care nursing.* 5th ed. St. Louis, MO: Elsevier Saunders.
[103]Cloherty, J., Eichenwald, E., & Stark, A. (2012). *Manual of neonatal care.* 8th ed. Philadelphia: Lippincott Williams & Wilkins.
[104]Gomella, T., Cunningham, D., & Eyal, F. (2013). *Neonatology: Management, on-call problems, diseases, and drugs.* 6th ed. New York, NY: McGraw Hill Education.
[105]Martin, R., Fanaroff, A., & Walsh, M. (2015). *Fanaroff & Martin's neonatal-perinatal medicine: Diseases of the fetus and infant.* 10th ed. Philadelphia: Elsevier Saunders.
[106]Cloherty, J., Eichenwald, E., & Stark, A. (2012). *Manual of neonatal care.* 8th ed. Philadelphia: Lippincott Williams & Wilkins.

2. Pharmacological support
   a) Sedation/analgesia (blocks stress response of infants)
      - Use of fentanyl, morphine, versed as needed (to maintain comfort and lower pain, thus allowing for decreased pulmonary vascular resistance [PVR])
      - Muscle relaxants/paralytics
        - Pancuronium or vecuronium prevents asynchronization of ventilation efforts and allows for muscle relaxation but it remains controversial.
3. Hemodynamic support
   - Volume expansion: normal saline or packed red blood cells (assists with stabilizing intravascular volume)
   - Vasopressors: dopamine, dobutamine, epinephrine, and milrinone (optimizes systemic blood pressure and cardiac output, thereby decreasing PVR and shunting)
4. Antibiotic therapy
   - Broad-spectrum antibiotics: ampicillin and gentamicin (possible sepsis association). Monitor CBC, CRP, blood cultures every 12 hours
5. Alkalotic therapy (reduction of acidosis)
   - Ventilation
   - Sodium bicarbonate
6. Nutritional support
   - Maintain adequate hydration via umbilical, central, or peripheral access
   - Provide excellent nutrition with hyperalimentation and intralipids
   - Maintain NPO status
   - Provide bowel decompression as needed

D. Nursing management
- Monitor vital signs, especially blood pressure, preductal and postductal saturations, and respiratory status
- Stabilize temperature
- Protect the airway, providing improved oxygenation; follow pulse oximetry to provide targeted oxygen saturations, suction as necessary
- Maintain sedation level
- Minimal handling, decrease noise, dim lighting
- Administer IV fluids and medication as ordered
- Monitor strict intake and output
- Support family; be a patient advocate

E. Complications
- Air leak (pneumothorax, pneumomediastinum)
- Persistent pulmonary hypertension

DID YOU KNOW?

Inhaled nitric oxide is used to treat pulmonary hypertension in infants. It causes vasodilation of the pulmonary vasculature.

VI. Small for Gestational Age and Intrauterine Growth Retardation

A. Small for gestational age (SGA)
SGA is defined as a fetus whose birth weight is less than the 10th percentile of infants born.[107,108,109]
1. Risk factors
   - Maternal genetic size
   - African American race
   - Postmaturity gestational age
   - High altitude
   - Inadequate maternal nutrition
   - Smoking
   - Drugs
   - Alcohol, amphetamines, corticosteroids, heroin, methadone, propanol, warfarin
   - Hypertension
   - Maternal diseases
     - Heart disease
     - Cystic fibrosis, asthma
     - Sickle cell
     - Lupus
     - Diabetes
     - Hyperthyroidism
       a) Multiple gestation
          - Placenta previa, abruption, abnormal cord insertion
          - Infection
          - Genetic anomalies
          - Skeletal anomalies
          - Cardiac anomalies
       b) Assessment findings
          - Reduced birth weight
          - Head proportional to rest of body size
          - Shrunken facial and abdominal appearance
          - Loose and dry skin
          - Decreased vernix
          - Overriding suture
          - Thin umbilical cord
          - Syndromic features (possible)
          - Heart murmurs and/or abnormal cardiac silhouette (possible)
2. Medical management
   Determine the underlying cause and treat accordingly.

[107]Cloherty, J., Eichenwald, E., & Stark, A. (2012). *Manual of neonatal care.* 8th ed. Philadelphia: Lippincott Williams & Wilkins.
[108]Gomella, T., Cunningham, D., & Eyal, F. (2013). *Neonatology: Management, on-call problems, diseases, and drugs.* 6th ed. New York, NY: McGraw Hill Education.
[109]Martin, R., Fanaroff, A., & Walsh, M. (2015). *Fanaroff & Martin's neonatal-perinatal medicine: Diseases of the fetus and infant.* 10th ed. Philadelphia: Elsevier Saunders.

3. Nursing management
   - Monitor vital signs
   - Perform a thorough physical examination
   - Stabilize temperature; prevent heat loss
   - Monitor strict intake and output
   - Support family; be a patient advocate
   - Plot growth curve with weight, head circumference, and length
   - Monitor glucose levels
   - Monitor respiratory distress, apnea
   - Monitor for murmurs, arrhythmias, pulses, and perfusion
   - Obtain laboratory work as ordered by the medical team
4. Complications
   - Perinatal asphyxia
   - Persistent pulmonary hypertension
   - Respiratory distress syndrome
   - Bronchopulmonary dysplasia
   - Patent ductus arteriosus
   - Hypoglycemia
   - Hypocalcemia
   - Hypothermia
   - Polycythemia
   - NEC
   - Cerebral palsy
   - Developmental delay[110,111]

B. Symmetric intrauterine growth restriction (IUGR)
Symmetric IUGR happens when an infant fails to gain the optimal growth while in utero. The symmetrical component of IUGR refers to the fact that the measurements of the head circumference, length, and weight are proportionally smaller for the gestational age.[112]
   1. Risk factors
      a) Chromosomal abnormalities
         - Gene defects
         - Short- and long-arm deletions
         - Trisomies 13, 18, 21
         - Silver-Russell syndrome
         - Skeletal abnormalities
           - Achondroplasia
           - Leprechaunism
      b) Congenital malformations
         - Anencephaly
         - Gastrointestinal atresia
         - Potter syndrome
         - Pancreatic agenesis

c) Cardiac anomalies
d) Congenital infections
   - TORCH: toxoplasmosis, rubella, cytomegalovirus, herpes simplex virus
e) Inborn errors of metabolism
   - Transient neonatal diabetes
   - Galactosemia
   - Phenylketonuria
2. Assessment findings
   - Reduced birth weight head circumference, and length
   - Head proportional to rest of body size
   - Shrunken facial and abdominal appearance
   - Loose and dry skin
   - Decreased vernix
   - Overriding suture
   - Thin umbilical cord
   - Syndromic features
   - Rashes or lesions
   - Abnormal CBC—low platelets, neutropenia, polycythemia, newborn state screen
   - Heart murmurs and/or abnormal cardiac silhouette
   - Enlarged liver or spleen
   - Short limbs
   - Hypoglycemia
   - Feeding intolerance with emesis
   - Lethargy, irritability
3. Medical management
   - Monitor vital signs
   - Perform a thorough physical examination
   - Stabilize temperature, prevent heat loss
   - Administer IV fluids and medication as ordered
   - Monitor strict intake and output
   - Support family; be a patient advocate
   - Plot growth curve with weight, head circumference, and length
   - Monitor glucose levels
   - Monitor respiratory distress, apnea
   - Monitor for murmurs, arrhythmias, pulses, and perfusion
   - Obtain laboratory work
   - Screening for abnormal skin lesions or rashes
   - Consideration of contact isolation (limit pregnant workers' viral exposure)
   - Assess feeding tolerance
   - Screen bacterial and viral infections
     - TORCH panel, titers
     - Blood, urine, cerebral spinal fluid cultures
     - Viral cultures—toxoplasmosis IgG, IgM; herpes polymerase chain reaction (PCR) and cytomegalovirus urine
   - Chest x-ray to assess lung disease, pulmonary hemorrhage, meconium aspiration, heart silhouette

110Gomella, T., Cunningham, D., & Eyal, F. (2013). *Neonatology: Management, on-call problems, diseases, and drugs.* 6th ed. New York, NY: McGraw Hill Education.
111Martin, R., Fanaroff, A., & Walsh, M. (2015). *Fanaroff & Martin's neonatal-perinatal medicine: Diseases of the fetus and infant.* 10th ed. Philadelphia: Elsevier Saunders.
112Cloherty, J., Eichenwald, E., & Stark, A. (2012). *Manual of neonatal care.* 8th ed. Philadelphia: Lippincott Williams & Wilkins.

- Echocardiogram, EKG, screening for cardiac anomalies and/or PPHN
- Abdominal x-ray to assess abnormal bowel gas pattern, perforation, malrotation, atresia
- Renal ultrasound to assess for renal anomalies
- Cranial ultrasound, MRI, CT scan
  - Intraventricular hemorrhage
  - Periventricular leukomalacia
  - Calcifications
    a) Laboratory work
      - CBC—low platelets, polycythemia, shift in differential count
      - Electrolytes, renal panels, and liver panels
      - Newborn screen
      - Infection screenings—blood, urine, cerebrospinal fluid (CSF) cultures, viral panels, TORCH panel
      - DNA microarray, karyotypes
    b) Nutrition
      (1) Need for increased caloric intake
        - Customized hyperalimentation with intralipids
        - Higher caloric formula or additives for breast milk
        - Medium-chain triglycerides
      (2) Increased dextrose requirements
        - Management of hypoglycemia
        - Increased dextrose level for increased caloric requirements
      (3) Increased electrolyte imbalances
        - Additives of sodium, potassium, calcium
      (4) Increased fluid volumes
        - Combat polycythemia
      (5) Consultations
        - Genetics
        - Orthopedics
        - Endocrinology
        - Cardiology
        - Gastroenterology
        - Neurology
        - Infectious disease department
4. Nursing management
   - Monitor vital signs
   - Perform a thorough physical examination
   - Stabilize temperature, prevent heat loss
   - Administer IV fluids and medication as ordered
   - Monitor strict intake and output
   - Support family; be a patient advocate
   - Plot growth curve with weight, head circumference, and length
   - Monitor glucose levels
   - Monitor respiratory distress, apnea
   - Monitor for murmurs, arrhythmias, pulses, and perfusion
   - Obtain laboratories as ordered
   - Screen for abnormal skin lesions or rashes
   - Consideration of contact isolation (limit pregnant workers' viral exposure)
   - Assess feeding tolerance
5. Complications
   - Prematurity
   - Perinatal asphyxia
   - Pulmonary hypertension
   - Bronchopulmonary dysplasia
   - Necrotizing enterocolitis
   - Retinopathy of prematurity
   - Cholestasis
   - Polycythemia
   - Cerebral palsy
   - Developmental delay[113]

C. Asymmetric intrauterine growth restrictions
Asymmetric IUGR typically results only in a reduction of the infant's weight but spares head circumference and length growth. This is a wasting effect or malnutrition state of the infant prior to birth.[114]
1. Risk factors
   a) Uteroplacental insufficiency
      - Pre-eclampsia
      - Abruptio placenta
      - Placenta previa
      - Inadequate cord insertion
      - Umbilical vascular thrombosis
      - Umbilical infarction
      - Placental mosaicism
      - Two-vessel cord
   b) Maternal factors
      - Hypertension (chronic and pregnancy-induced)
      - Renal disease
      - Diabetes mellitus
      - Hemoglobinopathies (sickle cell)
      - Lupus
      - Drugs and alcohol
        - Heavy smoking
        - Heroin use
        - Cocaine use
      - High altitude
      - Multiple pregnancies
      - Maternal malnutrition
      - Poor weight gain by mother
2. Assessment findings
   - Reduced birth weight body-wasting appearance
   - Large head in comparison to body

[113]Martin, R., Fanaroff, A., & Walsh, M. (2015). *Fanaroff & Martin's neonatal-perinatal medicine: Diseases of the fetus and infant.* 10th ed. Philadelphia: Elsevier Saunders.
[114]Cloherty, J., Eichenwald, E., & Stark, A. (2012). *Manual of neonatal care.* 8th ed. Philadelphia: Lippincott Williams & Wilkins.

- Shrunken facial and abdominal appearance
- Loose and dry skin
- Widened suture
- Thin and/or two-vessel umbilical cord
- Hypovolemic shock symptoms—hypotension, pallor, weakened pulses, decreased perfusion, increased heart rate
- Abnormal CBC—decrease platelet count
- Heart murmurs and/or abnormal cardiac silhouette, arrhythmias
- Extreme irritability, withdrawal symptoms, poor oral intake, excessive sucking, emesis, excoriation of buttocks, watery stools, abrasions to face and extremities, inconsolable screaming, tremors, jitteriness

3. Medical management
    - Resuscitation in delivery room—increased asphyxia, fetal distress
    - Respiratory support as indicated—chest x-ray to assess lung disease
    - Assess cardiac system—echocardiogram, EKG, screening for cardiac anomalies and/or PPHN
        a) Cranial ultrasound, MRI, CT scan
            - Intraventricular hemorrhage
            - Periventricular leukomalacia
            - Calcifications
        b) Laboratory work
            - CBC—low platelets, polycythemia, shift in differential count
            - Electrolytes, renal panels, and liver panels
            - Newborn screen
        c) Renal ultrasound for two-vessel cord
        d) Nutrition
            (1) Need for increased caloric intake
                - Customized hyperalimentation with intralipids
                - Higher caloric formula or additives for breast milk
                - Medium-chain triglycerides
            (2) Increased dextrose requirements
                - Management of hypoglycemia
                - Increased dextrose level for increased caloric requirements
            (3) Increased electrolyte imbalances
                - Additives of sodium, potassium, calcium
            (4) Increased fluid volumes
                - Combat polycythemia
        e) Screening for neonatal abstinence withdrawal syndrome
            - Drug screening
            - Medications for withdrawal—opioids, benzodiazepines

4. Nursing management
    - Monitor vital signs
    - Perform a thorough physical examination
    - Stabilize temperature, prevent heat loss
    - Administer IV fluids and medication as ordered
    - Monitor strict intake and output
    - Support family; be a patient advocate
    - Plot growth curve with weight, head circumference, and length
    - Monitor glucose levels
    - Monitor respiratory distress, apnea
    - Monitor for murmurs, arrhythmias, pulses, and perfusion
    - Obtain laboratory work as ordered by the medical team
    - Screen for abnormal skin lesions or rashes
    - Consideration of contact isolation (limit pregnant workers' viral exposure)
    - Assess feeding tolerance

5. Complications
    - Perinatal asphyxia
    - Persistent pulmonary hypertension
    - Respiratory distress syndrome
    - Bronchopulmonary dysplasia
    - Patent ductus arteriosus
    - Hypoglycemia
    - Hypocalcemia
    - Hypothermia
    - NEC
    - Cerebral palsy
    - Developmental delay[115]

VII. Large for Gestational Age

This is defined as a birth weight greater than the 90th percentile (Fig. 22.1).

A. Risk factors
- Maternal genetic size
- Postdelivery gestational age
- Infant of a diabetic mother
- Congenital syndromes/Beckwith–Wiedemann syndrome
- Hydrops fetalis
- Increased risk at delivery
- Difficulty births

B. Assessment findings
- Macrosomia
- Hairy ears
- Jitteriness
- Hypoglycemia
- Irritability
- Cyanosis
- Cardiac anomalies
- Polycythemia

[115]Martin, R., Fanaroff, A., & Walsh, M. (2015). *Fanaroff & Martin's neonatal-perinatal medicine: Diseases of the fetus and infant.* 10th ed. Philadelphia: Elsevier Saunders.

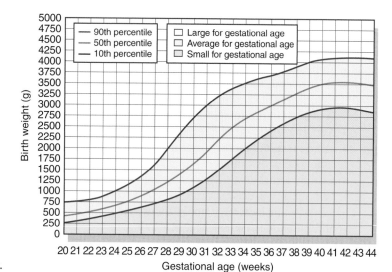

Fig 22.1 Gestational age measurement chart.

- Poor feeding or intolerance
- Respiratory distress
- Increased birth injuries
  - Brachial plexus injuries
  - Fractures of clavicles, arms
- Subdural, subgaleal cranial bleeds
- Jaundice

C. Medical management
- Resuscitation in delivery room—increased asphyxia, fetal distress
- Respiratory support as indicated
  - Chest x-ray to assess lung disease
  - Provide ventilation support as necessary
- Assess cardiac system
- Echocardiogram, EKG, screening for cardiac anomalies and/or PPHN
- Cranial ultrasound, MRI, CT scan
  - Intraventricular, subdural, subgaleal, hemorrhage
  1. Laboratory work
     - CBC—polycythemia
     - Electrolytes, cortisol, insulin, growth hormone factors, and glucose levels
  2. Nutrition
     - Need for increased caloric intake
       - Customized hyperalimentation with intralipids
       - Higher caloric formula or additives for breast milk
     - Increased dextrose requirements
       - Management of hypoglycemia
       - Increased dextrose level for increased caloric requirements
       - Insertion of central line for delivery of high dextrose
     - Increased electrolyte imbalances
       - Additives of sodium, potassium, calcium

- Increased fluid volumes
  - Assess for polycythemia

D. Nursing management
- Monitor vital signs
- Perform a thorough physical examination
- Administer IV fluids and medication as ordered
- Monitor strict intake and output
- Support family; be a patient advocate
- Plot growth curve with weight, head circumference, and length
- Monitor glucose levels, assess feeding intolerance
- Monitor respiratory distress, apnea
- Monitor for murmurs, arrhythmias, pulses, and perfusion
- Obtain laboratory work

E. Complications
- Birth trauma (brachial plexus injury)
- Perinatal depression
- Transient tachypnea of the newborn
- Hypoglycemia
- Polycythemia
- Beckwith–Wiedemann syndrome[116]

VIII. Hyperbilirubinemia

A. Physiological jaundice
This occurs when an infant's bilirubin level is elevated in the blood. Most infants are born with some elevation of bilirubin, and it is most noticeable at 2 to 5 days of life. Bilirubin is the by-product of the breaking down of old and dying red blood cells. This bilirubin is responsible for the yellow coloring of the skin due to

[116]Cloherty, J., Eichenwald, E., & Stark, A. (2012). *Manual of neonatal care.* 8th ed. Philadelphia: Lippincott Williams & Wilkins.

the immaturity of the liver. The liver is naturally able to convert and break down the excess bilirubin and get this by-product into stool so that it can be expelled. Most of the time it does not cause issues and dissipates from the body within the first 2 weeks of life.[117,118,119]

1. Risk factors
   - Family history of jaundice, liver disease.
   - Ethnicity—Asians, Greeks, American Indians.
   - Maternal illness—infection, diabetes, G6PD.
   - Delivery trauma—breech, vacuum extraction, forceps, asphyxia.
   - Cord-clamping delay.
   - Slow stooling pattern—since bilirubin is excreted in the stool, if the infant is not stooling well, the bilirubin will not be excreted effectively.
   - Sepsis.
   - Breastfeeding.
   - Prematurity.
2. Assessment findings
   - Yellow skin coloring—cephalocaudal progression
   - Hypotonia, lethargy
   - Poor feeding
   - Poor suck
   - High-pitched cry
   - Fever
   - Seizures
3. Medical management
   a) Laboratory work
      - Mother and infant blood type
      - Direct Coombs test
      - Total and direct bilirubin
      - RBC morphology
      - CBC
      - Reticulocyte count
      - G6PD
      - Liver panel
      - CRP
      - Blood culture
      - Thyroid test
      - Metabolic panels
      - Phototherapy
   b) Exchange transfusion
   c) Pharmacology
      - Phenobarbital
      - Intravenous immunoglobulin (IVIG)
   d) Nutrition
      - Encourage feeding frequently
      - Additional IV fluids—increase total fluids

4. Nursing management
   - Monitor vital signs.
   - Perform a thorough physical examination.
   - Administer IV fluids and medication as ordered. Ensure patency of IV site.
   - Monitor strict intake and output.
   - Support family; be a patient advocate.
   - Monitor glucose levels, assess feeding intolerance, encourage frequent feedings, supplement after breastfeedings.
   - Monitor respiratory distress, apnea.
   - Obtain laboratory work.
5. Complications
   - Kernicterus
   - Acute/chronic bilirubin encephalopathy

B. Pathological jaundice
This occurs when an infant's bilirubin level is high and remains elevated in the blood due to serious illness or the body's inability to rid itself of the by-product.[120,121,122]

1. Risk factors
   - ABO/Rh incompatibles
   - Bacterial and viral sepsis, TORCH
   - Inherited disorders of red cells—spherocytosis, elliptocytosis, G6PD
   - Immune or nonimmune hemolytic anemia
   - Continued polycythemia
   - Inherited disorders of bilirubin
     - Crigler-Najjar syndrome—autosomal recessive, affects metabolism of bilirubin, can lead to brain damage
     - Gilbert disease—constitutional hepatic dysfunction
   - Extravasation—cephalohematoma; pulmonary, cerebral, or retroperitoneal hemorrhage
   - Delayed feeding, intestinal obstructions
   - Decreased hepatic function—hypoxia, asphyxia, sepsis
   - Inborn errors of metabolism—galactosemia, tyrosinosis, antitrypsin deficiency
2. Assessment findings
   - Lethargy
   - Hypotonia
   - Tremors
   - Poor suck, no feeding
   - High-pitched cry
   - Irritability

[117]Cloherty, J., Eichenwald, E., & Stark, A. (2012). *Manual of neonatal care.* 8th ed. Philadelphia: Lippincott Williams & Wilkins.
[118]Gomella, T., Cunningham, D., & Eyal, F. (2013). *Neonatology: Management, on-call problems, diseases, and drugs.* 6th ed. New York, NY: McGraw Hill Education.
[119]Martin, R., Fanaroff, A., & Walsh, M. (2015). *Fanaroff & Martin's neonatal-perinatal medicine: Diseases of the fetus and infant.* 10th ed. Philadelphia: Elsevier Saunders.

[120]Cloherty, J., Eichenwald, E., & Stark, A. (2012). *Manual of neonatal care.* 8th ed. Philadelphia: Lippincott Williams & Wilkins.
[121]Gomella, T., Cunningham, D., & Eyal, F. (2013). *Neonatology: Management, on-call problems, diseases, and drugs.* 6th ed. New York, NY: McGraw Hill Education.
[122]Martin, R., Fanaroff, A., & Walsh, M. (2015). *Fanaroff & Martin's neonatal-perinatal medicine: Diseases of the fetus and infant.* 10th ed. Philadelphia: Elsevier Saunders.

- Hypertonia
- Fever
- Arching neck and back
- Severe yellow/green/bronze coloring to skin
- Petechiae
- Loose stools
- Dehydration
- Abdominal distention
- Thrombocytopenia

3. Medical management
   The following may be ordered by the health care team:
   a) Laboratory work
      - Mother and infant blood type
      - Direct Coombs test
      - Total and direct bilirubin
      - RBC morphology
      - CBC
      - Reticulocyte count
      - G6PD
      - Liver panel
      - CRP
      - Blood culture
      - Thyroid test
      - Metabolic panels
   b) Phototherapy
   c) Exchange transfusion—removing old RBC and replacing with fresh RBC through transfusion
   d) Pharmacology
      - Phenobarbital
      - IVIG
   e) Nutrition
      - Encourage feeding frequently
      - Additional IV fluids—increase total fluids
      - Insertion of central line
   f) Support breathing as needed

4. Nursing management
   - Monitor vital signs.
   - Perform a thorough physical examination.
   - Administer IV fluids and medication as ordered. Ensure patency of IV site.
   - Monitor strict intake and output.
   - Support family; be a patient advocate.
   - Monitor glucose levels, assess feeding intolerance, encourage frequent feeding schedules, supplement after breastfeedings.
   - Monitor respiratory distress, apnea.
   - Obtain laboratory work as ordered by the medical team.
   - Prep for central line placement for medication administration and exchange possibilities.[123,124]

5. Complications
   - Kernicterus
   - Acute/chronic bilirubin encephalopathy

IX. Central Nervous System Injuries

These injuries are usually the result of the birth process and can range from hemorrhages and nerve damage to the extreme case of encephalopathy.[125,126,127]

A. Risk factors
   - Shortened or prolonged labor
   - Large-sized infants
   - Disproportional size of birthing canal to size of infant
   - Prematurity
   - Malpositioned infant during birth (breech, transverse, facial)
   - Instrument-assisted birth (vacuum or forceps extraction)

B. Assessment findings
   1. Cephalohematoma—usually a unilateral subperiosteal hemorrhage that does not cross suture lines of the cranium. And enlarged and firm area on the cranium develops the first few days of life and can last for up to 2 weeks through 3 months of age before resolution.[128,129,130]

C. Medical management
   - Provide supportive care and education to family.
   - Observe for enlargement of area.
   - Observe for hyperbilirubinemia.
   - Observe neurological status.

D. Nursing management
   - Provide supportive care and education to family.
   - Follow daily head circumferences.
   - Observe for jaundice.
   - Obtain bilirubin levels as ordered.
   - Order neurological examinations.

E. Caput succedaneum
   This is a hemorrhagic edema that crosses suture lines and is a common finding postdelivery. It is noticeable

[123]Gomella, T., Cunningham, D., & Eyal, F. (2013). *Neonatology: Management, on-call problems, diseases, and drugs.* 6th ed. New York, NY: McGraw Hill Education.

[124]Martin, R., Fanaroff, A., & Walsh, M. (2015). *Fanaroff & Martin's neonatal-perinatal medicine: Diseases of the fetus and infant.* 10th ed. Philadelphia: Elsevier Saunders.

[125]Cloherty, J., Eichenwald, E., & Stark, A. (2012). *Manual of neonatal care.* 8th ed. Philadelphia: Lippincott Williams & Wilkins.

[126]Gomella, T., Cunningham, D., & Eyal, F. (2013). *Neonatology: Management, on-call problems, diseases, and drugs.* 6th ed. New York, NY: McGraw Hill Education.

[127]Martin, R., Fanaroff, A., & Walsh, M. (2015). *Fanaroff & Martin's neonatal-perinatal medicine: Diseases of the fetus and infant.* 10th ed. Philadelphia: Elsevier Saunders.

[128]Cloherty, J., Eichenwald, E., & Stark, A. (2012). *Manual of neonatal care.* 8th ed. Philadelphia: Lippincott Williams & Wilkins.

[129]Gomella, T., Cunningham, D., & Eyal, F. (2013). *Neonatology: Management, on-call problems, diseases, and drugs.* 6th ed. New York, NY: McGraw Hill Education.

[130]Martin, R., Fanaroff, A., & Walsh, M. (2015). *Fanaroff & Martin's neonatal-perinatal medicine: Diseases of the fetus and infant.* 10th ed. Philadelphia: Elsevier Saunders.

at birth as an enlarged discoloration over the sutures area. The size remains consistent postbirth.[131,132,133]

1. Medical management
   - Provide supportive care and education to family.
   - Observe for hyperbilirubinemia.
   - Perform no treatment.
2. Nursing management
   - Provide supportive care and education to family.
   - Observe for jaundice.
   - Obtain bilirubin levels as ordered.
3. Complications
   - Perinatal asphyxia
   - Encephalopathy
   - Seizures
   - Cerebral palsy
   - Developmental delay

F. Subgaleal hemorrhage

This is a rupture of the emissary veins (connections between the dural sinus and the sinus veins) that leads to an accumulation of blood under the scalp muscle and superficial to the periosteum. Clinical presentation is a boggy, fluctuant increasing swelling with superficial skin bruising. The condition develops over 1 to 72 hours after birth. It can become quickly serious as the bleeding continues to accumulate in large volumes, possibly to the point of complete exsanguination of the infant, leading to hemorrhagic shock and even death. This is most commonly associated with head trauma (e.g., vacuum extraction or forceps of head during the birth process.[134,135,136]

1. Medical management
   - Observe for enlargement of area.
   - Diagnosis of subgaleal hemorrhage via U/S, MRI.
   - Observation and treatment of shock and hypovolemia—hypotonia, pallor, tachycardia, hypotension, lethargy, seizures.
   - Obtain frequent serial CBC, coagulopathy.
   - Replacement of blood volume with PRBCs, normal saline (NS) boluses.
   - Observe for multiorgan failures.
   - Support respiratory status as needed with ventilation.
   - Provide supportive care and education to family.
   - Observe for hyperbilirubinemia and treatment with phototherapy.

- Observe neurological status—support seizures with Ativan and/or phenobarbital as needed.
2. Nursing management
   - Provide supportive care and education to family.
   - Frequently measure head circumferences.
   - Ensure infant receives vitamin K injection as soon as possible.
   - Monitor vital signs; check for signs and symptoms of shock—tachycardia, hypotension, decreased urine output, and neurological changes—seizure activity, lethargy.
   - Replacement of blood volume via transfusion and boluses.
   - Observe for jaundice.
   - Obtain bilirubin, CBC levels as ordered.
   - Order neurological examinations.
3. Complications
   - Severe anemia
   - Shock
   - Hypotension
   - Seizures
   - Hypotonia[137]

G. Injuries

Excessive stretching of brachial plexus during the birthing process. There are several different brachial plexus injuries, such as Erb's palsy, Klumpke paralysis, and Erb-Duchenne-Klumpke paralysis. Usually these injuries resolve spontaneously without treatment. If improvement is not noted, the infant may require surgical evaluation.[138,139,140]

- Erb's palsy—the affected arm is abducted and internally rotated with an absent Moro reflex but normal grasp in this arm.
- Klumpke paralysis—the shoulder and clavicle areas are affected, causing an absent grasp and claw hand deformity on that side.
- Erb-Duchene-Klumpke paralysis—the entire arm is affected and remains limp. Unable to appreciate a Moro or grasp reflex on the affected side.
1. Medical management
   Obtain x-rays on the affected side to evaluate for fractures or dislocations.
   - Obtain neurology and orthopedics consult.
   - Consult with PT/OT to prevent contractures and improve range of motion.
   - Provide family support and education.

[131]Cloherty, J., Eichenwald, E., & Stark, A. (2012). *Manual of neonatal care.* 8th ed. Philadelphia: Lippincott Williams & Wilkins.
[132]Gomella, T., Cunningham, D., & Eyal, F. (2013). *Neonatology: Management, on-call problems, diseases, and drugs.* 6th ed. New York, NY: McGraw Hill Education.
[133]Martin, R., Fanaroff, A., & Walsh, M. (2015). *Fanaroff & Martin's neonatal-perinatal medicine: Diseases of the fetus and infant.* 10th ed. Philadelphia: Elsevier Saunders.
[134]Cloherty, J., Eichenwald, E., & Stark, A. (2012). *Manual of neonatal care.* 8th ed. Philadelphia: Lippincott Williams & Wilkins.
[135]Gomella, T., Cunningham, D., & Eyal, F. (2013). *Neonatology: Management, on-call problems, diseases, and drugs.* 6th ed. New York, NY: McGraw Hill Education.
[136]Martin, R., Fanaroff, A., & Walsh, M. (2015). *Fanaroff & Martin's neonatal-perinatal medicine: Diseases of the fetus and infant.* 10th ed. Philadelphia: Elsevier Saunders.

[137]Gomella, T., Cunningham, D., & Eyal, F. (2013). *Neonatology: Management, on-call problems, diseases, and drugs.* 6th ed. New York, NY: McGraw Hill Education.
[138]Cloherty, J., Eichenwald, E., & Stark, A. (2012). *Manual of neonatal care.* 8th ed. Philadelphia: Lippincott Williams & Wilkins.
[139]Gomella, T., Cunningham, D., & Eyal, F. (2013). *Neonatology: Management, on-call problems, diseases, and drugs.* 6th ed. New York, NY: McGraw Hill Education.
[140]Martin, R., Fanaroff, A., & Walsh, M. (2015). *Fanaroff & Martin's neonatal-perinatal medicine: Diseases of the fetus and infant.* 10th ed. Philadelphia: Elsevier Saunders.

2. Nursing management
   - Provide supportive care and education to the family
   - Consistently and frequently perform prescribed exercises
   - Assess extremities, pulses, and reflexes
3. Complications
   - Flaccid arm
   - Immobility
   - Absent reflexes[141]

H. Hypoxic-ischemic encephalopathy (HIE)

HIE is a condition that arises when the fetus's brain is deprived, partially or completely, of oxygen to the point where areas of the brain experience ischemic insult and even cell death; this causes neurological dysfunction and multiorgan systems failure. There are three different classifications of HIE: mild, moderate, and severe encephalopathy.[142,143,144]

1. Risk factors
   - Pregnancy-induced hypertension
   - Maternal thyroid dysfunction
   - Fetal growth restriction
   - Postgestational age at time of birth
   - Malposition during birthing process
   - Acute intrapartum events—cord accidents, uterine rupture, abruption, decreased fetal heart rate, meconium staining, low Apgar score
2. Assessment findings
   a) Mild
      - Hyperalert state, hyperresponsiveness to stimulation
      - Normal muscle tone, strong Moro and grasp reflexes
      - Increased deep tendon reflexes
      - Dilated but reactive pupils
      - No seizure activity
   b) Moderate
      - Lethargy
      - Hypotonia, jitteriness
      - Increased deep tendon reflexes
      - Presence of seizure activity
      - Weak to absent suck and Moro reflex
      - Pupils constricted and reactive
      - Agonal or periodic breathing
   c) Severe
      - Obtunded, severe hypotonia; comatose
      - Apnea
      - Bradycardia
      - Seizures
      - Absence of all reflexes
      - Pupils unequal and nonreactive, poor light reflex
3. Medical management
   - Immediate and appropriate resuscitation
   - Cooling of body
   - Complete neurological examination
   - Support ventilation as needed
   - Treat acid deficits
   - Monitor blood volumes and treat hypovolemia and cardiac function
   - EEG with video
   - CT scan/MRI
   - Cranial ultrasound
   - Complete chemistry panel, CBC, coagulopathy studies, CSF analysis
   - Start antibiotic coverage
   - Support nutrition via total parenteral nutrition and intralipids, NPO, placement of central line access
   - Observe neurological status—support seizures with Ativan and/or phenobarbital as needed
   - Manage multiorgan system failures
   - Educate and support family
   - Neurology consultation
4. Nursing management
   - Provide supportive care and education to family
   - Cool the body as soon as possible per protocol (within 6 hours of delivery)
   - Monitor vital signs, signs and symptoms of shock—tachycardia, hypotension, decreased urine output, and neurological changes (seizure activity, lethargy)
   - Replacement of blood volume via transfusion and boluses
   - Observe for jaundice
   - Obtain bilirubin, CBC, chemistry levels as ordered
   - Frequent neurological examinations; give medications for seizure activity
   - Provide adequate nutrition as ordered
   - Maintain minimal stimulation and clustered care
5. Complications
   - Asphyxia
   - Cerebral edema
   - Neuronal necrosis
   - Hypotension
   - Metabolic acidosis
   - Hypoglycemia
   - Seizure activity
   - Multiorgan dysfunction

[141]Gomella, T., Cunningham, D., & Eyal, F. (2013). *Neonatology: Management, on-call problems, diseases, and drugs.* 6th ed. New York, NY: McGraw Hill Education.

[142]Cloherty, J., Eichenwald, E., & Stark, A. (2012). *Manual of neonatal care.* 8th ed. Philadelphia: Lippincott Williams & Wilkins.

[143]Gomella, T., Cunningham, D., & Eyal, F. (2013). *Neonatology: Management, on-call problems, diseases, and drugs.* 6th ed. New York, NY: McGraw Hill Education.

[144]Martin, R., Fanaroff, A., & Walsh, M. (2015). *Fanaroff & Martin's neonatal-perinatal medicine: Diseases of the fetus and infant.* 10th ed. Philadelphia: Elsevier Saunders.

- Microcephaly
- Developmental delay[145,146]

X. Newborns of Diabetic Mothers

This refers to an infant born to a mother with diabetes. The mother has had a higher level of blood sugar that her body has not been able to process properly, which has exposed the fetus to hyperglycemia throughout the pregnancy. These infants' bodies become accustomed to this increased glucose, and their bodies continue to produce a high level of insulin to break it down. The problem arises when the infant is born and the body continues to overproduce insulin for a normal level of glucose in the body. The anabolic effect of increased fetal insulin levels often leads to large for gestational age infants. The overproduction of insulin causes the infant to become hypoglycemic and not properly respond to glucose loads.[147,148,149]

A. Risk factors
  - Mothers with pregnancy-induced or type 1 or 2 diabetes during pregnancy
  - Mothers with uncontrolled blood sugar levels
  - Obesity
B. Assessment findings
  - Large infants/macrosomia
  - Blue, mottled, or ruddy skin
  - Heart murmurs, tachycardia
  - Respiratory distress, tachypnea
  - Jaundice
  - Poor feeding
  - Lethargy
  - Weak crying
  - Jitteriness/tremors
  - Puffy face
  - Consistently low blood sugars, unresponsive to given glucose loads
C. Medical management
  - Support respiratory system—intubation, ventilator support, surfactant administration
  - Echocardiogram to determine if cardiac anomalies are present
  - Septic workup with antibiotic coverage until no evidence of infection is present
  - Laboratory work—CBC, CRP, blood culture, glucose, insulin level, growth hormone level, cortisol

- Frequent blood sugar monitoring
- Nutrition
  - Supply central line or peripheral IV
  - Provide high level of dextrose as needed to maintain normal glucose levels
  - Wean IV fluids slowly so as not to cause rebound hypoglycemia
  - Encourage frequent high-caloric feedings; supplement after breastfeeding
  - Give glucagon as needed
  - Endocrine consultation
D. Nursing management
  - Monitor vital signs.
  - Perform thorough physical examination.
  - Administer IV fluids and medication as ordered. Ensure patency of IV site.
  - Monitor strict intake and output.
  - Support family; be a patient advocate.
  - Monitor glucose levels, assess feeding intolerance, encourage frequent feeding schedules, supplement after breastfeedings.
  - Monitor respiratory distress, apnea.
  - Obtain laboratory work.
  - Prep for central line placement for medication administration and exchange possibilities.
E. Complications
  - Hypoglycemia
  - Macrosomia
  - Congenital anomalies
  - Electrolyte abnormalities
  - Cardiomegaly
  - Respiratory distress/transient tachypnea of the newborn[150]

XI. Neonatal Infections

The infant's immune system can become infected by bacteria, viruses, or fungi while still in the uterus, during the birth process, within the first 72 hours of life (early-onset sepsis), or after the first 72 hours of life (late-onset sepsis).[151,152,153]

A. Risk factors
  - Inadequate prenatal care
  - Rupture of membranes, early or prolonged
  - Vaginal colonization of bacteria
  - Maternal infection, chorioamniotic, maternal fever
  - Prolonged birth
  - Prematurity
  - Maternal urinary tract infection

[145]Gomella, T., Cunningham, D., & Eyal, F. (2013). *Neonatology: Management, on-call problems, diseases, and drugs.* 6th ed. New York, NY: McGraw Hill Education.

[146]Martin, R., Fanaroff, A., & Walsh, M. (2015). *Fanaroff & Martin's neonatal-perinatal medicine: Diseases of the fetus and infant.* 10th ed. Philadelphia: Elsevier Saunders.

[147]Cloherty, J., Eichenwald, E., & Stark, A. (2012). *Manual of neonatal care.* 8th ed. Philadelphia: Lippincott Williams & Wilkins.

[148]Gomella, T., Cunningham, D., & Eyal, F. (2013). *Neonatology: Management, on-call problems, diseases, and drugs.* 6th ed. New York, NY: McGraw Hill Education.

[149]Martin, R., Fanaroff, A., & Walsh, M. (2015). *Fanaroff & Martin's neonatal-perinatal medicine: Diseases of the fetus and infant.* 10th ed. Philadelphia: Elsevier Saunders.

[150]Martin, R., Fanaroff, A., & Walsh, M. (2015). *Fanaroff & Martin's neonatal-perinatal medicine: Diseases of the fetus and infant.* 10th ed. Philadelphia: Elsevier Saunders.

[151]Cloherty, J., Eichenwald, E., & Stark, A. (2012). *Manual of neonatal care.* 8th ed. Philadelphia: Lippincott Williams & Wilkins.

[152]Gomella, T., Cunningham, D., & Eyal, F. (2013). *Neonatology: Management, on-call problems, diseases, and drugs.* 6th ed. New York, NY: McGraw Hill Education.

[153]Martin, R., Fanaroff, A., & Walsh, M. (2015). *Fanaroff & Martin's neonatal-perinatal medicine: Diseases of the fetus and infant.* 10th ed. Philadelphia: Elsevier Saunders.

- Invasive uterine procedures
- Birth depression
- Low birth weight
- Meconium staining
- Resuscitation
- Congenital anomalies
- Male infants
- Multiple births
- Subsequent abortions
- Hospital admission and length of stay
- Invasive procedures
- Prolonged use of antibiotics and resistance
- Exposure to sick families and hospital staff

B. Assessment findings
- Temperature instability (hypo- or hyperthermia)
- Lethargy/hypotonia
- Jitteriness
- Irritability/hypertonia
- Inconsolable crying
- Tachypnea, grunting, retractions, cyanosis, apnea
- Tachycardia, arrhythmias, hypotension
- Decreased perfusion
- Poor feeding
- Vomiting, residuals
- Distention
- Loose stools
- Beefy red or pale skin
- Jaundice, yellow or bronzed
- Rashes, lesions, petechiae, pustules
- Organomegaly
- Hypo- or hyperglycemia
- Increasing metabolic acidosis
- Positive blood, urine, tracheal, wound culture
- Shifted CBC; increased lactic acid, CRP, and ammonia levels

C. Medical management
- Obtain cultures—blood, urine, tracheal, wound, CSF, CBC, and CRP serial
- Serial CBC, CRP
- Obtain viral PCR, VDRL, HIV, hepatitis, IgM/IgG
- Collect CSF for analysis
- Assess absolute neutrophil count (ANC), immature to total neutrophil ration ratio
- Start broad-spectrum antibiotics and fine-tune to specific antibiotic coverage with microbiology findings
- Start antifungal or antiviral as indicated
- Support ventilation as needed
- Support nutrition and fluid resuscitation
- Consult with infection disease, neurology, ophthalmology, endocrinology

D. Nursing management
- Follow standard precautions—use of personal protective equipment
- Practice good hand hygiene
- Ensure clean environments

- Monitor vital signs
- Provide nutrition
- Support respiratory system
- Administer antibiotics and other medication on time
- Provide family with support and education.

E. Complications
1. Dependent on the organism, source of infection, gestational age of the infant, severity of disease, comorbidities[154]

XII. Substance Abuse Exposure

This occurs when an infant is exposed to drugs or alcohol in utero, usually for an extended period of time. These infants are born with numerous signs of substance withdrawal.[155,156,157]

A. Risk factors
- Poor demographic and socioeconomic status
- Poor prenatal care
- Teenaged mothers
- Prior drug/alcohol use
- Lower education

B. Assessment findings
- Hyperirritability
- Increased deep tendon reflexes
- Tremors, jitteriness
- High-pitched, inconsolable crying
- Seizures
- Hyperalertness
- Increased sucking and rooting
- Poor feeding coordination
- Vomiting, residuals
- Loose stools
- Tachypnea
- Yawning, hiccuping, sneezing
- Upper airway congestion
- Mottling
- Fever, sweating
- Poor weight gain
- Smooth philtrum
- IUGR

C. Medical management
- Urine and meconium drug screening
- Support ventilation as needed
- Support nutrition with sensitive formula or breast milk or IV nutrition as needed

[154]Martin, R., Fanaroff, A., & Walsh, M. (2015). *Fanaroff & Martin's neonatal-perinatal medicine: Diseases of the fetus and infant.* 10th ed. Philadelphia: Elsevier Saunders.

[155]Cloherty, J., Eichenwald, E., & Stark, A. (2012). *Manual of neonatal care.* 8th ed. Philadelphia: Lippincott Williams & Wilkins.

[156]Gomella, T., Cunningham, D., & Eyal, F. (2013). *Neonatology: Management, on-call problems, diseases, and drugs.* 6th ed. New York, NY: McGraw Hill Education.

[157]Martin, R., Fanaroff, A., & Walsh, M. (2015). *Fanaroff & Martin's neonatal-perinatal medicine: Diseases of the fetus and infant.* 10th ed. Philadelphia: Elsevier Saunders.

- Medications—opiates, benzodiazepines as needed to lessen withdrawal symptoms and decrease seizures
- Minimal stimulation
- Report to child protective services; consult social worker

D. Nursing management
- Provide minimal stimulation
- Perform NAS scoring
- Provide medications on time

- Practice swaddling and proper positioning
- Soothe crying and irritability by holding the infant or offering pacifier
- Support and provide education to family
- Provide nonjudgmental care

E. Complications
1. Largely dependent on the intrauterine drug exposure, length of exposure, gestational age of the infant. Data is inconclusive.

CASE STUDY: Putting It All Together

Subjective Data

A 28-year-old, Hispanic female is delivering an extremely premature infant at 25 weeks gestational age via spontaneous vaginal delivery. Ruptured membranes occurred 24 hours prior to the delivery, and the fluid was clear. Mother is febrile with a temperature of 102°F at the time of delivery. The mother has no other children, and this is her first pregnancy. She speaks only Spanish. Her husband is present with her for the delivery.

The mother reports taking the following medications during pregnancy:
- Prenatal vitamin once pregnancy test was confirmed until time of delivery; 1 capsule by mouth once a day with breakfast
- One dose of betamethasone given intramuscularly 4 hours prior to delivery

Objective Data

At delivery, the infant is limp, apneic, and cyanotic. His heart rate is 70. The infant is placed directly on the radiant warmer, where he is dried, bulb suctioned, and given face-mask positive-pressure ventilation. He is then intubated with a 2.5 ETT to a depth of 6.5 cm, and surfactant is given in the delivery room.

Nursing Assessment
1. Apgar scores: 5 at 1 minute and 8 at 5 minutes
2. Heart sounds: regular rate and rhythm
3. Respirations: congested and equal bilaterally, moderate retractions
4. Bowel sounds: hypoactive
5. Pulses: 2+ brachial, 1+ pedal, capillary refill sluggish
6. Anterior fontanel: soft and flat, sutures overriding
7. Skin: pale pink, mottled, cool to touch, with acrocyanosis present

Vital Signs
Heart rate: 160 bpm
Respiratory rate: 30 breaths per minute, assisted
Temperature: 96°F, axillary

Standard Health Care Provider Orders
1. Transfer to the neonatal intensive care unit once the infant is stable.
2. Obtain vital signs every 30 minutes for 4 hours, then every 2 hours when stable
3. Apply erythromycin eye ointment (if eyes are open).
4. Administer vitamin K IM per hospital policy.
5. Administer hepatitis B vaccine if infant is greater than 2,000 grams, with parental consent.

Case Study Questions

1. What *subjective* and *objective* data are most significant in the maternal history and labor for the neonatal nurse to know?

2. What data are most significant for the neonatal nurse to know about the neonate?

3. What interventions will be provided for the infant in the delivery room?

4. What nursing diagnoses would be priority for the neonate after delivery?

Continued

CASE STUDY: Putting It All Together (Continued)

Continuing Case Study

The infant arrives at the neonatal intensive care unit in the transport isolette. The infant is currently on a chemical mattress, in a polyethelene bag, on the transport high frequency jet ventilator (HFJV). The infant is transferred to a humidified isolette, where he is weighed and noted to be 600 grams. The parents were updated in the delivery room.

Objective Data

Physical Assessment of the Neonate

1. The infant is hypotonic in the isolette.
2. Cardiovascular: tachycardia, no murmur present
3. Respiratory: congested with crackles, equal bilateral breath sounds, moderate retractions
4. Bowel sounds: hypoactive
5. Urine output/stool: none at this time
6. Skin: pale pink, mottled
7. Capillary refill time: 4 to 5 seconds
8. Fontanels: soft, flat, overriding sutures

Vital Signs

Heart rate: 184 bmp
Respiratory rate: good chest wiggle on HFJV
Temperature: 96°F, axillary

Case Study Questions

5. What clinical presentations are a priority for the neonatal nurse to assess on this infant?

6. What interventions will be provided to this infant on admission?

7. What education should the neonatal nurse provide to the family at this time?

REVIEW QUESTIONS

1. Which of the following is the newborn at risk for during delivery due to green-stained amniotic fluid aspiration causing inflammation and respiratory distress?
   1. Atelectasis
   2. Meconium aspiration
   3. Bronchopulmonary dysplasia
   4. Patent ductus arteriosus

2. What term *best* describes an infant born with a birth weight below the 10th percentile for gestational age?
   1. Appropriate for gestational age
   2. Failure to thrive
   3. Small for gestational age
   4. Infant born to mother of gestational diabetes

3. Which tool provides the *best* assessment of neuromuscular and physical maturity correlating with gestational age of the newborn that the nurse can perform after birth?
   1. Apgar
   2. Ballard score
   3. Phenylketonuria (PKU)
   4. Length and weight measurements

4. Based on the following risk factors, which newborn is *least* at risk for developing persistent pulmonary hypertension? *Select all that apply.*
   1. Late or postdates delivery
   2. Born to a mother with gestational diabetes
   3. Appropriate for gestational age
   4. Meconium aspiration

5. Surfactant administration causes which of the following?
   1. Increased pulmonary vascular resistance
   2. Increased cerebral blood flow
   3. Decreased surface tension with increased lung compliance
   4. Increased blood viscosity

6. If the neonatal nurse is suspicious of necrotizing enterocolitis in the infant, which intervention should take place *first*?
   1. Stop feeds
   2. Obtain a blood gas
   3. Call the practitioner
   4. Check electrolytes

7. Which is the *most* common cause of patent ductus arteriosus in the neonate?
   1. Oxygen therapy
   2. Respiratory distress syndrome
   3. Genetic predisposition
   4. Necrotizing enterocolitis

8. Which causes infants of diabetic mothers to be large for gestational age?
   1. Maternal insulin crosses the placenta and makes the baby large.
   2. Blood flow across the placenta is greater than normal.
   3. Maternal doses of insulin are absorbed by the infant and cause increased body growth.
   4. Maternal glucose crosses the placenta and causes the infant to produce more insulin than usual, resulting in greater body growth.

9. Which factor places the premature infant at *greatest* risk for retinopathy of prematurity?
   1. 34 weeks gestation
   2. A weight of 2 kilograms
   3. A premature infant with bronchopulmonary dysplasia
   4. An infant does not receive erythromycin ointment at birth.

10. Which is the most common etiology for pathological jaundice in an infant?
    1. ABO incompatibility
    2. Physiological
    3. Inherited pathology
    4. Birth trauma

11. The neonate is placed on the radiant warmer in the delivery room. Which nursing intervention would take priority?
    1. Place pulse oximetry on the infant.
    2. Place leads on the infant.
    3. Place the infant in a polyurethane bag.
    4. Place temperature probe on the infant.

12. Which clinical sign is *most* concerning immediately following the delivery of a high-risk neonate?
    1. Axillary temperature of 97.8°F
    2. Blood glucose of 35 g/dL
    3. Oxygen saturation of 90%
    4. Blue-tinged hands and feet

13. Which maternal risk factor places the high-risk neonate at *greatest* risk for developing sepsis after delivery?
    1. Rupture of membranes at delivery
    2. Father has the flu
    3. Maternal fever
    4. History of herpes simplex virus (HSV) treated with Valtrex

14. Which infant is at *greatest* risk for developing hypoglycemia after birth?
    1. Severe small for gestational age infant
    2. Appropriate for gestational age infant
    3. Infant of a diabetic mother with maternal glucose control
    4. Cold-stressed term infant

15. A mother is taking methadone 85 mg. She has been told by her ob-gyn that her infant will not withdraw from this medication. At 3 days of life, the infant is jittery, inconsolable with poor feeding, and recent diarrhea. What is the *most* appropriate statement for the RN to make to the mother at this time?
    1. "Infants are often fussy during the newborn period."
    2. "Your infant is exhibiting signs and symptoms of withdrawal from the methadone and may need pharmacological intervention."
    3. "Your baby probably has hypoglycemia. I will get the practitioner."
    4. "Your baby is showing signs of colic and difficult temperament."

REVIEW QUESTION ANSWERS

1. ANSWER: 2
Rationale
1. Atelectasis is a collapse of the lung, creating low lung volumes and impaired gas exchange.
2. Meconium aspiration happens when the infant gasps for air and aspirates meconium into the lungs, creating blockage, pneumonitis, and atelectasis.
3. Bronchopulmonary dysplasia, also known as *chronic lung disease*, results from prolonged exposure to oxygen and mechanical ventilation.
4. Patent ductus arteriosus is a vessel that ideally closes after birth. In some infants, the vessel remains open, allowing oxygenated blood and deoxygenated blood to mix while allowing blood to flood the lungs, resulting in respiratory distress.
TEST-TAKING TIP: Recall the pathophysiology regarding the presence of meconium at delivery. The presence of meconium in the lungs creates inflammation, resulting in blockage, pneumonitis, and atelectasis.
Content Area: Newborn at Risk
Integrated Processes: Teaching/Learning; Nursing Process—Assessment
Client Need: Physiological Integrity; Physiological Adaptation; Pathophysiology
Cognitive Level: Comprehension
Concept: Critical Thinking
Reference: Nagtalon-Ramos, J. (2014). Best evidence-based practices: Maternal-newborn nursing care. Philadelphia: F.A. Davis Company.

2. ANSWER: 3
Rationale
1. Appropriate for gestational age illustrates an infant whose size is within the normal range for his or her gestational age.
2. Failure to thrive is the inability to gain weight at the same rate as other infants of similar age and gender.
3. Small for gestational age infants have a birth weight that is 10% less than other infants of the same gestational age.
4. Infants born to mothers of gestational diabetes are typically large for gestational age secondary to the increase in the mother's blood glucose, which passes to the infant through the placenta. The infant's body responds by producing more insulin, creating increased growth and fat deposits.
TEST-TAKING TIP: Recall percentages for growth related to gestational age. Categories include small for gestational age, appropriate for gestational age, and large for gestational age.
Content Area: Newborn at Risk
Integrated Processes: Nursing Process—Assessment
Client Need: Physiological Integrity; Physiological Adaptation; Pathophysiology
Cognitive Level: Comprehension
Concept: Assessment
Reference: Cloherty, J., Eichenwald, E., & Stark, A. (2012). Manual of neonatal care. 8th ed. Philadelphia: Lippincott Williams & Wilkins.

3. ANSWER: 2
Rationale
1. The Apgar score is a measure of the infant's physiological status in the first 5 minutes after birth.
2. The Ballard Score uses 12 criteria to assess for physical and neuromuscular maturity.
3. PKU is a newborn screen that detects for inborn errors of metabolism.
4. Length and weight are anthropometric measurements obtained after birth to help determine if the infant is appropriate size for gestational age.
TEST-TAKING TIP: Recall the gestational maturity assessment—the Ballard score.
Content Area: Newborn at Risk
Integrated Processes: Nursing Process—Assessment
Client Need: Physiological Integrity; Physiological Adaptation; Pathophysiology
Cognitive Level: Comprehension
Concept: Assessment
Reference: Nagtalon-Ramos, J. (2014). Best evidence-based practices: Maternal-newborn nursing care. Philadelphia: F.A. Davis Company.

4. ANSWER: 3
Rationale
1. Late or postdate infants may have abnormal development of pulmonary vasculature or decreased pulmonary vasodilation after birth resulting in PPHN. Premature infants rarely have sufficiently developed pulmonary vasculature to result in PPHN.
2. Infants born to mothers with gestational diabetes are at risk for anomalous development of pulmonary vasculature.
3. Infants who are appropriate for gestational age are at least risk for having factors to contribute to stress in utero or abnormal lung development.
4. Meconium aspiration can cause inflammation and increased pulmonary vasoconstrictions, resulting in PPHN.
TEST-TAKING TIP: Recall risk factors for the development of PPHN, resulting in pulmonary pressures that are higher than systemic pressure. The result of PPHN is characterized by an interruption in an infant's ordinary adaption from fetal circulation to that of neonatal circulation.
Content Area: Newborn at Risk
Integrated Processes: Nursing Process—Assessment
Client Need: Physiological Integrity; Physiological Adaptation; Pathophysiology
Cognitive Level: Comprehension
Concept: Promoting Health
Reference: Verklan, M., & Walden, M. (2010). Core curriculum for neonatal intensive care nursing. 5th ed. St. Louis, MO: Elsevier Saunders.

5. ANSWER: 3
Rationale
1. Surfactant increases pulmonary compliance.
2. Surfactant administration may decrease cerebral blood flow.
3. Exogenous surfactant is a lipoprotein containing phosphatidylcholine, which reduces surface tension in the lungs.
4. Surfactant should have no influence on blood viscosity.
TEST-TAKING TIP: Recall the pathophysiology of respiratory distress syndrome; surfactant increases lung compliance by decreasing surface tension in the lungs.
Content Area: Newborn at Risk
Integrated Processes: Nursing Process—Assessment
Client Need: Physiological Integrity; Physiological Adaptation; Pathophysiology

Cognitive Level: Comprehension
Concept: Medication
Reference: Martin, R., Fanaroff, A., & Walsh, M. (2015). Fanaroff & Martin's neonatal-perinatal medicine: Diseases of the fetus and infant. 10th ed. Philadelphia: Elsevier Saunders.

6. ANSWER: 1
Rationale
1. NEC is rare in infants who have not received enteral feeds. If one suspects an infant has NEC, feeds should be stopped immediately. If feeds are continued, the infant is at increased risk for developing pneumoperitoneum.
2. A blood gas may be performed on an infant displaying signs of NEC if signs of respiratory decomposition are present. However, this is a late sign. Initial signs begin with feeding intolerance, abdominal distention, and/or blood in the stool.
3. If there are signs of feeding intolerance in the infant, stop feeds and immediately notify the practitioner.
4. Electrolytes will be checked while the infant is unstable and NPO.
TEST-TAKING TIP: Recall the pathophysiology of NEC. Feedings should be stopped immediately if NEC is suspected; then the practitioner should be notified for further instruction.
Content Area: Newborn at Risk
Integrated Processes: Nursing Process—Assessment
Client Need: Physiological Integrity; Physiological Adaptation; Pathophysiology
Cognitive Level: Comprehension
Concept: Nursing Roles
Reference: Nagtalon-Ramos, J. (2014). Best evidence-based practices: Maternal-newborn nursing care. Philadelphia: F.A. Davis Company.

7. ANSWER: 2
Rationale
1. Infants with asymptomatic PDA often require oxygen therapy.
2. Respiratory distress syndrome, sepsis, fluid overload, high altitude, congenital heart defects, and genetic syndromes all increase the prevalence of PDA.
3. PDA is more likely a morbidity of prematurity than genetic predisposition.
4. PDA is associated with the development of NEC. Indocin is often given for PDA closure in premature infants, resulting in decreased blood flow to the gut.
TEST-TAKING TIP: Recall the pathophysiology of PDA. Respiratory distress is the most common cause of PDA in the neonate.
Content Area: Newborn at Risk
Integrated Processes: Nursing Process—Assessment
Client Need: Physiological Integrity; Physiological Adaptation; Pathophysiology
Cognitive Level: Comprehension
Concept: Assessment
Reference: Gomella, T., Cunningham, D., & Eyal, F. (2013). Neonatology: Management, on-call problems, diseases, and drugs. 6th ed. New York: McGraw Hill Education.

8. ANSWER: 4
Rationale
1. Maternal glucose crosses the placenta, causing the infant to produce higher levels of insulin.

2. Greater than normal blood flow across the placenta does not contribute to the development of LGA infants. Decreased blood flow across the placenta may cause IUGR.
3. The infant creates insulin in response to high maternal glucose levels.
4. The anabolic effect of increased fetal insulin levels often leads to large for gestational age infants.
TEST-TAKING TIP: Recall the pathophysiology of infants of diabetic mothers. As maternal glucose crosses the placenta, the infant produces more insulin to compensate for higher maternal glucose concentration, which results in accelerated growth.
Content Area: Newborn at Risk
Integrated Processes: Nursing Process—Assessment
Client Need: Physiological Integrity; Physiological Adaptation; Pathophysiology
Cognitive Level: Comprehension
Concept: Critical Thinking
Reference: Cloherty, J., Eichenwald, E., & Stark, A. (2012). Manual of neonatal care. 8th ed. Philadelphia: Lippincott Williams & Wilkins.

9. ANSWER: 3
Rationale:
1. Infants less than 31 weeks are at higher risk for developing ROP.
2. A weight of less than 1,250 grams places an infant at greater risk for developing ROP.
3. Hyperoxia contributes to abnormal development of retinal vessels in the premature infant. Infants with chronic lung disease (BPD) have prolonged exposure to oxygen. Primary risk factors for ROP include prematurity, length of mechanical ventilation, and bronchopulmonary dysplasia.
4. Erythromycin ointment is given for the prevention of ophthalmia neonatorum.
TEST-TAKING TIP: Recall the pathophysiology of retinopathy of prematurity. Increased exposure to mechanical ventilation and higher oxygen concentrations are linked to increased risk of ROP.
Content Area: Newborn at Risk
Integrated Processes: Nursing Process—Assessment
Client Need: Physiological Integrity; Physiological Adaptation; Pathophysiology
Cognitive Level: Comprehension
Concept: Promoting Health
Reference: Cloherty, J., Eichenwald, E., & Stark, A. (2012). Manual of neonatal care. 8th ed. Philadelphia: Lippincott Williams & Wilkins.

10. ANSWER: 1
Rationale
1. ABO incompatibility may develop from a type O mother who has a type A or B infant resulting in isoimmune hemolytic anemia; this causes pathological jaundice within the first 24 hours of life.
2. Physiologic jaundice appears between the 2nd and 5th day of life, causing a yellow hue to the infant's skin and sclera. It resolves with time.
3. Crigler-Najjar, Gilbert, Dubin-Johnson, and Rotor syndromes are four inherited hyperbilirubinemias. However, they are not the most common cause of pathological jaundice in an infant.

4. Birth trauma may result in significant bruising. As the old blood is reabsorbed and broken down, increased bilirubin may be produced.

TEST-TAKING TIP: Recall the pathophysiology of pathological jaundice. ABO incompatibility is the most common cause of pathological jaundice in an infant.

Content Area: Newborn at Risk
Integrated Processes: Nursing Process—Assessment
Client Need: Physiological Integrity; Physiological Adaptation; Pathophysiology
Cognitive Level: Comprehension
Concept: Assessment
Reference: Martin, R., Fanaroff, A., & Walsh, M. (2015). Fanaroff & Martin's neonatal-perinatal medicine: Diseases of the fetus and infant. 10th ed. Philadelphia: Elsevier Saunders.

11. ANSWER: 4
Rationale
1. Pulse oximetry would be the priority if the infant is showing signs of acute respiratory distress.
2. Leads are a priority if the infant is showing signs of cardiorespiratory decompensation.
3. Premature infants should be placed in a polyurethane bag to prevent heat loss after delivery.
4. Thermoregulation is the infant's ability to maintain body heat. After delivery, the infant is wet, causing heat loss. Placing a temperature probe on the infant will allow the radiant warmer to adjust heat in order to keep the infant in a thermoneutral environment.

TEST-TAKING TIP: Recall the pathophysiology of thermoregulation. If an infant is placed on a radiant warmer, the temperature probe should be placed first in order for the radiant warmer to help regulate the baby's temperature.

Content Area: Newborn at Risk
Integrated Processes: Nursing Process—Assessment
Client Need: Physiological Integrity; Physiological Adaptation; Pathophysiology
Cognitive Level: Comprehension
Concept: Critical Thinking
Reference: Nagtalon-Ramos, J. (2014). Best evidence-based practices: Maternal-newborn nursing care. Philadelphia: F.A. Davis Company.

12. ANSWER: 2
Rationale
1. Neonatal hypothermia is a temperature below 97.7°F. Infants should be dried and placed in a neutral thermal environment.
2. If the infant is symptomatic with a plasma glucose less than 40 g/dL, the infant should be treated with IV glucose. Prolonged hypoglycemia may result in brain cell death, leading to major adverse sequelae.
3. Oxygen saturations of 90% are acceptable in a newborn.
4. Blue-tinged hands and feet are known as *acrocyanosis*, a normal physical finding in newborns.

TEST-TAKING TIP: Recall appropriate vital signs in a high-risk neonate. A blood sugar of less than 40 requires treatment in a high-risk neonate.

Content Area: Newborn at Risk
Integrated Processes: Nursing Process—Assessment
Client Need: Physiological Integrity; Physiological Adaptation; Pathophysiology
Cognitive Level: Comprehension
Concept: Assessment
Reference: Gomella, T., Cunningham, D., & Eyal, F. (2013). Neonatology: Management, on-call problems, diseases, and drugs. 6th ed. New York: McGraw Hill Education.

13. ANSWER: 3
Rationale:
1. Rupture of membranes at delivery is not a risk factor for the development of sepsis in the neonate.
2. If the father of the baby has the flu, appropriate precautions should be taken to prevent the mother/infant dyad from developing the flu. Flu vaccination during pregnancy has been shown to protect the mother and infant from the flu.
3. Maternal fever indicates maternal infection or chorioamnionitis, which is a significant risk factor for neonatal sepsis.
4. Congenital HSV infection is associated with primary infections. Infants born vaginally to a mother with a primary infection are at highest risk of transmission. In this example, the history was known and the mother was being treated with Valtrex.

TEST-TAKING TIP: Recall maternal risk factors for neonatal infection. Maternal fever is an indication of chorioamnionitis, which places the infant at greatest risk for developing sepsis after delivery.

Content Area: Newborn at Risk
Integrated Processes: Nursing Process—Assessment
Client Need: Physiological Integrity; Physiological Adaptation; Pathophysiology
Cognitive Level: Comprehension
Concept: Promoting Health
Reference: Gomella, T., Cunningham, D., & Eyal, F. (2013). Neonatology: Management, on-call problems, diseases, and drugs. 6th ed. New York: McGraw Hill Education.

14. ANSWER: 1
Rationale
1. Small for gestational age infants are at highest risk for presenting with hypoglycemia due to their lack of subcutaneous fat.
2. Appropriate for gestational age infants should have normal glucose metabolism.
3. Infants of mothers whose diabetes is inadequately controlled are more likely to have hypoglycemia secondary to increased insulin production in the infant. The infant of a mother with adequate glucose control should not produce excessive insulin.
4. Term infants with prolonged cold stress can develop hypoglycemia; term infants have more reserve than a high-risk infant.

TEST-TAKING TIP: Recall complications of small for gestational age infants. These infants have less subcutaneous fat and higher plasma glucose and insulin ratios, making them more susceptible to hypoglycemia.

Content Area: Newborn at Risk
Integrated Processes: Nursing Process—Assessment
Client Need: Physiological Integrity; Physiological Adaptation; Pathophysiology
Cognitive Level: Comprehension
Concept: Promoting Health

Reference: *Cloherty, J., Eichenwald, E., & Stark, A. (2012).* Manual of neonatal care. *8th ed. Philadelphia: Lippincott Williams & Wilkins.*

15. ANSWER: 2

Rationale

1. The infant has been exposed to intrauterine opiates and is at risk for withdrawal.

2. Infants with intrauterine drug exposure may exhibit signs of withdrawal, including jitteriness, inconsolable crying, poor feeding, and diarrhea. Explaining withdrawal symptoms for this diagnosis would be the most appropriate statement for the RN to make.

3. Signs of hypoglycemia may include jitteriness, lethargy, apnea, poor feeding, and seizures. Infants may not exhibit any physical signs with confirmed hypoglycemia. The infant would be more likely to be lethargic than inconsolable if the diagnosis were hypoglycemia.

4. Colic is defined as an infant who cries more than 3 hours a day, 3 days a week, for 3 weeks or longer in an otherwise well-appearing infant. Poor feeding, diarrhea, and intrauterine drug exposure make this a less likely choice. Telling a parent their infant has a difficult temperament is nontherapeutic communication.

TEST-TAKING TIP: Recall assessment findings of infants with intrauterine drug exposure. Signs of withdrawal include jitteriness, inconsolable crying, poor feeding, and diarrhea.

Content Area: Newborn at Risk
Integrated Processes: Nursing Process—Assessment; Communication and Documentation
Client Need: Physiological Integrity; Physiological Adaptation; Pathophysiology
Cognitive Level: Comprehension
Concept: Nursing Roles
Reference: *Nagtalon-Ramos, J. (2014).* Best evidence-based practices: Maternal-newborn nursing care. *Philadelphia: F.A. Davis Company.*

Review

Chapter 23

Comprehensive Final Examination

1. A nurse is teaching a client with infertility about the medication cabergoline, which is effective in reducing prolactin levels. What are possible side effects of this medication? *Select all that apply.*
   1. Hypotension
   2. Nasal congestion
   3. Increased risk of endometriosis
   4. Increased risk of type 2 diabetes
   5. Increased risk of hypertrophic valvular heart disease

2. Which statements, if made by a male client with an X-linked recessive disorder, indicates correct understanding of transmission?
   1. "All of my sons will be affected."
   2. "My father had this disease and passed it on to me."
   3. "I have a 50% chance of passing the gene to a daughter."
   4. "If my daughter is a carrier, there is a 50% chance each of her sons will be affected."

3. A client, who is in the second trimester of pregnancy, tells the nurse that she has developed a reddish-pink skin color on the palm of her hands. Which of the following are other expected changes during pregnancy that the client may also notice? *Select all that apply.*
   1. Facial flushing
   2. Darkening that occurs across the nose and cheeks
   3. Darkening of the fingernails
   4. Thinning of hair
   5. Increase in acne on the face and back

4. The nurse is planning discharge care for a postpartum woman who has a body mass index (BMI) of 35. Because of the woman's BMI, which should the nurse plan on teaching this client?
   1. Breastfeeding
   2. Postpartum depression
   3. Heathy eating and exercise
   4. Signs and symptoms of heart failure

5. A newborn suffered from brachial nerve plexus injuries, and parents are concerned about the long-term impact. Which of the following is the best response by the nurse to the family?
   1. "These injuries require immediate surgery."
   2. "Your child will have permanent paralysis."
   3. "Injuries will generally heal spontaneously without treatment."
   4. "There really isn't anything we can do at this time."

6. A patient comes in requesting a hormone-free birth control option. Which is the most effective and easy-to-use form of hormone-free contraceptive?
   1. Copper intrauterine device
   2. Cervical cap
   3. Diaphragm
   4. Cervical ring

7. A 28-year-old G1 P0 client tells the nurse that she has a craving for chalk. What is the nurse's best response to her?
   1. "That is not normal for anyone. We need to refer you to a therapist."
   2. "Tell me more about why you have a craving for it."
   3. "You should consider eating foods that are white in color to steer your craving from chalk."
   4. "Tell me about your family history of psychiatric disorders."

8. In the male reproductive system, what internal structure secretes fluid into the semen and is responsible in shutting off the urethra at the bladder?
   1. Seminal vesicles
   2. Glans penis
   3. Seminiferous tubules
   4. Prostate gland

9. The nurse is caring for a 27-year-old G2 P1 at 36 weeks gestation. The client is receiving magnesium sulfate intravenously for pre-eclampsia. Which assessment requires immediate intervention?
   1. Blood pressure of 130/90 mm Hg
   2. Urine output of 20 mL in past hour
   3. Patellar reflexes 2+
   4. Respiratory rate of 16

10. A client with genital warts asks the nurse about what to expect with the infection. Which statement is most appropriate?
    1. "You might have to try several different medications before finding one that works."
    2. "Once you take the prescribed medication, you will be cured of the infection."
    3. "Even though you don't experience symptoms, you can still spread the infection."
    4. "You can expect additional outbreaks, each of which will be longer than the first."

11. Which of the following is true about the three layers of involuntary smooth muscles of the uterus?
    1. Designed to provide expansion of the growing fetus.
    2. Meant to inhibit the contraction of the uterus prior to the onset of labor.
    3. Located on the top of the uterus known as the fundus.
    4. Responsible for the dilation of the cervix.

12. The nurse is instructing a pregnant client on the best source of foods that supply vitamin B_{12}. Which foods should she discuss?
    1. Whole grains
    2. Meats
    3. Collard greens
    4. Carrots

13. What should be included in the discharge instructions for preventing sudden infant death syndrome? *Select all that apply.*
    1. Position newborns in the prone position to sleep.
    2. Avoid soft bedding or pillows in the newborn's sleeping area.
    3. Avoid smoking in the home.
    4. Encourage cosleeping to ensure the newborn is breathing.
    5. Use a room heater to prevent heat loss in the newborn.
    6. Offer a pacifier while sleeping.

14. A 23-year-old client comes to a community clinic for an annual Pap smear. Which infection is suspected with an abnormal result of this diagnostic test?
    1. Human papillomavirus (HPV)
    2. Chlamydia
    3. Trichomoniasis
    4. Syphilis

15. A client is being seen for the first time in a prenatal clinic. After taking an obstetric history, the nurse documents that the client is a G5T2P1A0L4. Which of the following statement would be consistent with this obstetrical history?
    1. The woman is not currently pregnant and has four living children.
    2. The woman is not currently pregnant and has had two term pregnancies.
    3. The woman is currently pregnant and has had two preterm pregnancies.
    4. The woman is currently pregnant and has had one set of twins.

16. The nurse is educating a client concerning the treatment for breast cysts. Which teachings should the nurse include? *Select all that apply.*
    1. Wear a good bra only during the day.
    2. Limit coffee, tea, and chocolate from your diet.
    3. Take 400 IU daily of vitamin E.
    4. Do not use oral contraceptives.
    5. Take acetaminophen for pain.

17. Which hormone is responsible for the increase in basal body temperature?
    1. Follicle-stimulating hormone
    2. Gonadotropin-releasing hormone
    3. Progesterone
    4. Estrogen

18. Placental circulation is dependent on maternal circulation. In which maternal circumstances is placental circulation impeded? *Select all that apply.*
    1. Hypotension
    2. Pre-eclampsia
    3. Ineffective or weak contractions
    4. Cervical dilation
    5. Hypertension
    6. Cocaine

19. The mother calls the newborn nursery nurse, screaming, "There is something wrong with my baby! Her head is swelling." What is the best response by the nurse to the mother?
    1. "This swelling occurred because of pressure on the cervix; it should resolve in a few days."
    2. "Swelling of the head is abnormal; the neurologist will need to discuss these findings."
    3. "Jaundice can cause swelling of the brain across suture lines; we will need to check the baby's blood work."
    4. "Molding can cause the baby's head to swell because the sutures are spread far apart."

20. A couple has just been told their child has an autosomal recessive inheritance disorder. Which statement by the nurse best describes this genetic disorder?
    1. "Your child has a disorder in which a single gene controls the particular trait."
    2. "Your child has a disorder in which the abnormal gene is carried on the X chromosome."
    3. "Your child has a disorder in which the abnormal gene for the disorder is expressed even when the other member of the pair is normal."
    4. "Your child has a disorder in which both genes of a pair must be abnormal for the disorder to be expressed."

21. A client in the infertility clinic is having her estrogen level tested. The nurse understands that estrogen is responsible for which effect?
    1. Inhibits the production of follicle-stimulating hormone (FSH)
    2. Inhibits the production of luteinizing hormone (LH)
    3. Increases endometrial secretions
    4. Inhibits hypertrophy of the myometrium

22. Which statement by the patient helps the nurse know she understands the teaching about condom use?
    1. "A condom can be worn for two sexual encounters as long as it does not break."
    2. "Condoms come in different sizes; it is important I get the right size to ensure proper protection."
    3. "I should make sure to get the latex condoms because they are the most reliable."
    4. "Condoms are only for males."

23. Which postoperative instruction should the nurse give to a client undergoing a mastectomy?
    1. Tylenol should be avoided after surgery.
    2. The affected arm should remain in a sling for 4 weeks.
    3. The client should expect the affected arm to be larger in diameter.
    4. The client should avoid blood draws and blood pressure in the affected arm.

24. Which instruction should the nurse provide a prenatal client with anemia?
    1. "Take your ferrous sulfate with food to avoid stomach upset."
    2. "Raisins are a good source of iron."
    3. "Your stools may be light brown on this medication."
    4. "Decrease your fiber intake to avoid the nausea associated with taking ferrous sulfate."

25. The nurse is teaching a class about cancer of the reproductive tract to women aged 60 to 70. What does the nurse inform this group that they are at highest risk for?
    1. Sexually transmitted diseases
    2. Uterine cancer
    3. Cervical cancer
    4. Ovarian cancer

26. The charge nurse is receiving a handoff communication on her postpartum clients. Which client has a high risk for postpartum hemorrhage? *Select all that apply.*
    1. Client who delivered vaginally at 40 weeks
    2. Client who delivered by cesarean delivery because of fetal distress
    3. Client who had induction of labor with oxytocin
    4. Client who delivered a large for gestational age newborn
    5. Client who delivered her fourth newborn

27. The nurse is interviewing a client with premenstrual dysphoric disorder. Which statement by the client would require immediate follow-up?
    1. "I have been crying the week of my period."
    2. "I am experiencing suicidal thoughts."
    3. "My menstrual cycle is 1 week late."
    4. "I smoke two cigarettes a day."

28. The nurse is educating a G1P0 client who is 34 weeks gestation and in her third trimester. Which of the following educational topics would be appropriate at this time? *Select all that apply.*
    1. Contraception options after delivery
    2. Group B strep (GBS) screen before onset of labor
    3. Maternal serum alpha-fetoprotein (MSAFP)
    4. Screening for gestational diabetes
    5. Pain management during labor

29. A nurse is doing genetic counseling with a couple. The mother has Down syndrome and the father has no chromosomal abnormalities. What is the chance of their offspring being affected by this disorder?
    1. 25%
    2. 50%
    3. 75%
    4. 100%

30. A 55-year-old client with a family history of ovarian cancer calls the nurse with several complaints. Which is most concerning to the nurse as an early sign of ovarian cancer?
    1. Bloating and/or feeling full after eating only a small amount
    2. Vomiting
    3. Headaches
    4. Vaginal bleeding

31. The fetal heart rate (FHR) monitor shows a deceleration in the FHR that is abrupt and appears to be in the shape of a W. What is the most likely cause of this?
    1. Compression of the fetal head
    2. Compression of the umbilical cord
    3. An abnormality in the placenta
    4. Premature labor

32. A patient is about to undergo an amniocentesis. Which procedures should the nurse perform? *Select all that apply.*
    1. Have the patient give verbal consent for the procedure.
    2. Assess for bleeding disorders.
    3. Be prepared to administer RhoD immune globulin to Rh-positive mothers to prevent isoimmunization.
    4. Monitor the temperature to assess for infection.
    5. Monitor for uterine contractions.

33. The nurse is educating a prenatal client about weight gain during pregnancy. Which statement by the client indicates effective understanding?
    1. "I should gain 2 to 4 pounds in the first trimester and half a pound per week in the last two trimesters."
    2. "I should gain 5 pounds in the first trimester, 10 pounds in the second trimester, and 15 pounds in the third trimester."
    3. "I should gain 3.5 to 5 pounds in the first trimester and 1 pound per week in the last two trimesters."
    4. "I should gain 10 pounds in the first trimester, 10 pounds in the second trimester, and 10 pounds in the third trimester."

34. The nurse observes a deceleration of the FHR from 140 to 90 bpm that begins with the contraction and gradually returns to the normal baseline rate when the contraction ends. Which is this related to?
    1. Uteroplacental insufficiency
    2. Umbilical cord compression
    3. Fetal head compression
    4. Mild hypoxemia

35. The nurse has recently instructed the client who was diagnosed with polycystic ovary syndrome on lifestyle modifications. Which statement by the client indicates an understanding of the instructions?
    1. "Exercise will decrease my metabolism and increase my glucose intolerance."
    2. "Starting on Glucophage will take the place of decreasing my sugar intake."
    3. "Weight loss will make me feel better, but it will not affect my ability to start ovulating."
    4. "Diet modifications and exercise will decrease my risk of developing cardiovascular disease."

36. Which statement is the most accurate to make to the parents of a newborn during discharge planning?
    1. "Meconium stools should be expected to resolve by the 2-week checkup appointment."
    2. "Breastfed babies usually only have one stool a day to every other day."
    3. "Report any stools that appear to have milk curds immediately to the infant's health care provider."
    4. "Stools will change from green to yellowish brown to golden yellow over the next several days."

37. Which risk is reduced by inducing labor within 48 hours of diagnosing a fetal demise?
    1. Coagulopathies
    2. Uterine atony
    3. Prolonged grief
    4. Hysterectomy

38. The nurse performs Leopold's maneuvers on a client admitted to labor and delivery. The nurse palpates the fetal head at the fundus and notices the presenting part is not engaged. Where should the ultrasound transducer be placed for optimal recording of the FHR?
    1. Right lower abdomen
    2. Near client umbilicus
    3. Lower pelvis
    4. Upper fundal area, along fetal back

39. A nurse is educating a prenatal client on pregnancy changes and her gastrointestinal system. Which statement is correct?
    1. Because of increased saliva production during pregnancy, the client should use a medium to hard toothbrush to prevent plaque.
    2. Heartburn may be relieved by sitting up after meals and elevating the head of the bed.
    3. Drinking adequate fluids and increasing fiber consumption lowers the risk for gallbladder problems.
    4. To avoid bloating and flatulence, the client should drink carbonated beverages.

40. A newborn is suspected of having substance abuse exposure. Which of the following assessment findings should the nurse expect? *Select all that apply.*
    1. Increased weight gain
    2. Seizures
    3. Tremors
    4. Decreased deep tendon reflexes
    5. Constipation
    6. Tachypnea

41. A nurse educator is teaching a class to nursing students about the highest risk group for gonorrhea. What is the age range of the clients?
    1. 36 to 45 years
    2. 14 to 25 years
    3. 26 to 35 years
    4. 46 to 55 years

42. A client in her third trimester complains of Braxton Hicks contractions. Which of the following interventions would help with this type of pain? Select all that apply.
    1. Drink four to six glasses of water per day.
    2. Rest until the contractions subside.
    3. Void regularly, keeping the bladder empty.
    4. Walk to help ease the pain.
    5. Do pelvic-tilt exercises.

43. The client is receiving intravenous oxytocin (Pitocin) for a contraction stress test (CST). Which is the most important nursing assessment of this client?
    1. FHR and uterine activity
    2. Maternal position and FHR
    3. Uterine activity and oxytocin titration rate
    4. Maternal vital signs and FHR

44. Which newborn is at highest risk of a skin infection?
    1. Infant born at 36 weeks who is being bottle fed
    2. Infant whose umbilical cord fell off on day 8 of life
    3. Term infant with multiple heel sticks in the healing phase
    4. Infant with bilirubin levels of 8 on day 4 of life

45. A G1P0 client calls the clinic and tells the nurse that she is experiencing a "whitish vaginal discharge." The nurse should:
    1. make an appointment for the client to be seen by the physician immediately.
    2. reassure the client that this is a normal change of pregnancy.
    3. ask the client if she has itching, irritation, pain, or foul odor in her vaginal area.
    4. tell the client that this type of discharge is usually seen after intercourse.

46. An infant was born prematurely and was lacking oxygen at delivery. For which diagnosis is the newborn most at risk?
    1. Phenylketonuria
    2. Hypertension
    3. Cerebral palsy
    4. Hypoxic ischemic encephalopathy

47. The nurse is assessing clients who are at risk for developing cervical cancer. Which client is at highest risk?
    1. Client with a Pap test and an HPV screen positive for type 12
    2. Client who is 40 years old and stopped smoking 15 years ago
    3. Client who was not sexually active until age 24
    4. Client with a Pap test and an HPV screen positive for type 16

48. The nurse is monitoring a client who is 34 weeks gestation with oligohydramnios. Which findings on a fetal monitor tracing are a priority for the nurse to notify the primary health care provider? *Select all that apply.*
    1. Baseline FHR 140, accelerations, late decelerations, minimal variability
    2. Baseline FHR 130, no accelerations, no decelerations, moderate variability
    3. Baseline FHR 140, occasional variable decelerations, moderate variability
    4. Baseline FHR 105, no accelerations, recurrent variable decelerations, minimal variability
    5. Baseline FHR 165, no decelerations, marked variability

49. A nurse is reviewing the prenatal laboratory results. Which of the following would indicate further action?
    1. Platelet count of 300,000 per µL of blood
    2. Red blood cell count of 4 million/microliter
    3. White blood cell count of 6,000/microliter
    4. Hematocrit 40%

50. A woman is trying the calendar rhythm method of natural family planning. After talking with the nurse, she understands she should subtract how many days from the end of her shortest cycle?
    1. 11
    2. 16
    3. 18
    4. 20

51. Which statement by the nurse would be appropriate to a client complaining about breast discomfort during pregnancy?
    1. "Your prepregnancy bras should be used during pregnancy to help with support."
    2. "You should go without a bra as much as possible."
    3. "Nipple stimulation will help with the increased breast sensitivity."
    4. "You should be fitted for a larger size bra to help with the increase in breast tissue."

52. A nurse educator is teaching a class to nursing students about the incidence of sexually transmitted infections (STIs) and their impact on public health. Which is the most commonly reported STI in the United States?
    1. Syphilis
    2. Gonorrhea
    3. Chlamydia
    4. Genital herpes

53. Which structure does the blastocyst become by dividing?
    1. Trophoblast or inner cell mass that becomes the placenta
    2. Embryoblast or inner cell mass that becomes the embryo
    3. Morula
    4. Gamete

54. A mother is learning how to breastfeed her newborn. The lactation nurse is assisting her with this process. Which technique is correct?
    1. Have the mother stroke the infant's mouth with her nipple so the infant will turn toward the mother's breast for feeding.
    2. Place a gloved finger in the newborn's mouth to elicit the sucking reflex and stimulate the infant to feed.
    3. Have the mother lean over the infant while feeding to facilitate gravity, thereby creating enhanced milk flow.
    4. Breastfeeding should not be attempted at this time because the baby was born prematurely and is not ready to learn.

55. The delivery room nurse caring for her patient in active labor determines that the second stage of labor has begun. What makes her determine this?
    1. The fetal membranes have just ruptured.
    2. The infant's head is engaged in the pelvis.
    3. The cervix is completely dilated.
    4. There is a lengthening of the umbilical cord from the vaginal introitus.

56. The nurse is counseling a client on the proper consumption of fish and fish products while pregnant. How much fish should the nurse instruct the client to eat?
    1. 8 to 12 ounces of a variety of fish every week
    2. 8 to 12 ounces of a variety of fish every month
    3. 12 to 16 ounces of a variety of fish every week
    4. 12 to 16 ounces of a variety of fish every month

57. Which of the following diagnoses would you expect in a preterm infant?
    1. Imbalanced nutrition, more than body requirements related to prematurity and a diabetic mother
    2. Ineffective breathing pattern related to immature lung development
    3. Risk for dysfunctional gastrointestinal motility related to birth before 38 weeks gestation
    4. Activity intolerance related to early gestational age

58. Which client would be at greatest risk for developing breast cancer?
    1. Client who had her first baby at the age of 24
    2. Client who did not breastfeed
    3. Client who is underweight after menopause
    4. Client who started menarche at the age of 14

59. A patient who is 16 weeks pregnant is about to undergo an amniocentesis, and an ultrasound is also going to be performed. For which purpose does the nurse understand that the ultrasound is being performed?
    1. To determine the fetus's gestational age
    2. To locate the best position to insert the needle
    3. To determine fetal lung maturity
    4. To measure the amount of amniotic fluid

60. A client with severe pre-eclampsia has been admitted to the labor and delivery unit for induction. A biophysical profile is performed, and the score is 6 out of 10. What should the nurse carefully monitor this client for during labor?
    1. Maternal hypotension
    2. Maternal hyperglycemia
    3. FHR, early decelerations
    4. FHR, late decelerations

61. A nurse is helping to perform an assessment on a client who suspects that she is pregnant and is checking the client for which diagnostic signs of pregnancy?
    1. Positive pregnancy test
    2. Visualization of embryo by transvaginal ultrasound
    3. Uterine enlargement
    4. Amenorrhea

62. A 35-year-old woman who 38 weeks pregnant is admitted to the labor and delivery unit complaining of "mild" contractions that are 10 minutes apart. After performing Leopold's maneuvers, the nurse determines that a hard round object is in the uterine fundus. What should the nurse do if green fluid is noted after rupture of the fetal membranes?
    1. Observe the fetal monitor for variable decelerations
    2. Prepare for imminent delivery
    3. Assess the pH of the fluid to determine if it is amniotic fluid
    4. Realize that this is normal with this type of presentation

63. A patient is trying to learn the cervical mucus detection natural family planning method. The patient understands that which type of cervical mucus is the most fertile?
    1. Scant
    2. Purulent
    3. Thick
    4. Wet/slippery with egg white consistency

64. The nurse on the postpartum unit is assessing a neonate of a mother with gestational diabetes. Based on prenatal history, what does the nurse note that the neonate is at risk for? *Select all that apply.*
    1. Respiratory distress syndrome
    2. Polycythemia
    3. Hypoglycemia
    4. Hydrops fetalis

65. The nurse-midwife performs an amniotomy on her patient, who is 38 years old and expecting her first child. What should the priority care for this patient be?
    1. Assess the uterine contraction pattern
    2. Check the maternal temperature
    3. Assess the FHR
    4. Check the color of the amniotic fluid

66. The nurse is caring for a postpartum client who is 1 day postcesarean birth. What assessment data would indicate infection? *Select all that apply.*
    1. Increased pulse
    2. Breast tenderness
    3. Uterine tenderness
    4. Temperature of 100°F
    5. Lethargy

67. The nurse is conducting a follow-up telephone post-partum assessment with a woman who is 4 days postpartum. The woman starts to cry and states to the nurse, "I don't know what's wrong. I seem to cry for no reason!" The nurse recognizes that the woman is experiencing which of the following?
    1. Letting-go phase
    2. Postpartum blues
    3. Postpartum depression
    4. Ineffective bonding and attachment

68. Upon assessment, the nurse finds that the infant's umbilical cord has one artery and one vein. What should the nurse do next?
    1. Record the findings on the flow sheet.
    2. Notify the practitioner of the findings.
    3. Discuss the findings with the parents of the infant.
    4. Transfer the infant to the neonatal intensive care unit.

69. A sterile vaginal examination is indicated for a patient admitted to the labor and delivery unit. Which are the indications for this exam? *Select all that apply.*
    1. Assess the fetal station
    2. Assess for rupture of the fetal membranes
    3. Determine dilation of the cervix
    4. Determine the stage of labor
    5. Assess for the amount of vaginal bleeding

70. What is the purpose of inserting a Foley catheter prior to cesarean section?
    1. To monitor hydration status
    2. To reduce the risk of bladder injury
    3. To prevent the patient from urinating during surgery
    4. To eliminate uterine displacement due to a full bladder

71. The infant nursery nurse knows that the infant who is experiencing increased oral mucus should provide parent education on which of the following?
    1. Correctly positioning the infant for feedings
    2. Initiating cardiopulmonary resuscitation
    3. Using the bulb syringe in the mouth and nose
    4. Performing the Heimlich maneuver on the infant

72. Persistent occiput posterior position during the first and second stage of labor is associated with which of the following?
    1. Increased risk for cord prolapse
    2. Extensive facial bruising
    3. Increased risk for abruption
    4. Increased lower back pain

73. Which circumstance is most likely to cause uterine atony and lead to excessive blood loss?
    1. Orthostatic hypotension
    2. Involution of the uterus
    3. Urine retention
    4. Afterpains

74. The nurse examines the breasts of a breastfeeding woman on postpartum day 2. What is an expected finding?
    1. Colostrum leaking from one breast
    2. Breast firm and hard when palpated
    3. A difference in the size of each breast
    4. Both breasts are warm and tender upon palpation

75. A woman in labor has received a dose of an opioid 45 minutes before delivery. Which medication should the labor nurse be prepared to administer to the neonate?
    1. Erythromycin
    2. Naloxone
    3. Nalbuphine
    4. Diphenhydramine

76. As the infant nursery nurse, you are assisting with a delivery. After the initial assessment of the baby, what is the next best action?
    1. Give the infant a bath
    2. Obtain footprints from the infant
    3. Administer medications to the infant
    4. Allow the mother to bond with her infant

77. Which of the following is an abnormal finding upon physical examination of an infant?
    1. Anterior fontanel that has a diamond-shaped open space
    2. Open spaces between the suture lines
    3. Ears that are below the outer canthus of the eyes
    4. One ear that is slightly smaller than the other

78. Which of the following should be implemented in management of hypovolemic shock due to postpartum hemorrhage? *Select all that apply.*
    1. IV fluid replacement with 5% dextrose
    2. Administration of oxygen with a nonrebreather face mask
    3. Instruct patient to use bed pan so strict intake and output can be obtained
    4. Placement of secondary IV access with 16- or 18-gauge needle
    5. Continued monitoring of blood loss by weight

79. A client is being educated about the in vitro fertilization procedure. Which statement is appropriate for the nurse to make?
    1. "A catheter is inserted through the cervix into the uterus and the prepared semen sample is injected into the uterus."
    2. "Sperm or ovarian tissue will be frozen for future use."
    3. "Fertilization will take place inside the woman's body."
    4. "Fertilization and maturation of the embryos occur in the laboratory prior to embryo transfer."

80. A 29-year-old low-risk primiparous patient has just begun the second stage of labor. In order to safely and efficiently support the patient, what should the nurse encourage the patient to do? *Select all that apply.*
    1. Use open-glottis pushing
    2. Take a deep breath and bear down for 20 to 30 seconds with breath held
    3. Use a birthing ball
    4. Wait until the urge to push is strong
    5. Perform FHR assessment every 30 minutes

81. Which of the following conditions is concerning to the infant nursery nurse?
    1. An infant who passes a thick, greenish to black stool with each bowel movement
    2. Hard, small, white papules on the face of the newborn
    3. A small, soft, painless protrusion next to the umbilicus
    4. Discharge from the umbilical cord 4 hours after delivery

82. The nurse is caring for a client who has anemia. Which should the nurse advise the client to do in order to increase her absorption of iron?
    1. Take her supplement with yogurt
    2. Take her supplement with full glass of orange juice
    3. Take her supplement after a meal
    4. Take her supplement with full glass of tea

83. The nurse is assessing the midline episiotomy on a woman who delivered 2 days ago. Which assessment findings should the nurse expect to see?
    1. Moderate drainage from the episiotomy site
    2. Approximated edges of episiotomy site
    3. Bruising distal to the episiotomy site
    4. Red swollen area around distal suture repair of episiotomy site

84. The nurse is discussing danger signs during pregnancy with a pregnant woman in her first trimester. Which of the following signs and symptoms would be appropriate at this time? *Select all that apply.*
    1. Severe headache and visual changes
    2. Persistent vomiting and nausea
    3. Decreased or absent movement
    4. Urinary frequency and urgency
    5. Abdominal pain/cramping

85. A placental abruption accompanied by abdominal tenderness, changes in FHR, and an estimated blood loss of 1,000 mL best describe which degree of placental abruption?
    1. Mild: Grade 1
    2. Moderate: Grade 2
    3. Marked: Grade 3
    4. Severe: Grade 4

86. Which hormonal shift occurs at the beginning of labor?
    1. Human chorionic somatomammotropin decreases
    2. Human chorionic gonadotropin increases
    3. Progesterone increases
    4. Estrogen increases

87. The nurse is caring for a client with placenta abruptio. The nurse recognizes which as a risk factor for placenta abruptio? *Select all that apply.*
    1. Use of alcohol
    2. Hypertension
    3. Preterm labor
    4. BMI of 36
    5. Intimate partner violence

88. Which of the following puts a client at risk for abnormal placental attachment?
    1. Nulliparity
    2. Preterm labor
    3. Previous surgery for uterine fibroids
    4. Family history of abnormal placental attachment

89. Which of the following serve as maternal risk factors to having a baby who may suffer from birth trauma? *Select all that apply.*
    1. Term delivery
    2. Scheduled cesarean delivery
    3. Cephalopelvic disproportion
    4. Delivery at 41 weeks
    5. Spontaneous delivery at 36+5 weeks
    6. Short labor process

90. The woman with the lowest risk for sexually transmitted pelvic inflammatory disease is one who uses which of the following?
    1. Oral contraceptives
    2. A barrier method of contraception
    3. An intrauterine device for contraception
    4. A birth control patch

91. A patient who is in active labor just received an epidural for pain management. What should the nurse be prepared to do? *Select all that apply.*
    1. Assess maternal vital signs
    2. Assess FHR
    3. Assist patient to the bathroom to void
    4. Place patient in supine position for the duration of labor
    5. Assess for maternal respiratory distress

92. What is the second stage of pathophysiology in an amniotic fluid embolism characterized by?
    1. Hemorrhage
    2. Hypoxia
    3. Capillary damage
    4. Immune modulator release

93. The nurse is evaluating a postpartum woman's perineal care technique. Which action of the client should cause the nurse to recognize the need for further instruction?
    1. Using soap and warm water to wash her perineum
    2. Changing her peri-pad with every void
    3. Applying her peri-pad from back to front with every void
    4. Using the peri-bottle to rinse her perineum after every void

94. A 39-year-old multigravida client asks the nurse for information about female sterilization with a tubal ligation. Which of the following client statements indicates effective teaching?
    1. "My fallopian tubes will be tied off through a small abdominal incision."
    2. "Reversal of a tubal ligation is easily done, with a pregnancy success rate of 80%."
    3. "After this procedure, I must abstain from intercourse for at least 3 weeks."
    4. "Both of my ovaries will be removed during the tubal ligation procedure."

95. A woman admitted to the labor and delivery unit in early labor gives the following obstetric history. She gave birth to her daughter at 38 weeks and her twin sons at 35 weeks. She also had a miscarriage at 10 weeks. All children born are still alive. Using the GTPAL system, which does the nurse calculate and document?
    1. G4 T1 P1 A1 L3 (4-1-1-1-3)
    2. G3 T1 P1 A1 L3 (3-1-1-1-3)
    3. G4 T1 P2 A1 L3 (4-1-2-1-3)
    4. G3 T1 P2 A1 L3 (3-1-2-1-3)

96. A patient who was diagnosed prenatally as having greater than 2,000 mL of amniotic fluid just delivered a 9 lb (4,082 g) baby girl. Her nurse is aware that she is now at risk for which condition?
    1. Infection
    2. Hemorrhage
    3. Hypotension
    4. Diabetes mellitus

97. The nurse is giving discharge instructions to a client on anticoagulant therapy due to a deep vein thrombosis, which occurred after giving birth. Which of the following instructions should the nurse include?
    1. "Take an herbal supplement such as St. John's wort to help increase the effect of the anticoagulant."
    2. "Avoid medications that contain aspirin."
    3. "Cranberry juice will increase the effect of the medication you are taking."
    4. "Take an antidepressant to help with the pain and help you to sleep."

98. For which condition should the nurse immediately notify the health care team?
    1. Periodic breathing in the newborn lasting approximately 3 to 5 seconds
    2. Blood sugar recording of 60 mg/dL in an infant born 6 hours ago
    3. Blue-green discolorations noted on the buttocks during physical assessment
    4. Asymmetrical chest movement in the preterm infant

99. Which of the following findings would indicate an infant who may be considered preterm?
    1. Labia minora are larger than labia majora
    2. Plantar creases cover two-thirds of foot
    3. Lanugo is mostly bald
    4. Ears with instant recoil

100. Upon assessment of a newborn, the nurse notices bruising over the shoulder area and an abrasion on the scalp. What are these markings most likely the result of?
    1. Suspected drug use during pregnancy
    2. Abuse by a caregiver
    3. Soft tissue injury during delivery
    4. Blue/gray macule (Mongolian spot)

1. **ANSWER: 1, 2, 5**
Rationale
1. Hypotension is a possible adverse effect of cabergoline.
2. Nasal congestion is a possible adverse effect of cabergoline.
3. Increased risk of endometriosis is not an adverse effect of cabergoline.
4. Increased risk of type 2 diabetes is not an adverse effect of cabergoline.
5. Increased risk of hypertrophic valvular heart disease is a possible adverse effect of cabergoline.
TEST-TAKING TIP: Review medication treatment options for infertility if you missed this question. It is very important for nurses to know adverse effects of all medications prescribed for their clients.
Content Area: Reproductive Health; Female Factor Infertility
Integrated Process: Nursing Process; Teaching/Learning
Client Need: Physiological Integrity
Cognitive Level: Application
Concept: Female Reproduction
Reference: *Fritz, M. A., & Speroff, L. (2011). Clinical gynecologic endocrinology and infertility. Philadelphia: Lippincott Williams & Wilkins.*

2. **ANSWER: 4**
Rationale
1. There is no male-to-male transmission of X-linked recessive disorders.
2. The client's father could not have passed the disease to him, as there is no male-to-male transmission.
3. All the client's daughters will inherit the X-linked recessive gene mutation from their father. They will be carriers of the X-linked recessive gene mutation and can pass the faulty gene on to their children.
4. The carrier mother of an X-linked recessive disorder has a 50% chance that each of her sons will be affected with the disorder. There is also a 50% chance that she will pass the normal gene to each of her sons and a 50% chance that each of her daughters will become carriers.
TEST-TAKING TIP: Females have two X chromosomes, while males have one X and one Y. So genes on the X chromosome can be recessive or dominant. The expression in females and males is not the same because the genes on the Y chromosome do not pair up with the genes on the X chromosome.
Content Area: X-Linked Recessive Disorders; Genetics
Integrated Process: Nursing Process—Evaluation
Client Need: Health Promotion and Maintenance; Health Promotion; Disease Prevention
Cognitive Level: Analysis
Concept: Family
Reference: *Lowdermilk, D. L., Perry, S. E., Cashion, K., & Alden, K. R. (2016). Maternity & women's health care. 11th ed. St. Louis, MO: Elsevier.*

3. **ANSWER: 1, 2, 5**
Rationale
1. Facial flushing is sometimes referred as the "glow" of pregnancy.
2. This hyperpigmentation is known as *melasma* or *chloasma*.
3. Darkening from hyperpigmentation may be noticed on the areolas and nipples, on the anal and vulvar skin, and other darkened skin such as moles.
4. In the last weeks of pregnancy, the hair follicles that are in a stage of growth increase in number. This limits the number of hairs that are shed, giving hair the appearance of more fullness.
5. Some women experience an increase in sebaceous oil production related to the increase in estrogens. This may cause acne that develops on the face or back.
TEST-TAKING TIP: The increase in hormones such as estrogen, progesterone, and alpha-melanocyte-stimulating hormone during pregnancy causes certain changes in the appearance of the integumentary system. The nurse should provide education and support concerning these changes.
Content Area: Integumentary System; Anatomy and Physiology of Pregnancy
Integrated Process: Nursing Process—Assessment
Client Need: Health Promotion and Maintenance: Ante/Intra/Postpartum and Newborn Care
Cognitive Level: Application
Concept: Pregnancy
Reference: *Ward, S. L., & Hisley, S. M. (2016). Maternal-child nursing care. 2nd ed. Philadelphia: F.A. Davis.*

4. **ANSWER: 3**
Rationale
1. The question does not indicate that the woman is breastfeeding.
2. Postpartum depression is important as far as discharge education. However, the question is referring to a high BMI, so this would be an incorrect answer.
3. A woman with a BMI is at high risk for diabetes and cardiac problems, including hypertension. Information on healthy eating and exercise is important to reduce long-term cardiovascular risk.
4. The question does not indicate that the woman has a preexisting heart condition.
TEST-TAKING TIP: A lot of information should be included in postpartum discharge education. However, the question is asking specifically to address discharge education pertaining to a BMI of 35.
Content Area: Diabetes; Antepartum at Risk
Integrated Process: Nursing Process—Implementation
Client Need: Physiological Integrity; Reduction of Risk Potential
Cognitive Level: Application
Concept: Metabolism
Reference: *Ward, S. L., & Hisley, S. M. (2016). Maternal-child nursing care. 2nd ed. Philadelphia: F.A. Davis.*

5. **ANSWER: 3**
Rationale
1. A brachial plexus injury may require surgery, but it is not immediate.
2. Paralysis of the entire arm rarely occurs in brachial plexus injury; reflexes are absent and the entire arm is hypotonic.
3. Usually these injuries resolve spontaneously without treatment. If improvement is not noted within 3 to 6 months, the infant may require surgical evaluation.
4. Providers will perform a physical evaluation, test reflexes, and possibly order radiological films to rule out clavicle fracture. Treatment will depend on the extent and severity of the injury and may include physical therapy, medication, and/or surgical intervention.

TEST-TAKING TIP: Recall treatment of brachial plexus injury. Most brachial plexus injuries will resolve spontaneously with time. These infants should be closely followed and if resolution does not occur, surgery may be an option.
Content Area: Newborn at Risk
Integrated Process: Nursing Process—Assessment
Client Need: Physiological Integrity; Physiological Adaptation; Pathophysiology
Cognitive Level: Comprehension
Concept: Nursing Roles
Reference: Gomella, T., Cunningham, D., & Eyal, F. (2013). Neonatology: Management, on-call problems, diseases, and drugs. 6th ed. New York: McGraw Hill Education.

6. **ANSWER: 1**
Rationale
1. The copper IUD would be the best to recommend to this client.
2. May be difficult to insert and remove.
3. May be difficult to insert and remove.
4. Vaginal ring (NuvaRing) is a small, flexible, plastic birth control ring that is inserted in the vagina. The ring contains the same hormones (progestin and estrogen) found in most birth control pills.
TEST-TAKING TIP: The copper IUD is 100% hormone free and can stay in place for 10 years.
Content Area: Barrier Method Contraceptive; Contraception
Integrated Process: Nursing Process—Planning
Client Need: Health Promotion and Maintenance
Cognitive Level: Analysis
Concept: Family
Reference: Ward, S. L., & Hisley, S. M. (2016). Maternal-child nursing care. 2nd ed. Philadelphia: F.A. Davis.

7. **ANSWER: 2**
Rationale
1. Having a craving for chalk is not a normal finding; however, it does not require therapy sessions.
2. This statement by the nurse is an open-ended question that will allow the nurse to obtain more information and provide adequate counseling.
3. This statement does not resolve the issue.
4. This will not help the patient's current situation.
TEST-TAKING TIP: An open-ended question is designed to encourage a full, meaningful answer using the subject's own knowledge and/or feelings. Open-ended questions also tend to be more objective and less leading than closed-ended questions.
Content Area: Eating Disorders Affecting Pregnancy; Maternal Nutrition
Integrated Process: Nursing Process—Implementation
Client Need: Health Promotion and Maintenance; High-Risk Behaviors
Cognitive Level: Application
Concept: Nutrition
Reference: Lowdermilk, D. L., Perry, S. E., Cashion, K., & Alden, K. R. (2016). Maternity & women's health care. 11th ed. St. Louis, MO: Elsevier.

8. **ANSWER: 4**
Rationale
1. Seminal vesicles are located at the base of the bladder and release a thick fluid that will nourish the sperm. Seminal vesicles do not shut the urethra off at the bladder.

2. The glans penis is the distal head of the penis.
3. Seminiferous tubules are located in the testes.
4. The prostate gland secretes fluid into the semen and is responsible for shutting off the urethra at the bladder.
TEST-TAKING TIP: Cowper's or bulbourethral glands, located at the base of the prostate gland, secrete a clear lubricant that serves to neutralize any uric acid remaining in the urethra. In order for sperm to remain healthy and mobile, they require a more alkaline environment.
Content Area: Male Reproduction; Internal Structures
Integrated Process: Nursing Process—Assessment
Client Need: Physiological Integrity
Cognitive Level: Knowledge
Concept: Male Reproduction
Reference: Ward, S. L., & Hisley, S. M. (2016). Maternal-child nursing care. 2nd ed. Philadelphia: F.A. Davis.

9. **ANSWER: 2**
Rationale
1. No immediate intervention required for this blood pressure. Reportable blood pressure is systolic 160 mm Hg or higher or diastolic 110 mm Hg or higher.
2. Magnesium sulfate is excreted in the urine. If renal function is not adequate, magnesium sulfate toxicity can occur.
3. No immediate intervention is required for this assessment; 2+ reflex is an expected response.
4. No immediate intervention is required for this assessment. Reportable respiratory rate is below 12 breaths/min.
TEST-TAKING TIP: When a client is receiving magnesium therapy for pre-eclampsia fluid intake should be no more than 125 mL/hr, and urine output should be at least 25 to 30 mL/hr.
Content Area: Pre-eclampsia; Antepartum at Risk
Integrated Process: Nursing Process—Evaluation
Client Need: Physiological Integrity; Pharmacological and Parenteral Therapies; Parenteral/Intravenous Therapies
Cognitive Level: Analysis
Concept: Medication
Reference: Lowdermilk, D. L., Perry, S. E., Cashion, K., & Alden, K. R. (2016). Maternity & women's health care. 11th ed. St. Louis, MO: Elsevier.

10. **ANSWER: 3**
Rationale
1. Genital warts respond well to treatment with client-applied topical antiviral medications.
2. Genital warts are controllable but not curable.
3. Most individuals with HPV never develop symptoms.
4. Subsequent episodes usually are shorter and less intense.
TEST-TAKING TIP: Read each answer to determine if it is a correct statement about genital herpes.
Content Area: Sexually Transmitted Infections
Integrated Process: Teaching/Learning
Client Need: Health Promotion and Maintenance
Cognitive Level: Knowledge
Concept: Sexuality
Reference: Centers for Disease Control and Prevention (2015). Sexually Transmitted Diseases. Retrieved from http://www.cdc.gov/std/; Pellico, L. H. (2013). Focus on adult health medical-surgical nursing. Philadelphia: Lippincott Williams and Wilkins.

11. ANSWER: 1

Rationale

1. These layers provide expansion to accommodate a growing fetus.
2. The three layers are responsible for contraction of the uterus.
3. This muscular layer extends through the entire uterus.
4. These three layers are located throughout the entire uterus not just the cervix.

TEST-TAKING TIP: The muscular layers extend through the entire uterus, extending into the fallopian tubes and the vagina. Though these structures have distinct functions, the continuity of the muscle serves to ensure that the system responds and functions as a whole.

Content Area: Female Reproduction—Internal Structures
Integrated Process: Nursing Process—Assessment
Client Need: Physiological Integrity
Cognitive Level: Knowledge
Concept: Female Reproduction
Reference: Ward, S. L., & Hisley, S. M. (2016). Maternal-child nursing care. *2nd ed. Philadelphia: F.A. Davis.*

12. ANSWER: 2

Rationale

1. Whole grains are a good source of thiamine.
2. Meats and dairy products are good sources of vitamin B_{12}.
3. Collard greens and other green leafy vegetables are good sources of niacin, folate, and carotenoids.
4. Carrots are a good source of vitamin A.

TEST-TAKING TIP: A vitamin B_{12} deficiency can lead to anemia, fatigue, and depression. Vitamin B_{12} can only be found naturally in animal products; however, synthetic forms are added to many foods like cereals.

Content Area: Vitamins; Maternal Nutrition
Integrated Process: Nursing Process—Teaching/Learning
Client Need: Health Promotion and Maintenance; Health Promotion; Disease Prevention
Cognitive Level: Application
Concept: Nutrition
Reference: Lowdermilk, D. L., Perry, S. E., Cashion, K., & Alden, K. R. (2016). Maternity & women's health care. *11th ed. St. Louis, MO: Elsevier.*

13. ANSWER: 2, 3, 6

Rationale

1. Newborns should be placed in the supine position to sleep.
2. Soft bedding, toys, loose blankets, or pillows should be removed from the sleeping area.
3. Smoking should be avoided near newborns.
4. Cosleeping should be discouraged, as this could lead to suffocation or smothering of the newborn.
5. The temperature in the room should be kept cool; overheating the newborn could increase the risk of SIDS.
6. Pacifiers are believed to help prevent SIDS; although at this time, the reason is not known.

TEST-TAKING TIP: Recall the risk factors that lead to SIDS. Recall proper positioning of the newborn for sleep.

Content Area: Newborns at Risk
Integrated Process: Teaching/Learning
Client Needs: Safe and Effective Care Environment; Safety and Infection Control; Accident/Injury Prevention

Cognitive Level: Application
Content: Critical Thinking
Reference: Ward, S. L., & Hisley, S. M. (2009). Maternal-child nursing care: Optimizing outcomes for mothers, children & families. *Philadelphia: F.A. Davis.*

14. ANSWER: 1

Rationale

1. A Pap test does not test directly for HPV, but dysplasia of cervical cells is strongly associated with HPV infection.
2. An abnormal Pap test is not indicative of chlamydia.
3. An abnormal Pap test is not indicative of trichomoniasis.
4. An abnormal Pap test is not indicative of syphilis.

TEST-TAKING TIP: Review the results from the virus effects on the skin and mucous membranes.

Content Area: Sexually Transmitted Infections
Integrated Process: Nursing Process—Diagnosis
Client Need: Health Promotion and Maintenance
Cognitive Level: Analysis
Concept: Sexuality
Reference: Centers for Disease Control and Prevention (2015). Sexually Transmitted Diseases. *Retrieved from http://www.cdc.gov/std/; Pellico, L. H. (2013).* Focus on adult health medical-surgical nursing. *Philadelphia: Lippincott Williams and Wilkins.*

15. ANSWER: 4

Rationale

1. The woman is currently pregnant and has four living children.
2. The woman is currently pregnant and had two term pregnancies.
3. The woman is currently pregnant and had only one preterm pregnancy.
4. The woman is currently pregnant and one of the term or preterm pregnancies was a set of twins because of the four living children. She has three previous pregnancies.

TEST-TAKING TIP: Remember when calculating an obstetric history that twins, triplets, and so forth count as one pregnancy and one birth.

Content Area: Birth History; Prenatal Care
Integrated Process: Nursing Process—Assessment
Client Needs: Health Promotion and Maintenance; Health Screening
Cognitive Level: Application
Concept: Prenatal
Reference: Lowdermilk, D. L., Perry, S. E., Cashion, K., & Alden, K. R. (2016). Maternity & women's health care. *11th ed. St. Louis, MO: Elsevier.*

16. ANSWER: 2, 3

Rationale

1. Wear a supportive bra during the day and night.
2. Eliminate products containing high doses of caffeine (coffee, tea, and chocolate) from the diet.
3. Vitamin E will help prevent breast cysts.
4. Oral contraceptives help prevent breast cysts.
5. NSAIDs are a prostaglandin inhibitor and help to prevent discomfort.

TEST-TAKING TIP: Breast cysts are small sacs filled with fluid. They can be of any size, feel like small lumps or grapes, can be soft or firm, and often fluctuate in size during the menstrual cycle, causing pain or tenderness.

Content Area: Disorders of the Breast
Integrated Process: Nursing Process—Implementation

Client Need: Physiological Integrity; Reduction of Risk Potential
Cognitive Level: Application
Concept: Female Reproduction
Reference: *Lowdermilk, D. L., Perry, S. E., Cashion, K., & Alden, K. R. (2016). Maternity & women's health care. 11th ed. St. Louis, MO: Elsevier.*

17. **ANSWER: 3**
Rationale
1. A gonadotrophic hormone is released by the anterior pituitary. This hormone is essential to the pubertal development and the growth of the ovarian follicle before the release of the egg from the follicle at ovulation.
2. This hormone stimulates the release of the gonadotropin FSH and LH from the anterior pituitary in a response to the decrease of estrogen and progesterone.
3. Progesterone is involved in the elevation of basal body temperature following ovulation.
4. Estrogen does not have a thermogenic effect on the basal body temperature.
TEST-TAKING TIP: When ovulation has occurred, the BBT typically rises 0.4°F to 1°F. This rise in temperature is caused by the increase in progesterone production during the ovarian luteal phase.
Content Area: Female Reproduction—Hormones
Integrated Process: Nursing Process—Assessment
Client Need: Physiological Integrity
Cognitive Level: Knowledge
Concept: Female Reproduction
Reference: *Ward, S. L., & Hisley, S. M. (2016). Maternal-child nursing care. 2nd ed. Philadelphia: F.A. Davis.*

18. **ANSWER: 1, 2, 5, 6**
Rationale
1. Placental circulation is affected by conditions that decrease blood flow through the placenta/umbilical cord. Maternal hypotension or low cardiac output causes low blood flow and decreases delivery of oxygen to the embryo/fetus.
2. Pre-eclampsia causes decreased blood flow through the placenta.
3. Ineffective or weak contractions do not decrease placental blood flow but strong or frequent contractions (tachysystole) do.
4. Cervical dilation does not decrease placental blood flow.
5. Hypertension causes vasoconstriction that decreases uterine blood flow and affects blood to the embryo or fetus.
6. Cocaine can cause vasoconstriction that decreases uterine blood flow and affects blood to the embryo or fetus.
TEST-TAKING TIP: If you were unable to answer the question correctly, review factors that affect utero-placental circulation. Recall the factors that increase vasoconstriction of placental blood vessels.
Content Area: Maternal Newborn
Integrated Process: Nursing Process—Analysis
Client Need: Health Promotion and Maintenance
Cognitive Level: Analysis
Concept: Pregnancy
Reference: *Lowdermilk, D. L., Perry, S. E., Cashion, K., & Alden, K. R. (2016). Maternity & women's health care. 11th ed. St. Louis, MO: Elsevier.*

19. **ANSWER: 1**
Rationale
1. Caput succedaneum occurs when there is increased pressure against the cervix; it causes an edematous area on the scalp and resolves in a few days. This answer is correct.
2. This answer is not appropriate and does not address the mother's concerns.
3. Jaundice can occur as a result of hyperbilirubinemia and may be a complication of cephalohematoma, which is a collection of blood between the skull and periosteum. It does not appear for a few days after delivery.
4. Molding occurs as a result of overriding sutures; this answer is incorrect.
TEST-TAKING TIP: Recall the reasons these conditions occur and address the mother's concerns in a holistic manner.
Content Area: Newborn
Integrated Process: Communication and Documentation; Nursing Process—Implementation
Client Need: Psychosocial Integrity; Therapeutic Communication
Cognitive Level: Application
Concept: Promoting Health
References: *Chapman, L., & Durham, R. (2010). Maternal-newborn nursing: The critical components of nursing care. Philadelphia: F.A. Davis.*

20. **ANSWER: 4**
Rationale
1. This would not be an autosomal inheritance.
2. This would be an X-linked inheritance. Autosomal inheritance would be any chromosome other than the sex (X and Y) chromosomes.
3. A child needs to inherit only one changed replica of the gene pair in order to be affected with an autosomal dominant disorder.
4. Autosomal recessive inheritance disorders exist when two mutated genes, one from each parent, are passed on to their offspring.
TEST-TAKING TIP: Unifactorial inheritance results when a specific trait or disorder is caused by a single gene. Single gene traits or disorders include autosomal dominant, autosomal recessive, X-linked dominant, and X-linked recessive modes of inheritance.
Content Area: Inheritance of Disease; Genetics
Integrated Process: Nursing Process—Teaching/Learning
Client Need: Physiological Integrity; Physiological Adaptation; Pathophysiology
Cognitive Level: Application
Concept: Family
Reference: *Murray, S. S., & McKinney, E. S. (2014). Foundations of maternal-newborn and women's health nursing. 6th ed. St. Louis, MO: Elsevier.*

21. **ANSWER: 1**
Rationale
1. Estrogen inhibits the production of FSH.
2. Progesterone inhibits the production of LH.
3. Progesterone increases endometrial secretions.
4. Estrogen causes hypertrophy of the myometrium.
TEST-TAKING TIP: Review the effects of estrogen and progesterone if you missed this question.

Content Area: Reproductive Health; Female Factor Infertility
Integrated Process: Nursing Process—Assessment
Client Need: Physiological Integrity
Cognitive Level: Comprehension
Concept: Female Reproduction
Reference: Lowdermilk, D. L., Perry, S. E., Cashion, K., & Alden, K. R. (2016). Maternity & women's health care. 11th ed. St. Louis, MO: Elsevier.

22. **ANSWER: 2**
Rationale
1. A condom should be used once and then discarded.
2. Condoms come in different sizes to ensure effectiveness.
3. Latex and nonlatex condoms provide adequate protection.
4. There is also a female condom called a *vaginal sheath*.

TEST-TAKING TIP: For condoms to be effective, the client must apply and remove the condom correctly. The nurse must educate the client about choosing the correct size, rolling the condom on an erect penis prior to intercourse, making sure there is a reservoir tip to allow for the collection of sperm, pulling the penis out of the vagina before it softens, holding the base of the condom snugly to prevent spillage of semen, and discarding the used condom.
Content Area: Barrier Method Contraceptives; Contraception
Integrated Process: Nursing Process—Evaluation
Client Need: Safe and Effective Care Environment
Cognitive Level: Application
Concept: Family
Reference: Lowdermilk, D. L., Perry, S. E., Cashion, K., & Alden, K. R. (2016). Maternity & women's health care. 11th ed. St. Louis, MO: Elsevier.

23. **ANSWER: 4**
Rationale
1. There is no contraindication in taking Tylenol after surgery.
2. The nurse should encourage early movement of the affected arm.
3. There should be no difference in the diameter in the affected arm. Any increase in size of this arm should be reported immediately.
4. Reinforce that there is a need to protect the affected arm from injury and infection. She should avoid blood draws and blood pressure measurements on that arm.

TEST-TAKING TIP: Postoperative care and special precautions must be used to prevent or minimize lymphedema in the affected arm.
Content Area: Disorders of the Breast
Integrated Process: Nursing Process—Implementation
Client Need: Physiological Integrity; Reduction of Risk Potential
Cognitive Level: Application
Concept: Cellular Regulation
Reference: Lowdermilk, D. L., Perry, S. E., Cashion, K., & Alden, K. R. (2016). Maternity & women's health care. 11th ed. St. Louis, MO: Elsevier.

24. **ANSWER: 2**
Rationale
1. Iron is best absorbed if taken without meals, but many women find it difficult to take iron on an empty stomach.
2. The treatment for iron deficiency anemia is to encourage intake of iron-rich foods such as green leafy vegetables, red meat, and raisins.
3. Stools are usually dark black on ferrous sulfate.

4. A diet high in fiber with adequate fluid intake will help to avoid constipation.

TEST-TAKING TIP: Most prenatal vitamins contain iron. For some women, the amount of iron in the prenatal vitamin may not be sufficient. If iron supplementation is needed, Fe sulfate 325 mg per day is usually prescribed.
Content Area: Anemia; Antepartum at Risk
Integrated Process: Nursing Process—Implementation
Client Need: Health Promotion and Maintenance; Ante/Intra/Postpartum and Newborn Care
Cognitive Level: Application
Concept: Hematologic Regulation
Reference: Durham, R. F., & Chapman, L. (2016). Maternal-child nursing care. 2nd ed. Philadelphia: F.A. Davis.

25. **ANSWER: 2**
Rationale
1. Sexually transmitted diseases are not risk factors.
2. Women aged 60 to 70 have the highest risk for developing uterine cancer.
3. Cervical cancer is not a risk factor.
4. Ovarian cancer is not a risk factor.

TEST-TAKING TIP: Women are at higher risk for certain cancers of the reproductive tract at different stages in their lives. It is important for the nurse to become aware of these risk factors by age to provide appropriate education. Postmenopausal women are at highest risk for uterine cancer, while the median age for developing ovarian cancer is 63. It is rare for women under 40 to develop ovarian cancer.
Content Area: Uterine Cancer; Care of the Woman Across the Life Span
Integrated Process: Nursing Process—Planning
Client Need: Health Promotion and Maintenance; Physiological Integrity
Cognitive Level: Application
Concept: Cellular Regulation
Reference: Ward, S. L., & Hisley, S. M. (2009). Maternal-child nursing care: Optimizing outcomes for mothers, children & families. Philadelphia: F.A. Davis.

26. **ANSWER: 3, 4, 5**
Rationale
1. Delivering at 40 weeks gestation is not a risk factor for postpartum hemorrhage.
2. Cesarean delivery is not a risk factor for postpartum hemorrhage.
3. Oxytocin receptors in the body become desensitized after continuous use of synthetic oxytocin.
4. A distended uterus from a large for gestational age infant can lead to uterine atony.
5. The uterus can become distended from multiple pregnancies.

TEST-TAKING TIP: Major causes of early postpartum hemorrhage include uterine atony, retained placenta, lacerations of the genital tract, hematomas, inversion of the uterus, and subinvolution of the uterus.
Content Area: Postpartum Complications
Integrated Process: Nursing Process—Assessment
Client Need: Physiological Integrity; Physiological Adaptation
Cognitive Level: Application
Concept: Perfusion
Reference: Murray, S. S., & McKinney, E. S. (2014). Foundations of maternal-newborn and women's health nursing. 6th ed. St. Louis, MO: Elsevier.

27. ANSWER: 2

Rationale

1. The client crying the week of her period is a normal finding in premenstrual dysphoric disorder.
2. If any client states she is having suicidal thoughts, it is a priority of the nurse to inform the health care provider and ensure proper follow-up is obtained.
3. The client whose menstrual cycle is 1 week late needs evaluation but does not take priority over the client with suicidal thoughts.
4. Smoking does not require immediate follow-up.

TEST-TAKING TIP: Any client who either threatens or has attempted suicide needs immediate intervention.

Content Area: Menstrual Disorders; Care of the Woman Across the Life Span
Integrated Process: Nursing Process; Planning
Client Need: Safe and Effective Care Environment; Psychosocial Integrity
Cognitive Level: Analysis
Concept: Female Reproduction
Reference: *Ladewig, P. A., London, M. L., & Davidson, M. R. (2010). Contemporary maternal-newborn nursing care. 7th ed. New York: Pearson.*

28. ANSWER: 1, 2, 5

Rationale

1. Contraception options after delivery is an appropriate educational topic during the third trimester.
2. Vaginal and rectal swab cultures to determine presence of group B strep bacterial colonization before onset of labor are appropriate.
3. MSAFP is offered and should be discussed in the first trimester.
4. Screening for gestational diabetes should be offered in the first trimester if high risk or at 28 weeks gestation if low risk.
5. Pain management during labor is an appropriate educational option during the third trimester.

TEST-TAKING TIP: Look for key words in the stem. In this stem, the key word is *third trimester.* Eliminate all answers that contain educational topics that should be discussed early in the pregnancy.

Content Area: Education and Counseling; Prenatal Care
Integrated Process: Nursing Process—Implementation
Client Needs: Health Promotion and Maintenance; Ante/Intra/Postpartum and Newborn Care
Cognitive Level: Application
Concept: Prenatal
Reference: *Lowdermilk, D. L., Perry, S. E., Cashion, K., & Alden, K. R. (2016). Maternity & women's health care. 11th ed. St. Louis, MO: Elsevier.*

29. ANSWER: 2

Rationale

1. The chance of their offspring inheriting the trait would not be 25%.
2. The chance of their offspring inheriting the trait would be 50%.
3. The chance of their offspring inheriting the trait would not be 75%.
4. The chance of their offspring inheriting the trait would not be 100%.

TEST-TAKING TIP: The Punnett square is used to predict the potential combinations and the odds of genotypes

that can occur in children by using the genotypes of their parents. Down syndrome is an abnormalities of chromosome number.

Carrier parent

		A	a
Carrier parent	**A**	AA Normal child	Aa Carrier child
	a	Aa Carrier child	aa Affected child

Content Area: Genetics and Reproduction; Genetics
Integrated Process: Nursing Process—Implementation
Client Need: Physiological Integrity; Reduction of Risk Potential
Cognitive Level: Application
Concept: Family
Reference: *Ward, S. L., & Hisley, S. M. (2016). Maternal-child nursing care. 2nd ed. Philadelphia: F.A. Davis.*

30. ANSWER: 1

Rationale

1. The complaints of feeling full after eating only a small amount and bloating with a family history of ovarian cancer is the highest concern for the nurse because these indicate early warning signs of ovarian cancer.
2. Vomiting is not an indication of ovarian cancer.
3. Headaches are not an indication of ovarian cancer.
4. Vaginal bleeding is not an indication of ovarian cancer.

TEST-TAKING TIP: Ovarian cancer may present with very subtle early warning signs such as bloating or the sensation of the clothing feeling tighter around the waist. The nurse's ability to synthesize the symptoms and risk factors of a disorder will help with developing priorities and providing appropriate care.

Content Area: Ovarian Cancer; Care of the Woman Across the Life Span
Integrated Process: Nursing Process—Assessment
Client Need: Safe and Effective Care Environment; Establishing Priorities; Physiological Adaptation
Cognitive Level: Synthesis
Concept: Cellular Regulation
Reference: *Durham, R. F., & Chapman, L. (2014). Maternal-newborn nursing: The critical components of nursing care. 2nd ed. Philadelphia: F.A. Davis.*

31. ANSWER: 2

Rationale

1. Compression of the fetal head results in early decelerations.
2. Compression of the umbilical cord either directly or with a nuchal cord may result in variable decelerations that are abrupt in nature and resemble a U, V, or W shape on the monitor strip.
3. An abnormality of the placenta usually results in late decelerations, which are gradual decreases from the baseline after the contraction is over.
4. Premature labor is diagnosed by patient history and sterile exam.

TEST-TAKING TIP: Review principles of FHR monitoring if you were unable to answer the question correctly.
Content Area: Variable Deceleration; Nursing Care During Labor and Birth
Integrated Process: Nursing Process—Analysis
Client Need: Physiological Integrity; Reduction of Risk Potential
Cognitive Level: Comprehension
Concept: Pregnancy
Reference: Lowdermilk, D. L., Perry, S. E., Cashion, K., & Alden, K. R. (2016). Maternity & women's health care. 11th ed. St. Louis, MO: Elsevier.

32. **ANSWER: 2, 4, 5**
Rationale
1. The patient should sign a written, informed consent prior to the procedure.
2. The woman should be assessed for bleeding abnormalities, as this can lead to complications with puncture of the abdomen.
3. RhoD immune globulin should be administered to Rh-negative mothers to prevent isoimmunization.
4. There is a risk for infection following the procedure, so temperature should be assessed.
5. There is a risk for uterine contractions following the procedure, so the woman should be assessed for uterine tone and abdominal pain.
TEST-TAKING TIP: Recall that an amniocentesis is an invasive procedure that has risks involved if not carried out correctly. Review the procedure, methods employed, reasons for the procedure, and risks associated with amniocentesis.
Content Area: Maternal Newborn
Integrated Process: Nursing Process—Implementation and Evaluation
Client Need: Physiological Integrity; Reduction of Risk Potential
Cognitive Level: Evaluation
Reference: Lowdermilk, D. L., Perry, S. E., Cashion, K., & Alden, K. R. (2016). Maternity & women's health care. 11th ed. St. Louis, MO: Elsevier

33. **ANSWER: 3**
Rationale
1. This is not the recommended weight gain during pregnancy.
2. This is not the recommended weight gain during pregnancy.
3. The normal pattern of weight gain is 3.5 to 5 pounds in the first trimester and 1 pound per week in the last two trimesters.
4. This is not the recommended weight gain during pregnancy.
TEST-TAKING TIP: When answers have options that contain two or more facts, identify a fact that is incorrect and eliminate that answer. By deleting distractors, you increase your chance of selecting the correct option.
Content Area: Weight Gain During Pregnancy; Maternal Nutrition
Integrated Process: Nursing Process—Evaluation
Client Need: Health Promotion and Maintenance; Health Promotion; Disease Prevention
Cognitive Level: Analysis
Concept: Pregnancy
Reference: Durham, R. F., & Chapman, L. (2016). Maternal-child nursing care. 2nd ed. Philadelphia: F.A. Davis.

34. **ANSWER: 3**
Rationale
1. A late deceleration indicates uteroplacental insufficiency.
2. A variable deceleration indicates umbilical cord compression.
3. An early deceleration indicates fetal head compression.
4. Mild hypoxemia may result from a late deceleration.
TEST-TAKING TIP: Early decelerations are caused by fetal head compression during uterine contraction, resulting in vagal stimulation and slowing of the heart rate. This type of deceleration has a uniform shape, with a slow onset that coincides with the start of the contraction and a slow return to the baseline that coincides with the end of the contraction. Thus, it has the characteristic mirror image of the contraction. Although these decelerations are not associated with fetal distress and thus are reassuring, they must be carefully differentiated from the other nonreassuring decelerations. Review interpretation of electronic fetal monitoring.
Content Area: Electronic Fetal Monitoring; Antepartum
Integrated Process: Nursing Process—Implementation
Client Need: Physiological Integrity; Reduction of Risk Potential
Cognitive Level: Application
Concept: Pregnancy
Reference: Perry, S. E., Hockenberry, M. F., Lowdermilk, D. L., & Wilson, D. (2014). Maternal child nursing care. 5th ed. St. Louis, MO: Elsevier.

35. **ANSWER: 4**
Rationale
1. Exercise is essential in women with polycystic ovary syndrome (PCOS) to increase their metabolism and decrease their glucose intolerance and is used in conjunction with Glucophage.
2. The client needs to change dietary habits as well as start Glucophage.
3. Weight loss is key to increasing menstrual cycle frequency and ovulation.
4. This statement best shows that the client understands the physiological changes that occur with PCOS.
TEST-TAKING TIP: Recall the pathophysiology of PCOS and apply this knowledge to select the correct response.
Content Area: Polycystic Ovary Syndrome; Care of the Woman Across the Life Span
Integrated Process: Nursing Process—Implementation
Client Need: Health Promotion and Maintenance; Psychosocial Integrity; Basic Care; Nutrition
Cognitive Level: Evaluation
Concept: Female Reproduction
Reference: Ladewig, P. A., London, M. L., & Davidson, M. R. (2010). Contemporary maternal-newborn nursing care. 7th ed. New York: Pearson.

36. **ANSWER: 4**
Rationale
1. Meconium stools should only appear for the first 48 hours and then begin to transition to a greenish brown stool known as the *transitional stool*.
2. Breastfed babies stool more often than those babies who are formula fed because the breast milk is more easily digestible. This answer is incorrect.

3. Milk curds are a normal and expected finding in the stools.
4. This answer is correct; the stools will change in color over the next several days.

TEST-TAKING TIP: Recall the stool patterns of the newborn.
Content Area: Newborn
Integrated Process: Communication and Documentation; Nursing Process—Planning
Client Need: Safe and Effective Care Environment; Management of Care; Continuity of Care
Cognitive Level: Application
Concept: Promoting Health
References: *Chapman, L., & Durham, R. (2010).* Maternal-newborn nursing: The critical components of nursing care. *Philadelphia: F.A. Davis.*

37. ANSWER: 1
Rationale
1. Expected management of a fetal demise can lead to sepsis, endometritis, and disseminated intravascular coagulation. Induction is started within 24 to 48 hours in an attempt to avoid these complications.
2. Induction does not prevent uterine atony. In fact, if the woman's labor is particularly lengthy, uterine atony may result.
3. Every family grieves differently and in their own time. Having the baby will not shorten the grief process.
4. Induction does not prevent a hysterectomy.

TEST-TAKING TIP: Many medical terms have synonyms. If there is not an answer that matches what you have studied, take a deep breath and see if one of the answers is a synonym.
Content Area: Labor and Birth at Risk—Fetal Demise
Integrated Process: Nursing Process—Analysis
Client Need: Health Promotion and Maintenance
Cognitive Level: Application
Concept: Pregnancy
Reference: *Durham, R. F., & Chapman, L. (2014).* Maternal-newborn nursing: The critical components of nursing care. *2nd ed. Philadelphia: F.A. Davis.*

38. ANSWER: 4
Rationale
1. The third maneuver, also called "Pallach's maneuver," identifies the presenting part and is performed with the clinician facing the woman. The middle finger and thumb are used to grasp the part of the fetus situated in the lower uterine segment or pelvic brim. In this question the clinician would determine that the buttock is the presenting part.
2. This area would be to locate the fetal spine. The second maneuver assesses the location of the fetal back. The clinician continues to face the woman. One hand is placed on the side of the abdomen to stabilize the fetus during palpation. The other hand is used to palpate the fetal spine down the side, which will feel firm and consistent. The small parts will feel irregular or protruding; fetal kicks may possibly be noted.
3. The fourth maneuver is performed with the clinician facing the woman's feet. Both hands are placed on the sides of the uterus moving in a downward motion toward the symphysis pubis. The fingertips are used to press deeply toward the pelvic inlet to feel for the fetal head (if the fetus is in a cephalic presentation). In this question, the presenting part would be moveable and engagement has not occurred.

4. The first maneuver is performed to determine whether the fetal head or buttocks are positioned in the uterine fundus. The practitioner faces the woman's head and positions the hands on the top and side of the fundus with focus on the upper region. In this question, the nurse would feel the firm and round head.

TEST-TAKING TIP: Leopold's maneuvers involve four specific steps in palpating the uterus through the abdomen in order to determine the lie and presentation of the fetus. It is important to know what is being assessed in each of the steps. Review Leopold's maneuver.
Content Area: Leopold's Maneuver; Antepartum
Integrated Process: Nursing Process—Assessment
Client Need: Physiological Integrity; Reduction of Risk Potential
Cognitive Level: Analysis
Concept: Pregnancy
Reference: *London, M. L., Ladewig, P. A., Davidson, M. R., Ball, J. W., Bindler, R. C., & Cowen, K. J. (2014).* Maternal & child nursing care. *4th ed. New Jersey: Pearson.*

39. ANSWER: 1
Rationales
1. Hyperemia of the gums is due to vascular congestion and may lead to gingival bleeding during brushing or flossing. Brushing with a soft toothbrush and flossing with a soft floss may help to avoid bleeding.
2. This helps to prevent the reflux of food/drink.
3. To avoid gallbladder problems, the client should avoid fried or other greasy foods.
4. This will not help bloating and flatulence.

TEST-TAKING TIP: The lower esophageal sphincter (cardiac sphincter) relaxes due to hormonal influences, leading to acid reflux or "heartburn." This relaxation prevents effective closure, allowing stomach contents to reflux into the esophagus, causing heartburn.
Content Area: Gastrointestinal System; Anatomy and Physiology of Pregnancy
Integrated Process: Nursing Process—Implementation
Client Need: Health Promotion and Maintenance: Ante/Intra/Postpartum and Newborn Care
Cognitive Level: Application
Concept: Pregnancy
Reference: *Ward, S. L., & Hisley, S. M. (2016).* Maternal-child nursing care. *2nd ed. Philadelphia: F.A. Davis.*

40. ANSWER: 2, 3, 6
Rationale
1. Infants experiencing withdrawal exhibit poor feeding and weight loss.
2. Infants experiencing withdrawal can develop seizures if not appropriately diagnosed and appropriately treated.
3. Tremors may be a physical sign of withdrawal.
4. Infants experiencing withdrawal are more likely to have increased deep tendon reflexes.
5. Infants experiencing withdrawal are more likely to have vomiting and diarrhea as opposed to constipation.
6. Tachypnea can be a physical sign of withdrawal.

TEST-TAKING TIP: Recall the assessment finding of infants exposed to drugs or alcohol. Signs of withdrawal include jitteriness, inconsolable crying, poor feeding, and diarrhea.

Content Area: Newborn at Risk
Integrated Process: Nursing Process—Assessment
Client Need: Physiological Integrity; Physiological Adaptation; Pathophysiology
Cognitive Level: Comprehension
Concept: Assessment
Reference: Gomella, T., Cunningham, D., & Eyal, F. (2013). Neonatology: Management, on-call problems, diseases, and drugs. 6th ed. New York: McGraw Hill Education.

41. ANSWER: 2
Rationale
1. Behavioral, biological, and cultural factors, such as sexual risk taking, put 14- to 25-year-olds at a higher risk.
2. Gonorrhea is the second most frequently reported communicable disease in the United States. Its highest incidence occurs in the 14- to 25-year-old age group.
3. Behavioral, biological, and cultural factors, such as sexual risk taking, put 14- to 25-year-olds at a higher risk.
4. Behavioral, biological, and cultural factors, such as sexual risk taking, put 14- to 25-year-olds at a higher risk.
TEST-TAKING TIP: Read each answer to determine the second most commonly reported STI in the United States. Review coinfection with gonorrhea and chlamydia.
Content Area: Sexually Transmitted Infections
Integrated Process: Nursing Process—Assessment
Client Need: Health Promotion and Maintenance
Cognitive Level: Knowledge
Concept: Sexuality
Reference: Centers for Disease Control and Prevention (2015). Sexually Transmitted Disease. Retrieved from www.cdc.gov/std/; Pellico, L. H. (2013). Focus on adult health medical-surgical nursing. Philadelphia: Lippincott Williams and Wilkins.

42. ANSWER: 1, 2, 4
Rationale
1. Adequate fluid will help to lessen irritability of the uterus.
2. Rest will not help to lessen the pain.
3. Keeping the bladder empty will help to lessen the irritability of the uterus.
4. Walking will help to lessen the pain.
5. Pelvic-tilt exercise is recommended for lower back pain, not Braxton Hicks contractions.
TEST-TAKING TIP: Braxton Hicks contractions start around the 16th week of pregnancy and help to prepare the uterus for labor. As the pregnancy advances, these contractions are more noticeable and uncomfortable.
Content Area: Reproductive System; Anatomy and Physiology of Pregnancy
Integrated Process: Nursing Process—Implementation
Client Need: Physiological Integrity; Basic Care and Comfort
Cognitive Level: Application
Concept: Comfort
Reference: Lowdermilk, D. L., Perry, S. E., Cashion, K., & Alden, K. R. (2016). Maternity & women's health care. 11th ed. St. Louis, MO: Elsevier.

43. ANSWER: 1
Rationale
1. The most critical component of the CST is the fetal heart assessment and response to uterine contractions.
2. Maternal position is important because of supine hypotension syndrome, but this would be a nursing action

placing the client in the side-lying position. FHR is one component, but the nurse must assess the fetal heart in response to uterine contractions.
3. Uterine activity is one component, but the nurse must assess the FHR in response to the uterine contractions.
4. The nurse would have taken maternal vital signs prior to the beginning of the CST. The ongoing assessment while administering the oxytocin would be FHR activity and uterine contractions.
TEST-TAKING TIP: Remember that the reason a CST is ordered is to evaluate the respiratory function (oxygen and carbon dioxide exchange) of the placenta and identify a fetus at risk for intrauterine asphyxia by observing the response of the FHR to the stress of uterine contractions.
Content Area: Contraction Stress Test; Antepartum
Integrated Process: Nursing Process—Assessment
Client Need: Safe and Effective Care Environment; Management of Care
Cognitive Level: Analysis
Concept: Pregnancy
Reference: Durham, R. F., & Chapman, L. (2014). Maternal-newborn nursing: The critical components of nursing care. 2nd ed. Philadelphia: F.A. Davis.

44. ANSWER: 3
Rationale
1. Although the infant is premature at 36 weeks, this alone does not place the baby at high risk of skin infection, and the fact that they are being bottle fed does not place them at a higher risk of a skin infection.
2. A baby whose umbilical cord fell off on day 8 of life is not at an increased risk of skin infection.
3. Multiple heel sticks place this baby at a high risk of skin infections.
4. This bilirubin level does not place the baby at a high risk of a skin infection.
TEST-TAKING TIP: Recognize the priority word in the stem is *highest risk* to determine which descriptor is either normal or places the infant at highest risk. It may be helpful to rank the findings in order of most risk.
Content Area: Newborns at Risk
Integrated Process: Nursing Process—Assessment
Client Need: Physiological Integrity; Reduction of Risk Potential; Potential for Alterations in Body Systems
Cognitive Level: Analysis
Concept: Critical Thinking
Reference: Ward, S. L., & Hisley, S. M. (2009). Maternal-child nursing care: Optimizing outcomes for mothers, children & families. Philadelphia: F.A. Davis.

45. ANSWER: 3
Rationale
1. Making an appointment may be appropriate if the client also complains of itching, irritation, pain, or foul order in her vaginal area. Further assessment is needed.
2. Leukorrhea is a normal change of pregnancy. However, the nurse should continue the assessment to see if the client is having any abnormal symptoms that could indicate a possible infection.
3. Further assessment is needed to rule out an infection.
4. This type of discharge is not seen after intercourse.
TEST-TAKING TIP: The tissues of the vagina experience changes because of the increased blood flow caused by

increased estrogen levels. The epithelial mucosa of the vaginal walls thicken and produce a whitish vaginal discharge. This leukorrhea is thicker than the secretions produced by nulliparous women and has a more acidic pH to discourage bacterial growth. If the amount, color, texture, or odor changes in vaginal secretions, the woman should call her health care provider because it could indicate a vaginal infection.

Content Area: Reproductive System; Anatomy and Physiology of Pregnancy
Integrated Process: Nursing Process—Implementation
Client Need: Health Promotion and Maintenance; Ante/Intra/Postpartum and Newborn Care
Cognitive Level: Analysis
Concept: Pregnancy
Reference: Ward, S. L., & Hisley, S. M. (2016). Maternal-child nursing care. 2nd ed. Philadelphia: F.A. Davis.

46. ANSWER: 4
Rationale
1. Phenylketonuria is an inherited disorder that causes an excessive amount of phenylalanine to build up in the body, leading to toxicity.
2. Hypertension is defined as high blood pressure. Values differ between newborns, children, and adults.
3. Cerebral palsy is a disorder of the nervous system affecting movement and coordination. Causes of CP include brain damage, trauma, and infection.
4. Hypoxic ischemic encephalopathy (HIE) develops from lack of oxygen and high carbon dioxide levels in the brain, causing inadequate gas exchange.

TEST-TAKING TIP: Recall the definition and pathophysiology of HIE. HIE results from lack of oxygen to the brain, resulting in cell death.

Content Area: Newborn at Risk
Integrated Process: Nursing Process—Assessment
Client Need: Physiological Integrity; Physiological Adaptation; Pathophysiology
Cognitive Level: Comprehension
Concept: Assessment
Reference: Gomella, T., Cunningham, D., & Eyal, F. (2013). Neonatology: Management, on-call problems, diseases, and drugs. 6th ed. New York: McGraw Hill Education.

47. ANSWER: 4
Rationale
1. HPV12 is not a high-risk HPV and is not a precursor to cervical cancer.
2. This client is not at a high risk for developing cervical cancer.
3. This client is not at a high risk for developing cervical cancer.
4. The nurse is aware that HPV types 16 and 18 are high risk and are the most common cause of cervical cancer. A client who tests positive for HPV16 and has an abnormal Pap test is at the highest risk.

TEST-TAKING TIP: Low-risk HPV infections are the cause of genital warts. The low-risk HPV types are not causes of cervical cancer. The high-risk HPV infections that are persistent are the most common cause of cervical cancer. More than 80% of women will be infected with one type

of HPV during their lives, but most resolve on their own in 1 to 2 years.

Content Area: Cervical Cancer; Care of the Woman Across the Life Span
Integrated Process: Nursing Process—Assessment
Client Need: Establishing Priorities; Health Promotion and Maintenance; Prevention of Disease
Cognitive Level: Analysis
Concept: Cellular Regulation
Reference: Ladewig, P. A., London, M. L., & Davidson, M. R. (2010). Contemporary maternal-newborn nursing care. 7th ed. New York: Pearson; National Cancer Institute. (2015). HPV and cancer. Retrieved from www.cancer.gov/about-cancer/causes-prevention/risk/infectious-agents/hpv-fact-sheet.

48. ANSWER: 1, 4, 5
Rationale
1. Late decelerations with minimal variability must be reported to the physician. Late decelerations are caused by uteroplacental insufficiency, resulting from decreased blood flow and oxygen transfer to the fetus through the intervillous spaces during contractions. Minimal variability is the best single indicator for determining fetal compromise.
2. This FHR activity falls within normal limits.
3. Variable decelerations indicate cord compression, so the nursing intervention would be to change the client's position. This tracing would not warrant the physician to be notified.
4. Baseline FHR of 105 is considered bradycardia and with minimal variability is the best single indicator for determining fetal compromise.
5. Baseline FHR of 165 is considered tachycardia and with marked variability may indicate fetal compromise.

TEST-TAKING TIP: Electronic fetal monitoring detects FHR baseline, variability, accelerations, and decelerations for clinicians to evaluate the status of fetal oxygenation. Another major purpose of electronic fetal monitoring is for clinicians to observe contraction patterns of pregnant women and to make decisions for appropriate intervention. Review all components of fetal monitoring.

Content Area: Fetal Monitoring; Antepartum
Integrated Process: Nursing Process—Assessment
Client Need: Physiological Integrity; Reduction of Risk Potential
Cognitive Level: Analysis
Concept: Pregnancy
Reference: Durham, R. F., & Chapman, L. (2014). Maternal-newborn nursing: The critical components of nursing care. 2nd ed. Philadelphia: F.A. Davis.

49. ANSWER: 4
Rationale
1. This is a normal value.
2. This indicates a possible problem with oxygen-carrying capacity.
3. This is a normal value.
4. This is a normal value.

TEST-TAKING TIP: Red blood cell count measures the number of red blood cells per mm³ of peripheral blood. A decrease could indicate anemia.

Content Area: Routine Laboratory; Diagnostic Studies; Prenatal Care
Integrated Process: Nursing Process—Assessment

Client Need: Health Promotion and Maintenance;
Ante/Intra/Postpartum and Newborn Care
Cognitive Level: Application
Concept: Prenatal
Reference: Durham, R. F., & Chapman, L. (2016). Maternal-child nursing care. 2nd ed. Philadelphia: F.A. Davis.

50. ANSWER: 3
Rationale
1. Subtract 11 from the total number of days in the longest cycle. This number represents the last fertile day of the cycle.
2. Subtract 18 from the total number of days in the shortest cycle.
3. Subtract 18 from the total number of days in the shortest cycle. This number represents the first fertile day of the cycle.
4. Subtract 18 from the total number of days in the shortest cycle.
TEST-TAKING TIP: The calendar method involves calculating the days that a woman is fertile or able to conceive.
Content Area: Natural Family Planning; Contraception
Integrated Process: Nursing Process—Evaluation
Client Need: Health Promotion and Maintenance
Cognitive Level: Application
Concept: Family
Reference: Lowdermilk, D. L., Perry, S. E., Cashion, K., & Alden, K. R. (2016). Maternity & women's health care. 11th ed. St. Louis, MO: Elsevier.

51. ANSWER: 4
Rationale
1. Because of the increase in breast tissue, a larger size bra is recommended.
2. This increase in breast tissue should be supported by a well-fitting bra. A soft supportive bra may be worn during sleep to help alleviate early sensitivity and discomfort.
3. Nipple stimulation during pregnancy is not recommended because it could lead to uterine stimulation and preterm labor.
4. Increased circulation to breast tissue causes breast enlargement, usually requiring a woman to utilize a larger bra cup size.
TEST-TAKING TIP: Breast sensitivity and enlargement results from the increased levels of estrogen and progesterone caused by pregnancy.
Content Area: Reproductive System; Anatomy and Physiology of Pregnancy
Integrated Process: Nursing Process—Implementation
Client Need: Physiological Integrity; Basic Care and Comfort
Cognitive Level: Application
Concept: Comfort
Reference: Ward, S. L., & Hisley, S. M. (2016). Maternal-child nursing care. 2nd ed. Philadelphia: F.A. Davis.

52. ANSWER: 3
Rationale
1. The incidence of syphilis increased by 10% from 2012 to 2013 but still remains below the reported rate of chlamydia.
2. Gonorrhea is the second most frequently reported communicable infection in the United States.
3. Chlamydia is the most commonly reported and fastest-spreading bacterial STI in the United States, with 1,401,906 cases reported in 2013.

4. Nursing considerations focus on educating individuals on the clinical signs and symptoms of HSV-2, as most infected individuals have not received a diagnosis.
TEST-TAKING TIP: Read each answer to determine the most commonly reported STI in the United States.
Content Area: Sexually Transmitted Infections
Integrated Process: Teaching/Learning
Client Need: Health Promotion and Maintenance
Cognitive Level: Knowledge
Concept: Sexuality
Reference: Centers for Disease Control and Prevention (2015). Sexually Transmitted Diseases. Retrieved from www.cdc.gov/std/; Pellico, L. H. (2013). Focus on adult health medical-surgical nursing. Philadelphia: Lippincott Williams and Wilkins.

53. ANSWER: 2
Rationale
1. The trophoblast is the outer cell mass of the blastocyst.
2. The embryoblast or inner cell mass becomes the embryo.
3. The morula stage (day 3) precedes the blastocyst stage (days 4 to 5).
4. A gamete (haploid) precedes the fertilization and the blastocyst stage (diploid).
TEST-TAKING TIP: Review the process of fertilization and early fetal development if you were unable to answer the question correctly.
Content Area: Maternal Newborn
Integrated Process: Nursing Process—Assessment
Client Need: Health Promotion and Maintenance
Cognitive Level: Application
Reference: Lowdermilk, D. L., Perry, S. E., Cashion, K., & Alden, K. R. (2016). Maternity & women's health care. 11th ed. St. Louis, MO: Elsevier.

54. ANSWER: 1
Rationale
1. This behavior will elicit the rooting reflex, which is encouraged for feeding.
2. This statement does describe the sucking reflex, but this does not aid in helping the mother to breastfeed.
3. Leaning over the infant to feed is not encouraged, as this will create unnecessary stress on the mother's back.
4. Babies born prematurely are encouraged to still have breast milk and breastfeed just as term babies.
TEST-TAKING TIP: Remember what the different primitive reflexes are and how they can aid in eliciting a response to assist with feeding.
Content Area: Newborn
Integrated Process: Teaching/Learning; Nursing Process—Evaluation
Client Need: Health Promotion and Maintenance; Principles of Teaching and Learning
Cognitive Level: Analysis
Concept: Nursing Roles
References: Chapman, L., & Durham, R. (2010). Maternal-newborn nursing: The critical components of nursing care. Philadelphia: F.A. Davis.

55. ANSWER: 3
Rationale
1. Fetal membranes may rupture at any time preceding labor or as late as delivery and does not define the stage of labor.

2. Engagement does not determine the stage of labor; cervical dilation does.

3. The second stage of labor commences with full dilation and ends with the birth of the infant.

4. Lengthening of the umbilical cord from the vaginal introitus signals the third stage of labor.

TEST-TAKING TIP: Review the signs and symptoms of the different stages of labor, fetal engagement, and rupture of membranes if you were unable to answer the question correctly.

Content Area: Stages of Labor; Nursing Care During Labor and Birth
Integrated Process: Nursing Process—Analysis
Client Need: Health Promotion and Maintenance
Cognitive Level: Comprehension
Concept: Pregnancy
Reference: Lowdermilk, D. L., Perry, S. E., Cashion, K., & Alden, K. R. (2016). Maternity & women's health care. 11th ed. St. Louis, MO: Elsevier.

56. ANSWER: 1
Rationale

1. Recommendation for consuming fish during pregnancy is 8 to 12 ounces of a variety of fish every week.

2. The correct recommendation is 8 to 12 ounces of a variety of fish every week.

3. The correct recommendation is 8 to 12 ounces of a variety of fish every week.

4. The correct recommendation is 8 to 12 ounces of a variety of fish every week.

TEST-TAKING TIP: Fish and shellfish are an important part of a healthy diet. They contain high-quality protein and other essential nutrients, are low in saturated fat, and contain omega-3 fatty acids. Pregnant women should eat up to 8 to 12 ounces (two average meals) a week of a variety of fish and shellfish that are lower in mercury. Five of the most commonly eaten fish that are low in mercury are shrimp, canned light tuna, salmon, pollock, and catfish. Another commonly eaten fish, albacore ("white") tuna has more mercury than canned light tuna. So, when choosing two meals of fish and shellfish, the pregnant client may eat up to 6 ounces (one average meal) of albacore tuna per week.

Content Area: Mercury; Maternal Nutrition
Integrated Process: Nursing Process—Teaching/Learning
Client Need: Health Promotion and Maintenance; Health Promotion; Disease Prevention
Cognitive Level: Application
Reference: Ward, S. L., & Hisley, S. M. (2016). Maternal-child nursing care. 2nd ed. Philadelphia: F.A. Davis.

57. ANSWER: 2
Rationale

1. The infant born prematurely is not at risk to have imbalanced nutrition more than body requirements simply because of prematurity and a diabetic state of the mother.

2. Premature infants are at risk to have respiratory distress syndrome because of low surfactant production if born less than 36 weeks gestational age.

3. The infant's gastrointestinal motility is not necessarily affected by early gestational age.

4. The infant should not have any activity intolerance due to early gestational age.

TEST-TAKING TIP: Recall that full lung maturity is not complete at less than 36 weeks of gestational age, increasing the risk for respiratory distress.

Content Area: Newborns at Risk
Integrated Process: Nursing Process—Analysis
Client Need: Health Promotion Process; Developmental Stages and Transitions
Cognitive Level: Analysis
Concept: Critical Thinking
Reference: Ward, S. L., & Hisley, S. M. (2009). Maternal-child nursing care: Optimizing outcomes for mothers, children & families. Philadelphia: F.A. Davis.

58. ANSWER: 2
Rationale

1. Nulliparity or first pregnancy after age of 30 is a risk factor.

2. Not breastfeeding is a modifiable risk factor.

3. Obesity after menopause is a risk factor.

4. Early menarche (under 12 years of age) is a risk factor.

TEST-TAKING TIP: Important assessment questions regarding the risk for breast cancer should include the client's age, number of first-degree relatives diagnosed with breast cancer, age at menarche, age at first live birth, number of breast biopsies, and history of atypical hyperplasia in biopsy.

Content Area: Disorders of the Breast
Integrated Process: Nursing Process—Assessment
Client Need: Physiological Integrity; Reduction of Risk Potential
Cognitive Level: Application
Concept: Female Reproduction
Reference: Lowdermilk, D. L., Perry, S. E., Cashion, K., & Alden, K. R. (2016). Maternity & women's health care. 11th ed. St. Louis, MO: Elsevier.

59. ANSWER: 2
Rationale

1. An amniocentesis is not done to determine gestational age.

2. It is important for the practitioner to locate the fetus, placenta, and amniotic fluid pocket in order to perform the amniocentesis safely.

3. Amniocentesis can be performed to determine fetal lung maturity but not this early in the gestation.

4. Amniotic fluid volume is determined by ultrasound.

TEST-TAKING TIP: Recall that an amniocentesis is an invasive procedure that has risks involved if not carried out correctly. Review the procedure, methods employed, reasons for the procedure, and risks associated with amniocentesis.

Content Area: Maternal Newborn
Integrated Process: Nursing Process—Analysis
Client Need: Physiological Integrity Reduction of Risk Potential
Cognitive Level: Comprehension
Concept: Pregnancy
Reference: Lowdermilk, D. L., Perry, S. E., Cashion, K., & Alden, K. R. (2016). Maternity & women's health care. 11th ed. St. Louis, MO: Elsevier.

60. ANSWER: 4
Rationale

1. For severe pre-eclampsia, the client would have elevated blood pressure, not hypotension.

2. There is nothing in the stem that indicates the client is at risk for hyperglycemia.
3. Early decelerations indicate fetal head compression and are benign. This should not warrant careful monitoring.
4. The fetus is at high risk for late decelerations secondary to severe pre-eclampsia.

TEST-TAKING TIP: A fetal biophysical profile is a prenatal test used to check on a baby's well-being. The test combines FHR monitoring (nonstress test) and fetal ultrasound. During a biophysical profile, a baby's heart rate, breathing, movements, muscle tone, and amniotic fluid level are evaluated and given a score. A biophysical profile of 8 or lower indicates that the fetus is at a high risk for being compromised. Review scoring interpretation for biophysical profile.
Content Area: Biophysical Profile; Antepartum
Integrated Process: Nursing Process—Assessment
Client Need: Physiological Integrity; Reduction of Risk Potential
Cognitive Level: Application
Concept: Pregnancy
Reference: Perry, S. E., Hockenberry, M. F., Lowdermilk, D. L., & Wilson, D. (2014). Maternal child nursing care. 5th ed. St. Louis, MO: Elsevier.

61. **ANSWER: 2**
Rationale
1. This is a probable (objective) sign of pregnancy.
2. This is a positive (diagnostic) sign of pregnancy.
3. This is a probable (objective) sign of pregnancy.
4. This is a presumptive (subjective) sign of pregnancy.

TEST-TAKING TIP: Positive or diagnostic signs of pregnancy are objective signs that cannot be caused by a pathological state and are a definite confirmation of a pregnancy.
Content Area: Signs of Pregnancy; Prenatal Care
Integrated Process: Nursing Process—Assessment
Client Needs: Health Promotion and Maintenance; Ante/Intra/Postpartum and Newborn Care
Cognitive Level: Application
Concept: Prenatal
Reference: Durham, R. F., & Chapman, L. (2016). Maternal-child nursing care. 2nd ed. Philadelphia: F.A. Davis.

62. **ANSWER: 4**
Rationale
1. Variable decelerations are generally caused by compression of the umbilical cord. There is no evidence here that there is umbilical cord compression.
2. There is no evidence that delivery is imminent since uterine contractions are 10 minutes apart. The patient will likely be considered for a cesarean section due to malpresentation.
3. The presence of meconium fluid would make the diagnosis of rupture of membranes, so assessment of fluid is not needed.
4. It is a common occurrence for a fetus in breech presentation to pass meconium before birth due to pressure on the fetus from uterine contractions.

TEST-TAKING TIP: Review assessment of rupture of membranes if you answered this question incorrectly. Recall that a hard, round object in the fundus is suggestive of the fetal head and a breech presentation.

Content Area: Process of Labor and Birth
Integrated Process: Nursing Process—Implementation
Client Need: Physiological Integrity; Reduction of Risk Potential
Cognitive Level: Analysis
Concept: Pregnancy
Reference: Lowdermilk, D. L., Perry, S. E., Cashion, K., & Alden, K. R. (2016). Maternity & women's health care. 11th ed. St. Louis, MO: Elsevier.

63. **ANSWER: 4**
Rationale
1. Scant or no visible mucus is seen during the preovulatory phase.
2. Purulent cervical discharge indicates infection.
3. Thick cervical mucus acts as a barrier to sperm. This is seen during the postovulatory phase.
4. So-called egg white cervical mucus is the most fertile of all cervical mucus types because it allows the sperm to swim easily into the cervix. Its consistency is similar to raw egg whites, and it can stretch an inch or two without breaking in the middle.

TEST-TAKING TIP: The cervical mucus method involves a woman evaluating her cervical mucus to determine the days that she is fertile or able to conceive.
Content Area: Natural Family Planning; Contraception
Integrated Process: Nursing Process—Assessment
Client Need: Health Promotion and Maintenance
Cognitive Level: Application
Concept: Family
Reference: Murray, S. S., & McKinney, E. S. (2014). Foundations of maternal-newborn and women's health nursing. 6th ed. St. Louis, MO: Elsevier.

64. **ANSWER: 1, 2, 3**
Rationale
1. High circulating insulin impedes the glucocorticoid effect, producing adequate surfactant and resulting in delayed fetal lung maturation, premature birth, increased incidence of cesarean section and thus respiratory distress syndrome.
2. Episodic fetal hypoxia stimulated by episodic maternal hyperglycemia leads to an outpouring of adrenal catecholamines, which can cause hyperbilirubinemia and polycythemia.
3. Episodic fetal hypoxia stimulated by episodic maternal hyperglycemia leads to an outpouring of adrenal catecholamines, which can cause hyperbilirubinemia and polycythemia.
4. Hydrops fetalis occurs when fetal hemolysis in severe cases of Rh isoimmunization.

TEST-TAKING TIP: It is important to know the maternal and fetal risk factors resulting from diabetes.
Content Area: Diabetes; Antepartum at Risk
Integrated Process: Nursing Process—Assessment
Client Need: Physiological Integrity; Physiological Adaptation; Pathophysiology
Cognitive Level: Application
Concept: Metabolism
Reference: Durham, R. F., & Chapman, L. (2016). Maternal-child nursing care. 2nd ed. Philadelphia: F.A. Davis.

65. ANSWER: 3

Rationale

1. Although uterine contractions may be enhanced after rupture of membranes, it is not the first priority to assess them.
2. Although temperature needs to be assessed to rule out infection, it is not the first priority.
3. The priority during labor and especially after rupture of the membranes is status of the fetus by assessing the fetal heart rate.
4. Although the color of the fluid needs to be assessed, it is not the first priority.

TEST-TAKING TIP: Review assessment before and after rupture of membranes if you answered this question incorrectly. Fetal assessment is a top priority.

Content Area: Process of Labor and Birth
Integrated Process: Nursing Process—Evaluation
Client Need: Physiological Integrity; Physiological Adaptation
Cognitive Level: Application
Concept: Pregnancy
Reference: Lowdermilk, D. L., Perry, S. E., Cashion, K., & Alden, K. R. (2016). Maternity & women's health care. 11th ed. St. Louis, MO: Elsevier.

66. ANSWER: 1, 3, 5

Rationale

1. Increased pulse is a clinical sign of endometritis.
2. Breast tenderness would be a sign of mastitis and would not be present 1 day postdelivery.
3. Uterine tenderness is a clinical sign of endometritis.
4. Temperature of 100°F is not considered a fever.
5. Lethargy is a clinical sign of endometritis.

TEST-TAKING TIP: Postpartum infection is the presence of fever 100.4°F or higher 24 hours after birth.

Content Area: Postpartum Complications
Integrated Process: Nursing Process—Assessment
Client Need: Physiological Integrity
Cognitive Level: Application
Concept: Infection
Reference: Lowdermilk, D. L., Perry, S. E., Cashion, K., & Alden, K. R. (2016). Maternity & women's health care. 11th ed. St. Louis, MO: Elsevier.

67. ANSWER: 2

Rationale

1. The letting-go phase is the last phase. In this phase, the woman is trying to realize and accept the physical separation from the infant and to adjust her life to dependency of her infant and the additional workload.
2. The woman may experience postpartum "baby blues" caused by hormonal changes that occur during the postpartal period. Common manifestations may be irritability, tears, loss of appetite, and difficulty sleeping. The woman may feel guilty about her emotional displays because she cannot identify why she is crying.
3. Postpartum depression onset is typically 6 weeks to 1 year. Physical symptoms may include marked weight loss or gain, changes in sleeping patterns, crying spells, withdrawal, despair, avoiding the infant, numbness, chest pains, and heart palpitations.
4. Negative bonding/attachment signs shown by the mother can be refusing to look at the infant, refusing to touch or hold the infant, refusing to name the infant, finding the infant unattractive or ugly, or refusing to

respond or responding negatively to infant cues such as crying or smiling.

TEST-TAKING TIP: The nurse should provide privacy for a crying mother. Let her know there is nothing wrong with her behavior. Crying may even be therapeutic for postpartum blues.

Content Area: Psychological Postpartum Adaptations; Nursing Care of the Postpartum Woman
Integrated Process: Nursing Process—Assessment
Client Need: Health Promotion and Maintenance
Cognitive Level: Application
Concept: Pregnancy
Reference: London, M. L., Ladewig, P. A., Davidson, M. R., Ball, J. W., Bindler, R. C., & Cowen, K. J. (2014). Maternal & child nursing care. 4th ed. New Jersey: Pearson.

68. ANSWER: 2

Rationale

1. This is not a normal finding; the umbilical cord should have two arteries and one vein. The findings need to be reported immediately because the newborn could have renal or cardiac anomalies.
2. This is the correct course of action by the nurse.
3. The practitioner needs to be notified first, and then he or she should discuss the findings.
4. The practitioner should first be notified, and then they may decide to transfer the newborn.

TEST-TAKING TIP: Recognize the key word *next* in the stem and whether the finding is normal or abnormal.

Content Area: Newborns
Integrated Process: Nursing Process: Implementation
Client Need: Physiological Integrity; Reduction of Risk Potential
Cognitive Level: Synthesis
Concept: Critical Thinking
Reference: Ward, S. L., & Hisley, S. M. (2009). Maternal-child nursing care: Optimizing outcomes for mothers, children & families. Philadelphia: F.A. Davis.

69. ANSWER: 1, 2, 3, 4

Rationale

1. Determining the presenting part assesses fetal position and evaluates fetal descent.
2. Rupture of membrane usually occurs spontaneously at full term either during or at the beginning of labor.
3. Assessment of dilation is important in determining stage of labor and nursing care.
4. Determining the stage of labor by performing an SVE is important in developing nursing care.
5. Observing blood draining from the introitus can assess vaginal bleeding, and a vaginal examination is contraindicated with bleeding.

TEST-TAKING TIP: Review assessment of a sterile vaginal examination if you answered this question incorrectly. Recall the parameters that can be assessed with this exam.

Content Area: Process of Labor and Birth
Integrated Process: Nursing Process—Assessment
Client Need: Health Promotion and Maintenance
Cognitive Level: Application
Concept: Pregnancy
Reference: Durham, R. F., & Chapman, L. (2014). Maternal-newborn nursing: The critical components of nursing care. 2nd ed. Philadelphia: F.A. Davis.

70. ANSWER: 2
Rationale
1. Since a cesarean section is a relatively short surgery, hydration status is not a priority assessment.
2. The Foley catheter keeps the bladder deflated. This decreases the likelihood that the surgeon will nick the bladder accidentally during the surgery.
3. Accidental urination is not a priority concern during cesarean section.
4. Uterine displacement is desired and is accomplished by positioning the mother in a left tilt position.
TEST-TAKING TIP: Bladder injury is one of the primary complications of a cesarean section. Hematuria due to the forces of delivery and organ manipulation are not uncommon. The presence of mild transient hematuria in the Foley catheter is not a concern if clear yellow urine follows.
Content Area: Labor and Birth at Risk—Cesarean Section
Integrated Process: Nursing Process—Analysis
Client Need: Health Promotion and Maintenance
Cognitive Level: Application
Concept: Pregnancy
Reference: Durham, R. F., & Chapman, L. (2014). Maternal-newborn nursing: The critical components of nursing care. 2nd ed. Philadelphia: F.A. Davis.

71. ANSWER: 3
Rationale
1. Although it is important to position the baby correctly for feedings, the infant needs help removing the additional secretions from the mouth.
2. It is important for the parents to know cardiopulmonary resuscitation, but knowing how to correctly use the bulb syringe is the priority. The infant is having trouble managing secretions, so removing them is necessary.
3. Using the bulb syringe is the priority.
4. Performing the Heimlich maneuver is an important technique for the parents to know, but the infant would benefit from using the bulb syringe to remove the increased secretions.
TEST-TAKING TIP: Understand which action is most appropriate for the parents to perform based on the stem: *increased oral mucus.*
Content Area: Newborns
Integrated Process: Nursing Process—Evaluation
Client Need: Physiological Integrity; Reduction of Risk Potential
Cognitive Level: Synthesis
Concept: Critical Thinking
Reference: Ward, S. L., & Hisley, S. M. (2009). Maternal-child nursing care: Optimizing outcomes for mothers, children & families. Philadelphia: F.A. Davis.

72. ANSWER: 4
Rationale
1. Breech and shoulder positions are at increased risk for cord prolapse.
2. Extensive facial bruising is associated with face presentation.
3. Occiput posterior is not a risk factor for placental abruption.
4. The pressure the occiput exerts on the maternal sacrum results in increased low back pain.

TEST-TAKING TIP: When studying for an examination, tables and boxes can provide you with additional information that does not fit into the flow of text. Just because it is not part of the main dialogue does not mean that it does not contain important and testable material. Boxes and tables often enhance learning by providing comparisons that are not easy to isolate from paragraphs.
Content Area: Labor and Birth at Risk—Malpresentations
Integrated Process: Nursing Process—Analysis
Client Need: Health Promotion and Maintenance
Cognitive Level: Application
Concept: Pregnancy
Reference: Durham, R. F., & Chapman, L. (2014). Maternal-newborn nursing: The critical components of nursing care. 2nd ed. Philadelphia: F.A. Davis.

73. ANSWER: 3
Rationale
1. Orthostatic hypotension is a sudden drop in blood pressure when standing up from a sitting position or when standing up after lying down. This does not cause uterine atony.
2. Involution of the uterus is the return of the uterus to a prepregnant state after birth. This process begins immediately after expulsion of the placenta with contraction of the uterine smooth muscle.
3. Urine retention causes a distended bladder, which can displace the uterus above the umbilicus and to the side. This displacement prevents the uterus from contracting, which can result in hemorrhage.
4. Contractions called *afterpains* aid in the involution of the uterus. These contractions resemble menstrual cramps and help to prevent excessive bleeding by compressing the blood vessels in the uterus.
TEST-TAKING TIP: Some questions are factual, with only one correct answer. The student should always narrow the options down to two; go with your gut response. You have a 50% chance of guessing the right answer at this point.
Content Area: Uterus; Nursing Care of the Postpartum Woman
Integrated Process: Nursing Process—Assessment
Client Need: Physiological Adaptation
Cognitive Level: Analysis
Concept: Pregnancy
Reference: Durham, R. F., & Chapman, L. (2014). Maternal-newborn nursing: The critical components of nursing care. 2nd ed. Philadelphia: F.A. Davis.

74. ANSWER: 1
Rationale
1. Breasts are unchanged for the first 2 to 3 days after birth. Colostrum is present and may leak from the nipples.
2. The breasts become full, warm, and tender between postpartum days 3 and 4.
3. The breasts are unchanged at this time and should be the same size.
4. This does not happen until milk production begins, usually on the 3rd or 4th day.
TEST-TAKING TIP: Breast assessment should include inspection for size, symmetry, shape of breasts and nipples, taking note of erection, flatness, redness, bruising, open wounds, and presence of mastitis and colostrum. The nurse

should palpate the breasts for fullness, firmness, and lumps and to determine if they are soft or engorged. A pain assessment should also be included in the assessment.
Content Area: Breast; Nursing Care of the Postpartum Woman
Integrated Process: Nursing Process—Assessment
Client Need: Physiological Adaptation
Cognitive Level: Application
Concept: Pregnancy
Reference: *Durham, R. F., & Chapman, L. (2014).* Maternal-newborn nursing: The critical components of nursing care. *2nd ed. Philadelphia: F.A. Davis.*

75. **ANSWER: 2**
Rationale
1. Erythromycin is administered to the neonate, but it is indicated for prevention of ophthalmia neonatorum, an eye infection.
2. Naloxone is an opioid antagonist that may be administered to either the mother or the infant to treat side effects from opioids, specifically respiratory depression.
3. Nalbuphine may be used for pain relief or pruritus in the mother.
4. Diphenhydramine is an antihistamine used in the mother for treatment of pruritus.
TEST-TAKING TIP: Review opioid pain medications commonly used in labor if you were unable to answer the question correctly. Eliminate medications that although commonly used in the perinatal period are not opioids.
Content Area: Pain Management; Nursing Care During Labor and Delivery
Integrated Process: Nursing Process—Analysis
Client Need: Physiological Integrity; Pharmacological and Parenteral Therapies
Cognitive Level: Application
Concept: Pregnancy
Reference: *Anderson, D. (2011). A review of systemic opioids commonly used for labor pain relief.* Journal of Midwifery and Women's Health *56(3), 222-239.*

76. **ANSWER: 4**
Rationale
1. The infant should be bathed, but establishing a strong family unit or mother–newborn bond is the first step.
2. Footprints can be done after the mother has had a chance to hold her baby to establish bonding.
3. Medications should be given after delivery, but not before the mother and newborn have had a chance to bond.
4. Establishing a strong bond or maternal–newborn attachment is important.
TEST-TAKING TIP: Recall that once the initial assessment is done after the delivery and the baby appears to be in no distress, the mother should be given the opportunity to hold her newborn.
Content Area: Newborns
Integrated Process: Nursing Processes—Evaluation
Client Need: Physiological Integrity; Basic Care and Comfort
Cognitive Level: Synthesis
Concept: Family
References: *Ward, S. L., & Hisley, S. M. (2009).* Maternal-child nursing care: Optimizing outcomes for mothers, children & families. *Philadelphia: F.A. Davis.*

77. **ANSWER: 3**
Rationale
1. The anterior fontanel should be diamond shaped and open.
2. Open spaces between the suture lines allow for molding during the birth process and are normal.
3. Ears that are slightly lower than the outer canthus of the eye may indicate abnormalities such as Down syndrome; this is the correct answer.
4. Normal findings may indicate that one ear could be slightly lower than the other ear.
TEST-TAKING TIP: Recognize the normal and abnormal findings of a newborn's physical assessment and signs that are found in a newborn with Down syndrome.
Content Area: Newborns at Risk
Integrated Process: Assessment
Client Needs: Physiological Integrity; Physiological Adaptation; Alterations in Body Systems
Cognitive Level: Comprehension
Concept: Assessment
Reference: *Ward, S. L., & Hisley, S. M. (2009).* Maternal-child nursing care: Optimizing outcomes for mothers, children & families. *Philadelphia: F.A. Davis.*

78. **ANSWER: 2, 3, 5**
Rationale
1. IV fluid replacement with crystalloids, such as Lactated Ringer's normal saline
2. Oxygen administration treats compromised tissue perfusion.
3. Placement of indwelling urinary catheter will prevent bladder distention, uterine displacement, and potential additional bleeding, as well as allow for monitoring of urine output.
4. Provides access for blood products
5. Measuring gives accurate estimation of blood loss.
TEST-TAKING TIP: Remember, 1 gram in weight equals 1 mL in volume of blood. A fully saturated perineal pad can hold between 50 to 80 mL.
Content Area: Postpartum Complications
Integrated Process: Nursing Process—Implementation
Client Need: Safe and Effective Care Environment: Management of Care
Cognitive Level: Application
Concept: Perfusion
Reference: *Ward, S. L., & Hisley, S. M. (2016).* Maternal-child nursing care. *2nd ed. Philadelphia: F.A. Davis.*

79. **ANSWER: 4**
Rationale
1. This technique requires collection of the sperm sample and preparation of the sample in the laboratory prior to injecting into the uterus.
2. Cryopreservation involves sperm or ovarian tissue to be frozen for future use.
3. Fertilization does not take place inside the woman's body.
4. In vitro fertilization involves fertilization and maturation of the embryos in the laboratory prior to embryo transfer.
TEST-TAKING TIP: Review treatment options for infertility if you missed this question.
Content Area: Reproductive Health: Female Factor Infertility

Integrated Process: Nursing Process—Teaching/Learning
Client Need: Physiological Integrity
Cognitive Level: Application
Concept: Female Reproduction
Reference: Ward, S. L., & Hisley, S. M. (2016). Maternal-child nursing care. 2nd ed. Philadelphia: F.A. Davis.

80. **ANSWER: 1, 3, 4**
Rationale
1. Open-glottis pushing and self-directed pushing are more effective, decrease fatigue, enhance confidence and comfort, and result in less time actively pushing.
2. The use of closed-glottis pushing triggers the Valsalva maneuver and increases intrathoracic pressure, which decreases maternal blood flow and placental perfusion.
3. The use of a birthing ball simulates the action of squatting.
4. This urge to push assists with the expulsion of the fetus.
5. FHR should be assessed every 15 minutes in the second stage of this low-risk patient.
TEST-TAKING TIP: Review the maternal positioning and care during the second stage of labor if you answered this question incorrectly.
Content Area: Process of Labor and Birth
Integrated Process: Nursing Process—Intervention
Client Need: Physiological Integrity; Physiological Adaptation
Cognitive Level: Analysis
Concept: Pregnancy
References: Lowdermilk, D. L., Perry, S. E., Cashion, K., & Alden, K. R. (2016). Maternity & women's health care. 11th ed. St. Louis, MO: Elsevier.

81. **ANSWER: 4**
Rationales
1. Meconium stools are thick, greenish to black in color. They are an expected finding in a newborn and aid in ridding the body of bilirubin, thus preventing jaundice.
2. This is called *milia,* which is a normal finding in a newborn and will go away without treatment.
3. Umbilical hernias are common in newborns and are seen at the umbilicus as soft, painless protrusions that often go away without surgical intervention.
4. Discharge from the umbilicus is abnormal and could be a sign of infection; this should be reported to the practitioner for further investigation.
TEST-TAKING TIP: Recognize the normal and abnormal findings associated with newborn assessment and signs of possible infection.
Content Area: Newborns
Integrated Process: Nursing Process—Evaluation
Client Need: Physiological Integrity; Reduction of Risk Potential
Cognitive Level: Analysis
Concept: Critical Thinking
References: Ward, S. L., & Hisley, S. M. (2009). Maternal-child nursing care: Optimizing outcomes for mothers, children & families. Philadelphia: F.A. Davis.

82. **ANSWER: 2**
Rationale
1. Dairy products such as yogurt, cheese, and milk interfere with the absorption of iron in the body.

2. Vitamin C (ascorbic acid) assists the absorption of iron.
3. Taking an iron supplement with food may decrease how much iron is absorbed by the body by up to 50%.
4. Avoid drinking tea or wine within 30 to 45 minutes of taking iron supplements. The tannin in both these drinks can bind iron, which prevents iron absorption in the stomach.
TEST-TAKING TIP: Iron is absorbed best on an empty stomach. Yet, iron supplements can cause stomach cramps, nausea, and diarrhea in some people. You may need to take iron with a small amount of food to avoid this problem. Remember if a client is having trouble with their stomach after taking an iron supplement, the nurse should advise against eating high-fiber foods, such as whole grains, raw vegetables, and bran, and foods or drinks with caffeine with their iron supplement.
Content Area: Iron; Maternal Nutrition
Integrated Process: Nursing Process—Teaching/Learning
Client Need: Health Promotion and Maintenance; Health Promotion; Disease Prevention
Cognitive Level: Application
Concept: Hematologic Regulation
Reference: Ward, S. L., & Hisley, S. M. (2016). Maternal-child nursing care. 2nd ed. Philadelphia: F.A. Davis.

83. **ANSWER: 2**
Rationale
1. If healing appropriately, there should be no drainage.
2. If healing appropriately, the wound edges should be well approximated.
3. If healing appropriately, there should be no bruising.
4. If healing appropriately, the wound area should not be swollen or red.
TEST-TAKING TIP: The acronym REEDA is often used to assess an episiotomy or laceration of the perineum. REEDA stands for redness, edema, ecchymosis, discharge, approximation.
Content Area: Episiotomy; Nursing Care of the Postpartum Woman
Integrated Process: Nursing Process—Assessment
Client Need: Health Promotion and Maintenance
Cognitive Level: Analysis
Concept: Pregnancy
Reference: London, M. L., Ladewig, P. A., Davidson, M. R., Ball, J. W., Bindler, R. C., & Cowen, K. J. (2014). Maternal & child nursing care. 4th ed. New Jersey: Pearson.

84. **ANSWER: 2, 4, 5**
Rationale
1. Possible indication of a hypertensive disorder, such as pre-eclampsia. Pre-eclampsia does not develop until after 20 weeks.
2. Possible indication of hyperemesis gravidarum.
3. Fetal movement is not felt until the second trimester.
4. Possible indication of urinary tract infection.
5. Possible indication of threatened abortion or urinary tract infection.
TEST-TAKING TIP: All the choices are danger signs during pregnancy. However, the question asked for the danger signs during the first trimester.

Content Area: Education Related to Danger Signs During Pregnancy; Prenatal Care
Integrated Process: Nursing Process—Implementation
Client Needs: Health Promotion and Maintenance; Health Promotion; Disease Prevention
Cognitive Level: Application
Concept: Prenatal
Reference: *Lowdermilk, D. L., Perry, S. E., Cashion, K., & Alden, K. R. (2016). Maternity & women's health care. 11th ed. St. Louis, MO: Elsevier.*

85. **ANSWER: 2**
Rationale
1. In mild, or grade 1, abruptions, abdominal tenderness is absent, there are no FHR changes, and estimated blood loss (EBL) is less than 500 mL.
2. Moderate, or grade 2, abruptions are characterized by abdominal tenderness, changes in FHR, and EBL of 1,000 to 1,500 mL. In addition, the woman will begin to show signs of mild shock.
3. Grade 3 is a severe abruption with greater than 50% separation, constant tearing, knifelike pain, rigid abdomen, dark vaginal bleeding greater than 1,500 mL, low blood pressure, and pronounced tachycardia.
4. Severe is a type of abruption and recorded as Grade 3 not Grade 4.
TEST-TAKING TIP: Answers 3 and 4 can be eliminated immediately because those are not accurate descriptions of placental abruption degrees. If part of the answer is incorrect, then all of it is incorrect.
Content Area: Labor and Birth at Risk—Placenta-Related Complications
Integrated Process: Nursing Process—Assessment
Client Need: Physiological Integrity
Cognitive Level: Application
Concept: Pregnancy
Reference: *Durham, R. F., & Chapman, L. (2014). Maternal-newborn nursing: The critical components of nursing care. 2nd ed. Philadelphia: F.A. Davis.*

86. **ANSWER: 4**
Rationale
1. Human chorionic somatomammotropin does not affect labor onset.
2. Human chorionic gonadotropin does not affect labor onset.
3. Progesterone maintains the pregnancy. A decrease in progesterone, not an increase, occurs before the onset of labor.
4. Estrogen increases contractility and increases prior to the onset of labor.
TEST-TAKING TIP: Review the four major hormones of pregnancy and their functions if you were unable to answer the question correctly.
Content Area: Maternal Newborn
Integrated Process: Physiological Integrity; Physiological Adaptation
Client Need: Health Promotion and Maintenance
Cognitive Level: Comprehension
Concept: Pregnancy
Reference: *Lowdermilk, D. L., Perry, S. E., Cashion, K., & Alden, K. R. (2016). Maternity & women's health care. 11th ed. St. Louis, MO: Elsevier*

87. **ANSWER: 1, 2, 5**
Rationale
1. Substance abuse, including alcohol, puts the patient at risk of abruption.
2. Hypertension during pregnancy is a risk factor for abruption.
3. Preterm labor is not a risk factor.
4. Obesity is not a risk factor for placental abruption.
5. Trauma resulting from intimate partner violence is a risk factor for abruption.
TEST-TAKING TIP: It is important for the nurse to recognize the risk factors for placental abruption.
Content Area: Placental Abruption; Antepartum at Risk
Integrated Process: Nursing Process—Assessment
Client Need: Health Promotion and Maintenance; Health Screening
Cognitive Level: Application
Concept: Perfusion
Reference: *Association of Women's Health, Obstetric and Neonatal Nurses; K. R. Simpson, & P. A. Creehan (Eds.). (2014). Perinatal nursing. 4th ed. Philadelphia: Wolters Kluwer Health Lippincott Williams & Wilkins; Lowdermilk, D. L., Perry, S. E., Cashion, K., & Alden, K. R. (2016). Maternity & women's health care. 11th ed. St. Louis, MO: Elsevier.*

88. **ANSWER: 3**
Rationale
1. Multiparity is a predisposing factor.
2. Preterm labor is not a predisposing factor.
3. Uterine surgery for fibroids is a predisposing factor.
4. Family history is not a predisposing factor.
TEST-TAKING TIP: Remember predisposing factors for abnormal placental attachment include previous cesarean delivery, previous uterine surgery, fibroids or other endometrial defects, advanced maternal age, placenta previa, or multiparity.
Content Area: Postpartum Complications
Integrated Process: Nursing Process—Assessment
Client Need: Physiological Integrity
Cognitive Level: Comprehension
Concept: Pregnancy
Reference: *Ward, S. L., & Hisley, S. M. (2016). Maternal-child nursing care. 2nd ed. Philadelphia: F.A. Davis.*

89. **ANSWER: 3, 4, 5**
Rationale
1. A term delivery is not a risk factor for birth trauma.
2. Having a scheduled cesarean section is not a risk factor for birth trauma.
3. A mother with cephalopelvic disproportion is a known maternal risk factor for birth trauma because it will be difficult to deliver the baby.
4. Delivery postdates is a known risk factor for birth trauma.
5. Delivery of a preterm baby is known to cause birth trauma.
6. Having a prolonged labor, not short labor, is a risk factor for birth trauma.
TEST-TAKING TIP: Recall the maternal factors that can cause birth trauma and lead to physical injury of the newborn. Some of these injuries may require intervention.
Content Area: Newborn
Integrated Process: Teaching/Learning; Nursing Process—Analysis

Client Need: Health Promotion and Maintenance; Health Screening
Cognitive Level: Synthesis
Concept: Safety
References: Chapman, L., & Durham, R. (2010). Maternal-newborn nursing: The critical components of nursing care. Philadelphia: F.A. Davis.

90. **ANSWER: 2**
    Rationale
    1. Current data on use of oral contraception and risk of lower- and upper-genital-tract infection and sequelae are inconsistent.
    2. Preventive measures include abstinence and consistent use of barrier methods of birth control (e.g., condoms, diaphragms, and vaginal spermicides).
    3. Women who use IUDs are probably at increased risk of pelvic inflammatory disease (PID) that may not be STI-related.
    4. The hormones in the patch are the same hormones as in the birth control pill—estrogen and progestin—and are not effective in preventing PID.
    TEST-TAKING TIP: Read each answer to determine if it is a correct preventative measure for PID.
    Content Area: Sexually Transmitted Infections
    Integrated Process: Nursing Process—Planning
    Client Need: Health Promotion and Maintenance
    Cognitive Level: Comprehension
    Concept: Sexuality
    Reference: Centers for Disease Control and Prevention (2015). Sexually Transmitted Disease. Retrieved from www.cdc.gov/std/; Pellico, L. H. (2013). Focus on adult health medical-surgical nursing. Philadelphia: Lippincott Williams and Wilkins.

91. **ANSWER: 1, 2, 4**
    Rationale
    1. Priority assessments immediately after the administration of an epidural include checking maternal vital signs for hypotension.
    2. The FHR is also a high-priority assessment.
    3. The patient will have limited mobility after the epidural, and ambulation is not encouraged or possible due to the effect of the anesthetic.
    4. The patient is initially placed in a supine position with a wedge under her right hip to prevent maternal supine hypotension.
    5. Priority assessments immediately after the administration of an epidural include checking maternal vital signs for hypotension and respiratory rate and effort for possible high spinal block.
    TEST-TAKING TIP: Review the effects of neuraxial anesthesia, including side effects. Recall priority interventions performed during neuraxial anesthesia.
    Content Area: Epidural; Nursing Care During Labor and Birth
    Integrated Process: Nursing Process—Analysis
    Client Need: Physiological Integrity; Pharmacological and Parenteral Therapies
    Cognitive Level: Application
    Concept: Pregnancy
    Reference: Lowdermilk, D. L., Perry, S. E., Cashion, K., & Alden, K. R. (2016). Maternity & women's health care. 11th ed. St. Louis, MO: Elsevier.

92. **ANSWER: 1**
    Rationale
    1. Hemorrhage resulting from disseminated intravascular coagulation characterizes the second stage of amniotic fluid embolism and is the ultimate cause of maternal death.
    2. Hypoxia presents in the first stage.
    3. Capillary damage also presents in the first stage.
    4. Immune modulator release is the first response to fetal cell presence in maternal circulation.
    TEST-TAKING TIP: It is difficult to remember processes with multiple steps. In this case it would be easier to remember the two-component second stage of amniotic fluid embolism. Then the first-stage factors could be identified by process of elimination.
    Content Area: Labor and Birth at Risk—Amniotic Fluid Embolism
    Integrated Process: Nursing Process—Assessment
    Client Need: Physiological Integrity
    Cognitive Level: Application
    Concept: Pregnancy
    Reference: Durham, R. F., & Chapman, L. (2014). Maternal-newborn nursing: The critical components of nursing care. 2nd ed. Philadelphia: F.A. Davis.

93. **ANSWER: 3**
    Rationale
    1. The woman should use soap and warm water when washing her perineum.
    2. The peri-pad should be changed with every void and bowel movement.
    3. Peri-pads should be applied from front to back.
    4. The peri-bottle should be used to rinse her perineum after every void.
    TEST-TAKING TIP: Proper perineal care is important in preventing infection of the episiotomy, bladder, and uterus. Proper hand washing is an important aspect in the prevention of infection. The nurse must also instruct the woman to always wash her hands thoroughly before and after going to the bathroom or changing a sanitary pad.
    Content Area: Perineal Care; Nursing Care of the Postpartum Woman
    Integrated Process: Nursing Process—Intervention
    Client Need: Health Promotion and Maintenance
    Cognitive Level: Application
    Concept: Pregnancy
    Reference: Perry, S. E., Hockenberry, M. F., Lowdermilk, D. L., & Wilson, D. (2014). Maternal child nursing care. 5th ed. St. Louis, MO: Elsevier

94. **ANSWER: 1**
    Rationale
    1. Tubal ligation is the surgical procedure to interrupt the patency of the fallopian tubes.
    2. It's possible to reverse a tubal ligation, but reversal requires major surgery and isn't always effective.
    3. The client can have sexual intercourse as soon as she feels like it and it does not cause pain, which is usually 1 week after surgery.
    4. Tubal ligation is a surgical procedure consisting of severance and/or burning of fallopian tubes, not removing them.

TEST-TAKING TIP: Tubal ligation is performed by either inserting a needle or making an incision just under the navel so the abdomen can be inflated with gas (carbon dioxide or nitrous oxide). Then a laparoscope is inserted into the abdomen.
Content Area: Operative Sterilization; Contraception
Integrated Process: Nursing Process—Evaluation
Client Need: Physiological Integrity
Cognitive Level: Analysis
Concept: Female Reproduction
Reference: Ward, S. L., & Hisley, S. M. (2016). Maternal-child nursing care. 2nd ed. Philadelphia: F.A. Davis.

95. **ANSWER: 1**
Rationale
1. The correct response is G4 T1 P1 A1 L3 (4-1-1-1-3). This woman is a gravida 4, which includes the current pregnancy, the miscarriage, her daughter, and her sons. Remember twins count as one G.
Her para is broken down as follows:
T = 1 for her daughter born at 38 weeks.
P = 1 for her twins who were born at 35 weeks. Remember twins count as one P.
A = 1 for her miscarriage at 10 weeks.
L = 3 for live children: 1 daughter and 2 sons.
2. Gravida 3 is incorrect. In determining the gravida the current pregnancy must always be included.
3. Preterm is incorrect. Twins count as one preterm pregnancy.
4. The gravida and preterm are incorrect in this calculation.
TEST-TAKING TIP: Recall that G (gravida) is the total number of pregnancies, including the present one. The length of gestation, the outcome (live birth or not), or the number of fetuses (single, twin, etc.) does not affect this number.
Para, the number of deliveries, is subdivided into TPAL.
T = delivery between 37 and 42 weeks.
P = delivery between 20 and 37 weeks.
A = delivery before 20 weeks, miscarriage, ectopic pregnancy, induced abortion.
L = living children. Review gravida, para, and GTPAL if you answered this question incorrectly.
Content Area: Process of Labor and Birth
Integrated Process: Nursing Process—Assessment
Client Need: Health Promotion and Maintenance
Cognitive Level: Analysis
Concept: Pregnancy
Reference: Lowdermilk, D. L., Perry, S. E., Cashion, K., & Alden, K. R. (2016). Maternity & women's health care. 11th ed. St. Louis, MO: Elsevier.

96. **ANSWER: 3**
Rationale
1. There is no increased incidence of infection or hydramnios.
2. Hydramnios (or polyhydramnios) is diagnosed when the amniotic fluid amount is greater than 2,000 mL. Postpartum hemorrhage is a risk in women who have an overdistended uterus, which would occur in this case.
3. The patient is not at risk for hypotension.
4. Diabetes may have caused the hydramnios but will not be caused by it.

TEST-TAKING TIP: Review the causes and untoward effects of an overdistended uterus if you were unable to answer the question correctly.
Content Area: Hemorrhage; Nursing Care During Labor and Birth
Integrated Process: Nursing Process—Analysis
Client Need: Physiological Integrity; Reduction of Risk Potential
Cognitive Level: Analysis
Concept: Pregnancy
Reference: Lowdermilk, D. L., Perry, S. E., Cashion, K., & Alden, K. R. (2016). Maternity & women's health care. 11th ed. St. Louis, MO: Elsevier.

97. **ANSWER: 2**
Rationale
1. St. John's wort will decrease the effects.
2. Aspirin may increase bleeding.
3. Cranberry will decrease the effects.
4. Antidepressants are contraindicated because of the risk of increasing the effects of anticoagulants.
TEST-TAKING TIP: Aspirin is an antiplatelet agent and prevents blood from clotting. Taking it will prolong blood clotting and increase bleeding.
Content Area: Postpartum Complications
Integrated Process: Nursing Process—Implementation
Client Need: Physiological Integrity: Reduction of Risk Potential
Cognitive Level: Application
Concept: Pregnancy
Reference: Lowdermilk, D. L., Perry, S. E., Cashion, K., & Alden, K. R. (2016). Maternity & Women's Health Care. 11th ed. St. Louis, MO: Elsevier.

98. **ANSWER: 4**
Rationale
1. Periodic breathing lasting 3 to 5 seconds is normal in the newborn. Apnea lasting 15 to 20 seconds would be concerning and require immediate intervention.
2. Blood sugar levels of 60 mg/dL is a normal finding.
3. These blue-green discolorations are Mongolian spots or macular spots that are common in certain ethnicities.
4. Asymmetrical chest movement may indicate pneumothorax or diaphragmatic hernia and requires immediate intervention.
TEST-TAKING TIP: Recall the normal and abnormal findings of a newborn assessment.
Content Area: Newborns at Risk
Integrated Process: Nursing Process—Assessment
Client Need: Physiological Integrity; Physiological Adaptation; Medical Emergencies
Cognitive Level: Synthesis
Concept: Critical Thinking
Reference: Ward, S. L., & Hisley, S.M. (2009). Maternal-child nursing care: Optimizing outcomes for mothers, children & families. Philadelphia: F.A. Davis.

99. **ANSWER: 1**
Rationale
1. In a preterm infant, the labia minora and clitoris will be larger than the labia majora.
2. A full-term infant is expected to have plantar creases on two-thirds of the foot.
3. In a full-term infant, lanugo should have bald areas.

4. Ear recoil in a full-term infant should be instant with thick cartilage or stiffness.

TEST-TAKING TIP: Recall normal findings in a preterm infant upon physical exam.

Content Area: Newborns
Integrated Process: Nursing Process—Assessment
Client Need: Physiological Integrity; Reduction of Risk Potential; System Specific Assessments
Cognitive Level: Analysis
Concept: Assessment
Reference: *Ward, S. L., & Hisley, S.M. (2009). Maternal-child nursing care: Optimizing outcomes for mothers, children & families. Philadelphia: F.A. Davis.*

100. ANSWER: 3
Rationale
1. Drug use in pregnancy does not explain why the newborn has these markings.

2. The nurse is speculating that abuse occurred when these markings can be indicative of a soft tissue injury occurring during the delivery process.
3. Soft tissue injuries can result in skin changes such as bruising, petechiae, abrasions, lacerations, and edema.
4. Blue/gray macules, or Mongolian spots, typically appear on the buttocks area.

TEST-TAKING TIP: Recall the reason for soft tissue injuries of the newborn.

Content Area: Newborn
Integrated Process: Caring; Nursing Process—Evaluation
Client Need: Physiological Integrity; Physiological Adaptation; Unexpected Responses to Therapies
Cognitive Level: Synthesis
Concept: Critical Thinking
References: *Chapman, L., & Durham, R. (2010). Maternal-newborn nursing: The critical components of nursing care. Philadelphia: F.A. Davis.*

Putting It All Together Case Study Answers

Chapter 1

1. Julia's growth is within normal limits according to Centers for Disease Control and Prevention (CDC) charts. Her body mass index (BMI) is approximately in the 20% percentile. Her vital signs are within expected parameters. She has been involved in sports, so would appear to get adequate physical activity. However, it would be important to review her prior medical records to ensure normal growth patterns. She should receive the meningococcal (MCV4) vaccine if she has not yet received it and verify that a Tdap booster is up-to-date. It is Julia's choice to receive the human papillomavirus (HPV) vaccine, but the nurse should provide standardized literature regarding the facts and purpose for the vaccine.

2. Though blood work is not usually included in typical teen physical checkups, her complaints of heavier menses and increased discomfort did warrant the Hgb and HCT measurement. Her results are on the low side of normal, though she is not clinically anemic. It would be good for the nurse to review her diet and eating patterns and offer suggestions for increasing her dietary intake of iron. Many young women do not get adequate amounts of iron or calcium; both are important as she enters her 20s and future childbearing years.

   It is not possible to relate the heavier menses to her test results without getting more specific information about the heavier menstrual flow. Questions such as "How many days does your period last?" "How many pads or tampons do you need on your heavier days?" will elicit more information for the nurse to determine if further assessment is needed in regard to heavy menstrual bleeding. Questions regarding the pain and other physical symptoms will help the nurse determine if there may be cause for greater concern. Additional assessment of Julia's complaints would determine whether the symptoms are likely due to premenstrual syndrome, dysmenorrhea, or a combination of these two conditions. The nurse can explain in simple terms how Julia's hormones and reproductive anatomy contribute to her symptoms.

3. The nurse can share that many women experience the symptoms associated with normal cyclical changes in the female body. Some recommendations would be to limit sodium (salt) and caffeine intake in the week prior to her menses, continue her exercise routines, consume plenty of water, and keep a routine sleep schedule. Some women find that taking vitamin B_6 and vitamin E supplements can help with the cramping. In addition to over-the-counter pain medications (e.g., NSAIDs), warm packs to the sacral and pelvic regions, or a warm bath or shower may offer relief.

   According to the American Congress of Obstetricians and Gynecologists (ACOG; www.acog.org/Resources-And-Publications/Committee-Opinions/Committee-on-Gynecologic-Practice/Well-Woman-Visit), an annual physical exam for young women under age 21 should not include a pelvic exam unless there are concerning symptoms involving the genitals or rectum. An external exam by a trained examiner offers the opportunity to further assess and provide education for the young woman. Breast self-examination teaching is not recommended at this age (American Cancer Society; www.cancer.org/cancer/breastcancer/moreinformation/breastcancer earlydetection/breast-cancer-early-detection-acs-recs-bse). As the possibility for becoming sexually active increases with age, the nurse should ask if Julia has any questions related to pregnancy and sexually transmitted infection protection, and offer resources.

Chapter 2

1. Subjective symptoms include irregular menses, acne, hair loss, male pattern hair growth, failure to conceive. Objective symptoms include acne, male pattern hair growth, overweight, acanthosis nigricans, skin tags. Assessment findings are consistent with a diagnosis of polycystic ovary syndrome (PCOS) with insulin resistance. Lifestyle changes are considered the first line of treatment for PCOS.

2. Provide instructions for obtaining diagnostic labs and ultrasound. Collection of sperm for sperm analysis

should follow 2 to 3 days of abstinence. The sample should be collected by masturbation in a clean container and delivered to the laboratory within 1 hour. Client laboratories to be drawn following an overnight fast and on the third day of the menstrual cycle.

The nurse should provide education on lifestyle modifications to maximize reproductive health, such as eating healthy, getting regular exercise, controlling weight, avoiding heat to scrotum, avoiding substance use (including alcohol and tobacco), managing stress, avoiding exposure to environmental toxins, taking folic acid supplements, timing of intercourse, and using water-soluble lubricants.

The nurse should also complete a psychosocial assessment to determine cultural, religious, psychological, and financial factors impacting the treatment plan for this client and her partner.

3. The client and partner should complete diagnostic testing and should verbalize their understanding of how lifestyle impacts reproductive health.

Chapter 3

1. Yes, Richard can be a carrier. Because his sister had cystic fibrosis (CF), his parents both must be carriers. Richard has a two in four chance he will not have cystic fibrosis but will be a carrier (by inheriting a CF gene from one parent but the normal gene from the other parent).

2. There would not be any chance their child would have CF. To have an autosomal recessive disorder, a child must inherit two mutated genes, one from each parent. Autosomal recessive disorders are passed on by two carriers. The carrier's health is rarely affected because they have one mutated gene (recessive gene) and one normal gene (dominant gene) for the condition.

3. If two people carry the CF gene and have a child, there is a one in four chance that the child will have CF (by inheriting the CF gene from both parents); a two in four chance that the child will not have CF but will be a carrier (by inheriting a CF gene from one parent but the normal gene from the other parent); a one in four chance that the child will not have CF and will not be a carrier (by inheriting the normal gene from both parents).

4.

Father's alleles

	C	c
C	CC	Cc
c	Cc	cc

(Mother's alleles)

Explanation: The possible offspring outcomes for parents who are both carriers of a CF gene mutation.
n = normal allele
C = allele with CF mutation
In this example, each child would have a:
25% chance of being unaffected with CF (CC).
50% chance of being a carrier of CF (Cn).
25% chance of being affected with CF (nn).

5.

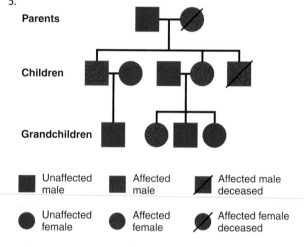

■ Unaffected male	■ Affected male
● Unaffected female	● Affected female

Affected male deceased
Affected female deceased

6. The nurse is responsible for educating the parents on the inheritance possibility when both parents carry the mutated recessive gene. The nurse should also provide education and emotional support to include the nature of CF, extent of risk, and consequences if the child inherits the disorder; discuss options available, including genetic testing and continuing or not continuing the pregnancy if the child is affected; discuss use of reproductive technology or adoption; be sensitive to cultural and religious beliefs; encourage expression of feelings; and refer the couple for further counseling or support groups.

Chapter 4

1. Anxiety
2. Forty-pound increase in weight from prepregnancy weight; anxiety as evidenced by the patient expressing anxiety, relaxed facial expression, stable vital signs, ability to concentrate and interact with others
3. Risk for complicated *grieving* related to loss of prior pregnancy; risk for *powerlessness* related to situational crisis; *anxiety* related to unknown pregnancy outcome.
4. The nurse should assess for level of anxiety; maternal vital signs and maternal temperature postprocedure; baseline fetal heart rate before and after procedure; and uterine contractions. The nurse should also administer RhoD immune globulin (RhoGAM) and educate mother about its need. Educate patient regarding the inheritance pattern of cystic fibrosis. If she is not a carrier, then the baby will have no chance of inheriting the disease but may become a carrier. After the

amniocentesis is complete and patient's anxiety is diminished, discuss need for dietary changes.
5. Patient is able to identify stressors and methods of coping; absence of signs of infection, as evidenced by no maternal fever and no fetal tachycardia; absence of uterine contractions; the patient understands the method of inheritance for cystic fibrosis; anxiety is decreased and patient would benefit from dietary teaching. This should be reinforced at the next prenatal visit.

Chapter 5

1. The client is actively seeking a reliable birth control method. She has a boyfriend but is not considering marriage at this time. She would have difficulty remembering scheduled birth control methods because of her busy schedule.
2. Vital signs are normal. She has an appropriate weight for her height. All general assessments are within normal limits. Pelvic exam and Pap smear are also normal.
3. An intrauterine device (IUD) may be the best choice for this client.
4. The IUD is placed by the health care provider (HCP) and is left in place for an extended length of time (3 to 10 years, depending on the type of IUD). The effectiveness rate is around 98% to 99% and is recommended for women who have never been pregnant, adolescents, and women who have children. It may be inserted anytime during the menstrual cycle.

Chapter 6

1. Her periods have been regular until recently, when she noted some "spotting between periods."
2. The cervix appears inflamed, bleeds easily with swab insertion for diagnostic testing, and there is a purulent discharge coming from the cervical opening. NAAT for *Chlamydia trachomatis* is positive.
3. Knowledge is deficient related to sexually transmitted infections (STIs) and transmission.
4. She should refer her sex partners for evaluation, testing, and treatment (chlamydia is often asymptomatic in men and women). She should abstain from intercourse until she and her sex partners have completed treatment. Discuss individual risk reduction and prevention strategies, including abstinence, monogamy, and condoms (condoms, when used consistently and correctly, can reduce the risk of chlamydia transmission). If a hormonal contraceptive method is prescribed, inform the patient that these methods of birth control offer no protection from STIs and HIV infection. Effective treatment of chlamydia may reduce HIV transmission and susceptibility.
5. A repeat chlamydia test returned positive. The client stated that her partner went to get tested, but the test result was negative, so he was not treated. She began to use condoms consistently and correctly to reduce the risk of transmission.

Chapter 7

1. Breast cancer risk factors for Judy include female, age, race, family history that includes first-degree relatives diagnosed with breast cancer, early onset menarche, high BMI.
2. Diagnostic ultrasound and fine-needle biopsy.
3. Surveillance: Women at high risk benefit from additional screening. Yearly mammography beginning at age 25 years, clinical breast exam performed twice yearly, MRI, and ultrasound. Chemoprevention is the main method used to prevent this disease. Both Tamoxifen and Raloxifene (Evista) are currently used as chemo preventative agents in high-risk women. Prophylactic mastectomy may be used as a primary prevention strategy and has been shown to reduce breast cancer by 90%. Prophylactic mastectomy consists of a total mastectomy (removal of breast tissue only) followed by breast reconstruction if desired. Candidates for this procedure include women with a strong family history of breast cancer, women with a diagnosis of lobular carcinoma in situ, women with atypical hyperplasia, women found to have a mutation in the BRCA gene, and women with a history of a previous breast cancer in one breast.

Chapter 8

1. Irregular periods, only one every 3 months; unable to conceive a child after 2 years; tearful; does not understand the diagnosis of PCOS
2. BMI of 32 (obese); blood pressure is elevated 140/90 mm Hg; skin is pale and dry; hirsutism; acne; elevated fasting glucose higher than 200; elevated triglycerides
3. (1) Infertility related to obesity: The nurse should ensure the client is aware that weight loss can improve fertility. A weight-loss plan should be developed with the client that includes both diet changes and an exercise plan. Exercise should start with 3 days per week and slowly increase to 5 days per week. Encouraging her to keep a food diary can help improve accountability as she begins her lifestyle modifications.
(2) Knowledge deficit: The client stated she did not understand the diagnosis of PCOS and was visibly upset by the confirmation of the diagnosis by the HCP. The nurse should assess the client's learning needs and prioritize them prior to client teaching. The client will not be able to retain all information in one visit. An alternative would be giving resources for her to explore and making a follow-up visit to reassess her knowledge.

(3) Risk for type 2 diabetes: The client has an elevated fasting glucose (210) and elevated triglycerides. Obesity can cause an increased glucose level as well as insulin resistance and hyperinsulinemia. All these factors can contribute to the development of type 2 diabetes. The nurse should reinforce the weight management plan and discuss how weight loss can reverse the insulin resistance and hyperinsulinemia and improve fertility. The client was also started on Glucophage. An explanation of the benefits of Glucophage in lowering the blood glucose and the potential side effects should be discussed.

4. (1) Causes an increase in the frequency of ovulation and menstruation and therefore an increase in fertility; (2) lowers lipids, which will decrease the risk of cardiovascular disease; (3) increases glucose metabolism and decrease hyperinsulinemia; (4) decreases androgen levels, which decreases clinical features of hyperandrogenemia (hirsutism, acne, male-patterned baldness) and increases the frequency of ovulation and menstruation, which then increases fertility.

Chapter 9

1. Continuing to travel throughout the pregnancy will depend on the time spent inactive during travel and the mode of transportation. She should be taught about the increased risk for blood clot formation for any pregnant woman. Moving around every hour during a flight will help, as will wearing nonbinding compression socks or stockings. Traveling long distances away from the primary HCP from weeks 28 to 36 may not be wise; the risk of delivering a preterm infant in an unfamiliar place is a consideration, but not necessarily prohibitive. Some health care providers may discourage plane travel during the last month of pregnancy. The law requires that reasonable accommodations be afforded pregnant women in the workplace. At some point, she should meet with a company representative to discuss a modified travel schedule and distance meeting alternatives. She should discuss her status with her HCP at each prenatal visit.

2. Most women find that they become less fatigued toward the end of the first trimester, at 12 to 14 weeks. Until then, she should plan rest periods when possible during the day. Pace activities and avoid becoming overtired. Keep well hydrated with 8 to 10 glasses of fluid per day, avoiding caffeine use for stimulation.

3. Any exercise that the woman is used to and enjoys may be acceptable. However, exercise that requires exceptional balance or risks falls should be avoided. The nurse can explain the musculoskeletal changes that affect center of gravity as the pregnancy progresses. Ms. Chang should understand that the changes in joint flexibility related to ligament softening may require some adjusting in her routines to prevent injury. Good warm-up and cool-down periods will help exercise to be safe and effective.

4. The fluid recommendation does not change due to trying to limit trips to the bathroom. She can make sure that she is wearing comfortable nonrestrictive clothing. It may help to plan fluid intake during times when she has more flexibility to excuse herself to a restroom (e.g., not during a 2-hour meeting).

5. As previously stated, her pregnancy is currently low risk. She should be told about the recommended prenatal visit schedule. It is important for her to know that there is still a slight risk of spontaneous miscarriage. If she has any concerns, a 24-hour triage number should be provided. Her risk during the next trimester will relate to her travel and normal hypercoagulopathy of pregnancy. Optimal fluid intake, regular activity, and promoting lower-extremity circulation will help reduce the possibility of deep vein thrombosis.

6. So far, it appears that she is following typical recommendations—small, frequent meals consisting of foods that are familiar, palatable favorites for her. Getting plenty of rest will give her body the energy to make the changes associated with the pregnancy.

7. During the first trimester, unless the woman cannot keep down any nourishment, the ideal balance of nutrients is not deleterious. As her appetite returns and she desires a wider variety of foods, nutrient needs should be met. If needed, a dietitian consult might be suggested.

8. The health and reproductive history results indicate that there are no apparent historical factors that place her in a high-risk pregnancy category. The symptoms she describes are common for the first trimester of pregnancy. The nurse can reassure Ms. Chang that so far, her pregnancy appears to be within expectations.

Chapter 10

1. Gravida 3, para 2; gravida 3, term 2, preterm 0, abortions 1, living 2

2. Last menstrual period: June 1, 2015
   Minus 3 months plus 7 days: March 8
   Adjust the year: March 8, 2016

3. 10 weeks

4. Amenorrhea, nausea, fatigue, breast tenderness

5. Goodell's sign and Chadwick's sign

6. Menstrual period: menarche, regularity, frequency, duration of menses; medical history: past illnesses, surgeries, and current prescribed medications, over-the-counter medications, or herbal supplements; family history to also include family history

of pregnancies; genetic history; domestic violence screening; assess for tobacco, alcohol, drug use; depression screening

7. First the nurse should explain that a pelvic exam is done for evaluation of uterine size. Palpation of the pelvic contents is done to identify any abnormal masses or tumors. A Pap smear will be done if the patient has not had one in a year. A Pap smear checks for abnormal cervical cells. Cervical cultures will be taken to check for diseases that can infect the fetus during birth.

  The nurse should instruct the patient to empty her bladder so she is more comfortable. It is easier for the examiner to evaluate the size of the uterus when the bladder is empty. Have the patient remove her clothing and put on a patient gown. Allow for privacy while changing. The patient should be positioned on the exam table in the lithotomy position with a drape to cover her.

8. Blood typing: determines the client's blood type, Rh type, and antibody factor.
  Antibody screen: detects unusual antibodies that may have arisen in a prior pregnancy or from a blood transfusion.
  CBC (complete blood count): test the client's blood to determine if anemic. Women usually become slightly anemic as the pregnancy progresses, but very low levels of iron will need to be treated. Platelet levels are also assessed.
  Rubella test (German measles): an antibody test to determine if protected from rubella. If nonimmune, a vaccination will be given during the postpartum period before discharge.
  Syphilis screening (RPR/VDRL): tests for exposure to syphilis. If present, treatment can be initiated so that the fetus is not harmed.
  Hepatitis B (HBSAG): checks for infection with the hepatitis B virus, which can be passed to an unborn child.
  HIV: test for the AIDS virus will be offered. This test is recommended for all women at the first prenatal visit. It is very important for the nurse to educate the patient that if she has HIV infection, it can be treated during pregnancy. This treatment will reduce the chances of passing the virus to their unborn child.
  Cystic fibrosis carrier screening: screening should be offered to all couples regardless of ethnicity. Genetic counseling is recommended for individuals with a family history of cystic fibrosis or those found to be carriers.
  Hemoglobin electrophoresis: tests for sickle cell anemia and other genetic causes of chronic anemia. Couples at risk for having a child with sickle cell or thalassemia should be offered genetic counseling to review prenatal testing and reproduction options.

9. Stephanie is considered at this time to be a low-risk pregnancy. She should return in 4 weeks.

Chapter 11

1. Amanda offers a history of anxiety and worries that she will "gain a lot of weight during the pregnancy." As you collect her health history, you document a history of mild depression as a teenager treated with therapy and medication. She offers a history of iron deficiency anemia as a child and recalls taking iron tablets daily. She runs about 4 miles daily as her form of exercise. She offers that she has tried a number of diets in the past to keep her weight down and has succeeded. She has been struggling to maintain her current weight of 105 pounds. She says her significant other does not want her to "gain weight." Occasionally feels out of breath and tired during running, but pushes herself to continue her goal. She also states she drinks an "adequate" amount of water.

2. Pulse 50; respiratory rate 16; blood pressure 90/60; height 5´4˝; weight 105 pounds; BMI 18.4; integumentary: skin is cool to the touch, no apparent lesions or aberrations, decreased skin turgor, lips and mucous membranes pink, nail beds pallor; HEENT: hair thinning and short

3. Risk for imbalanced nutrition related to fear of gaining weight. Risk for fluid and electrolyte imbalance related to daily exercising and drinking "adequate" amount of water. Self-concept disturbance (self-image) related to desire to remain same weight during pregnancy.

4. Discuss her needs for a healthy pregnancy and instructions on how to eat healthy, gain an appropriate amount of weight during the pregnancy. Review MyPlate with the patient to ascertain her realistic view on diet and proper nutrition. Anticipate referring to a registered dietitian to maintain a healthy eating regimen. Monitor weight gain at each visit and demonstrate positive reinforcement with successful gain. Anticipate referring to psychosocial secondary to history of depression and possible return of symptoms.

5. Amanda is able to verbalize importance of diet during pregnancy and gaining of weight. She demonstrates successful weight gain during pregnancy with proper fetal growth.

Chapter 12

1. The fetal nonstress test (NST) is a simple, noninvasive test performed in pregnancies over 28 weeks gestation. The test is named "nonstress" because no stress is placed on the fetus during the test. An NST may be performed if there is a decrease in fetal movement, a

reason to suspect inadequate placental functions, or high-risk reason such as gestational diabetes. The test can indicate if the baby is not receiving enough oxygen because of placental or umbilical cord problems; it can also indicate other types of fetal distress. The primary goal of the test is to measure the heart rate of the fetus in response to its own movements. Healthy babies will respond with an increased heart rate during times of movement, and the heart rate will decrease at rest. The concept behind a nonstress test is that adequate oxygen is required for fetal activity and heart rate to be within normal ranges.

2. This fetal tracing would be classified as a nonreactive fetal heart rate. The criteria for a reactive fetal heart rate tracing would be if there are two or more fetal heart rate accelerations within a 20-minute period, with or without fetal movement discernible by the woman. The nonreactive stress test lacks sufficient fetal heart rate accelerations over a 40-minute period.

3. Biophysical profile. The biophysical profile is an NST plus four observations made by real-time ultrasonography. The five components of the biophysical profile are (1) NST; (2) fetal breathing movements—one or more episodes of rhythmic fetal breathing movements of 30 seconds or more within 30 minutes; (3) fetal movement—three or more discrete body or limb movements within 30 minutes; (4) fetal tone—one or more episodes of extension of a fetal extremity with return to flexion, or opening or closing of a hand; and (5) determination of the amniotic fluid volume—a single vertical pocket of amniotic fluid exceeding 2 cm is considered evidence of adequate amniotic fluid.

4. Mrs. Martin should be instructed to count all fetal movements over a specific amount of time and to contact her care provider if a minimum amount of movements are not felt. She should be instructed to lie on her side and count all movements over 1 to 2 hours. If she feels a minimum of four movements in 1 hour, the assessment is reassuring. If fetal movement is decreased, she should be instructed to eat and rest. Mrs. Martin should be taught about factors that may affect fetal activity: exercise, chronic maternal anxiety or stress, smoking, and caffeine use. Mrs. Martin should be instructed how to record fetal movements and when to report concerns to their care providers.

Chapter 13

1. CBC to detect for anemia or other dyscrasias, adequate WBC, and platelet count; blood type to confirm Rh-negative status and to have on file in case transfusion is needed; HIV screening to determine if patient is HIV positive; syphilis testing; gonorrheal culture;

urinalysis and urine culture; varicella and rubella titers to make sure there is immunity (vaccine would not be given at this time, since both are live attenuated viruses, so vaccination postpartum would be recommended); hepatitis B screening to determine if mother is positive; illicit drug screen; Pap smear; sickle screen for women of African American or Latino descent.

2. Nutrition: woman should be given information on four food groups and suggested servings. Recommended increase of 300 kcal/day; recommended weight gain based on her BMI should be discussed. Need to limit sweets and high-fat foods. Need to limit fish high in mercury and abstain from eating raw or undercooked meats to prevent transmission of cytomegalovirus. Discussion of current exercise and if appropriate with care provider. Reinforce need to wear seat belts. Need to abstain from smoking, alcohol, and drugs, including marijuana, throughout pregnancy due to effects on fetus. If patient is currently abusing substances, referral for treatment such as Mom's Quit Connection should be provided.

3. First pregnancy.

4. Abruptio placenta; preterm delivery; hypertension after pregnancy.

5. Patient will need to monitor blood pressure, usually two times a day and record readings. Patient will weigh herself daily at the same time on the same scale. She will report to her doctor an increase of 3 pounds in 1 day or 4 pounds over 3 days. She should report visual changes, headache, upper gastric pain, and difficulty reading. Patient will be told to rest on her left side as much as possible and refrain from strenuous activities. She will be asked to record fetal kick counts and notify the care provider if they decrease. Patient will be told to go for NST at least once a week.

6. The patient's lungs should be assessed at least hourly to detect pulmonary edema. Respiratory rate and level of consciousness should be assessed at least every hour. Vital signs, especially blood pressure, should be monitored continuously. The patient should have urine output measured hourly. Her reflexes should be checked to identify hyper- or hyporeflexia. She should be asked about upper quadrant pain, headache, and visual changes.

7. Notify the physician of the blurred vision and 3 plus urine. In case of impending seizure, make sure suction equipment and oxygen are available. Lower the lights and noise in the room.

Chapter 14

1. Subjective changes include the client reporting irregular uterine contractions every 6 minutes and

complaining of dark bloody mucus since yesterday. The fetus is not considered full term because she is 38 weeks. The client is a primigravida.

2. Objective data include vertex position. The first Leopold's maneuver is performed to determine whether the fetal head or buttocks are positioned in the uterine fundus. The practitioner faces the woman's head and positions the hands on the top and side of the fundus with focus on the upper region. The head feels firm and round and the buttocks feel soft and less defined. The external fetal monitor should be in either the right or left lower quadrant if fetus is in the vertex position. The sterile vaginal exam reveals that the client has cervical change and is in active labor because the client is 4 cm dilated.

3. The nurse should plan for a normal vaginal delivery because no high-risk complications have been noted. She should explore with the client her decision for pain management. The nurse should note that this is the first pregnancy for this client, so anxiety may be a factor throughout her labor and delivery. Client goals should include increased knowledge concerning labor, birth, and active participation.

Chapter 15

1. Complaints of leaking "urine," which may be amniotic fluid; abdominal "tightening," which is assumed to be uterine contractions.

2. Confirmation of premature rupture of membranes with sterile speculum exam, ferning, and use of immunoassay test; presence of uterine contractions via external fetal monitor; preterm labor at 34 weeks evidenced by history and diagnosed by change in cervical status

3. Risk for infection related to possible ruptured amniotic membranes, invasive procedures; anxiety related to threat to fetus; anticipatory grieving related to possibility of birth to preterm infant.

4. Assess maternal temperature, pulse, respirations, and WBC to rule out infection. Closely monitor maternal blood pressure for continued elevation; may consider pre-eclampsia. Assess hydration status and administer IV fluids as ordered. Maintain intake and output. Maintain NPO status. Position patient on side to prevent maternal supine hypotension. Provide continuous external fetal monitoring. Limit vaginal exams to prevent infection. Administer betamethasone to mother to improve fetal lung maturation and other morbidities. Urinalysis and urine culture to rule out urinary tract infection. Determine last dose of levothyroxine. Assess thyroid function status and administer medications as ordered, being mindful of NPO status. Prepare the neonatal intensive care unit for possible admission. Be prepared to

administer RhoGAM if infant is delivered and is Rh positive. Provide physical and emotional support to mother and support person.

5. Patient remains afebrile with vital signs within normal limits. Assessment of blood pressure reveals no further elevation and no other signs of illness. Patient remains well hydrated with urine output exceeding oral/IV intake. Intake and output monitored and charted. Maternal supine hypotension avoided. Patient understands need for proper positioning. Continuous external fetal monitoring to determine fetal heart rate, variability, and decelerations. Assess uterine contractions for frequency, duration, and strength. No signs of infection noted: maternal temp, heart rate, respiratory rate, and WBC count are within normal limits. Fetal heart rate shows no tachycardia. Vaginal exams performed only when clinical picture warrants. Betamethasone administered. Urinalysis shows no signs of infection, and urine culture demonstrates no bacterial growth. Thyroid function studies are within normal limits; medication administered as necessary. Appropriate hospital staff and units prepare for possible admission of newborn. RhoGAM administered if infant is delivered and is Rh positive. Patient and her support person(s) are able to cope with their situation.

Chapter 16

1. The patient has a pain score of 3/10 compared to 0/10 earlier in the day. This may indicate that labor is imminent. The patient also reports that her water has broken.

2. The variable decelerations to the 50s with each contraction. The patient is also now contracting every 3 to 4 minutes compared to every 5 minutes previously.

3. The nurse should be concerned that the variable decelerations with every contraction are indicative of a cord prolapse. This patient has multiple risk factors, including preterm gestation, breech presentation, polyhydramnios, and a high fetal station.

4. Independent: Trendelenburg position, hand-and-knees position, counter pressure on the fetal presenting part. Collaborative: Emergent cesarean section delivery is indicated.

Chapter 17

1. The nurse's priority assessment at this time should be the firmness of uterine fundus and amount of lochia. Her assessment findings of the fundus, lochia, and small clots are normal. It is common for

the lochia to contain small clots, which occur when the lochia has been pooling in the lower uterine segment because of the woman being in a supine position. Small clots (less than the size of a nickel) should be documented in the patient's chart. The nurse should understand that Mrs. Smith is a multipara and she is at a high risk for uterine atony, which could lead to excessive uterine bleeding. A full bladder can impede contraction of the uterus. If the uterus does not contract, then Mrs. Smith has a high risk for excessive bleeding. Since Mrs. Smith has feeling and movement in her leg, then the nurse should help her to the bathroom to void. Care should be taken when getting her out of bed because of orthostatic hypotension. The nurse should assist the woman to a sitting position, then slowly assist her out of the bed. The nurse should explain orthostatic hypotension to Mrs. Smith and instruct her to call for assistance when getting out of bed for the first few times. The nurse should assess Mrs. Smith again in 30 minutes.

2. Mrs. Smith's pain score of 6 out of 10 should be addressed. Pain medication should be administered as ordered by the physician/midwife. Nonpharmacological measures should also be implemented. The nurse can apply an ice pack to the perineum, which can decrease the pain from her repaired laceration. The nurse can fill a plastic bag with crushed ice and wrap the ice pack in a washcloth. She should then place the ice bag in the perineal area for 15 to 20 minutes; remove it for at least 10 minutes before replacing it again. The nurse should understand and provide support and rest during this taking-in phase. During this phase, the mother is focused primarily on her own needs, especially sleeping and eating. She will exhibit a behavior of being passive and dependent. Nursing activities should be planned so that the woman can rest as much as possible. Failure to allow the woman to receive adequate rest may lead to irritability, fatigue, and general interference with the normal restorative process.

The nurse should begin educating Mrs. Smith on how to monitor and assess her uterus for firmness and about the natural process of involution. For heavy bleeding or a boggy uterus, the nurse should instruct Mrs. Smith on how to properly perform fundal massage and to notify the nurse if she experiences heavy bleeding in which she saturates a pad within 1 hour. The nurse should also instruct Mrs. Smith to void frequently to aid in the effectiveness of uterine involution. The nurse can recommend (if ordered by the physician/midwife) the use of ibuprofen for the cramping (afterbirth pains) she is experiencing. Women who have given birth

two or more times experience more uterine relaxation and vigorous contractions, resulting in moderate to severe cramping. Afterpains typically resolve in 3 to 7 days.

Breastfeeding and exogenous oxytocin usually intensify afterpains because both stimulate uterine contractions. Because of the intense pain, Mrs. Smith may choose to stop breastfeeding. It is very important for the nurse to educate and support her so that she will be successful with breastfeeding. The nurse should advise Mrs. Smith to request pain medication 30 minutes prior to breastfeeding to minimize afterpains. The nurse should also advise Mrs. Smith to apply a heating pad or to lie prone to relieve afterpain. Warm blankets and relaxation techniques help to interfere with the transmission of pain sensations.

Chapter 18

1. External fundal massage: The uterus can be massaged externally by placing a hand just above the pubic bone and cupping the uterus to give it support. The other hand is placed on the fundus and massaged in a circular fashion until it firms up and contracts. The uterus should feel firm after massage; if it does not contract, the uterus remains soft and boggy below the hands. External fundal massage is performed as the primary nursing intervention when managing uterine atony.
2. Mrs. Miller's risk factors for uterine atony/ hemorrhage include a large, oxytocin augmentation; grand-multiparity; use of magnesium sulfate or tocolytics; forceps-assisted vaginal delivery; fetal malpresentation; macrosomia; and laceration.
3. Methergine—0.2 mg IM every 2 to 4 hours or Hemabate 250 mcg IM every 15 to 90 minutes. Mrs. Miller has no contraindications for receiving either of these drugs.

Chapter 19

1. Time of delivery; type of delivery; afebrile mother at delivery; no support system present; gestational age; parity; medications taken during pregnancy; prenatal vitamins started at 6 weeks; Apgar scores; assessment findings
2. The mother having no support; her age; postdates; prenatal vitamin started at 12 weeks
3. Administer prescribed medications—vitamin K, eye prophylaxis, hepatitis B (if consent given), and triple dye; assess vital signs according to orders; feed infant; perform hearing screen.
4. Risk for altered nutrition, less than body requirements related to inadequate formula intake; risk

for altered body temperature related to evaporative, conductive, radiant, and connective heat losses; risk for ineffective airway clearance related to excessive secretions in the airway; risk for ineffective thermoregulation related to an immature thermoregulatory system; risk for infection related to parents' lack of knowledge concerning umbilical cord care; risk for injury related to lack of parental knowledge about normal newborn needs.

5. The mother has asked not to be disturbed at this time; the newborn has been fed only one time; the mother does not appear to want to see the baby; there are no visitors present to offer support for the mother; the mother's temperature increased after delivery, warranting antibiotics.

6. Meconium stools are normal and expected during the first few days of life; the infant needs to eat every 2 to 3 hours if breastfeeding and every 3 hours if formula fed; maintain temperature of the newborn by always covering the infant's head, swaddling the baby in blankets, or providing skin-to-skin contact. Measures should be taken to avoid drafts or heat loss; support systems are important to have during this time; medicines administered in the nursery (vitamin K, hepatitis B, eye prophylaxis, triple dye); blue/gray macules in some darker pigmented ethnicities cause bluish/gray discolorations around the buttocks area that will fade after a few years of life.

Chapter 20

1. Risk for infection, readiness for enhanced immunization status, ineffective protection, ineffective infant feeding pattern, risk for neonatal jaundice, ineffective breastfeeding, interrupted breastfeeding, readiness for enhanced breastfeeding, risk for impaired parenting, risk for impaired attachment.

2. Care should focus on instructing parents how to use a bulb syringe, using proper bathing techniques, taking a temperature, diapering, feeding, caring for circumcision, swaddling, and caring for cord.

3. The parents should be informed about when to follow up with the pediatrician, immunization status, bonding, car seat safety, and avoidance of cosleeping/SIDS risks. Review the proper techniques for bathing, temperature taking, diapering, feeding, caring for circumcision and cord, and swaddling. They should also discuss what to do if the infant appears sick and/or risk factors to look for such as respiratory distress, fever, color change.

4. The newborn should receive a hepatitis B vaccine, vitamin K, triple dye, and erythromycin ointment.

5. The first visit will be within 3 to 4 days of discharge.

Chapter 21

1. Jaundice related to Chinese descent, which can be increased and stay increased for a longer time frame; Pitocin, which can influence bilirubin levels; use of forceps, which may increase bruising and lead to the destruction of red blood cells; maternal fever, which can place the infant at risk of infection.

2. Altered health maintenance related to separation from the maternal support system; risk for infection related to the newborn's immature immunological system; risk for ineffective airway clearance related to excessive fluid present in lungs during neonatal transition; risk for pain related to increased environmental stimuli; risk for ineffective thermoregulation related to the newborn's immature temperature regulation system; altered nutrition: less than body requirements related to limited nutritional and fluid intake and increased caloric expenditure.

3. Breastfeeding, parental support, maternal/infant attachment and bonding, general care of the infant that includes swaddling, bathing, feeding, diapering, illness protection, immunizations.

4. Interventions based on the findings would include possible antibiotics, phototherapy, breastfeeding support/education or lactation consult, and social worker consult to talk about father not present at this time.

Chapter 22

1. Gestational age of the infant; maternal fever; maternal infectious history (serologies); length of rupture of membranes; medications during pregnancy; type of delivery

2. Vital signs; neonatal resuscitation measures; Apgar scores; respiratory measures (intubation, oxygen saturations, ventilator settings)

3. Dry/stimulate the infant; bulb suction; place hat; assist with intubation; place leads and pulse oximeter on infant; place in transport bag on warming mattress

4. Impaired gas exchange related to immature pulmonary function; ineffective thermoregulation related to prematurity, secondary to lack of subcutaneous fat

5. Evaluate vital signs and respiratory status; check blood glucose.

6. Take temperature and vital signs; place leads and pulse oximeter; administer vitamin K (based on weight) and erythromycin; maintain thermoneutral environment; start peripheral intravenous catheter assist with line placement; administer intravenous fluids; administer antibiotics.

7. Clinical status; plan of care; education on technologies such as ventilator, lines, IVF, monitors; anticipatory guidance related to gestational age, clinical status, and discharge planning.

Bibliography

Chapter 2

American Society for Reproductive Medicine (2011). Assisted reproductive technology: A guide for patients. Retrieved from www.reproductivefacts. org/uploadedFiles/ASRM_Content/Resources/ Patient_Resources/Fact_Sheets_and_Info_ Booklets/ART.pdf.

American Society for Reproductive Medicine (2012). Medications for inducing ovulation: A guide for patients. Retrieved from www.reproductivefacts.org/ BOOKLET_Medications_for_Inducing_Ovulation/.

Durham, R. F., & Chapman, L. (2014). *Maternal-newborn nursing: The critical components of nursing care.* Philadelphia: F.A. Davis.

Fritz, M. A., & Speroff, L. (2011). *Clinical gynecologic endocrinology and infertility.* Philadelphia: Lippincott Williams & Wilkens.

Perry, S. E., Hockenberry, M. F., Lowdermilk, D. L., & Wilson, D. (2014). *Maternal child nursing care.* St. Louis, MO: Elsevier.

Venes, D., & Thomas, C. L. (Eds.) (2001). *Taber's cyclopedic medical dictionary.* 19th ed. Philadelphia: F.A. Davis.

Ward, S. L., & Hisley, S. M. (2011). *Maternal-child nursing care: Optimizing outcomes for mothers, children, and families.* Philadelphia: F.A. Davis.

Chapter 9

Durham, R., & Chapman, L. (2014). *Maternal-newborn nursing: The critical components of nursing care.* 2nd ed. Philadelphia: F.A. Davis.

London, M. L., Ladewig, P. A. W., Davidson, M. R., Ball, J. W., Bindler, R. C., & Cowen, K. J. (2014). *Maternal & child nursing care.* 4th ed. Boston: Pearson.

Simpson, K. R., & Creehan, P. A. (2014). *Perinatal nursing.* 4th ed. Philadelphia: Wolters Kluwer/Lippincott Williams & Wilkens.

Ward, S. L., & Hisley, S. M. (2009). *Maternal-child nursing care.* Philadelphia: F.A. Davis.

Chapter 11

American Congress of Obstetricians and Gynecologists (ACOG) Committee Opinion #614 (2014).

Management of pregnant women with presumptive exposure to Listeria monocytogenes. *Obstetrics and Gynecology, 124*(6), 1241–1244.

American Congress of Obstetricians and Gynecologists (2015). FAQ001, Nutrition during pregnancy. Retrieved from www.acog.org/Patients/FAQs/ Nutrition-During-Pregnancy.

Corbett, R. W., & Kolasa, K. M. (2014). Pica and weight gain in pregnancy. *Nutrition Today, 49*(3), 101–108.

Greer, L. (2013). Pregnant with anorexia nervosa. *International Journal of Childbirth Education, 28*(4), 68–71.

Harris, J. (2012). Be cautious with herbal therapy in pregnancy. *International Journal of Childbirth Education, 27*(3), 95–99.

Institute of Medicine (2009). Weight gain during pregnancy: Reexamining the guidelines. Washington, DC: National Academies Press.

Kaiser, L. (2008). Position of the American Dietetic Association: Nutrition and lifestyle for a healthy pregnancy. *Journal of American Dietetic Association, 108*(3), 61.

Linna, M. S., Raevuori, A., Haukka, J., Suvisaari, J. M., Suokas, J. T., & Gissler, M. (2014). Pregnancy, obstetric and perinatal health outcomes in eating disorders. *American Journal of Obstetrics and Gynecology, 211*, 392.

Mills, M. E. (2007). Craving more than food: The implications of pica in pregnancy. *Nursing for Women's Health, 11*(3), 266–273.

Mitchell, A. M., & Bulik, C. M. (2006). Eating disorders and women's health: An update. *Journal of Midwifery and Women's Health, 51*(3), 193–201.

Peters, K., Rhoades, S., Ezzell, D. A., Holland, J., & Weatherspoon, D. (2012). Environmental mercury exposure. *International Journal of Childbirth Education, 28*(4), 19–26.

Shinde, P., Patil, P., & Bairagi, V. (2012). Herbs in pregnancy and lactation: A review appraisal. *International Journal of Pharmaceutical Sciences and Research, 3*(9), 3001–3006.

Tyree, S., Baker, B. R., & Weatherspoon, D. (2012). On veganism and pregnancy. *International Journal of Childbirth Education, 27*(3), 43–49.

United States Department of Agriculture (2015). Choose MyPlate. Retrieved from www.choosemyplate.gov/about.

U.S. Food and Drug Administration (2014). Fish: What pregnant women and parents should know. Retrieved from www.fda.gov/downloads/Food/FoodborneIllnessContaminants/Metals/UCM 400358.pdf.

White, C. (2014). Eating right during pregnancy. *U.S. National Library of Medicine*. Retrieved from https://www.nlm.nih.gov/medlineplus/ency/patientinstructions/000584.htm.

Chapter 13

American Congress of Obstetricians and Gynecologists (ACOG) (2007). ACOG practice bulletin no. 82: Clinical management guidelines for obstetrician-gynecologists. Management of herpes in pregnancy. *Obstetrics & Gynecology, 109*(6),1489–1498.

American Congress of Obstetricians and Gynecologists (ACOG). (2013). Task force on hypertension in pregnancy. *Hypertension in Pregnancy*. Retrieved from www.acog.org/Resources-And-Publications/Task-Force-and-Work-Group-Reports/Hypertension-in-Pregnancy.

Connelly, C. D., Hazen, A. L., Baker-Ericzén, M. J., Landsverk, J., & Horwitz, S. M. (2013). Is screening for depression in the perinatal period enough? The co-occurrence of depression, substance abuse, and intimate partner violence in culturally diverse pregnant women. *Journal of Women's Health, 22*(10), 844–852.

Dean, C. (2014). Helping women prepare for hyperemesis gravidarum. *British Journal of Midwifery, 22*(12), 847–852.

Donnelly, M., & Davies, J. K. (2014). Contemporary management of human immunodeficiency virus in pregnancy. *Obstetrics and Gynecology Clinics of North America, 41*(4), 547–571.

Gaskins, A. J., Rich-Edwards, J. W., Hauser, R., et al. (2014). Maternal prepregnancy folate intake and risk of spontaneous abortion and stillbirth. *Obstetrics & Gynecology, 124*(1), 23–31. doi:10.1097/AOG. 0000000000000343.

Horowitz, K. M., Ingardia, C. J., & Borgida, A. F. (2013). Anemia in pregnancy. *Clinics in Laboratory Medicine, 33*(2), 281–291.

Jaques, S. C., Kingsbury, A., Henshcke, P., Chomchai, C., Clews, S., Falconer, J., & Oei, J. L. (2014). Cannabis, the pregnant woman and her child: Weeding out the myths. *Journal of Perinatology, 34*(6), 417–424. doi:10.1038/jp.2013.180.

Klauser, C. K., Briery, C. M., Martin, R. W., Langston, L., Magann, E. F., & Morrison, J. C. (2014). A comparison of three tocolytics for preterm labor: A randomized clinical trial. *Journal of Maternal-Fetal & Neonatal Medicine, 27*(8), 801–806. doi:10.3109/14767058. 2013.847416.

Randis, T. M., Gelber, S. E., Hooven, et al. (2014). Group B streptococcus [beta]-hemolysin/cytolysin breaches maternal fetal barriers to cause preterm birth and intrauterine fetal demise in vivo. *Journal of Infectious Diseases, 210*(2), 265–273. doi:10. 1093/infdis/jiu067.

Warnes, C. A. (2015). Pregnancy and delivery in women with congenital heart disease. *Circulation Journal, 79*(7), 1416–1421.

Zilberman, D., Williams, S. F., Kurian, R., & Apuzzio, J. J. (2014). Does genital tract GBS colonization affect the latency period in patients with preterm premature rupture of membranes not in labor prior to 34 weeks? *Journal of Maternal-Fetal & Neonatal Medicine, 27*(4), 338–341.

Chapter 18

Alvarez-Ramirez, P., Trial, J., Hoff, B., & Scott, A. (2015). Quantifying blood loss at birth saves lives: Proceedings of the 2015 AWHONN convention. *Journal of Obstetric, Gynecologic & Neonatal Nursing, 44*(6), 45.

American Congress of Obstetricians and Gynecologists (ACOG) (2006). ACOG practice bulletin no. 76: Clinical management guidelines for obstetrician-gynecologists: Postpartum hemorrhage. *Obstetrics & Gynecology, 108*(4), 1039–1047.

American Congress of Obstetricians and Gynecologists (ACOG) (2008). ACOG practice bulletin no. 92: Clinical management guidelines for obstetrician-gynecologists. Use of psychiatric medications during pregnancy and lactation. *Obstetrics & Gynecology, 111*(4), 1001–1020. doi: 10.1097/AOG.0b013e31816fd910.

Anderson, J., & Etches, D. (2007). Prevention and management of postpartum hemorrhage. *American Family Physician, 75*(6), 875–888.

Bateman, B., Huybrechts, K., Hernandez-Diaz, S., Liu, J., Ecker, J., & Avorn, J. (2013). Methylergonovine maleate and the risk of myocardial ischemia and infarction. *American Journal of Obstetrics & Gynecology, 209*(5), 459.

Beck, C. T. (2006). Postpartum depression: It isn't just the blues. *American Journal of Nursing, 105*(5), 40–51.

Bhati, S., & Richards, K., (2015). A systematic review of the relationship between postpartum sleep disturbance and postpartum depression. *Journal of Obstetric, Gynecologic & Neonatal Nursing, 44*(3), 350–357.

Black, L. P., Hinson, L., & Duff, P. (2012). Limited course of antibiotic treatment for chorioamnionitis. *Obstetrics & Gynecology, 119*(6), 1102–1105.

Borra, C., Iacovou, M., & Sevilla, A. (2015). New evidence on breastfeeding and postpartum depression: The importance of understanding women's intentions. *Maternal & Child Health Journal, 19*(4), 897–907.

Brady, M., Carroll, A., Cheang, K., Straight, C., & Chelmow, D. (2015). Sequential compression device compliance in postoperative obstetrics and gynecology patients. *Obstetrics & Gynecology, 125*(1), 19–25.

Burgazli, K., Bilgin, M., Ertan, A., et al. (2011). Diagnosis and treatment of deep-vein thrombosis and approach to venous thromboembolism in obstetrics and gynecology. *Journal of the Turkish-German Gynecological Association, 12*(3), 168–175.

California Maternal Quality Care Collaborative, CMQCC. (2014). Planning for and responding to obstetric hemorrhage. *Obstetric hemorrhage toolkit Version 2.* California Department of Public Health.

Cooper, S., Bulle, B., Endacott, R., et al. (2012). Managing women with acute physiological deterioration: Student midwives performance in a simulated setting. *Women & Birth, 25*(3), 27–36.

Corrigan, C. P., Kwasky, A. N., & Groh, C. J. (2015). Social support, postpartum depression, and professional assistance: A survey of mothers in the Midwestern United States. *Journal of Perinatal Education, 24*(1), 48–60.

Cunningham, F. G., Leveno, K. J., Bloom, S. L., Haxth, J. C., Rouse, D. J., & Sprong, C.Y. (2010). *Williams obstetrics.* 23rd ed. New York: McGraw-Hill.

Dahlke, J., Mendez-Figueroa, H., Rouse, D., et al. (2015). Prevention and management of postpartum hemorrhage: A comparison of 4 national guidelines. *American Journal of Obstetrics & Gynecology, 213*(1), 1–76.

Debost-Legrand, A., Riviere, O., Dossou, M., & Vendittelli, F. (2015). Risk factors for severe secondary postpartum hemorrhages: A historical cohort study. *Birth: Issues in Perinatal Care, 42*(3), 235–241.

Dennis, C., & Chung-Lee, L. (2006). Postpartum depression help seeking barriers and maternal treatment preferences: A qualitative systematic review. *Birth, 33*(4), 323–331.

Dossou, M., Debost-Legrand, A., Dechelotte, P., Lemery, D., & Vendittelli, F. (2015). Severe secondary postpartum hemorrhage: A historical cohort. *Birth: Issues in Perinatal Care, 42*(2), 149–155.

Doucet, S., Dennis, C. L., Letourneau, N., & Blackmore, E. R. (2009). Differentiation and clinical implications of postpartum depression and postpartum psychosis.

Journal of Obstetric, Gynecologic, and Neonatal Nursing, 38(3), 269–279.

Driscoll, J. (2006). Postpartum depression: How nurses can identify and care for women grappling with this disorder. *AWHONN Lifelines, 10*(5), 400–409.

Ducarme, G., Hamel, J., Bouet, P., Lengendre, G., Vandenbroucke, L., & Sentilhes, L. (2015). Neonatal morbidity after attempted operative vaginal delivery according to fetal head station. *Obstetrics & Gynecology, 126*(3), 521–529.

Edmonds, D. K. (2012). Puerperium and lactation. In D. K. Edmonds (Ed.), *Dewhurst's textbook of obstetrics & gynecology* (365–376). 8th ed. Oxford: John Wiley & Son.

Engqvist, I., Ferszt, G., Ahlin, A., & Nilsson, K. (2009). Psychiatric nurses' descriptions of women with postpartum psychosis and nurses' response—an exploratory study in Sweden. *Issues in Mental Health Nursing, 30*, 23–30.

Heron, J., Gilbert, N., Dolman, C., et al. (2012). Information and support needs during recovery from postpartum psychosis. *Archives of Women's Mental Health, 15*(3), 155–165.

Holt, J. (2015). Multidisciplinary care of a woman experiencing obstetric hemorrhage. *Journal of Obstetric, Gynecologic &Neonatal Nursing, 44*(6), 85–86.

Houston, K. A., Kaimal, A. J., Nakagawa, S., Gregorich, S. E., Yee, L. M., & Kuppermann, M. (2015). Mode of delivery and postpartum depression: The role of patient preferences. *American Journal of Obstetrics & Gynecology, 212*(2), 229.

Jaiyeoba, O. (2012). Postoperative infections in obstetrics and gynecology. *Clinical Obstetrics & Gynecology, 5*(4), 904–913.

Jones, V. A., & Henderson, J. (2011). Gestational complications. In K. J. Hurt, M. W. Guile, J. L. Bienstock, et al. (Eds.), *The Johns Hopkins manual of gynecology and obstetrics* (110–121). 4th ed. Philadelphia: Lippincott Williams & Wilkins.

Kaplan, H., & Sadock, B. (2005). *Kaplan & Sadock's comprehensive textbook of psychiatry.* Philadelphia: Lippincott Williams & Wilkins.

Ko, J. Y., Farr, S. L., Dietz, P. M., & Robbins, C. L. (2012). Depression and treatment among U.S. pregnant and nonpregnant women of reproductive age, *Journal of Women's Health, 21*(8), 830–836.

Lagana, A. S., Sofo, V., Salmeri, F. M., Chiofalo, B., Ciancimino, L., & Triolo, O. (2015). Post-partum management in a patient affected by thrombotic thrombocytopenic purpura: Case report and review of literature. *Clinical and Experimental Obstetrics and Gynecology, 42*(1), 90–94.

Liu, C., & Tronick, E. (2013). Rates and predictors of postpartum depression by race and ethnicity: Results from the 2004 to 2007 New York City PRAMS survey

(Pregnancy Risk Assessment and Monitoring System). *Maternal & Child Health Journal, 17*(9), 1599–1610.

McPeak, K. E., Sandrock, D., Spector, N. D., & Pattishall, A. E. (2015). Important determinants of newborn health: Postpartum depression, teen parenting, and breast-feeding. *Current Opinion in Pediatrics, 27*(1), 138–144.

Meaney-Delman, D., Bartlett, L., Gravett, M., & Jamieson, D. (2015). Oral and intramuscular treatment options for early postpartum endometritis in low-resource settings: A systematic review. *Obstetrics & Gynecology, 125*(4), 789–800.

Newton, E. (2007). Breastfeeding. In S. Gabbe, J. Niebyl, & J. Simpson (Eds.), *Obstetrics: Normal and problem pregnancies.* 5th ed. Philadelphia: Churchill Livingstone.

O'Connor, D. J., Scher, L. A., & Gargiulo, N. J. (2011). Incidence and characteristics of venous thromboembolic disease during pregnancy and the postnatal period: A contemporary series. *Annals of Vascular Surgery, 25*(1), 9–14.

Ogston-Tuck, S. (2014). Patient safety and pain in IV therapy. *British Journal of Nursing, 23*(2), 23.

Oliveira, S., Silva, F., Riesco, M., Latorre, M., & Nobre, M. (2012). Comparison of application times for ice packs used to relieve perineal pain after normal birth: A randomized clinical trial. *Journal of Clinical Nursing, 21*(23), 3382–3391.

Silveira, M., Ertel, K., Dole, N., & Chasan-Taber, L. (2015). The role of body image in prenatal and postpartum depression: A critical review of the literature. *Archives of Women's Mental Health, 18*(3), 409–421.

Snohomish County, Washington, Government Document Center (2011). Family guide to involuntary treatment. County informational brochure and pdf. View 5722, 1–3.

Vatne, M., & Naden, D. (2012). Finally, it became too much—experiences and reflections in the aftermath of attempted suicide. *Scandinavian Journal of Caring Sciences, 26*(2), 304–312.

Werner, E., Miller, M., Osborne, L., Kuzava, S., & Monk, C. (2015). Preventing postpartum depression: Review and recommendations. *Archives of Women's Mental Health, 18*(1), 41–60.

Chapter 19

American Academy of Pediatrics (2012). Ages and Stages: Apgar score. Retrieved from www.healthychildren.org/English/ages-stages/prenatal/delivery-beyond/Pages/Apgar-Scores.aspx?nfstatus=401&nftoken=00000000-0000-0000-0000-000000000000&nfstatusdescription=ERROR%3a+No+local+token.

American Congress of Obstetricians and Gynecologists (2015). Ob-gyns redefine meaning of "term pregnancy." Retrieved from www.acog.org/About-ACOG/News-Room/News-Releases/2013/Ob-Gyns-Redefine-Meaning-of-Term-Pregnancy.

Durham, R., & Chapman, L. (2014). *Maternal-infant nursing: The critical components of nursing care.* Philadelphia: F.A. Davis.

March of Dimes Foundation (2014). Pregnancy complications. Retrieved from www.marchofdimes.com/pregnancy/umbilical-cord-abnormalities.aspx.

MedlinePlus (2014a). Foramen ovale. Retrieved from www.nlm.nih.gov/medlineplus/ency/article/001113.htm.

MedlinePlus (2014b). Transient tachypnea-newborn. Retrieved from www.nlm.nih.gov/medlineplus/ency/article/007233.htm.

Ward, S. L., & Hisley, S. M. (2009). *Maternal-child nursing care: Optimizing outcomes for mothers, children & families.* Philadelphia: F.A. Davis.

Chapter 20

American Academy of Pediatrics (n.d.). AAP updates recommendation on car seats. Retrieved from www.aap.org/en-us/about-the-aap/aap-press-room/Pages/AAP-Updates-Recommendation-on-Car-Seats.aspx.

American Academy of Pediatrics (2012a). Healthy children ages and stages: Reduce the risk of SIDS. Retrieved from https://www.healthychildren.org/English/ages-stages/baby/sleep/Pages/Preventing-SIDS.aspx.

American Academy of Pediatrics (2012b). Healthy children: Listen up about why newborn screening is important. Retrieved from https://www.healthychildren.org/English/ages-stages/baby/Pages/Listen-Up-About-Why-Newborn-Hearing-Screening-is-Important.aspx.

American Academy of Pediatrics (2012c). Where we stand: Circumcision. Retrieved from www.healthychildren.org/English/ages-stages/prenatal/decisions-to-make/Pages/Where-We-Stand-Circumcision.aspx.

Centers for Disease Control and Prevention (n.d.). Screening and diagnosis. Retrieved from www.cdc.gov/ncbddd/hearingloss/screening.html.

Centers for Disease Control and Prevention (2012). Sudden unexpected infant death and sudden infant death syndrome. Retrieved from www.cdc.gov/SIDS/index.htm.

Durham, R., & Chapman, L. (2014). *Maternal-newborn nursing: The critical components of nursing care.* Philadelphia: F.A. Davis.

International Hip Dysplasia Institute (2012). Newborn and child hip dysplasia. Retrieved from www.hipdysplasia.org/developmental-dysplasia-of-the-hip/tips-for-parents/pavlik-harness-tips/.

London, M. L., Ladewig, P. A., Davidson, M. R., Ball, J. W., Bindler, R. C., & Cowen, K. J. (2014). *Maternal & child nursing care*. 4th ed. Upper Saddle River, NJ: Pearson.

March of Dimes Foundation (2014). Baby care 101. Retrieved from www.marchofdimes.org/baby/caring-for-your-baby.aspx.

Mayo Foundation for Medical Education and Research (2013). Clubfoot. Retrieved from www.mayoclinic.org/diseases-conditions/clubfoot/home/ovc-20198067.

MedlinePlus (2013). Developmental dysplasia of the hip. Retrieved from www.nlm.nih.gov/medlineplus/ency/article/000971.htm.

MedlinePlus (2014). Nevus flammeus. Retrieved from www.nlm.nih.gov/medlineplus/ency/article/001475.htm.

National Highway Traffic Safety Administration (n.d.). Car seat types. Retrieved from www.safercar.gov/parents/CarSeats/Car-Seat-Types.htm?view=full.

Nugent, P. M, & Vitale, B. A. (2014). *Fundamentals of nursing: Content review plus practice questions*. Philadelphia: F.A. Davis.

Rudd, K., & Kocisko, D. (2014). *Pediatric nursing: The critical components of nursing care*. Philadelphia: F.A. Davis.

Ward, S. L., & Hisley, S. M. (2009). *Maternal-child nursing care: Optimizing outcomes for mothers, children & families*. Philadelphia: F.A. Davis.

Chapter 21

American Academy of Pediatrics (n.d.). AAP updates recommendation on car seats. Retrieved from www.aap.org/en-us/about-the-aap/aap-press-room/Pages/AAP-Updates-Recommendation-on-Car-Seats.aspx.

American Academy of Pediatrics (2012a). Healthy children ages and stages: Reduce the risk of SIDS. Retrieved from https://www.healthychildren.org/English/ages-stages/baby/sleep/Pages/Preventing-SIDS.aspx.

American Academy of Pediatrics (2012b). Healthy children: Listen up about why newborn screening is important. Retrieved from https://www.healthychildren.org/English/ages-stages/baby/Pages/Listen-Up-About-Why-Newborn-Hearing-Screening-is-Important.aspx.

American Academy of Pediatrics (2012c). Where we stand: Circumcision. Retrieved from www.healthychildren.org/English/ages-stages/prenatal/decisions-to-make/Pages/Where-We-Stand-Circumcision.aspx.

Centers for Disease Control and Prevention (n.d.). Screening and diagnosis. Retrieved from www.cdc.gov/ncbddd/hearingloss/screening.html.

Centers for Disease Control and Prevention (2012). *Sudden Unexpected Newborn Death (SUID)*. Retrieved from www.cdc.gov/SIDS/index.htm.

Durham, R., & Chapman, L. (2014). *Maternal-newborn nursing: The critical components of nursing care*. Philadelphia: F.A. Davis.

International Hip Dysplasia Institute (2012). Newborn and child hip dysplasia. Retrieved from www.hipdysplasia.org/developmental-dysplasia-of-the-hip/tips-for-parents/pavlik-harness-tips/.

London, M. L., Ladewig, P. A., Davidson, M. R., Ball, J. W., Bindler, R. C., & Cowen, K. J. (2014). *Maternal & child nursing care*. 4th ed. Upper Saddle River, NJ: Pearson.

March of Dimes Foundation (2014). Baby care 101. Retrieved from www.marchofdimes.org/baby/caring-for-your-baby.aspx.

Mayo Foundation for Medical Education and Research (2013). Clubfoot. Retrieved from www.mayoclinic.org/diseases-conditions/clubfoot/home/ovc-20198067.

MedlinePlus (2013). Developmental dysplasia of the hip. Retrieved from www.nlm.nih.gov/medlineplus/ency/article/000971.htm.

MedlinePlus (2014). Nevus flammeus. Retrieved from www.nlm.nih.gov/medlineplus/ency/article/001475.htm.

National Highway Traffic Safety Administration (n.d.). Car seat types. Retrieved from www.safercar.gov/parents/CarSeats/Car-Seat-Types.htm?view=full.

Nugent, P. M, & Vitale, B. A. (2014). *Fundamentals of nursing: Content review plus practice questions*. Philadelphia: F.A. Davis.

Rudd, K., & Kocisko, D. (2014). *Pediatric nursing: The critical components of nursing care*. Philadelphia: F.A. Davis.

Ward, S. L., & Hisley, S.M. (2009). *Maternal-child nursing care: Optimizing outcomes for mothers, children & families*. Philadelphia: F.A. Davis.

Chapter 22

American Academy of Pediatrics, Committee on Fetus and Newborn (2011). Postnatal glucose homeostasis in late-preterm and term infants. *Pediatrics, 127*, 575–579. doi: 10.1542/peds.2010-3851.

Cloherty, J., Eichenwald, E., & Stark, A. (2012). *Manual of neonatal care*. 8th ed. Philadelphia: Lippincott Williams & Wilkins.

Fanaroff, A., & Fanaroff, J. (2013). *Klaus & Fanaroff's care of the high-risk neonate*. Philadelphia: Elsevier Saunders.

Gomella, T., Cunningham, D., & Eyal, F. (2013). *Neonatology: Management, on-call problems, diseases, and drugs*. 6th ed. New York: McGraw Hill Education.

Martin, R., Fanaroff, A., & Walsh, M. (2015). *Fanaroff & Martin's neonatal-perinatal medicine: Diseases of the fetus and infant.* 10th ed. Philadelphia: Elsevier Saunders.

Nagtalon-Ramos, J. (2014). *Best evidence-based practices: Maternal-newborn nursing care.* Philadelphia: F.A. Davis.

NeoFax (2016). Retrieved from http://micromedex.com/neofax-pediatric.

Tappero, E., & Honeyfield, M. (2015). *Physical assessment of the newborn: A comprehensive approach to the art of physical examination.* 5th ed. Petaluma, CA: NICU.

Verklan, M., & Walden, M. (2010). *Core curriculum for neonatal intensive care nursing.* 5th ed. St. Louis, MO: Elsevier Saunders.

Index

Note: Page numbers followed by *b* indicate boxes, *t* tables, and *f* figures.